DISCOVERY LIBRARY
LEVEL 5 SWCC
DERRIFORD HOSPITAL
DERRIFORD ROAD
PLYMOUTH
PL6 8DH

D1345747

Dental Materials and Their Selection

Fourth Edition

Dental Materials and Their Selection

Fourth Edition

Edited by

William J. O'Brien, PhD, FADM

Professor, Department of Biologic and Materials Sciences
Director, Dental Materials Laboratory
School of Dentistry
University of Michigan
Ann Arbor, Michigan

Quintessence Publishing Co, Inc
Chicago, Berlin, Tokyo, London, Paris, Milan, Barcelona,
Istanbul, São Paulo, Mumbai, Moscow, Prague, and Warsaw

This book is not for patient use. The material presented herein is intended for use by professionals only. Patients should contact their personal dentist to discuss their treatment options.

Library of Congress Cataloging-in-Publication Data

Dental materials and their selection / [edited by] William J. O'Brien. --
4th ed.
    p. ; cm.
Includes bibliographical references and index.
ISBN 978-0-86715-437-5 (hardcover)
1. Dental materials. I. O'Brien, William J. (William Joseph), 1940-
[DNLM: 1. Dental Materials. WU 190 D4152 2008]
RK652.5.D454 2008
617.6'95--dc22

                              2008014998

quintessence
books

© 2008 Quintessence Publishing Co, Inc

Quintessence Publishing Co, Inc
4350 Chandler Drive
Hanover Park, IL 60133
www.quintpub.com

Editor: Bryn Goates
Design: Annette McQuade
Production: Sue Robinson

Printed in Canada

Table of Contents

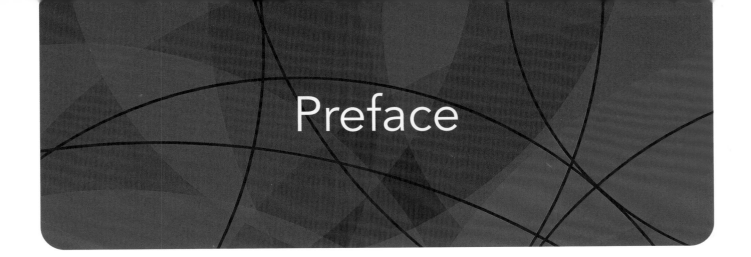

Preface

This fourth edition of *Dental Materials and Their Selection* continues the objective of presenting a concise consensus of information on basic and applied dental materials. This text is envisioned as a review of basic principles and an update on current dental products for predoctoral and graduate dental students along with dental practitioners, dental hygienists, and dental technicians. Keeping this text comprehensive yet concise is a challenge. The field of dental materials has grown significantly, but the time available for teaching and studying this subject has not. Therefore, the approach maintained since the very first edition of this book has been to stress basic principles and limit the coverage of historic techniques and materials in order to keep the size of the book relatively constant.

The main purpose of this fourth edition is to update chapters, especially on the following topics: color and appearance, surface phenomena and adhesion to tooth structure, polymeric restorative materials, dental amalgams, dental porcelains, orthodontic wires, and implant and bone augmentation materials. This edition also includes updated references and revision of some clinical decision scenarios. I welcome and appreciate comments on the technical coverage and educational application of this edition.

I would like to thank the many people who, in addition to the contributors, have made this fourth edition possible: Elizabeth Rodriguiz for her invaluable efforts in manuscript preparation, Chris Jung for his excellent illustrations (especially Fig 3-19), and Dr Sumant Ram for his indispensable assistance. I would also like to welcome Drs Joseph B. Dennison and Peter X. Ma as authors in this fourth edition with their contributions on polymeric restorative materials and polymers and polymerization, respectively. Several contributors to the third edition are also recognized for their valuable contributions: Dr Raymond L. Bertolotti, Dr Gerald N. Glickman, Dr Eugene F. Huget, Dr Ann-Marie L. Neme, and Dr Denis C. Smith. Finally, I want to acknowledge the staff at Quintessence for their expert assistance in preparing this book for publication.

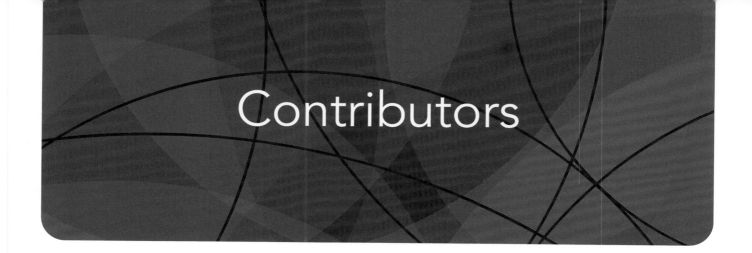

Contributors

Kenzo Asaoka, BS, PhD, FADM
Professor
Department of Biomaterials and Bioengineering
Institute of Health Biosciences
The University of Tokushima Graduate School
Tokushima, Japan
Ch 19 • High-Temperature Investments

William A. Brantley, PhD
Professor
Division of Restorative and Prosthetic Dentistry
College of Dentistry
Ohio State University
Columbus, Ohio
Ch 21 • Orthodontic Wires

Joseph B. Dennison, DDS, MS
Marcus L. Ward Professor
Department of Cariology, Restorative Sciences and
   Endodontics
School of Dentistry
University of Michigan
Ann Arbor, Michigan
Ch 8 • Polymeric Restorative Materials

Richard G. Earnshaw, PhD, MDSc
Professor Emeritus
Faculty of Dentistry
University of Sydney
Sydney, Australia
Ch 4 • Gypsum Products

Ibrahim Jarjoura, DDS, MS
Private Practice
Grand Blanc, Michigan
Ch 9 • Dental Cements

David H. Kohn, PhD
Professor
Department of Biologic and Materials Sciences
School of Dentistry
Department of Biomedical Engineering
College of Engineering
University of Michigan
Ann Arbor, Michigan
Ch 23 • Implant and Bone Augmentation Materials

Peter X. Ma, MS, PhD
Professor
Department of Biologic and Materials Sciences
School of Dentistry
University of Michigan
Ann Arbor, Michigan
Ch 6 • Polymers and Polymerization

J. Rodway Mackert, Jr, DMD, PhD
Professor of Dental Materials
Department of Oral Rehabilitation
School of Dentistry
Medical College of Georgia
Augusta, Georgia
Ch 1 • A Comparison of Metals, Ceramics, and Polymers
Ch 2 • Physical Properties and Biocompatibility

Peter C. Moon, MS, PhD
Professor of General Practice
School of Dentistry
Medical College of Virginia
Virginia Commonwealth University
Richmond, Virginia
Ch 11 • Structure and Properties of Metals and Alloys

Osamu Okuno, PhD
Professor
Division of Dental Biomaterials
Graduate School of Dentistry
Tohoku University
Sendai, Japan
Ch 19 • High-Temperature Investments

Kenneth W. Stoffers, DMD, MS
Clinical Associate Professor
Department of Cariology, Restorative Sciences,
 and Endodontics
School of Dentistry
University of Michigan
Ann Arbor, Michigan
Clinical Decision-Making Scenarios

John A. Tesk, BS, MS, PhD, FADM
Biomedical Materials and Devices Consultant
Highland, Maryland
Ch 19 • High-Temperature Investments

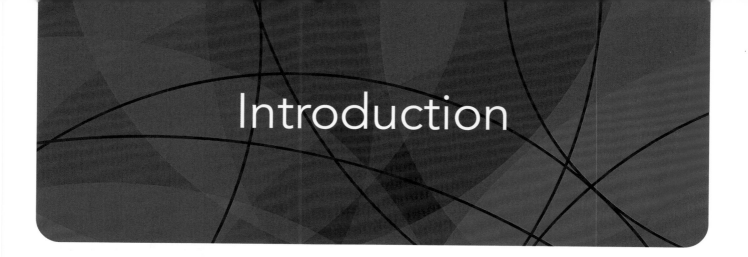

Introduction

Dental materials textbooks have evolved significantly over the past century. An early textbook on dental materials provided recipes for a handful of materials (three cements, amalgam alloys, gold foil, vulcanized rubber, and gold casting materials) and emphasized formulation, techniques, and crude testing. Then came the research and development period, when dental materials properties were optimized by the dentist according to the results of laboratory testing and the American Dental Association (ADA) standards were developed. Dental materials have been further refined to offer simpler techniques for clinicians and to meet the increasing esthetic demands of middle-class patients in developed countries.

Another dimension to proliferation is the large number of products and techniques available for each type of material, which only intensifies the need for clinicians to stay current with the literature. To ease this burden, publications such as *Clinical Research Associates Newsletter*, *Dental Advisor*, and *Reality* compile new information and provide monthly updates for dental practitioners. Perhaps the greatest drawback of proliferation is that many new materials are not sufficiently tested prior to full-scale marketing, thereby increasing the risk of clinical failures.

As a result of this product explosion, dental materials education has an opportunity to become a more integral part of the overall curriculum but, to do so, the way in which it has been taught must be revised. A long-standing problem is that dental materials courses are grouped with basic sciences, which tends to encourage memorization of facts rather than understanding of clinical application. A new approach (Fig 1) would be more pragmatic, integrating problem-based learning and evidence-based dentistry with the traditional overview of clinical materials and materials science concepts, which is still important. Table 1 summarizes the characteristics and indications of current restorative materials. An understanding of the properties and behavior of materials is essential for selection and clinical service. Problem-based learning and evidence-based dentistry would be the links between basic science and clinical practice.

◼ Problem-Based Learning

Problem-based learning is an approach that focuses students on developing the skills they will need as practicing dentists. In the dental materials curriculum, this includes selecting restorative materials as part of treatment planning, explaining their application to patients, handling materials for optimal results, and correcting problems in their clinical performance. A well-designed dental materials course will present not only a materials science framework but also the most current information on available materials. It should emphasize the selection of competing materials for a given clinical situation, taking into account material properties as well as factors such as patient goals and financial situations. The clinical scenarios that were first introduced in the second edition of this book proved to be helpful exercises in choosing the most appropriate materials. They present many facts about materials and promote an understanding of the clinical application. Though experts may disagree with some of the outcomes of these scenarios, their purpose is to reinforce the rational decision-making process necessary for treatment planning.

Evidence-Based Approach

The concept behind evidence-based dentistry originated in medicine about 25 years ago, the premise being to base clinical decisions on factual evidence from scientific studies. In the area of dental materials, evidence-based dentistry is used to evaluate and determine the clinical application of new materials. A hierarchy of the different types of evidence available for assessing the clinical performance of new biomaterials is shown in Box 1. The most rigorous type of evidence is published data from large-scale, long-term clinical trials. Publication in a peer-reviewed journal gives assurance that the design and results of a study have been reported according to acceptable statistical approaches. Because the life cycles of dental materials are growing shorter, both critical thinking and knowledge of basic materials science are necessary to make competent, rational choices. This edition incorporates the hierarchy of evidence as a tool for material selection.

The level of evidence needed to evaluate a new material or technology depends on the level of innovation or the level of risk as compared with the conventional material or technology. The higher the level of innovation and the greater the potential for harm or financial loss to the patient or clinician, the higher the standard for evidence. Materials and technology that are entirely new for a given application have the highest level of innovation and risk. For example, dentin etching for the purpose of bonding composite materials to dentin was highly innovative and had many risks when it was first introduced. The next, lower level of innovation includes major product changes in a conventional material, such as with high-copper amalgam alloys in the 1970s or hybrid ionomer cements in the 1990s. Decreasing levels of innovation and risk include minor product improvements (eg, more shades for a resin restorative material). The majority of "new products" fall into this last category.

Each category in the hierarchy of evidence is described below.

Large-scale, long-term clinical trials

A well-designed clinical trial will have a clearly stated hypothesis about the clinical performance of a new material when compared with a control material. It will have a large number of subjects to be sufficiently definitive. A good design will also reduce subjectivity by using meth-

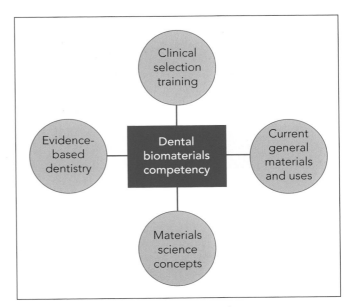

Fig 1 New paradigm for dental materials competency.

ods such as calibration of observers, double-blind procedures, and randomization, and the institutional review board of the organization will protect the study participants. These studies are indicated for adoption of brand new innovations and major product changes.

Other clinical studies

Other types of clinical study generally are not as decisive as full clinical trials, but they nevertheless provide valuable information. A cohort study would follow a group of patients who receive biomaterials, for instance, and record successes and failures related to the biomaterials' characteristics. Follow-up studies evaluate product longevity and causes of failure in patients who are treated in a clinic. A significant finding might be one in which a researcher discovers a high failure rate of a new biomaterial as patients return for replacement within a short period of time. Short-term clinical studies performed for new dental restorative materials by manufacturers are common and useful, but they miss long-term effects and less frequent problems that are usually only evident in larger groups of patients. Studies in this category are indicated for product improvements and new techniques.

Animal experiments

Several of the biocompatibility tests for new materials involve animal testing. Animal tests are valuable, but they

Table 1 Longevity of restorations commonly used in dentistry*

MATERIAL	INDICATIONS	CONTRAINDICATIONS	STRENGTHS	WEAKNESSES
Amalgam, silver (14 y approx)	Incipient, moderate-sized, and some large lesions in adolescents and adults	Large intracoronal restorations (cusp replacement); endodontically treated teeth	Good marginal seal; strength; longevity; manipulability; cariostatic activity	Objectionable color; stains tooth; marginal breakdown; alleged health challenges
Cast gold: inlays, onlays, and crowns (20 y approx)	Large lesions; teeth requiring additional strength or used in rebuilding or changing occlusion	Adolescents; high caries activity; patients who object to gold display	Reproduces anatomy well; onlays and crowns may increase strength of tooth; longevity; wears occlusally similar to enamel	Time required for placement; high fee; poor esthetics; thermal sensitivity
Ceramic crowns (15 y approx)	Restoration of teeth requiring good appearance and moderate strength	Heavy occlusal stress; bruxism; fixed prosthesis longer than three teeth	Esthetics; no metal content	Moderate strength; required resin bonding for strength
Ceramic inlays and onlays, fired or pressed (10 y approx)	Class 2 and 5 locations where high esthetics is desired	Teeth that are grossly broken down and require crowns	Esthetic potential extremely high; properly etched tooth and restoration may increase strength of tooth; onlays stronger than inlays	Tooth sensitivity possible if bonding agents are not used properly; fracture possible during service
Compacted golds: gold foil, powdered gold, mat gold (24 y approx)	Initial Class 3 and 5 lesions for patients of all ages	Periodontally unstable teeth; high caries activity; patients who object to gold display	Marginal integrity; longevity	Time-consuming; poor esthetics
Compomer (10 y approx)	Moderate to high caries activity; repair of crowns; pediatric lesions	Occlusal stress; locations where color stability is necessary	Moderate fluoride release; easy to use	Color degradation
Glass ionomer (8 y approx)	Class 1 and 2 lesions; high caries activity; crown repairs	Areas of high esthetic need or difficult moisture control	High fluoride release	Fair esthetics; difficult and time-consuming to place
Hybrid ionomer (10 y approx)	High caries activity; repair of crowns; pediatric Class 1 and 2 lesions	Occlusal stress; locations where color stability is necessary	High fluoride release; tricured; sets in dark	Somewhat difficult to use; color degradation
Porcelain-fused-to-metal crowns (20 y approx)	Teeth that require full coverage and are subject to heavy occlusal forces; fixed prosthesis	Heavy occlusal stress; bruxism	Strength; good marginal fit; acceptable to excellent esthetics	Mediocre esthetics; possible wear of opposing teeth
Resin composite: Class 1 and 2 restorations (10 y approx)	Class 1 and 2 lesions in areas of high esthetic need; patients sensitive to metal	Bruxism and clenching	Esthetics; may strengthen tooth with acid-etch concept	Wear of restoration during service; no cariostatic activity; tooth sensitivity possible if bonding agents are not used adequately
Resin composite: Class 3, 4, and 5 restorations (15 y approx)	Incipient to large Class 3, 4, and 5 lesions	Teeth where coronal portion is nearly gone	Esthetics; ease of use; strength	Marginal breakdown over time; sometimes becomes rough; wear; no cariostatic activity

*Courtesy of G. J. Christensen, DDS, MSD, PhD.

are often difficult to interpret. Cytotoxicity screening tests with cell cultures will detect gross toxicity of a material, but subtle effects require expert interpretation. Animal tests are required for new compositions or techniques with questionable biocompatibility.

Physical properties data

The publication of physical properties data on new biomaterials is essential for predicting successful performance, as compared with a standard material. However, since conditions in the body are highly complex, data from laboratory tests cannot always be extrapolated to clinical performance. For example, a new material may be strong when tested in the laboratory, but it may deteriorate more rapidly in body fluids and thus may not be an improvement when compared with a standard material. It is important to evaluate all applicable physical properties of a new material alongside its clinical trials. Physical properties data are usually necessary for minor improvements in materials, but they are insufficient for products with a higher level of innovation.

In vitro experiments

The biomaterials literature has many examples of laboratory experiments designed to simulate the clinical situation. For instance, the wear resistance of biomaterials is often assessed with toothbrushing machines that use thousands of cycles to simulate years of daily brushing. Although useful, these experiments are tricky to interpret. In one such study using a toothbrushing test, a new porcelain glaze was reported to be more resistant to wear than the current glazes. It was later disclosed that no dentifrice had been used. Thermocycling, marginal leakage, adhesion testing, and corrosion testing are a few examples of in vitro tests. They are useful for all new products and techniques.

Deductions from clinical experiments and scientific theories

Deductive reasoning is frequently used to support the superiority of new materials, but it can be unreliable without supporting data. One example is the conclusion that the caries rate will be reduced when fluoride-containing materials are used. Original clinical research on fluoride-containing silicate cements reported that these materials were associated with a low caries rate. The deduction that other fluoride-containing restorative materials provide equal caries protection is often unsupported by clin-

---

Box 1 Hierarchy of evidence

Scientific/Published
- Long-term clinical trials
- Other clinical studies
- Animal studies
- In vitro studies
- Physical properties data

Speculative/Unpublished
- Deductions from clinical literature
- Deductions from scientific theories
- Product manufacturer literature
- Popular media
- Rumors and myths

---

ical data. Another example is the claim that a new high-strength ceramic will have a low clinical failure rate for posterior crowns. It may be strong, but dental laboratory fabrication and the oral environment may contribute to clinical failure. This type of evidence is useful during product development but very speculative for new products.

Product literature from the manufacturer

There are too many fallacies and extreme claims in dental advertising for this to be a reliable source of evidence. Advertisements that provide references to the published literature are more reliable than those that do not cite published studies.

Popular media, rumors, and myths

None of these is reliable.

■ Recommended Reading

Niederman R, Badovinac R. Tradition-based dental care and evidence-based dental care. J Dent Res 1999;78:1288–1291.

Sackett DL, Straus SE, Richardson WS, Rosenberg W, Haynes RB. Evidence-Based Medicine: How to Practice and Teach EBM, ed 2. New York: Churchill-Livingstone, 2000.

CHAPTER 1

A Comparison of Metals, Ceramics, and Polymers

When a clinician considers the type of restoration to place in a patient's mouth, the choice may be between different varieties of the same material (eg, different types of amalgam), or between two kinds of the same basic material, such as two kinds of metal (eg, amalgam and cast gold). With the rapid developments in dental materials over the past several years, it is more common that the clinician's choice is between two basic materials, such as between a metal amalgam and a polymer-and-ceramic composite, or between a metal crown and an all-ceramic crown.

Each of the three basic material categories has its own wide spectrum of properties; nevertheless, there is a "family resemblance" among the varieties of materials in each category. For example, although **metals** exhibit a range of strengths, melting ranges, and so on, they resemble one another in their ductility, thermal and electric conductivity, and metallic luster. Similarly, **ceramics** can be characterized as strong yet brittle, and **polymers** tend to be flexible (low elastic modulus) and weak. Understanding just one key concept for each of the three basic materials gives us significant insight into their ability to function as restorative dental material, as well as their potential if some of their limitations can be overcome. The relationships among the three basic materials are shown in Fig 1-1.

■ Selection of Material

Table 1-1 summarizes the general characteristics of the three basic materials discussed in this chapter: metals, ceramics, and polymers. Each of these main categories

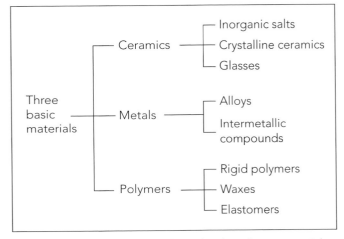

Fig 1-1 A tree diagram classifying the three basic materials.

has certain inherent properties that determine its usefulness in dentistry. For example, metals are inherently strong and have good stiffness (**modulus of elasticity**), which are ideal properties of a restorative material. However, metals conduct heat rapidly and are opaque (nonesthetic), limiting their usefulness in restorative dentistry. Ceramics and polymers are thermally insulating and tend to be more translucent. Hence, these materials insulate the pulp from extremes of heat and cold and provide better esthetic results than metals. Nevertheless, they tend to have lower toughness than metals, and polymers have much lower strength than metals.

Because no one class of materials possesses all of the desired properties, it is not surprising that materials tend to be used in combination. A porcelain-fused-to-metal (PFM) restoration combines the strength and ductility of metal with the esthetics of porcelain. A ceramic or

Table 1-1 A comparison of the properties of metals, ceramics, and polymers

| PROPERTIES | METALS | | CERAMICS | | | POLYMERS | |
	ALLOYS	INTERMETALLIC COMPOUNDS	INORGANIC SALTS	CRYSTALLINE	GLASSES	RIGID	RUBBERS
Hardness	Medium to hard	Hard	Medium to hard	Hard	Hard	Soft	Very soft
Strength	Medium to high	Medium	Medium	High	High	Low	Low
Toughness	High	Low	Low	Most low, some high	Low	Low	Medium
Elastic modulus	High	High	High	High	High	Low	Very low
Electric conductivity	High	High	Low	Low	Low	Low	Low
Thermal conductivity	High	High	Low	Low	Low	Low	Low
Thermal expansion	Low	Low	Low	Low	Low	High	High
Density	High	High	Medium	Medium	Medium	Low	Low
Translucency	None	None	Medium	High	High	High	Low
Examples	Gold-copper	Amalgam phases	Gypsum, zinc phosphate	SiO_2, Al_2O_3	Dental porcelain	Poly(methyl methacrylate)	Impression materials

polymer base is used to insulate the pulp from a thermal-conductive metallic restoration. A high-thermal-expansion, low-strength, low-elastic-modulus polymer is reinforced with a low-thermal-expansion, high-strength, high-elastic-modulus ceramic filler to form a dental resin composite material. An understanding of the advantages and limitations of the various types of materials enables clinicians to make selections based on the best compromise of desired properties versus inherent limitations.

■ Predicted Versus Actual Strengths

It is possible to predict the strength of a material from the strengths of the individual bonds between the atoms in the material. The values of strength obtained by such a prediction are typically 7 to 21 GPa (about 1 to 3 million psi). Actual strengths of most materials are 10 to 100 times lower.

Why do materials fail to exhibit the strengths one would expect from the bonds between atoms? Why do ceramics break suddenly without yielding, whereas metals often yield and distort to 120% or more of their original length before fracturing? Why are polymers so much weaker and more flexible than metals and ceramics? Why do metals conduct heat and electricity, whereas polymers and ceramics do not? There is one key concept, for example, that will not only explain the tendency for ceramics to be brittle, but will also explain all of the methods used to strengthen ceramics. Similarly, one key concept will explain why polymers expand about 10 times as much as metals or ceramics when heated to the same temperature, why polymers are generally weak, why they are 10 times more flexible than metals or ceramics, and why they tend to absorb water and other fluids.

■ Ceramics

Stress concentration and ceramic strength

Consider a block of material as depicted in Fig 1-2a. If this block is stretched by applying a force *F*, the stress at any point on cross section *A* will be the same as the average stress, σ_{ave}. For example, if the cross-sectional dimensions of the block are 1.0 cm × 1.0 cm = 1.0 cm² (0.394 inch × 0.394 inch = 0.155 inch²), and a force of 10.0 kN (2,250 lbs) is applied, the average stress along

Fig 1-2 Stress raisers and the effect of their shape on stress concentration. *(a)* If no stress raiser is present, the stress is constant across cross section A. *(b)* If a rounded notch is present, the stress is constant over most of the cross section. *(c)* As the notch becomes sharper, the stress concentration becomes greater.

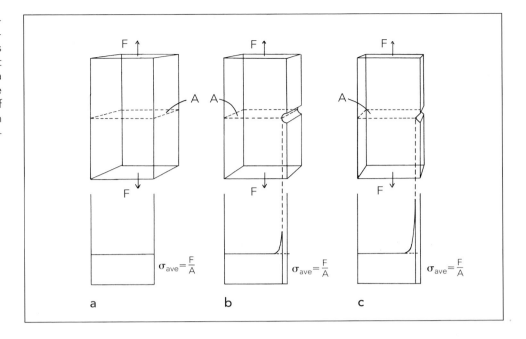

cross section *A* is 100 MPa (14,500 psi). However, if a semicircular groove were machined across one side of the block of material as depicted in Fig 1-2b, the stress at each point of a plane passing through this groove would not be the same as the average stress. The stress would be constant over most of the cross section, but near the groove the stress would suddenly rise and reach a maximum at the edge of the groove. This phenomenon occurs around any irregularity in a block of material. The groove or other irregularity is called a **stress raiser**. The stress around a stress raiser can be many times higher than the average stress in the body. The amount of increased stress depends on the shape of the stress raiser. For example, if the stress raiser in our block of material were a sharp notch rather than a semicircular groove, the stress would increase greatly at the tip of the notch (Fig 1-2c). The minute scratches on the surfaces of nearly all materials behave as sharp notches whose tips are as narrow as the spacing between atoms in the material. Thus, the stress concentration at the tips of these scratches reaches the theoretic strength of the material at relatively low average stress. When the theoretic strength of the material is exceeded at the tip of the notch, the bonds at the tip break (Fig 1-3a). The adjacent bonds now at the tip of the notch are at the point of greatest stress concentration (Fig 1-3b). As the crack propagates

through the material, the stress concentration is maintained at the crack tip until the crack moves completely through. This stress concentration phenomenon enables us to understand how materials can fail at stresses far below their expected strength, such as in the technique in glass cutting, where a shallow line is scribed on one surface with a diamond point or a hardened steel glass-cutting wheel. Although the scribed line is a mere shallow scratch or crack in comparison with the thickness of the glass, it acts as a stress raiser, concentrating the stress at the tip of the crack. (Please note that the exceeding of the theoretic strength of the material at the crack tip is a necessary but insufficient condition for crack propagation. The remaining condition involves a balance between the surface energy required to form the two new surfaces of the crack, and the elastic strain energy arising from the applied stress. This phenomenon is called the *Griffith energy balance,* the discussion of which is beyond the scope of this book.)

Understanding the effect of stress concentration is the key to understanding the failure of brittle materials, such as ceramics, which tend to fail at stresses far below the theoretic strengths of these materials because of the stress concentration at surface scratches and other defects. Most of the techniques for strengthening ceramics can also be understood by virtue of this concept.

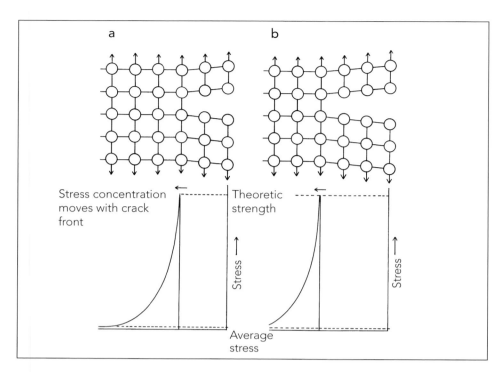

Fig 1-3 Role of stress raisers in achieving localized stresses as great as the theoretic strength of the material. The stress at the tip of the notch reaches the theoretic strength of the material even though the average stress is many times lower. As the most highly stressed bond breaks (a), the stress is transferred to the next bond (b).

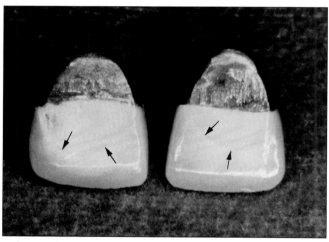

Fig 1-4 Brittle fracture (arrows) of ceramic (dental porcelain) due to mismatch in the coefficient of thermal expansion between porcelain and metal. (Photo courtesy of R. P. O'Connor, DMD.)

Clinical applications of ceramics

Ceramics are inherently brittle and must be used in such a way as to minimize the effect of this property. To avoid catastrophic failure, ceramic restorations must not be subjected, for example, to large tensile stresses. A method for reducing the brittleness of ceramics is to fuse them to a material of greater toughness (eg, metal), as is done with PFM restorations. Ceramics also may be reinforced with dispersions of high-toughness materials, as is the case with the alumina (Al_2O_3)-reinforced porcelain used in porcelain jacket crowns. Figure 1-4 shows brittle fractures in the porcelain of two PFM crowns due to the

mismatch in thermal expansion between the porcelain and metal.

■ Metals

Effect of ductility on stress concentration

In a ductile material, an intervening factor acts before the theoretical strength of the material is reached at the tip of the stress raiser. While a sharp notch or scratch on the surface of a brittle material will cause a stress concentration like that shown in Fig 1-5a, on a ductile metal, the material at the tip of the stress raiser will deform under stress so that the sharp notch becomes a rounded groove, as shown in Fig 1-5b. Because the tip of the stress raiser is now rounded rather than sharp, the stress concentration at the tip of this stress raiser is much lower.

There are two important facts to recognize in this process:

1. As with brittle materials, the actual strengths of ductile materials are many times less than those predicted from strengths of bonds between atoms.
2. Unlike the behavior around the notch in a brittle material, the stress concentration blunts the sharp tip of the stress raiser, thus lowering the stress concentration.

Mechanism of ductile behavior

A schematic of the arrangement of atoms in a piece of metal is shown in Fig 1-6. If this piece of metal is subjected to a tensile stress as shown, this stress can be resolved into two components when considered relative to the plane A-A'. One component tends to move the rows of atoms on either side of the plane A-A' apart from each other, and the other component tends to cause the planes to slide past one another along the plane A-A'.

The component of the stress that tends to cause the planes to slide past one another is the one that causes a material to deform plastically. Scientists are able to calculate, from the bond strengths between the atoms, the stresses that would be required to make one plane of atoms slide past another plane, although these stresses are 100 or more times higher than those actually observed. If, however, the bonds were to break one at a time and re-form immediately with the adjacent atom, one plane could move past the other at very low stress levels.

The mechanism of this process is shown in Fig 1-7. Figures 1-7a through 1-7f show how, by breaking and re-forming bonds, an extra plane of atoms can move along plane A-A' until this "ripple" in the crystal lattice passes completely through the material. Multiple repetitions of this process along many planes similar to A-A' allow a metal to yield to an applied stress without fracturing. This ripple in the lattice structure is called a **dislocation**, and it is responsible for the ductile behavior of metals.

Metals can be hardened and strengthened by a variety of treatments that make it more difficult for dislocations to move through the metal lattice. Alloying, cold-

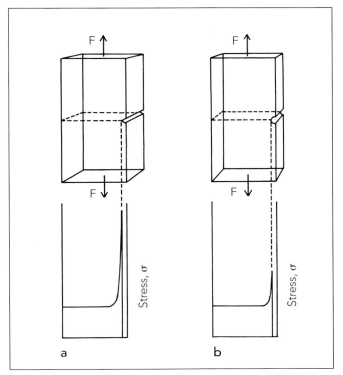

Fig 1-5 Rounding or blunting of stress raisers that occurs in ductile materials. Stress concentration is self-limiting in ductile materials because the region under greatest stress, the tip of the sharp stress raiser (a), yields to round or blunt the stress raiser and lower the stress (b).

working, and formation of second phases in a metal are all ways of impeding dislocation motion. Some crystal structures of metals, such as intermetallic compounds, make it difficult for the dislocations to move. The passage of a dislocation through the ordered structure of an intermetallic compound would result in an unfavorable atomic arrangement, so dislocations move only with difficulty. With metals, it is important to remember that their ability to yield without fracturing, as well as all of the methods for making metals harder and stronger, is understandable in light of the concept of dislocations in the metal structure.

Other properties of metals, such as their electric and thermal conductivity, can be understood as resulting from **metallic bonds**. In a metallic bond, some of the electrons are free to move rapidly through the lattice of metal ions. This unusual aspect of metallic bonds enables metals to conduct heat and electricity. The electronic structure of the metallic bond also accounts for the opacity of metals. Figure 1-8 illustrates the metallic bond with its lattice of

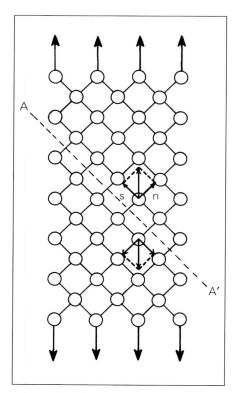

Fig 1-6 Tensile stress on a piece of material can be considered stress normal (n) (perpendicular) to plane A-A', together with stress parallel (s) to plane A-A'. The stress parallel to plane A-A' tends to cause the atoms along the plane to slide (shear) past each other.

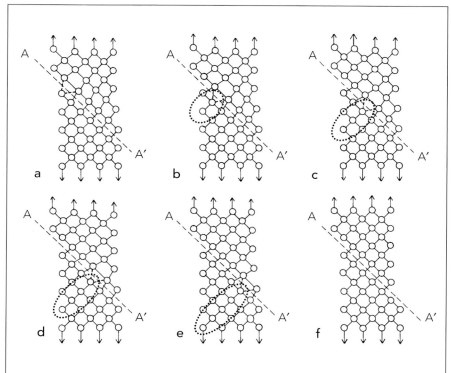

Fig 1-7 Shearing stress can cause a dislocation to pass through the network of atoms. *(a)* The leftmost atom below the plane A–A' is induced by the shear stress to partially break its bond with its corresponding atom above the plane and partially reform a bond with the next atom to the right. The partial bonds are represented by dashed lines. *(b to f)* This process continues, where the extra plane of atoms created in the lattice is circled with a dotted outline. The region where one atom is partially bonded to two atoms above the plane is a kind of "ripple" in the ordered lattice structure of the material. For the atoms along plane A-A' to slip past one another all at once would require enormous stress. Dislocations allow this slip to occur at much lower stresses.

positively charged metal ion cores and electrons that are free to move between the ion cores.

Dislocations in ceramic materials and in intermetallic compounds

Why do ceramic materials not yield in the same manner as metals? The answer to this question involves consideration of the characteristics of two types of ceramic materials:

1. **Amorphous** materials (glasses)—Glassy materials do not possess an ordered crystalline structure as do metals. Because dislocations of a crystalline lattice cannot exist in glassy materials, glasses have no mechanism for yielding without fracture.
2. **Crystalline** ceramic materials—Dislocations exist in crystalline ceramic materials, but their mobility is se-

verely limited, because their movement would require that atoms of like charge be brought adjacent to one another, as seen in Fig 1-9. The energy required for this movement is so large that dislocations are essentially immobile in crystalline ceramic materials.

Intermetallic compounds, unlike ordinary metal **alloys**, have a specific formula (eg, Ag_3Sn, the main component of dental amalgam alloy powder) and an ordered arrangement of atoms. The movement of a dislocation through this ordered structure would produce a disruption of the order similar to that shown in Fig 1-9 for crystalline ceramic materials. Hence, dislocations move only with difficulty in intermetallic compounds, and this property renders them more brittle than ordinary metal alloys.

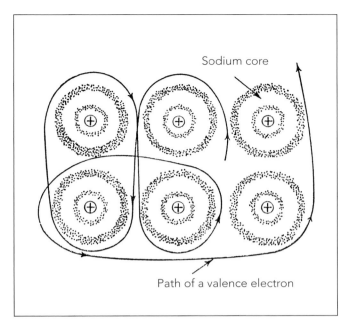

Fig 1-8 Representation of the metallic bond showing the metal ion cores surrounded by free electrons. (After Lewis and Secker.[1])

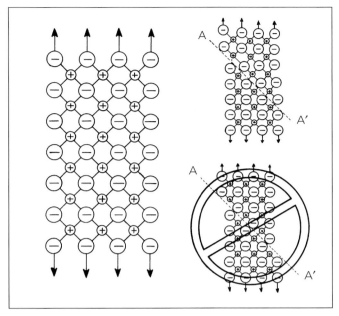

Fig 1-9 The alternating charges of an ionic structure (crystalline ceramic) do not allow dislocations to move along plane A-A'. If a dislocation were to pass through such a structure, it would result in ions of like charge coming into direct contact, which would require too much energy.

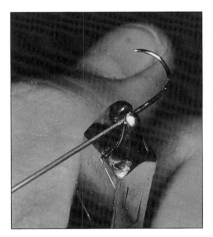

Fig 1-10 Ductility of metal as illustrated by the adaptation (bending) of a partial denture wrought wire clasp.

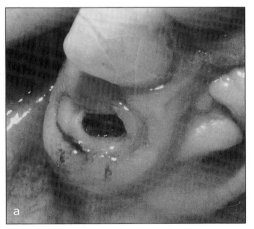

Fig 1-11 Brittle fracture of (a) an amalgam post and core that had supported (b) a PFM crown. Set dental amalgam is a mixture of several intermetallic compounds. Intermetallic compounds tend to be brittle rather than ductile. (Photo courtesy of R. P. O'Connor, DMD.)

Clinical applications of metals

Metals are generally ductile and tough when compared with ceramics, although a few types of metals, such as dental amalgams, are markedly more brittle than others. This ductility allows the margins of castings to be burnished, orthodontic wires to be bent, and partial denture clasps to be adjusted. Figure 1-10 shows how the ductility of metal allows the wire clasp for a partial denture framework to be bent permanently to provide the desired retention. The ductile behavior of the partial denture alloy can be contrasted with the brittle behavior of the intermetallic dental amalgam, as shown in Fig 1-11.

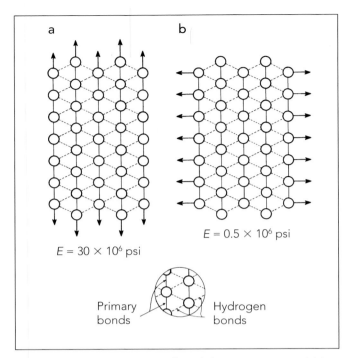

Fig 1-12 (*a*) Strong (primary) bonds between atoms within a polymer chain result in a high stiffness (modulus of elasticity) when aligned chains are stretched along their lengths. (*b*) Weak (hydrogen) bonds between atoms in adjacent chains result in a low modulus of elasticity when aligned chains are stretched perpendicular to their lengths.

■ Polymers

The behavior of polymers is fundamentally different from that of ceramics and metals. To understand this difference, it is useful to consider the modulus of elasticity and the strength of polymers at a molecular level.

Modulus of elasticity

When chains of polyethylene are aligned parallel to one another and are subjected to a tensile stress along their long axis, as shown in Fig 1-12a, the stress required to stretch the atoms in the chains farther apart is surprisingly high. The modulus of elasticity of polyethylene when measured in this way is 200 GPa, about the same as steel! However, if the applied stress is perpendicular to the long axis of the chains, the modulus of elasticity is only about 3 GPa. The high modulus of elasticity in the first case results from the strong bonds between the atoms *within* polymer chains. The low elastic modulus (3 GPa) in the second case results from the weak bonds between atoms in *adjacent* chains.

The molecules of bulk polymers are in a more random, tangled arrangement, and hence there are somewhat fewer secondary bonds between chains than when the chains are perfectly aligned. The tangling and coiling of the polymer molecules make polymers even more flexible, because of the lower stress required to straighten out a coiled molecule compared with the stress necessary to stretch the atoms in a molecule farther apart.

Strength

The low strength of polymers when compared with that of ceramics and metals can also be understood in terms of the strong bonds within polymer chains and the weak bonds between polymer chains. If the rule-of-thumb value for theoretic strength, 0.1 *E* (modulus of elasticity), is applied to the oriented polyethylene fiber shown in Fig 1-12b, a value of 20 GPa is obtained for the theoretic strength of polyethylene. Typical bulk polymers, however, seldom have tensile strengths of more than 70 MPa. The weak secondary bonds between polymer chains allow these chains to slide past one another at much lower stresses than those required to break the bonds within the chains.

Thermal expansion

Increases in the temperature of a material are the result of increased atomic vibration. This atomic vibration is limited by the bonds between atoms in a material such that when strong bonds are present between atoms, the atoms vibrate over a small amplitude, and when weak bonds are present, the atoms vibrate over a large amplitude. Ceramics and metals are characterized by strong bonds between atoms, and the secondary bonds play an insignificant role in their properties. As a result, most ceramics and metals expand relatively little when heated—that is, their coefficients of thermal expansion are relatively low. Polymers, however, are characterized by strong bonds within polymer chains and weak bonds between polymer chains. Thus, the vibration of carbon atoms within the polymer chain is restricted in the directions parallel to the long axis of the chain, but the atoms are free to vibrate in the two directions perpendicular to the long axis of the polymer chain. As a result, when a polymer is heated, the chains must move farther apart to allow for the larger-amplitude vibration, which occurs perpendicular to the long axes of the polymer chains. This phenomenon accounts for the large coefficient of thermal expansion exhibited by polymers. Figure 1-13

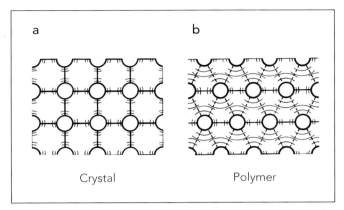

Fig 1-13 The different thermal expansion behaviors of a polymeric material and a crystalline material. (a) The crystalline material has strong bonds to all neighboring atoms, so the amplitude of thermal vibration is small during heating. (b) The polymeric material has strong bonds within polymer chains (ie, with the corresponding small amplitude of thermal vibration) and weak bonds between polymer chains (ie, with the corresponding large amplitude of thermal vibration). The large amplitude of thermal vibration forces the chains apart as the polymer is heated and results in the higher thermal expansion of polymers.

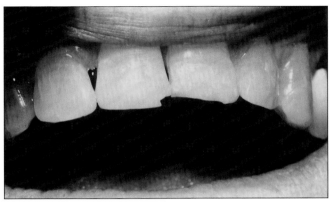

Fig 1-14 Fracture of a Class 4 microfilled composite restoration. The low filler content of most microfills leaves the polymer matrix bearing the majority of the stress. Polymers are generally too weak for bearing large stresses. (Photo courtesy of C. D. Smith, DDS.)

illustrates the different thermal expansion behaviors of a polymeric material and a crystalline material.

Water absorption

Because of the weak secondary bonds in polymers, water molecules are able to penetrate between the polymer chains in a process called **water absorption**. Water absorption has both positive and negative aspects. On the positive side, it is the main factor in correcting the 0.5% processing shrinkage that occurs during the fabrication of heat-cured denture bases. When the acrylic resin polymer absorbs water, the polymer molecules are forced apart slightly, causing the denture base to expand. This expansion during water absorption compensates for the processing shrinkage. On the negative side, water is responsible for the hydrolytic degradation of polymers. In addition, the ions carried by the water may cause the polymer to break down more quickly or to become stained or malodorous.

Effect of cross-linking

Because many of the undesirable properties of polymers are due to weak bonds between polymer chains, it would seem that a way to improve them would be to link chains together with primary chemical bonds. This method, called **cross-linking**, is widely used to improve strength,

resistance to water absorption, abrasion resistance, and other properties of polymers. Because of the small number of primary bonds in a given volume of polymer material as compared with ceramics or metals, however, polymer properties remain generally inferior even with cross-linking.

The key to understanding polymers is that the low strengths and elastic moduli of polymers, as well as many other distinctive properties, can be seen in light of the concept of strong bonds within polymer chains and weak bonds between polymer chains.

Clinical applications of polymers

Polymers have had limited use as restorative materials by themselves because of their low strength and high thermal expansion. Some of the unfavorable properties of polymers have been mitigated by the incorporation of inorganic fillers to form composite materials. In general, the higher the filler loading (volume %), the better the properties of the resulting composite. The incisal fracture of a Class 4 microfilled composite restoration is shown in Fig 1-14. Microfilled resin composites tend to have considerably lower levels of the stronger inorganic filler, and so the stresses are borne more heavily by the weaker resin matrix. In Class 4 restorations, microfills generally have insufficient strength to withstand the stresses that may be encountered. By using blends of different-sized particles, manufacturers have been able to create hybrid composites that offer polishability close to microfilled composites, yet filler loading approaching or even exceeding the larger particle composites. Manufacturers have taken advantage of the unique properties of nano particles to create nano-hybrid composites with workable viscosities and extremely high filler loads (over 70 volume %).

◼ Glossary

alloy A material that exhibits metallic properties and is composed of one or more elements—at least one of which is a metal. For example, steel is an alloy of iron and carbon, brass is an alloy of copper and zinc, and bronze is an alloy of copper and tin.

amorphous Literally, "without form." Atoms in crystalline solids exhibit an ordered arrangement, whereas atoms in amorphous solids lack this long-range periodicity.

ceramic In the broadest sense, a compound of metallic and nonmetallic elements. By this definition, materials ranging from aluminum oxide (Al_2O_3) to table salt (NaCl) are classified as ceramics. In dentistry, gypsum ($CaSO_4 \cdot 2H_2O$), many dental cements (eg, zinc phosphate), and porcelains are examples of ceramic materials.

cross-linking A method for making a polymer stronger and more rigid by creating chemical bonds between the molecular chains in the polymer.

crystalline Having atoms or molecules arranged in a regular, repeating three-dimensional pattern. Metals are nearly always crystalline; ceramics and polymers can be crystalline or noncrystalline (amorphous).

dislocation A defect in a crystal that is caused by an extra plane of atoms in the structure (see Fig 1-7). The movement of dislocations is responsible for the ability of metals to bend without breaking.

intermetallic compound A chemical compound whose components are metals. The γ phase of amalgam, Ag_3Sn, is an example of an intermetallic compound.

metal A crystalline material that consists of positively charged ions in an ordered, closely packed arrangement and bonded with a cloud of free electrons. This type of bond, called a *metallic bond*, is responsible for many of the properties of metals—electric and thermal conductivity, metallic luster, and (usually) high strength.

metallic bond One of the three types of primary (strong) chemical bond. (Ionic and covalent are the other two.) Metallic bonds involve the sharing of valence electrons among all atoms in the metal. Metallic bonds are responsible for many of the distinctive properties of metals, including electric conductivity.

modulus of elasticity A measure of the stiffness or flexibility of a material. A stiff material has a high modulus of elasticity, and a flexible material has a low modulus of elasticity. Also called the *Young modulus*. (See chapter 2 for more detail.)

polymer A material that is made up of repeating units, or *mers*. Most polymers are based on a carbon backbone (ie, –C–C–C–C–) in the polymer chain, although a silicone backbone (ie, –O–Si–O–Si–O–) is important in many polymers.

stress raiser An irregularity on the surface or in the interior of an object that causes applied stress to concentrate in a localized area of the object. Other characteristics being equal, the sharper the stress raiser, the greater the localized stress around it.

water absorption The penetration of water into the structure of a material. Water absorption by polymers can help offset the effects of processing or polymerization shrinkage (as in heat-processed denture bases), but it can also have detrimental effects, such as discoloration and leaching of unreacted components. For water to be absorbed into the structure of a material, it must first be *ad*sorbed onto the surface. Because both phenomena occur when water is *ab*sorbed, the process is often referred to simply as *water sorption*.

◼ Discussion Questions

1. Although metals have had a long history of application as restorative materials, which properties of metals are causing a decline in their use? Which properties will promote their use for dental applications for many more years?

2. Which physical properties are related to the large differences in wear resistance of polymers and ceramics?

3. Although the strength values of materials based on testing and reported in research publications are often high, dental devices may fail at low levels of stress. Explain and indicate how materials need to be used in dentistry to achieve the full strength potential of the materials used.

4. Why are the mechanical properties of materials so important in restorative dentistry?

5. How does the atomic bonding of materials determine many of the observed properties of materials?

Study Questions

(See appendix E for answers.)

1. Characterize the three basic materials (metals, ceramics, and polymers) in regard to modulus of elasticity, strength, ductility, and coefficient of thermal expansion.

2. Describe the relationship between the shape of a stress raiser and the concentration of stress around it.

3. Discuss the key concept for each of the three basic materials and show how it explains the properties of each.

Reference

1. Lewis TJ, Secker PE. Science of Materials. London: Harrap, 1965.

Recommended Reading

Callister WD. Materials Science and Engineering: An Introduction, ed 5. New York: John Wiley & Sons, 2000.

Kittel C. Introduction to Solid State Physics, ed 7. New York: John Wiley & Sons, 1996.

Marder MP. Condensed Matter Physics. New York: John Wiley & Sons, 2000.

Roylance D. Mechanics of Materials. New York: John Wiley & Sons, 1996.

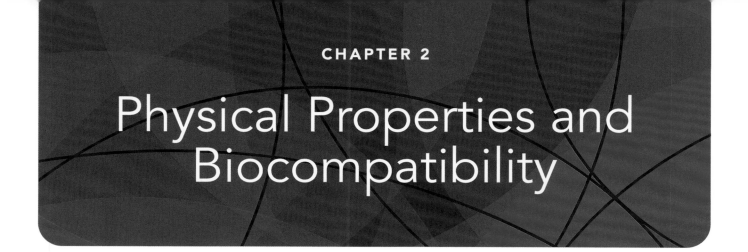

Physical Properties and Biocompatibility

Physical properties determine how materials respond to their environment, and *biocompatibility* relates to the effect a material has on the surrounding tissue. Physical properties are classified according to the scheme in Fig 2-1.

◼ Mechanical Properties

The concepts of stress, strain, modulus of elasticity, plastic deformation, and other properties were introduced in chapter 1, and are discussed here in greater depth.

Stress

Consider again the block of material described in the previous chapter (see Fig 1-2), which measured 1.0 cm × 1.0 cm = 1.0 cm² (0.394 in × 0.394 in = 0.155 in²) in cross section and was subjected to a 10.0-kN (2,250-lb) load. As was pointed out previously, the stress experienced by that block is 100 MPa (14,500 psi). Stress (σ) is the force (F) divided by the cross-sectional area (A):

$$\sigma = \frac{F}{A}$$

Consider now a similar block but with smaller dimensions—0.50 cm × 0.50 cm (0.197 in × 0.197 in) in cross section (area = 0.25 cm² or 0.0388 in²). If this new block is subjected to the same 10.0-kN (2,250-lb) tensile load, the stress is 10 kN (2,250 lb) divided by 0.25 cm² (0.0388 in²) = 400 MPa (58,000 psi).

The usefulness of the concept of **stress** is apparent. It is not sufficient merely to state the load or force that is being applied to a dental material, because the stress

that is produced in the material depends just as much on the cross-sectional area on which the load is acting as it does on the load itself. For instance, if the block that measured 1.0 cm × 1.0 cm in cross section is subjected to a load of 40 kN (9,000 lb) instead of 10 kN (2,250 lb), the stress is 400 MPa (58,000 psi). If the cross-sectional area is made four times smaller (one-fourth as large), or if the load is made four times larger, the stress is increased by a factor of four. Thus, the stress is said to be inversely proportional to the cross-sectional area and directly proportional to the load.

The basic types of stresses produced in dental structures under a force are **tensile**, **compressive**, and **shear**. All three are active in a beam loaded in the center. If the value of these stresses exceeds the strength of the material, the structure will fail. It is therefore important to know the strength values of materials. It is rare that an object will be subject to the pure tensile, compressive, or shear stresses experienced by test specimens in a materials testing laboratory. As shown in Fig 2-2, however, wherever bending forces are present, tensile stresses are also present in critical areas, which could result in failure.

Strain

When a block of material is subjected to a tensile stress as described in the preceding paragraph, it temporarily becomes longer. This temporary increase in length is called **strain**. The following examples illustrate conditions of strain. Consider the block with the cross section of 0.50 cm × 0.50 cm = 0.25 cm² (0.197 in × 0.197 in = 0.0388 in²), and assume it has a length of 25.0 cm (9.843 in) when no load is applied. If the length is measured while the 10.0-kN (2,250-lb) tensile load is being applied and the

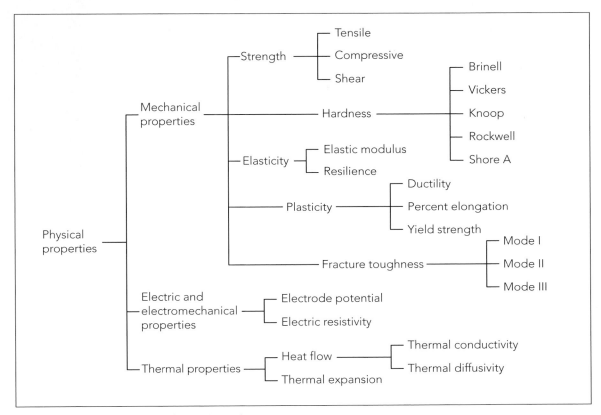

Fig 2-1 A tree diagram classifying physical properties.

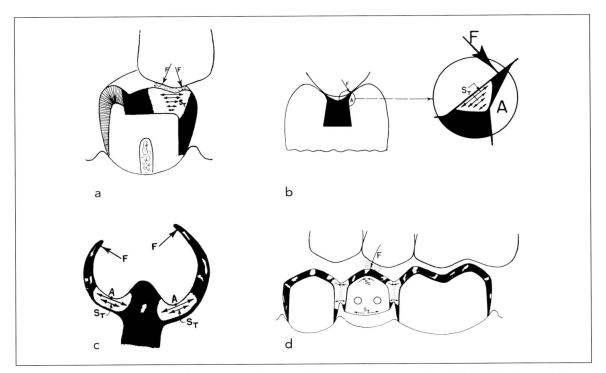

Fig 2-2 (a) Tensile stress (S_T) at the isthmus of a two-surface amalgam restoration. (b) Tensile stress at the occlusal surface of a beveled amalgam restoration. (c) Tensile stress at the junctions of a partial denture clasp. (d) Tensile and compressive stresses (S_C) in a soldering bridge. F = force; A = area. (Reprinted with permission from Mahler and Terkla.[1])

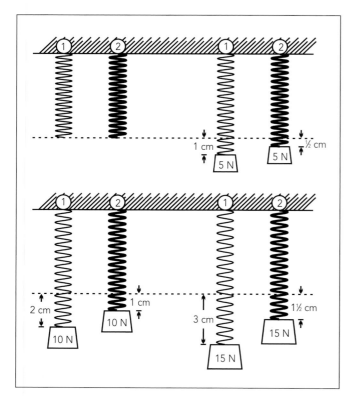

Fig 2-3 The concept of modulus of elasticity (*E*) using the analogy of springs. Spring 1 is a flexible spring, representing a material with a low modulus of elasticity. Spring 2 is a stiff spring, representing a material with a high modulus of elasticity. When the same load is applied to both springs, they stretch different amounts. The weight applied to the spring is analogous to the stress (σ), the amount the spring stretches is analogous to the strain (ε), and the stiffness of the spring is analogous to the modulus of elasticity.

new length is 25.04 cm (9.859 in), the strain is computed by dividing the increase in length (0.04 cm [0.016 in]) by the original length (25.00 cm [9.843 in]) to obtain 0.0016. Strain is a dimensionless quantity, because unit length is being divided by unit length, but sometimes it is written as "cm/cm" or "in/in." Strain can also be expressed as a percentage where the dimensionless value is multiplied by 100%, which in the given example would be 0.16%.

If a piece of the same material with the same cross section but a length of 27.500 cm (10.827 in) were subjected to the same load (10.0 kN [2,250 lb]), and the length of the block of material was measured while the load was being applied, it would be 27.544 cm (10.844 in) long. To compute the strain produced, the change in length (0.044 cm [0.017 in]) is divided by the original length (27.500 cm [10.827 in]), which yields a strain of

0.0016 (or 0.16%), the same value obtained above for the block of material measuring 25.00 cm (9.843 in) long. Thus, it can be seen that strain is independent of the length of the specimen.

Now consider a bar of high-strength steel measuring 0.50 cm × 0.50 cm = 0.25 cm² (0.197 in × 0.197 in = 0.0388 in²) in cross section and 25.00 cm (9.843 in) in length that is capable of supporting a tensile load of 20.0 kN (4,500 lb). The length of this bar under this load would be 25.08 cm (9.874 in), and the strain would be the change in length (0.08 cm [0.031 in]) divided by the original length (25.00 cm [9.843 in]), which is 0.0032 or 0.32%. Hence, if the cross-sectional area of the block of material is kept the same and the load applied is doubled, the strain experienced by the material is doubled.

Elasticity

The preceding examples showed that both stress and strain are directly proportional to the load applied when the cross-sectional area is kept the same, and if the load is doubled, both the stress and the strain will be doubled. The ratio between stress (σ) and strain (ε) is the same, thus:

$$\frac{\sigma}{\epsilon} = \frac{2\sigma}{2\epsilon} = \frac{3\sigma}{3\epsilon}$$

The property of having a constant ratio of stress to strain is called **elasticity**, and this constant is called the **modulus of elasticity**. To gain a clearer understanding of the concept of elasticity and to see what it means for two materials to have different moduli of elasticity, it is helpful to consider the analogy of two springs of different stiffnesses, as shown in Fig 2-3. Spring 2 is stiffer than spring 1; therefore, when they support equal weights, the stiffer spring is extended a smaller amount. Increasing the load from 5 N (1.12 lb) to 10 N (2.25 lb) causes each spring to extend twice as much as it did under the 5-N (1.12-lb) load. Subjecting both springs to a 15-N (3.37-lb) load causes each one to extend three times as much as it did under a 5-N (1.12-lb) load, and so on. It can be seen that, irrespective of the load applied for either spring 1 or spring 2, the ratio of the extension to the load is a constant for that spring. However, the constants for the two springs are different. In this analogy, the extension of the spring corresponds to strain, the load or weight on the spring corresponds to stress, and the spring constant corresponds to the modulus of elasticity.

Weight cannot be added to a spring indefinitely and still have the extension increase proportionately. At some point the spring will become "stretched out" and will not return to its original size when the weight is removed. In the same way, when a material is stressed above a certain point, stress is no longer proportional to strain. The greatest stress at which stress is proportional to strain is called the *elastic limit*, or the **proportional limit**. Because this stress is difficult to determine precisely, as it would entail looking for an infinitely small deviation from proportionality, it is customary to designate a certain permanent deformation or offset (usually 0.002, or 0.2%) and to report the **yield strength** of the material at this strain. The yield strength of a material is always slightly higher than the elastic limit.

If a material continues to have more and more weight applied to it, it will of course eventually break. If the material is being stretched (tensile loading), the stress at the point of breakage is called the **ultimate tensile strength** (UTS). When many types of metals are stressed further than their proportional limits, they undergo a process called **work hardening**, through which they become stronger and harder. But with the increased strength comes increased brittleness. Too much bending back and forth of a wire or a partial denture clasp will make it harder and more brittle.

The modulus of elasticity is an inherent property of a material and cannot be altered appreciably by heat treatment, work hardening, or any other kind of conditioning. This property is called *structure insensitivity*, because it is not sensitive to any alteration to the structure (meaning the microstructure) of the material. The modulus of elasticity is one of the few physical properties that have this characteristic. The yield strength of a material, for example, is sensitive to work hardening and will increase with increasing amounts of work hardening.

Plasticity

When the elastic or proportional limit is exceeded in a material, it is said to exhibit "plastic behavior." (The term *plastic* means moldable, but it has come to be associated with polymers.) Materials that experience a large amount of plastic behavior or permanent deformation are said to be **ductile**. Materials that undergo little or no plastic behavior are said to be **brittle**. If stress is plotted against strain, with stress as the ordinate (y-axis) and strain as the abscissa (x-axis), a diagram such as the one in Fig 2-4 is the result. Stress is proportional to strain up to the elastic (or proportional) limit. If a material is stressed into the plastic region or region of permanent deformation

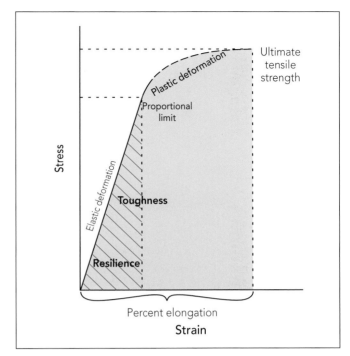

Fig 2-4 Measurement of stress and strain on an object being stretched. In the region labeled *elastic deformation*, stress is proportional to strain, whereas in the region labeled *plastic deformation*, stress and strain are no longer proportional (strain increases faster than does stress). The highest stress at which stress and strain are still proportional is called the *proportional limit*, and the maximum stress just before the object breaks is called the *ultimate tensile strength*. The total amount that the object stretches (ie, the total strain), which is the sum of the elastic deformation and the plastic deformation, is called the *percent elongation*.

and then the stress is removed, the material will have a permanent set, or deformation. If stress is continuously increased, the material will undergo more and more plastic deformation and will ultimately fracture. The highest stress achieved during this process is called the *ultimate tensile strength* of the material, as mentioned previously. The total strain at fracture (elastic strain + plastic strain) is called **elongation**. When one is burnishing the margin of a crown, this property is of greatest value, although the yield strength is also important. For example, gold alloys are generally easy to burnish because they have a lower yield strength. Nickel-chromium and cobalt-chromium alloys may have adequate elongation for burnishing, but their yield strengths are so high that they make burnishing difficult. Another example of the importance of elongation in dentistry is the bending of a partial denture clasp to adjust the retention.

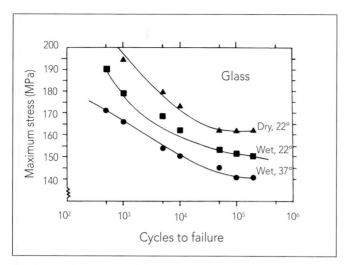

Fig 2-5 Fatigue curves for glass-filled resin composite restorative material. (Courtesy of R. A. Draughn, PhD.)

The entire area under the stress-strain curve is a measure of the energy required to fracture the material, or its **toughness**. The area under only the elastic region of the stress-strain curve, called **resilience**, is a measure of the ability of the material to store elastic energy (the way a compressed spring does).

Tabulated data for the Young modulus of elasticity, yield strength, ultimate tensile strength, percent elongation, and other mechanical properties are listed in appendix A.

Fatigue

When materials are subjected to cycles of loading and unloading, as during mastication, they may fail due to **fatigue** at stresses below the ultimate tensile strength. Usually, small cracks at the surface or within the material gradually grow larger on cycling, and eventually the material fails. Fatigue curves, such as the one depicted in Fig 2-5, show the experimentally determined number of cycles to failure at different stress levels. The higher the stress placed on and off the material, the fewer the number of cycles until failure.

Viscous flow

Many dental materials are in a fluid state when they are formed, and **viscous** flow characteristics are important

considerations. The behavior of impression materials and amalgam involve **viscoelastic** phenomena. When shear stress–strain rate (flow rate) plots are obtained, they enable viscous materials to be classified in several ways. A newtonian fluid shows a constant viscosity, η, which is independent of strain rate:

$$\eta = \frac{\sigma}{\epsilon} = \text{constant}$$

where η is the viscosity in poise, σ is the shear stress acting on the fluid, and ϵ is the strain or flow rate.

Actual fluids differ from these in their flow responses to the level of stress applied. Plastic fluids (eg, putty) do not flow until a minimum stress is applied. Pseudoplastic fluids (eg, fluoride gels) show an instantaneous decrease in apparent viscosity or consistency (become more free-flowing) with increasing shear rate. Dilatant fluids (eg, fluid denture base resins) show an increase in rigidity as more pressure is applied. Thixotropic fluids (eg, fluoride gels, house paints) flow more freely when vibrated, shaken, or stirred than if allowed to sit undisturbed. Formulation of the various suspensions and gels used in dentistry to impart one or more of these properties can make them easier to handle. For example, impression materials that do not run off impression trays but are less viscous under pressure in a syringe have a definite advantage.

Viscoelastic behavior

Many materials, including elastic impression materials, waxes, and even hardened amalgam, show a combination of elasticity and viscous flow. Figure 2-6 is a model of how a viscoelastic material acts under stress, the so-called spring-and-dashpot (or Voigt) model. (A dashpot is an oil-filled cylinder with a loosely fitted piston—most automobile shock absorbers are of a dashpot design.) As the model is stretched, the spring component on the left stretches, and the piston of the dashpot also moves through the viscous liquid. The strain under stress and after release of the stress is time-dependent. The strain gradually builds up until the release of stress, and then it gradually goes back to zero as the spring element returns to its original length but is dampened by the dashpot element. Elastic impression materials are viscoelastic; initially they are strained on removal from the mouth and require a short period of time to recover before models or dies are poured.

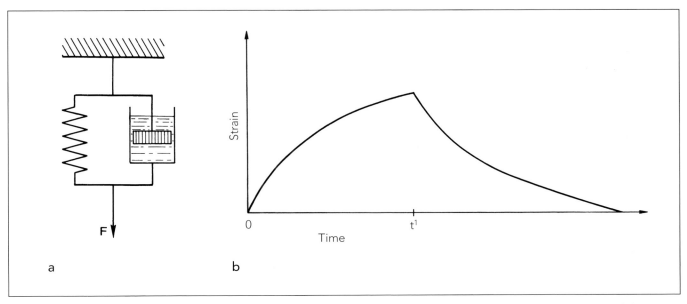

Fig 2-6 *(a)* Voigt model for viscoelastic behavior. *(b)* Response of Voigt model to stress. Strain increases with time and decreases after force (F) is released at t[1] but is slow because of the damping effect of the dashpot or the elastic action of the spring element. (Reprinted with permission from O'Brien and Ryge.[2])

Fig 2-7 Relative hardnesses of a variety of dental materials and tooth substances.

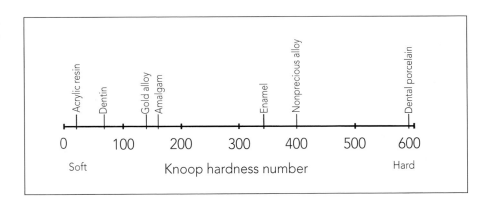

Hardness

The technical definition of **hardness** varies little, if at all, from the familiar definition: the resistance of a material to indentation or penetration. Most of the methods for measuring hardness consist of making a dent in the surface of a material with a specified force in a controlled and reproducible manner and measuring the size of the dent. For the measurement methods discussed in this section, as the hardness increases, the respective hardness number also increases. Figure 2-7 shows the relative positions of a variety of dental and other materials on a Knoop hardness scale ranging from soft on the left to hard on the right.

Brinell hardness number (BHN)

The indenter for the Brinell hardness test is a small, hardened steel ball that is forced into the surface of a material under a specified load. This indentation process leaves a round dent in the material, and hardness is determined by measuring the diameter of the dent. BHNs for selected metals are listed in appendix A.

Vickers hardness number (VHN)

The Vickers hardness indenter is a pyramid-shaped diamond with a square base. Hardness is determined by measuring the diagonals of the square-shaped indentation and taking the average of the two dimensions. The Vickers hardness test is also called the *diamond pyramid hardness test.*

The hardness values on alloy packages are expressed in either BHN or VHN. To compare the two values, use the following equation:

$$VHN = 1.05 \times BHN,$$

$$or\ BHN = \frac{VHN}{1.05}$$

For example, if a package of casting alloy lists a VHN of 242 and you want to compare it with a different brand that lists the BHN, you would divide the VHN by 1.05 to obtain a BHN of 230. VHNs for several types of materials are listed in appendix A.

Knoop hardness number (KHN)

The indenter for the Knoop hardness test is also shaped like a diamond, but one diagonal is much longer than the other. Only the long diagonal is measured to determine the KHN. Appendix A lists KHNs for a variety of materials.

Rockwell hardness

The Rockwell hardness test is used primarily to determine the hardness of steels and is the most widely used hardness test in the United States. The Vickers, Brinell, and Knoop hardness tests are more commonly used for dental materials, however. The Rockwell test uses different types of hardened steel balls or diamond cones and different loads. Each combination forms a specific Rockwell scale (A, B, and C scales are the most common). The different scales are used for materials of different hardness ranges.

Shore A durometer

The Shore A hardness test is used to measure the hardness of rubbers and soft plastics. The Shore A scale is between 0 and 100 units, with complete penetration of the material by the indenter yielding a value of 0, and no penetration yielding a value of 100. Shore A hardness values for several polymeric materials are listed in appendix A.

Fracture Toughness

Resistance of a material to brittle fracture

As discussed in chapter 1, the strength of a block of material is governed by flaws in that block of material, particularly on its surface. This phenomenon is called *stress concentration*. Brittle materials are particularly susceptible to stress concentration because, unlike metals, they

have no mechanism to "blunt" the crack tip and reduce the stress concentration level at that crack tip. Brittle materials are variable, however, in the ease at which a crack can propagate through the material. The resistance of a material to brittle fracture when a crack is present in (or at the surface of) the material is called **fracture toughness**. Fracture toughness is a measure of the amount of energy absorbed during propagation of a crack. In highly brittle materials such as window glass, a crack travels easily because the only process absorbing energy at the tip of the advancing crack is the rupture of the bonds between atoms in the material. In a tougher material, other processes beyond mere bond rupture absorb energy at the tip. In metals, plastic deformation of the metal around the crack tip is by far the most important process for absorbing energy from the crack and slowing its progress. The fracture toughness of a metal is essentially a measure of the extent of this *plastic zone* around the advancing crack. In ceramics, polymers, and composite materials, the situation is much more complicated, with many different toughening mechanisms operating to deplete energy from a crack and slow its progress. Many of these materials are described as having a *fracture process zone* around the tip of the advancing crack that is analogous to the plastic zone in metals.

Fracture toughness is one of the most important properties of a material, because virtually all objects contain interior and surface flaws when they are made, and they develop additional flaws during service. In a material with low fracture toughness, these flaws will more likely grow (under stress) into failure-inducing cracks than they are in a material with high fracture toughness, even if the basic strengths of the two materials are the same. Fracture toughness is expressed in the unusual units of $MPa \cdot m^{1/2}$. These units derive from a parameter called the *stress intensity factor*, *K*, which is used to characterize the distribution of stress around the tip of a crack in a material. The stress intensity factor is a function of the product of the applied stress and the square root of the crack length:

$$k = Y\sigma\sqrt{\pi a}$$

where *Y* is a dimensionless parameter on the order of 1, σ is the applied stress, and *a* is the crack length—hence the unusual units of $MPa \cdot m^{1/2}$. When the stress intensity factor reaches a critical value (by an increase either in the stress or the crack length), the crack will begin to propa-

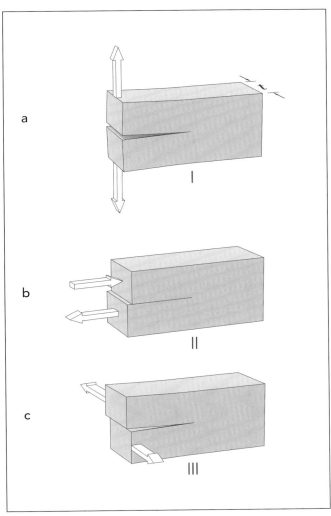

Fig 2-8 The three modes of crack propagation in materials. *(a)* Mode I, *tensile* or *opening* mode. *(b)* Mode II, *in-plane shear* or *sliding* mode. *(c)* Mode III, *anti-plane shear* or *tearing* mode. All three modes tend to cause the crack to advance toward the right.

Table 2-1 Fracture toughness of some materials relevant to dentistry

MATERIAL	K_{IC} (MPA · M$^{\frac{1}{2}}$)
Titanium alloy[3]	55
Aluminum oxide	2.7–5.0
Poly(methyl methacrylate)	0.7–1.6
Amalgam[4]	1.5
Posterior resin composite restorative[5]	1.2–1.3
Packable resin composite restorative[5]	0.7–1.7
Flowable resin composite restorative[6]	1.15–1.65
Zirconia[7]	4.9
Yttria-partially-stabilized-zirconia (YPSZ)[8]	9–10
Human enamel[9]	0.6–0.7
Human dentin[10]	3.1
Human cortical bone[11]	3–6
Dental luting cements[12]	0.27–0.72
Conventional glass ionomer core material[4]	0.72
Resin-modified glass ionomer core material[4]	0.75

gate unstably, and catastrophic failure will occur. This critical value of the stress intensity factor, K_c, is a measure of the fracture toughness of the material.

Stress and propagation of cracks in a material

There are three modes by which stresses can operate on a crack to cause it to propagate. Mode I is called *tensile* or *opening* mode, the crack is "pulled" open (Fig 2-8a). Mode II is called *in-plane shear* or *sliding* mode (Fig 2-8b), and mode III is called *anti-plane shear* or *tearing* mode (Fig 2-8c). Mode I behavior is most commonly encoun-

tered. Published tables of fracture toughness values of materials generally list fracture toughness data for the most commonly encountered situation—mode I crack propagation in an object whose thickness (*t* in Fig 2-8a) is large compared with the dimensions of the crack and its associated plastic zone or fracture process zone. These fracture toughness values are denoted by the parameter K_{Ic}, which is the critical stress intensity factor (K_c) in mode I, as designated by the *I* subscript. Under these crack propagation conditions, K_{Ic} remains constant as the specimen thickness increases. Because of the state of stress and strain around the crack under these conditions, K_{Ic} is also termed *plane strain* fracture toughness.

Plane strain fracture toughness (K_{Ic}) values of selected materials relevant to dentistry are presented in Table 2-1. Materials with a lower fracture toughness are more prone to fail catastrophically during service than those with higher fracture toughness.

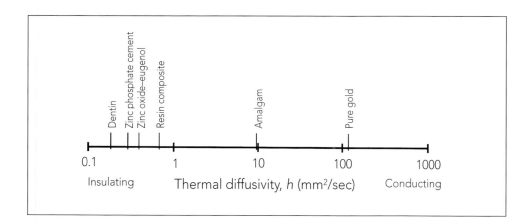

Fig 2-9 Thermal diffusivities of restorative materials.

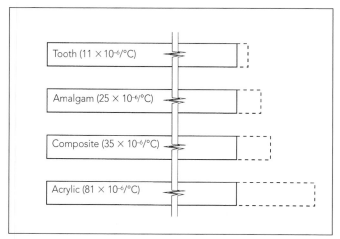

Fig 2-10 Relative thermal expansions of several restorative materials and tooth structure. The relative amounts that the materials expand when heated to the same temperature are represented by the dashed lines. The degree of expansion is magnified to make it visible for comparison.

● Thermal Properties

Heat flow through a material

Metals tend to be good conductors of heat, and this property must be taken into consideration when placing metallic restorations. Dentin is a thermal insulator (poor conductor of heat); thus, when a sufficient thickness of dentin is present, the patient feels no sensitivity to heat and cold through a metallic restoration. However, when only a thin layer of dentin remains, some thermal protection must be provided for the pulp. A good rule of thumb in determining the thickness of cement base necessary in a given situation is to visualize how much dentin would have to be present in the excavation site so that no base would be necessary and then to apply base up to this level. The rate at which heat flows through a material is expressed as **thermal conductivity** or **thermal diffusivity**.

Thermal conductivity

Thermal conductivity (k) is a measure of the speed at which heat travels (in calories per second) through a given thickness of material (1 cm) when one side of the material is maintained at a constant temperature that is 1°C higher than the other side. Thermal conductivity is expressed in units of cal/cm · sec ·°C. Thermal conductivity values for a variety of materials are listed in appendix A.

Thermal diffusivity

Thermal conductivity gives an idea of the relative rates at which heat flows through various materials, but it fails to take into account that various materials require different amounts of heat (calories) to raise their temperatures an equal amount. For example, 1 g of water requires 1.00 cal to raise its temperature 1°C, whereas 1 g of dentin requires only 0.28 cal, and 1 g of gold requires only 0.031 cal to produce a 1°C temperature increase. Thus, thermal conductivity alone will not tell us, for instance, how rapidly the interior surface under a crown will heat up when the exterior surface is heated. To know how quickly the interior of the crown will approach the temperature of the exterior, we need to know the thermal diffusivity of the alloy. The thermal diffusivity (h) of a material (expressed in units of mm²/sec) is dependent on its thermal conductivity, heat capacity (C_p), and density (ρ):

$$h = \frac{k}{(C_p \times \rho)}$$

The relative thermal diffusivities of several dental materials are shown in Fig 2-9, and tabular data on a variety of materials are included in appendix A.

Thermal expansion

Some restorative materials have coefficients of thermal expansion that are markedly different from tooth structure. In such cases, temperature fluctuations that occur in the mouth can cause **percolation** at the tooth-restoration interface as the restoration contracts and expands. To avoid the buildup of large residual stresses, the porcelain and metal in a porcelain-fused-to-metal restoration must contract at the same rate on cooling from the firing temperature. The cooling of a denture base from the processing temperature to room temperature is primarily responsible for the processing shrinkage that occurs. The thermal expansion behavior of dental wax, gold alloy, investment, and so on are important factors to consider in producing properly fitting castings. Figure 2-10 illustrates the relative values of **linear coefficient of thermal expansion** for tooth, amalgam, composite, and acrylic resin. The diagram is only schematic—the expansion has been magnified to make it visible; the actual thermal expansion would be too small to see. The thermal expansion coefficients, or the fractional changes in length per degree Celsius, are given in parentheses. Appendix A lists tabular thermal expansion data on a variety of materials.

Table 2-2 Standard electrode potentials

HALF-REACTION	E⁰ (VOLTS)
$Li^+ + e = Li$	−3.04
$K^+ + e = K$	−2.93
$Ca^{2+} + 2e = Ca$	−2.87
$Na^+ + e = Na$	−2.71
$Mg^{2+} + 2e = Mg$	−2.37
$Al^{3+} + 3e = Al$	−1.662
$Zn^{2+} + 2e = Zn$	−0.762
$Cr^{3+} + 3e = Cr$	−0.744
$Fe^{2+} + 2e = Fe$	−0.447
$Ni^{2+} + 2e = Ni$	−0.257
$Sn^{2+} + 2e = Sn$	−0.1375
$Pb^{2+} + 2e = Pb$	−0.1262
$Fe^{3+} + 3e = Fe$	−0.037
$H^+ + e = H$	0.000 (reference)
$Cu^{2+} + 2e = Cu$	+0.342
$Cu^+ + e = Cu$	+0.521
$Ag^+ + e = Ag$	+0.800
$Hg^{2+} + 2e = Hg$	+0.851
$Pt^{2+} + 2e = Pt$	+1.118
$Au^+ + e = Au$	+1.692

◼ Electric and Electrochemical Properties

Electrode potentials

An electrochemical series is a listing of elements according to their tendency to gain or lose electrons in a solution. The reference standard for this series is the potential of a standard hydrogen electrode, which is arbitrarily assigned a value of 0.000 V. If the elements are listed according to the tendency of their atoms to lose electrons, the potentials are termed *oxidation potentials*. If they are listed according to the tendency of their ions to gain electrons, they are termed *reduction potentials*. Reduction potentials at 25°C and 1 atm are called *standard electrode potentials* (Table 2-2). Metals with a large positive electrode potential, such as platinum and gold, are more resistant to oxidation and corrosion in the oral cavity. If there is a large difference between the electrode potentials of two metals in contact with the same solution, such as between gold and aluminum, an electrolytic cell may develop. In the mouth, this reaction will cause the patient to experience discomfort.

The exact nature of tarnish and corrosion of restorative materials in vivo is extremely complex and involves much more than electrode potentials of materials. A possible source of the corrosion of gold alloys is accidental contamination of the surface with copper during pickling, and subsequent tarnishing in saliva (Fig 2-11).

Electric resistivity

The resistance of a material to the flow of an electric current is **electric resistivity**. The relationship between the resistance (R) in ohms, the resistivity (ρ), the length (l), and the cross-sectional area (A) is as follows:

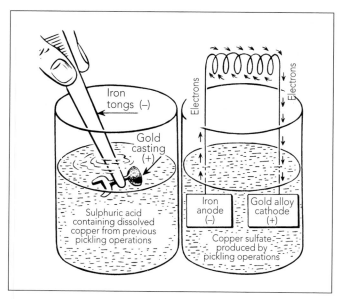

Fig 2-11 Accidental plating of copper during pickling of gold casting. The model of the cell is formed by iron tongs and gold alloy (*right*). (Reprinted with permission from O'Brien.[13])

Table 2-3 Electric resistivity of several materials

MATERIAL	RESISTIVITY (OHM-CM)
Copper	1.7×10^{-6}
SiO₂ (glass)	$> 10^{14}$
Human enamel	-4×10^{6}
Human dentin	-3×10^{4}
Zinc phosphate cement	2×10^{5}
Zinc oxide–eugenol	5×10^{9}

$$R = \rho \left(\frac{l}{A} \right)$$

Electric resistivity values for several materials are presented in Table 2-3. The low resistivity of metallic restorative materials is responsible for pulpal discomfort if dissimilar metals generate a voltage. The insulating properties of cements help to reduce this problem.

● Biocompatibility

A material that is designed to be implanted in the body for the repair or replacement of a diseased or damaged tissue is called a **biomaterial**, and these materials must be **biocompatible**. All materials used in dentistry interact with tissues, producing changes in both the materials and the surrounding tissues; there is no such thing as an "inert material."

Several factors affect the biocompatibility of a material. The chemical composition and structure of the material affect the type and quantities of chemicals released. However, the relative abundance of chemicals in a material will not reliably predict the amounts or even the proportions of the chemicals released. For this reason, the biocompatibility of a material is usually determined empirically. The characteristics of the site of use also influence a material's biocompatibility. For example, many variables in the oral environment affect the release of components from dental materials. Chemical factors, such as bacterial metabolic products, water, enzymes, and polar and nonpolar solvents, can accelerate the release of components. Mechanical factors in the site of use can also affect the biocompatibility of a material. For example, under most conditions, high-molecular-weight polyethylene elicits little if any tissue reaction when implanted. When it is used for the acetabular (socket) side of a total hip replacement, however, it can generate wear debris over time, producing an inflammatory response that eventually causes loosening of the prosthesis and failure of the implant.

For new products that will be used in the body, data must first be presented to government agencies that document possible adverse reactions the material might cause. This information includes the history of the material, its chemical composition, and results from a series of biocompatibility tests. A new version of an old composition used successfully in similar applications may be classified under the Food and Drug Administration (FDA) classification 510(k), which requires less extensive testing for premarket clearance. Another strategic qualification is whether the new product has temporary or long-term contact with the body. The FDA has different categories for materials with short-term contact, such as an impression materials, than for materials used for the long-term, such as a cemented crown or an implant. The more potential for harm, the greater the burden of testing required. The testing required depends on many factors, including the results of initial minimal screening tests. A brief description of these tests is provided in appendix B.

Glossary

biocompatible A material is considered biocompatible if it does not produce harmful or toxic reactions in the tissues it contacts or adverse systemic reactions as a result of elements, ions, and/or compounds it releases.

biomaterial A material that is designed to be implanted in the body for the repair or replacement of a diseased or damaged tissue.

brittle Characteristic of a material that tends to fracture without appreciable plastic deformation.

compressive stress Two forces applied toward one another in the same straight line.

ductile Characteristic of a material to be plastically strained in tension.

elasticity Ability to sustain deformation without permanent change in size or shape.

electric resistivity Ability of a material to resist conduction of an electric current.

elongation Overall deformation (elastic + plastic) as a result of tensile force application.

fatigue Tendency to fracture under cyclic stresses.

fracture toughness The resistance of a material to brittle fracture when a crack is present in (or at the surface of) the material. Fracture toughness is a measure of the amount of energy absorbed during propagation of a crack. Materials with lower fracture toughness are more prone to fail catastrophically during service than those with higher fracture toughness.

hardness Resistance to permanent indentation on the surface.

linear coefficient of thermal expansion Change in length per unit of original length for a 1°C temperature change.

modulus of elasticity Stiffness of a material within the elastic range. Numerically, it is the ratio of stress to strain.

percolation The pumping of oral fluids in and out at the tooth-restoration interface as the restoration contracts and expands with temperature changes. Percolation occurs when the thermal expansion coefficient of the restoration is markedly different from that of tooth structure.

proportional limit (elastic limit) The maximum stress at which the straight-line relationship between stress and strain is valid.

resilience Energy needed to deform a material to the proportional limit.

shear stress Two forces applied toward one another but not in the same straight line.

strain (nominal) Change in length per unit of original length.

stress (nominal) Force per unit area.

tensile stress Two forces applied away from one another in the same straight line.

thermal conductivity The quantity of heat passing through a material 1 cm thick with a cross section of 1 cm^2, having a temperature difference of 1°C.

thermal diffusivity Measure of the heat transfer of a material in the time-dependent state.

toughness Amount of energy needed for fracture.

ultimate tensile strength The maximum strength obtained based on the original dimensions of the sample.

viscoelastic Having both elastic and viscous properties.

viscous Resistant to flow (referring to a fluid).

work hardening The increase in strength and hardness, with accompanying decrease in ductility, that occurs in a ductile metal as it is plastically deformed. Also called *strain hardening.*

yield strength Strength measured at the stress at which a small amount of plastic strain occurs. Also called *yield point.*

Discussion Questions

1. What is galvanic action in the mouth, and how can it be minimized?

2. Why is thermal diffusivity more relevant to insulation of the pulp than thermal conductivity?

3. Explain why fixed partial dentures may fail under tensile stresses due to biting forces that appear to be compressive.

4. Explain how two materials with the same measured tensile strength could have markedly different fracture toughness values.

5. How is the leakage of oral fluids around a composite restoration related to the coefficient of thermal expansion and temperature changes in the mouth?

6. Why is time so important in the behavior of viscoelastic materials such as impression materials and waxes?

7. Why is there a hierarchy of biocompatibility tests?

8. Why can biocompatibility tests be difficult to interpret?

■ Study Questions

(See appendix E for answers.)

1. Discuss why a knowledge and understanding of the physical and mechanical properties of biomaterials is important in dentistry.

2. Explain why the thermal diffusivity of a material is more applicable to behavior in vivo than is its thermal conductivity.

3. Draw and label a stress-strain diagram including the proportional limit, yield point, and ultimate tensile strength.

4. Define *hardness* and its relation to other mechanical properties.

5. Compare materials *a* and *b* on the basis of the two stress-strain curves below obtained by pulling the materials in tension.

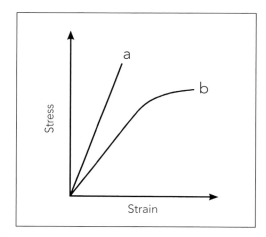

6. Explain what is meant by *fracture toughness* and how it differs from *strength*.

7. Why are laboratory biocompatibility tests run prior to clinical trials?

■ References

1. Mahler DB, Terkla LG. Analysis of stress in dental structures. Dent Clin North Am 1958:789–798.
2. O'Brien WJ, Ryge G. Outline of Dental Materials. Philadelphia: WB Saunders, 1978.
3. Callister WD. Materials Science and Engineering: An Introduction. New York: John Wiley & Sons, 1994.
4. Bonilla ED, Mardirossian G, Caputo AA. Fracture toughness of various core build-up materials. J Prosthodont 2000;9:14–18.
5. Knobloch LA, Kerby RE, Seghi R, Berlin JS, Clelland N. Fracture toughness of packable and conventional composite materials. J Prosthet Dent 2002;88:307–313.
6. Bonilla ED, Yashar M, Caputo AA. Fracture toughness of nine flowable resin composites. J Prosthet Dent 2003;89:261–267.
7. Quinn JB, Sundar V, Lloyd IK. Influence of microstructure and chemistry on the fracture toughness of dental ceramics. Dent Mater 2003;19:603–611.
8. Christel P, Meunier A, Heller M, Torre JP, Peille CN. Mechanical properties and short-term in-vivo evaluation of yttrium-oxide-partially-stabilized zirconia. J Biomed Mater Res 1989;23:45–61.
9. Okazaki K, Nishimura F, Nomoto S. Fracture toughness of human enamel. Shika Zairyo Kikai 1989;8:382–387.
10. El Mowafy OM, Watts DC. Fracture toughness of human dentin. J Dent Res 1986;65:677–681.
11. Zioupos P, Currey JD. Changes in the stiffness, strength, and toughness of human cortical bone with age. Bone 1998;22:57–66.
12. Ryan AK, Orr JF, Mitchell CA. A comparative evaluation of dental luting cements by fracture toughness tests and fractography. Proc Inst Mech Eng [H] 2001;215(1):65–73.
13. O'Brien WJ. Electrochemical corrosion of gold alloys. Dent Abstracts 1962;7:46.

■ Recommended Reading

Practice for direct contact cell culture evaluation of materials for medical devices. In: 1995 Annual Book of ASTM Standards. West Conshohocken, Pa: American Society for Testing and Materials, 1995: 13.01, F813, 233–236.

Standard test method for agar diffusion cell culture screening for cytotoxicity. In: 1995 Annual Book of ASTM Standards. West Conshohocken, Pa: American Society for Testing and Materials, 1995: 13.01, F895, 247–250.

Babich H, Borenfreund E. Structure-activity relationship (SAR) models established in vitro with the neutral red cytotoxicity assay. Toxicol In Vitro 1987;1:3–9.

Billmeyer FW Jr. Textbook of Polymer Science, ed 3. New York: John Wiley & Sons, 1984.

Borenfreund E, Puerner JA. Short-term quantitative in vitro cytotoxicity assay involving an S-9 activating system. Cancer Lett 1987; 34:243–248.

Callister WD Jr. Materials Science and Engineering: An Introduction, ed 5. New York: John Wiley & Sons, 1999.

Chappell RP, Spencer P, Eick JD. The effects of current dentinal adhesives on the dentinal surface. Quintessence Int 1994;25:851–859.

Chiang Y-M, Birnie D III, Kingery WD. Physical Ceramics. New York: John Wiley & Sons, 1997.

Dieter GE. Mechanical Metallurgy, ed 3. New York: McGraw-Hill, 1986.

Doremus RH. Glass Science, ed 2. New York: John Wiley & Sons, 1994.

Ferracane JL, Condon JR. Rate of elution of leachable components from composites. Dent Mater 1990;6:282–287.

Hanks CT, Wataha JC, Sun Z. In vitro models of biocompatibility: A review. Dent Mater 1996;12:186–193.

International Standards Organization. "In vitro" Method of Test for Cytotoxicity of Medical and Dental Materials and Devices. Pforzheim, Germany: International Standards Organization, 1992: 10993–10995.

Rathbun MA, Craig RG, Hanks CT, Filisko FE. Cytotoxicity of a bis-GMA dental composite before and after leaching in organic solvents. J Biomed Mater Res 1991;25:443–457.

Ratner BD, Schoen FJ, Lemons JE (eds). Biomaterials Science: An Introduction to Materials in Medicine. San Diego: Academic Press, 1996.

Reed-Hill RE, Abbaschian R. Physical Metallurgy Principles. Boston: PWS-Kent, 1991.

Tyas MJ. A method for the in vitro toxicity testing of dental restorative materials. J Dent Res 1977;56:1285–1290.

Williams D (ed). Concise Encyclopedia of Medical and Dental Materials. Oxford: Pergamon Press, 1990.

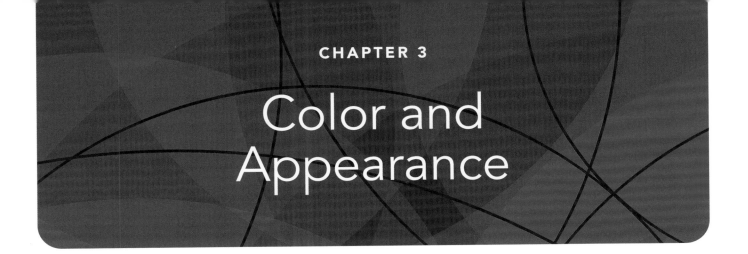

CHAPTER 3

Color and Appearance

Among the important factors that influence the esthetic qualities of restorations are color, translucency, gloss, and fluorescence. Each of these factors, as perceived by an observer, is influenced by *(1)* the illuminant (light source), *(2)* the inherent optical parameters of the restorative materials that dictate the interaction of the light from the illuminant with the material, and *(3)* the interpretation of the observer (Fig 3-1). An understanding of these factors and proper consideration of and communication of this information to the patient is necessary to ensure the appropriate selection and fabrication of esthetic restorations.

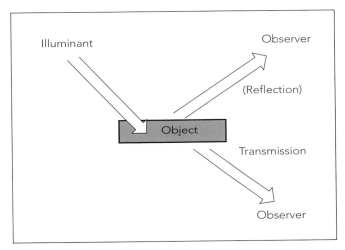

Fig 3-1 Illuminant, object, and observer interaction.

◼ Illuminant

The appropriate illuminant needs to be used in shade selection and matching. The intensity of light emitted at each wavelength (spectral distribution), or **color content**, varies according to the type of illuminant (Fig 3-2). White light contains a mixture of wavelengths (colors). It is dispersed into components when it passes through a prism, as shown in Fig 3-3. Different illuminants have different intensity distributions, or spectra, with respect to wavelength, as illustrated in Figs 3-4a and 3-4b.

Illuminants are sometimes described by their color temperature (in kelvin) based on the equivalence of the illuminant compared with a radiating body having a temperature equal to the color temperature.

The characteristics of an illuminant are important in color evaluation because the intensity distribution, with respect to wavelength, identifies the light spectrum available to interact with the object. Illuminants that closely approximate daylight are preferred because color con-

siderations for restorations, when seen under these illuminants, are close to those seen under natural light. Several "daylight" sources intended for use in dental operatories are available. Representative spectral distributions of some of these illuminants are shown in Figs 3-5a and 3-5b.

Color-rendering index

Color rendering of a light source is the effect that the illuminant has on the color appearance of objects in comparison with their color appearance under a reference source. The *color-rendering index* is a measure of the degree to which the illuminant can impart the color of an object compared with that achieved by the reference source. A color-rendering index of 100 is considered

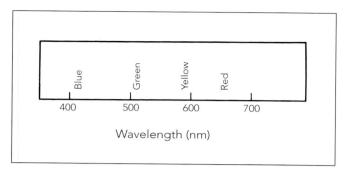

Fig 3-2 Wavelength and hue. (Adapted with permission from Billmeyer and Saltzman.[1])

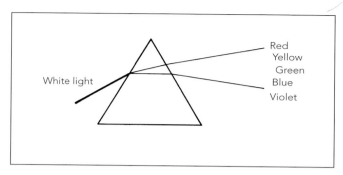

Fig 3-3 Dispersion of white light by a prism.

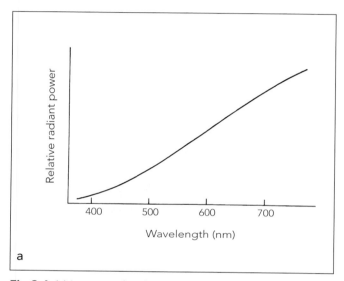

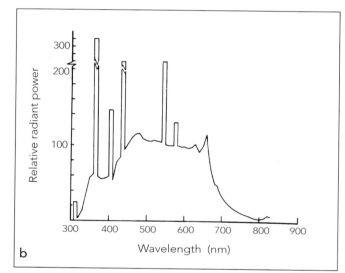

Fig 3-4 (*a*) Intensity distributions of standard illuminant A. (*b*) Intensity distributions of fluorescent light.

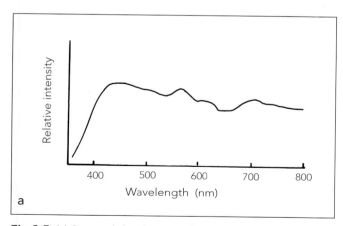

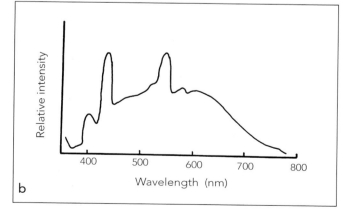

Fig 3-5 (*a*) Spectral distribution of Neylite (J.M. Ney), a device used for dental shade matching. (*b*) Spectral distribution of Vita-Lite (Duro-Test Lighting), a fluorescent lamp for dental operatories.

ideal. For an adequate color-matching environment, the illuminant should have a color-rendering index of 90 or above.[2] A summary of color-rendering indices of some illuminants used in dentistry is shown in Table 3-1.

Surroundings in a dental operatory may modify the actual light reaching the object. Colors of walls, clothing, and soft tissues such as lips contribute to the color of the light incident on teeth, shade guides, and restorative materials.

Table 3-1 Color-rendering indices of illuminants

ILLUMINANT (MANUFACTURER)	COLOR-RENDERING INDEX
Chroma 50 (General Electric)	92
Chroma 75 (General Electric)	94
Cool white (General Electric)	65
Hanau Viewing Lamp (Teledyne Hanau)	93
Neylite (J.M. Ney)	98
Verilux (Verilux)	93
Vita-Lite (Duro-Test)	87, 91

◗ Object

The inherent color property of an object is its characteristic interactions with the light from an illuminant. These interactions include reflection, transmission, and the absorption involved in both processes.

Reflection

A material gains its reflective color by reflecting the part of the spectrum of light incident upon it and absorbing the other parts of the light spectrum. A blue surface reflects only the blue part of the light spectrum and absorbs all of the other colors (Fig 3-6). A **white object** reflects all incident wavelengths, whereas a **black object** absorbs all wavelengths and reflects none. An object that is not black may appear black when no light is reflected from it; for example, a blue object appears black when viewed in red light. Materials of different **reflected color** have different **color reflectance** spectra (Fig 3-7). Reflection spectra of objects are usually obtained using a spectrophotometer.

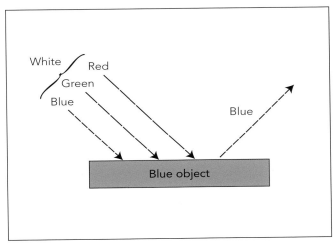

Fig 3-6 Reflected color. A blue object reflects only blue light and absorbs all other colors.

Mixing of reflected colors

To obtain a desired esthetic appearance for a restoration, it is often necessary to use more than one colorant. Each colorant has its own characteristic reflected color because of its reflection spectrum and its absorption of other parts of the spectrum. The mixing of two colorants with different reflected colors and therefore different absorptions results in a reflection of the part or parts of the light spectrum common to both colorants. In other words, each colorant will absorb the part of the light spectrum as if it were by itself. The parts of the light spectrum that are not absorbed by either colorant are, therefore, the resultant reflected color of the mixture of the two.

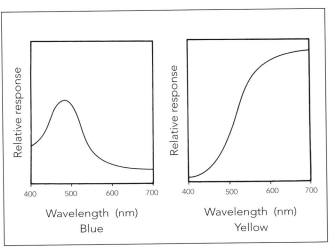

Fig 3-7 Color reflectance of a blue object and a yellow object. (Adapted with permission from Billmeyer and Saltzman.[1])

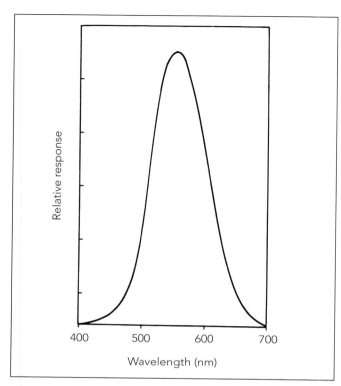

Fig 3-8 Relative response of a human eye at different wavelengths. (Adapted with permission from Billmeyer and Saltzman.[1])

Transmission

A translucent material gains its transmitted color by the spectrum it transmits. As a beam of light passes through a translucent material (eg, glass), it can be changed by the color of the material or scattered by fine particles, giving a milky appearance. Wavelengths that are not transmitted are absorbed. For example, a green filter transmits light in the green wavelength region of the light spectrum and absorbs all other wavelengths.

◉ Observer

The observer receives the light reflected or transmitted by the object and then interprets the results. In many cases, the observer uses the human eye, whose response varies with wavelength. It is most sensitive in the green color region (Fig 3-8) and is best in detecting color differences by comparison.

The detection of color by the human eye results from stimuli received by cone-shaped cells in the retina. Color blindness—the inability to distinguish certain colors—is due to abnormalities in these cells. Constant stimulus of one color decreases the response of the eye to that color, resulting in **color fatigue**. After removal of the stimulus, a complementary color image may persist.

Other detectors may be used as an observer in place of the human eye. Photodetectors, such as spectrophotometers or colorimeters, vary in their responses depending on the type. Color-measuring devices are designed to minimize the effect of photodetector responses. In color measurements and parametric color determinations, the CIE (Commission Internationale de l'Eclairage) Standard Colorimetric Observer is often referenced.

◉ Color Systems

Color systems are used to describe the color parameters of objects. The following are examples of some color systems used in describing the color of dental materials.

Munsell color system

The Munsell color system uses a three-dimensional system with hue, value, and chroma as coordinates (Fig 3-9). **Hue** is the attribute of color that makes it appear blue, yellow, or red. **Value** is the lightness or darkness of a color; a tooth of low value appears gray and nonvital. Value is the most important color factor in tooth color matching. **Chroma** is the intensity of a color, that is, the amount of hue saturation. An example is a beaker of water containing 1 drop of colorant; it is lower in chroma than a beaker of water containing 10 drops of the same colorant.

Color differences between shades in the Munsell system may be calculated using the hue, value, and chroma parameters of the two shades using the equation developed by O'Brien.[3]

CIE color systems

The CIE tristimulus values system uses three parameters, X, Y, and Z, which are based on the spectral response functions defined by the CIE observer. A CIE chromaticity diagram is also sometimes used to define color.

Another CIE color system (CIE L*a*b*) uses the three parameters L*, a*, and b* to define color. The L*, a*, and b* values can be calculated from the tristimulus X, Y, and Z values. The advantage of this color system is that its arrangement is an approximately uniform three-dimensional color space whose elements are equally spaced on the

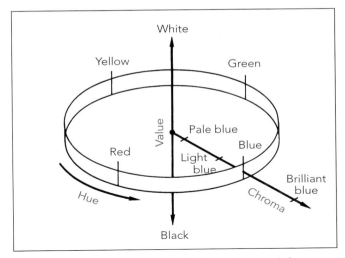

Fig 3-9 Munsell color system with hue, value, and chroma as coordinates.

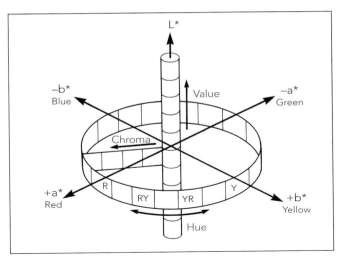

Fig 3-10 CIE and Munsell color arrangements. (Reprinted with permission from Seghi et al.[4])

basis of visual color perception. A unit change in each of the three color parameters is approximately equally perceived. The quality L* correlates to lightness, similar to value in the Munsell system. The a* and b* coordinates describe the chromatic component (Fig 3-10).

The color difference, ΔE*, in the CIE L*a*b* system is defined as:

$$\Delta E^* = [(\Delta L^*)^2 + (\Delta a^*)^2 + (\Delta b^*)^2]1/2$$

where ΔL*, Δa*, and Δb* are the differences between the CIE L*a*b* color parameter of two samples. An advantage of ΔE* is that it can serve as a tolerance for color matching. Clinical color matching between teeth and restorations may be rated according to ΔE* values, as presented in Table 3-2, based on clinical studies. Shade guides are held to a tolerance of an ΔE* of 1, according to an American Dental Association standard. Although these ΔE* values can serve as approximate tolerances, some patients perceive color differences as low as 0.5, whereas others do not see differences of 4. The perception of color is often a source of disagreement among patients, dentists, and laboratory technicians. The reason that a perfect match is not necessary for an acceptable clinical match of a restoration with adjacent natural teeth is that natural teeth in a given patient's arch do not match perfectly. Also, there is a natural color variation in the three regions of each tooth.[5] Indeed, complete dentures with teeth perfectly matching often look artificial.

Table 3-2 Clinical color-matching tolerances

COLOR DIFFERENCE (ΔE*)	CLINICAL COLOR MATCH
0	Perfect
0.5–1	Excellent
1–2	Good
2–3.5	Clinically acceptable
> 3.5	Mismatch

◼ Color Measurements

Apart from visual comparison using color standards such as Munsell color chips, color measurements can be made using either spectrophotometric or colorimetric methods.

Spectrophotometers measure the amount of light reflected at each wavelength. A double-beam spectrophotometer compares the responses from the object with a reference standard. From the spectral response, color parameters for the object can be calculated. Spectrophotometric measurements have been used to evaluate the color parameters for restorative resins, denture teeth, porcelains, shade guides, and color changes in dental materials. Figure 3-11 shows one model of a spectrophotometer.

Colorimeters measure the amount of light reflected at selected colors (eg, red, green, blue). The selections

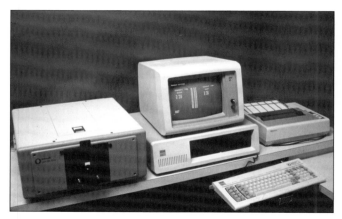

Fig 3-11 Coloreye spectrophotometer for laboratory measurement of color parameters (Macbeth).

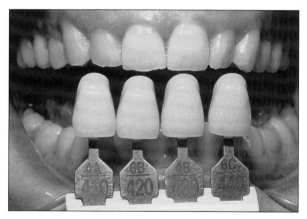

Fig 3-12 Photograph of patient's teeth compared with the closest-matching shade guide teeth.

are based on the CIE tristimulus value standard observers. There are several instruments available, and applications of their measurement methods for dental materials have been reported.[6–8] The instruments give readings in tristimulus values (X, Y, Z) or CIE L*a*b* values.

The major technical problem in using such instruments to measure the color parameters of teeth is the **edge effect**. Dental enamel is a translucent material that scatters the incident light from the instrument at many angles. As a result, the light reflected back into the instrument for analysis is not reliable and presents major errors in shade selection.

Another approach to tooth shade selection is the use of photography in combination with a spectrophotometer. Although accurate instrumental measurements of color parameters of translucent materials are difficult to use, color measurements on photographs are routine. This procedure of photocolorimetry involves the following steps:

1. The clinician or assistant holds the three or four closest-matching shade guide teeth next to the patient's teeth and photographs them with a 35-mm camera under a balanced light source (Fig 3-12).
2. The photograph is sent to the dental laboratory along with the impression, and the laboratory technician measures the color of the patient's teeth and shade guide teeth in the photograph. A computer program then aids in selecting the closest match.

This approach was tested in a clinical study[9] in comparison with visual matching of 40 patients. The difference in color parameters between shades selected by experienced observers and those selected by photocolorimetry resulted in an ΔE* within the color tolerance of an ΔE* of 2.00 for shade guide teeth.

Several chairside colorimeters and spectrophotometers have been introduced in the past several years (Fig 3-13). These instruments determine tooth shade by direct application to a patient's tooth. Their accuracy is difficult to assess and, for some instruments, depends on the angle at which the instrument is positioned and other operator variables. Recent studies[10–12] show considerable differences in reliabilities and accuracies among the different commercial instruments. A dental professional who can match shades well (eg, two shade guides at 90%) is still the standard, but technology is improving. The high cost of these instruments limits their use in most practices.

■ Metamerism

The change in color matching of two objects under different light sources is called **metamerism**. Two objects that are matched under one light source but not under other light sources form a **metameric pair** (Fig 3-14). Their different color reflectance curves cause this phenomenon. An example of metamerism is when a shade-guide tooth matches the fabricated tooth under fluorescent light but not under incandescent light. Metamerism results from possible differences in illumination between the dental clinic and the dental laboratory, causing poor matching of a fabricated restoration, such as a porcelain crown.

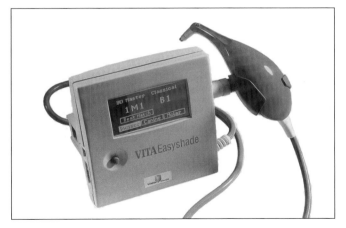

Fig 3-13 Chairside EasyShade spectrophotometer (Vident).

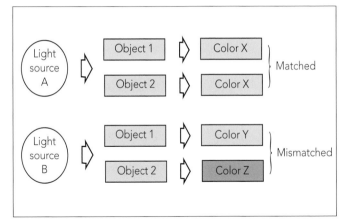

Fig 3-14 Metamerism. Objects 1 and 2 match under light source A but do not match under light source B.

Fig 3-15 Schematic of diffuse and specular reflection. (*a*) High gloss; (*b*) low gloss. (Reprinted with permission from O'Brien et al.[17])

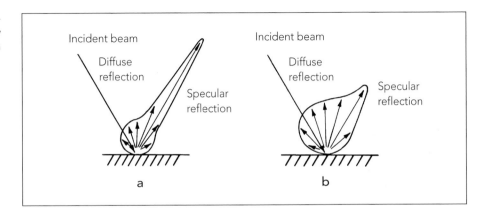

Standardization of illuminations (usually similar to the patient's environment) in color matching diminishes the effect of metamerism in shade matching. Ideally, of course, the objects would be an **isomeric pair**, possessing the same color reflectance curve and thus able to be color matched under all light sources.

◼ Translucency

The **translucency** of an object is the amount of incident light transmitted and scattered by that object. A color with high translucency appears lighter and reveals more of the backing in the color. Translucency decreases with increasing scattering.

The opposite of translucency is **opacity**. Light scattering in a material is the result of scattering centers that cause the incident light to be scattered in all directions. Examples of scattering centers include air bubbles and

opacifiers such as titanium dioxide, or the filler particles in a resin composite matrix. The effect of scattering depends on the size, shape, and number of scattering centers. Scattering is also dependent on the difference in **refractive indices** between the scattering centers and the matrix in which the centers are located.

Measurements of translucency may be performed using transmission spectrophotometers, reflection spectrophotometers, light meters, or colorimeters. Measurements of translucency of dental porcelains and human enamel have been published in the dental literature.[13–16]

◼ Gloss

Surface **gloss** is the optical property that produces a lustrous appearance. Contrast gloss, or *luster*, is the proportion of specular reflection to diffuse reflection (Fig 3-15). The amount of collimated incident light that is specularly

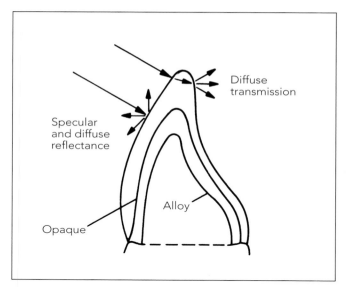

Fig 3-16 Optical considerations for a porcelain-fused-to-metal restoration. (Reprinted with permission from O'Brien et al.[15])

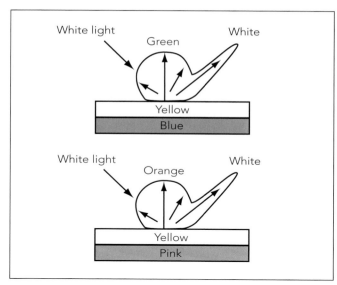

Fig 3-17 Double-layer effect. (Modified with permission from O'Brien.[18])

reflected is another factor that affects gloss. In specular reflection, the angle of incidence is equal to the angle of reflectance. When the incident beam is scattered by the object, there is a decrease in gloss as a larger portion of the incident beam is diffuse-scattered.

A high surface gloss is usually associated with smooth surfaces. In resin composite, surface gloss decreases with increasing surface roughness. Differences in gloss between multiple restorations or between restorations and teeth can be easily detected even in colors that are matched. In addition, high gloss reduces the effect of a color difference, because the color of the reflected light is more prominent. In a restorative material, high gloss also lightens the color appearance.

■ Fluorescence

Fluorescence is the emission of light by an object at wavelengths different from those of incident light. The emission ceases immediately on removal of the incident light. Natural teeth fluoresce in the blue region when illuminated by ultraviolet light. Dental porcelains are also fluorescent under ultraviolet light. The quality of the fluorescence depends on the brand of porcelain, some of

which fluoresce in colors different from those of natural teeth.

■ Double-Layer Effects on Esthetics

The color of a tooth is strongly influenced by the thickness of the enamel and the color of the underlying dentin. Similar considerations apply to restorations that are of layered structure, such as porcelain restorations composed of body porcelain over an inner opaque porcelain (Fig 3-16) and resin composites over more opaque resins. In these layered structures, diffuse reflectance and the relationship between the translucency and thickness of the outer layer and the color and reflectance of the inner layer pose challenges to esthetic concerns. The outer translucent layer acts as a light-scattering filter over the inner layer (Fig 3-17). As the thickness of the outer layer increases, the effect of the inner layer is diminished. Similar situations exist when the translucency of the outer layer decreases. Models of diffuse reflectance in dental porcelain systems using the Kubelka-Munk equation have shown excellent agreement between experimentally observed and theoretically calculated color parameters.[15,19]

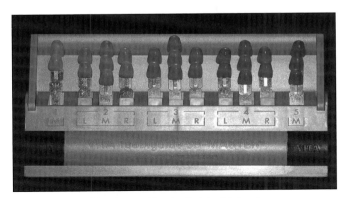

Fig 3-18 Vita 3D Master Shade Guide (Vident).

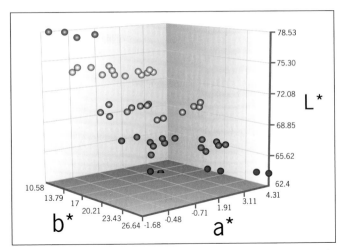

Fig 3-19 Plot of CIE L*a*b* values of Vita 3D Master Shade Guide. Twenty-six shades are plotted according to lightness (L*), red value (a*), and yellow value (b*).

Dental Shade Guides

Shade guides are used in determining the color of natural teeth so that artificial substitute restorations will possess similar color and esthetics. Preferred characteristics of a shade guide include logical arrangement and adequate distribution in color space, matching with natural teeth, inherent consistency among shade guides, and matching between shade guides and the dental materials such as porcelains and resin composites or denture teeth. Not all of these properties are met by the shade guides currently available. Furthermore, not all shade guides are fabricated from the dental materials to which they will be matched.

Most shade guides use a designation to denote the shade and color, but the same designation may not be comparable among brands. Furthermore, the distribution of shades within a shade guide is not necessarily evenly partitioned in color space. Some attempts have been made to use a more logical approach and an even distribution in shade guides, but only a limited number of products follow this approach. The Vita 3D Master Shade Guide (Vident) is based on hue, value, and chroma in a logical arrangement (Figs 3-18 and 3-19). The **coverage error** is an estimate of the color difference error between the shades of a given shade guide and the closest matching tooth from clinical studies of tooth colors. Therefore, the coverage error of the Vita 3D Master Shade Guide

has a lower value than the Vita Classical guide because it has more shades that are more logically distributed in the natural tooth color space.[20]

Shade Matching in the Dental Operatory

Shade matching is complex. It is important to remember the triadic interactions of illuminant, object, and observer described previously. Considerations should also include metamerism, gloss, translucency, and fluorescence. Recognition of the factors influencing shade match improve the result of the match.

The most important factor in shade matching is the illuminant. A color-corrected light source with a color temperature of 5,500 K and a color-rendering index of 90 or above is recommended. If possible, the shade matching should also be checked under a different light condition, for example, a warm white fluorescent light. In cases where the patients may have specific requirements, such as extensive activity under certain lighting conditions, shade-matching checks under those conditions are also recommended. The color environment of the dental operatory is another important factor in shade matching. A neutral, light gray background color reduces modification of color perception.

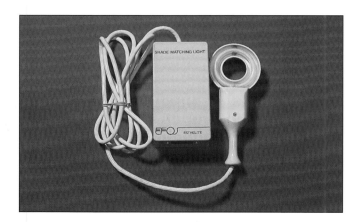

Fig 3-20 Ring light to simulate daylight for shade matching.

Some recommendations in shade matching are as follows:

1. Match shades under lights of similar spectral distribution and intensity, both in the dental operatory and the laboratory. Lighting conditions should be similar to daylight. A dental ring light is one such option (Fig 3-20).
2. Consider the effects of translucency and position. A high translucency and a more distal position in the natural dentition cause a darker gray appearance.
3. Use the manufacturer's shade guide for fabricating the restoration.
4. Follow the manufacturer's recommendations for preparing the surface of the tooth for shade matching. A diffuse-reflection condition is usually used.
5. Remove the individual shade tab from the guide and hold it close to the tooth for shade matching.
6. Match the surface texture of the restoration to that of the remaining dentition as closely as possible.

■ Communication of Shade-Matching Information to the Laboratory

The shade prescription given to the laboratory should accurately transmit the shade information as well as any characterization. The shade tab used should be specific for the fabrication material, and the type of lighting used to match the shades should be specified to decrease the effect of metamerism. A map indicating the approximate shade, its depth, and information about its location is shown in Fig 3-21.

The sequential steps in the transmission of information and the final clinical acceptance of the fabricated restoration have been described by O'Brien[22]; a schematic is shown in Fig 3-22. The *source spectrum* is the color and translucency information of the tooth to which the fabricated restoration is to be matched. The shade taking is the *encoding* process, and the information is *decoded* in the dental laboratory. The *simulation* is the fabricated restoration, which is then delivered to the dentist *observer* for evaluation and acceptance. Additional data may be given to enhance the matching until the *final simulation* is reached. The final simulation should reflect a clinically acceptable degree of shade matching to adjacent teeth.

■ Glossary

black object An object that reflects no incident color lights.

chroma Color intensity.

color content Relative intensity at each wavelength.

color fatigue Decrease in response to one color due to constant stimulus.

colorimeter A device used to measure the amount of light reflected by selected colors.

color reflectance Relative amount of each color reflected.

color system A three-dimensional system for defining color.

coverage error An estimate of the error of a shade guide based on how well it matches natural tooth colors measured in a large natural tooth color study.

Fig 3-21 Illustration of a map supplied to a ceramist to communicate color. (Reprinted with permission from Seluk and La Londe.[21])

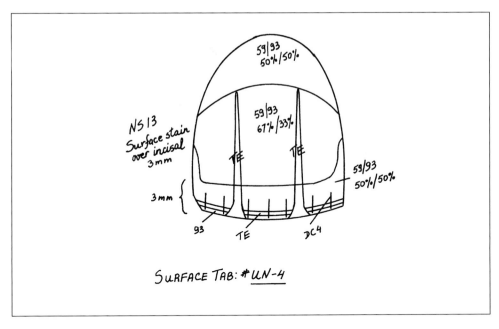

Fig 3-22 Schematic of transmission of shade-matching information.

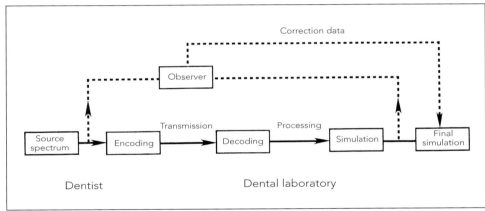

edge effect Lateral scattering of a light beam on entering a translucent material; causes an error in color measurement.

fluorescence Glow of an object when illuminated.

gloss Shininess; relative amount of light reflected.

hue The attribute of color that makes it appear as, eg, blue or yellow. Associated with wavelength.

isomeric pair Two objects that match color under different light sources.

metameric pair Two objects that exhibit metamerism.

metamerism Change in color matching of two objects under different light sources.

opacity $\text{Opacity} = \dfrac{\text{Intensity of incident light}}{\text{Intensity of transmitted light}}$

High opacity is associated with low intensity of transmitted light.

reflected color Color reflected by an object.

refractive index

$\text{Refractive index (n)} = \dfrac{\text{Velocity of light in air}}{\text{Velocity of light in medium}}$

Refractive index of dental porcelain is 1.5. Refractive index of tin dioxide (an opacifier) is 2.0.

spectrophotometer A device used to measure the amount of light reflected at each wavelength.

translucency Amount of light transmitted; the rest of the light is scattered.

value Lightness or darkness of a color; a measurement of the amount of gray.

white object An object that reflects all incident wavelengths.

■ Discussion Questions

1. How would a dental clinic need to be changed in order to be a better environment for color matching?

2. Why is it not necessary that a dental restoration match adjacent tooth structure exactly? About how far off in color can it be?

3. Why is it necessary to send the selected shade guide sample to the dental laboratory rather than just the shade guide number?

4. Besides color, which other appearance properties are important in creating an esthetic restoration?

5. Why do some dentists use more than one brand of shade guide in matching a patient's teeth?

6. How could a dentist who has poor color matching skills compensate in an effort to get better results clinically?

■ Study Questions

(See appendix E for answers.)

1. Name the coordinates required to define a color in a color system.

2. A porcelain crown may appear gray and nonvital; which variable is involved?

3. Why does a green object appear black in blue light?

4. What factors affect color appearance?

5. How does translucency affect color appearance?

6. What does gloss do to color appearance?

7. What is metamerism?

8. How does metamerism affect the appearance of dental restorations?

9. Why do dental porcelains appear different under different lighting environments?

■ References

1. Billmeyer FW Jr, Saltzman M. Principles of Color Technology. New York: Interscience, 1960.
2. Preston JD, Ward LC, Bobrick M. Light and lighting in the dental office. Dent Clin North Am 1978;22:431–451.
3. O'Brien WJ, Groh CL, Boenke KM. A new, small-color-difference equation for dental shades. J Dent Res 1990;69:1762–1764.
4. Seghi RR, Johnston WM, O'Brien WJ. Spectrophotometric analysis of color differences between porcelain systems. J Prosthet Dent 1986;56:35–40.
5. O'Brien WJ, Hemmendinger H, Boenke KM, Linger JB, Groh CL. Color distribution of three regions of extracted teeth. Dent Mater 1997;13:179–185.
6. Powers JM, Fan PL, Raptis CN. Color stability of new composite restorative materials under accelerated aging. J Dent Res 1980;59:2071–2074.
7. O'Brien WJ, Nelson D, Lorey RE. The assessment of chroma sensitivity to porcelain pigments. J Prosthet Dent 1983;49:63–66.
8. Stanford WB, Fan PL, Wozniak WT, Stanford JW. Effect of finishing on color and gloss of composites with different fillers. J Am Dent Assoc 1985;110:211–213.
9. Dancy WK, Yaman P, Dennison JB, O'Brien WJ, Razzoog ME. Color measurements as quality criteria for clinical shade matching of porcelain crowns. J Esthet Restor Dent 2003;15:114–121; discussion 122.
10. Kim-Pusateri S, Brewer S, Wee AG, Monaco EA, Davis EL. Reliability and accuracy of electronic shade matching instruments [abstract]. Presented at the International Association of Dental Research General Session, Baltimore, 9–12 March, 2005.
11. Dozi A, Kleverlaan CJ, El-Zohairy A, Feilzer AJ, Khashayar G. Performance of five commercially available tooth color-measuring devices. J Prosthodont 2007;16:93–100.
12. Chu SJ. Use of a reflectance spectrophotometer in evaluating shade change resulting from tooth-whitening products. J Esthet Restor Dent 2003;15:S42–S48.
13. Brodbelt RHW, O'Brien WJ, Fan PL. Translucency of dental porcelains. J Dent Res 1980;59:70–75.
14. Brodbelt RHW, O'Brien WJ, Fan PL, Frazier-Dib JG, Yu R. Translucency of human dental enamel. J Dent Res 1981;60:1749–1753.
15. O'Brien WJ, Johnston WM, Fanian F. Double-layer color effects in porcelain systems. J Dent Res 1985;64:940–943.
16. Spitzer D, ten Bosch JJ. The absorption and scattering of light in bovine and human enamel. Calcif Tissue Res 1975;17:129–137.
17. O'Brien WJ, Johnston WM, Fanian F, Lambert S. The surface roughness and gloss of composites. J Dent Res 1984;63:685–688.
18. O'Brien WJ. Double layer effect and other optical phenomena related to esthetics. Dent Clin North Am 1985;29:667–672.
19. Ragain JC Jr, Johnston WM. Accuracy of Kubelka-Munk reflectance theory applied to human dentin and enamel. J Dent Res 2001;80:449–452.
20. O'Brien WJ, Boenke KM. Coverage error of a new three dimensional shade guide[abstract]. Presented at the International Association of Dental Research General Session, Vancouver, BC March, 1999.
21. Seluk LW, La Londe TD. Esthetics and communication with a custom shade guide. Dent Clin North Am 1985;29:741–751.
22. O'Brien WJ. Optical phenomena at interfaces. Presented at the International Association of Dental Research Symposium on Biomaterials and Interfaces, Chicago, 1987.

Recommended Reading

Bergen SF, McCasland J. Dental operatory lighting and tooth color discrimination. J Am Dent Assoc 1977;94:130–134.

Cook WD, Chong MP. Color stability and visual perception of dimethacrylate based dental composite resins. Biomaterials 1985;6:257–264.

Cook WD, Vryonis P. Spectral distributions of dental colour-matching lamps. Aust Dent J 1985;30:15–21.

Dennison JB, Powers JM, Koran A. Color of dental restorative resins. J Dent Res 1978;57:557–562.

Dickson G, Forziati AF, Lawson MS, Schoonover IC. Fluorescence of teeth: A means of investigating their structure. J Am Dent Assoc 1956;45:661–667.

Ecker GA, Moser JB, Wozniak WT, Brinsden GJ. Effect of repeated firing on fluorescence of porcelain-fused-to-metal porcelains. J Prosthet Dent 1985;54:207–214.

Hall JB, Hefferen JJ, Olsen H. Study of fluorescence characteristics of extracted human teeth by the use of a clinical fluorometer. J Dent Res 1978;49:1431–1436.

Johnston WM, O'Brien WJ, Tien TY. The determination of optical absorption and scattering in translucent porcelain. Color Res Application 1986;11:125–130.

Johnston WM, O'Brien WJ, Tien TY. Concentration additivity of Kubelka-Munk optical coefficients of porcelain mixtures. Color Res Application 1986;11:131–137.

Jørgenson MW, Goodkind RJ. Spectrophotometric study of five porcelain shades relative to the dimensions of color, porcelain thickness and repeated firings. J Prosthet Dent 1979;42:96–105.

Judd DB, Wyszecki G. Color in Business, Science and Industry. New York: John Wiley & Sons, 1975.

McPhee ER. Light and color in dentistry. I. Nature and perception. J Mich Dent Assoc 1978;60:565–572.

McPhee ER. Extrinsic coloration of ceramometal restorations. Dent Clin North Am 1985;29:645–666.

Miller L. Organizing color in dentistry. J Am Dent Assoc 1987;(special issue):26E–40E.

Miyagawa Y, Powers JM, O'Brien WJ. Optical properties of direct restorative materials. J Dent Res 1981;60:890–894.

O'Brien WJ. Double layer effect and other optical phenomena related to esthetics. Dent Clin North Am 1985;29:667–672.

O'Brien WJ. Research in esthetics related to ceramic systems. Ceramic Eng Sci 1985;6:57–65.

O'Brien WJ. Fraunhofer diffraction of light by human enamel. J Dent Res 1988;67:484–486.

O'Brien WJ, Boenke KM, Groh CL. Coverage errors of two shade guides. Int J Prosthodont 1991;4:45–50.

O'Brien WJ, Groh CL, Boenke KM. A one-dimensional color order system for dental shade guides. Dent Mater 1989;5:371–374.

O'Brien WJ, Kay K-S, Boenke KM, Groh CL. Sources of color variation on firing porcelain. Dent Mater 1991;7:170–173.

Peplinski DR, Wozniak WT, Moser JB. Spectral studies of new luminophors for dental porcelain. J Dent Res 1980;59:1501–1506.

Powers JM, Dennison JB, Koran A. Color sensitivity of restorative resins under accelerated aging. J Dent Res 1978;57:964–970.

Powers JM, Dennison JB, Lepeak PJ. Parameters that affect the color of direct restorative resins. J Dent Res 1978;57:876–880.

Powers JM, Yeh CL, Miyagawa Y. Optical properties of composites of selected shades of white light. J Oral Rehabil 1983;10:319–324.

Preston JD. Current status of shade selection and color matching. Quintessence Int 1985;16:47–58.

Shotwell JL, Johnston WM, Swarts RG. Color comparison of denture teeth and shade guides. J Prosthet Dent 1986;56:31–34.

Spitzer D, ten Bosch JJ. The total luminescence of bovine and human dental enamel. Calcif Tissue Res 1976;20:201–208.

Sproull RC. Color matching in dentistry. I. The three-dimensional nature of color. J Prosthet Dent 1973;29:416–424.

Sproull RC. Color matching in dentistry. II. Practical applications of the organization of color. J Prosthet Dent 1973;29:556–566.

Sproull RC. Color matching in dentistry. III. Color control. J Prosthet Dent 1974;31:146–154.

Woolsey GD, Johnston WM, O'Brien WJ. Masking power of dental opaque porcelains. J Dent Res 1981;63:936–939.

Wozniak WT, Fan PL, McGill SB, Stanford JW. Color comparisons of composite resins of various shade designations. Dent Mater 1985;1:121–123.

Wozniak WT, Moore BK. Luminescence spectra of dental porcelain. J Dent Res 1978;57:971–974.

Wozniak WT, Moser JB. Council on Dental Materials, Instruments and Equipment. How to improve shade matching in the dental operatory. J Am Dent Assoc 1981;102:209–210.

Wyszecki G, Stiles WS. Color Science. New York: John Wiley & Sons, 1967.

Yeh CL, Powers JM, Miyagawa Y. Color of selected shades of composites by reflection spectrophotometry. J Dent Res 1982;61:1176–1179.

Zhao Y, Zhu J. In vivo color measurements of 410 maxillary anterior teeth. Chin J Dent Res 1998;1:49–51.

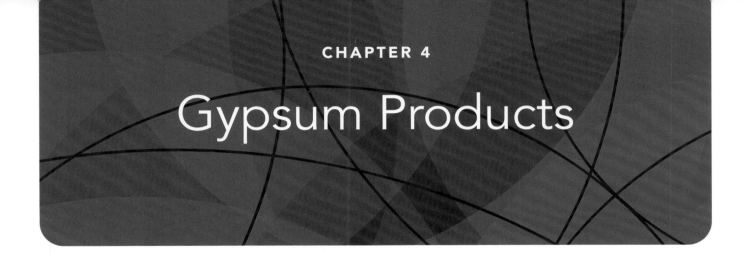

CHAPTER 4

Gypsum Products

In general, *gypsum products* refers to various forms of calcium sulfate, hydrous and anhydrous, that are manufactured by the **calcination** of calcium sulfate dihydrate ($CaSO_4 \cdot 2H_2O$), which occurs as the mineral gypsum. Calcination can be controlled to produce partial or complete dehydration. Gypsum products can also be obtained by calcining "synthetic" or "chemical" gypsum, a by-product of the manufacture of phosphoric acid. Industrially, all of these materials are known as *gypsum plasters*.

Although not directly used in dental restorations, gypsum products are important accessory materials in many clinical and laboratory procedures. Their correct use contributes to the success of these procedures. They are classified by the International Organization for Standardization (ISO)[1] into five types:

Type 1: Impression plaster
Type 2: Plaster
Type 3: Stone
Type 4: Stone, high-strength, low-expansion
Type 5: Stone, high-strength, high-expansion

This classification is illustrated in Fig 4-1. Both types of plaster are based on ordinary commercial gypsum plaster (plaster of Paris), while the three types of stone are based on high-strength gypsum plasters. Types 4 and 5 are commonly referred to as *die stones*. Table 4-1 lists typical materials.

Gypsum products can also include gypsum-bonded investments, because calcium sulfate hemihydrate is an essential component in forming the bond in the set material. These materials will be dealt with separately later in this chapter.

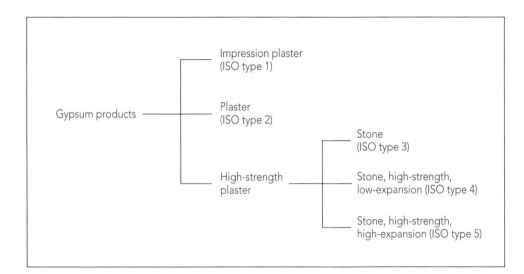

Fig 4-1 Classification of gypsum products.

▪ Plaster and Stone

Both plaster and stone are the products of partial dehydration of gypsum, which produces calcium sulfate hemihydrate ($CaSO_4 \cdot \frac{1}{2}H_2O$). Differences in properties result from differences in the physical nature of the powders, which in turn are a result of differences in manufacturing methods.

▪ Chemistry

In the temperature range 20°C to 700°C, which is of importance in the dental manipulation of gypsum products, three phase transformations occur in the calcium sulfate–water system. The first two represent the two stages in the dehydration of gypsum, and these are followed by a further transformation into anhydrous calcium sulfate:

$CaSO_4 \cdot 2H_2O$ calcium sulfate dihydrate $\underset{40°C \text{ to } 45°C}{\rightleftharpoons}$ $CaSO4 \cdot \frac{1}{2}H_2O$ (+ water) calcium sulfate hemihydrate

$\underset{90°C \text{ to } 100°C}{\rightleftharpoons}$ $\gamma\text{-}CaSO_4$ (+ water) hexagonal calcium sulfate (soluble anhydrite)

$\underset{300°C \text{ to } 400°C}{\rightleftharpoons}$ $\beta\text{-}CaSO_4$ orthorhombic calcium sulfate (insoluble anhydrite)

It is not possible to give unequivocal temperatures for these transformations; the given ranges summarize the results of several different determinations. In the first transformation, from dihydrate to hemihydrate, the temperature limits were determined by weight loss measurements on specimens heated isothermally in dry air for 2.5 years and would represent an equilibrium value.[2] The transformation from calcium sulfate hemihydrate to hexagonal calcium sulfate involved isothermal heating for periods up to a maximum of 22 days,[3,4] so the true equilibrium temperature for this transformation is probably a little lower than shown. Gay[5,6] identified hexagonal calcium sulfate by x-ray diffraction in specimens of hemihydrate heated in the range of 75°C to 105°C. Hexago-

Table 4-1 Typical gypsum products

TYPE	EXAMPLE
Impression plaster (ISO type 1)	Impression Plaster (Modern Materials Manufacturing)
Plaster (ISO type 2)	Snow White Plaster no. 1 (Kerr/Sybron)
Stone (ISO type 3)	Microstone (Whip Mix)
Stone, high-strength, low-expansion (ISO type 4)	Vel Mix Stone (Kerr/Sybron)
Stone, high-strength, high-expansion (ISO type 5)	Suprastone (Kerr/Sybron)

nal calcium sulfate is unstable below about 80°C, and, if cooled to lower temperatures and exposed to the environment, it rapidly rehydrates to form the hemihydrate. The temperature range given for the third transformation, hexagonal to orthorhombic calcium sulfate, is based on measurements made on specimens heated at a rate of 5 K/min,[7] so again the true equilibrium temperature for this transformation would be lower than shown here. Orthorhombic calcium sulfate is the stable anhydrous form in this system and exists as the mineral insoluble anhydrite.

Theoretically, hemihydrate is the stable hydrous form of calcium sulfate only in the approximate temperature range of 45°C to 90°C. It exists as a metastable phase under dry conditions at lower temperatures, including ambient, although it has been shown that hydration can occur if particles are exposed to the atmosphere under conditions where the water vapor pressure is high.[8]

▪ Manufacture

From the transformation temperatures given in the previous section, it can be seen that calcium sulfate hemihydrate would be produced by heating gypsum to temperatures between 45°C and 90°C. However, at these temperatures, the reaction is slow; even at 90°C, complete conversion takes about 12 hours.[3] Therefore, in commercial processes, temperatures higher than this are used for shorter times. The stable phase at these higher temperatures is hexagonal calcium sulfate, so the initial product of calcination is at least partly in this anhydrous form. However, on cooling to temperatures below 80°C

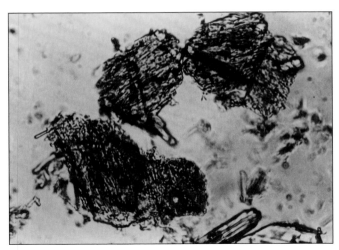

Fig 4-2 Particles of plaster. (Original magnification ×400.)

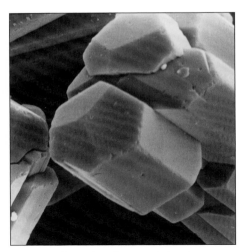

Fig 4-3 Crystals of wet-calcined gypsum plaster before grinding. (Scanning electron micrograph, original magnification ×3,000.)

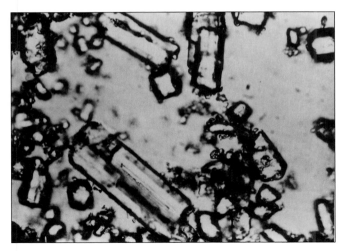

Fig 4-4 Particles of high-strength stone. (Original magnification ×400.)

and exposure to the atmosphere, the hexagonal calcium sulfate rehydrates to form the hemihydrate.

Plaster of Paris

This traditional hemihydrate plaster is produced by the dry calcination of ground gypsum in open containers (pans, kettles, or rotary kilns) at temperatures in the range of 120°C to 180°C. In the absence of liquid water, there is no opportunity for reorganization of crystal morphology, so although the **crystal structure** of the final product after exposure to air is that of calcium sulfate hemihydrate, the powder particles retain the rough irregular shape of the original ground gypsum. Loss of water under dry conditions leaves parallel channels in these particles (Fig 4-2), so hemihydrate plasters produced by dry calcination are powders with a low **apparent density**, a high **relative surface area**, and a poor packing ability.

Medium- and high-strength plasters (stones)

Plasters manufactured by wet calcination have a stronger set mass. In this process, sufficient liquid water is present to allow through-solution conversion, so recrystallization produces dense prismatic crystals of hexagonal calcium sulfate. These crystals then rehydrate to the hemihydrate on cooling, but this secondary conversion cannot be accompanied by recrystallization. The final powder particles are **pseudomorphic**, having the monoclinic crystal structure of hemihydrate, but retaining the hexagonal crystal habit of the anhydrous calcium sulfate precursor (Fig 4-3).

Hemihydrate powders produced by wet calcination therefore have a higher apparent density and a smaller relative surface area than those resulting from dry calcination. A controlled amount of grinding rounds off the crystals and produces a proportion of fines, both factors improving the packing ability of the powder and further increasing the apparent density. Particles of a typical dental stone are shown in Fig 4-4.

Medium-strength plasters

These are typified by Hydrocal (United States Gypsum), which is the basis of many ordinary dental stones. It is produced by autoclaving lump gypsum in superheated steam at a pressure of 117 kPa, giving a temperature of 123°C, for 5 to 7 hours. After drying at 100°C or higher and grinding, a hemihydrate powder is produced that gives a set mass considerably stronger than that produced by dry-calcined materials.

High-strength plasters

Modifications to the wet process yield hemihydrate powders that give even stronger set products, such as Densite (Georgia-Pacific) and Crystacal (British Gypsum). In these processes, wet calcination takes place in the presence of **crystal habit** modifiers, producing crystals that are shorter and thicker than those resulting from autoclaving in steam. After controlled grinding, these powders have even higher apparent densities and yield even stronger set masses than Hydrocal-type stones: they form the basis of most dental die stones. Densite is produced by boiling lump gypsum in a 30% calcium chloride solution, and Crystacal is produced by autoclaving finely ground gypsum in the presence of small amounts (< 1%) of sodium succinate.

Apparent density

The *apparent density* of a powder is the reciprocal of its bulkiness and so gives a measure of its packing ability. The low apparent density of hemihydrate powders produced by dry calcination is caused in part by the rough irregular shapes of the individual particles (see Fig 4-2). A more important factor, however, is a high adhesion of particles to their neighbors, caused by a high surface-free energy resulting from crystal imperfections and adsorption of gases during calcination.[9] This adhesiveness of particles makes it likely that they will stick together at first contact, establishing bridges in the powder and creating a structure with many voids and a low apparent density. In contrast, powder particles produced by wet calcination are smooth and dense (see Fig 4-4). They show less crystallographic strain and therefore have a lower surface free energy. As a result, they have a better packing ability and a higher apparent density.

▪ The Setting Process

The setting reaction

When the hemihydrate powder is mixed with water in the correct proportions, it forms a thick slurry. The hemihydrate is sparingly soluble in water (6.5 g/L at 20°C), so only a small amount can dissolve. Initially, therefore, the mix is a two-phase suspension of hemihydrate particles in a saturated aqueous solution. The stable hydrate at temperatures below 40°C is the dihydrate (gypsum), which is even less soluble (2.4 g/L at 20°C) than the hemihydrate. The aqueous phase is therefore supersaturated with respect to the dihydrate, which crystallizes out at suitable **nucleation centers** in the suspension. These gypsum crystals normally are **acicular** in habit and often radiate out from nucleation centers in the form of **spherulitic** aggregates.

These nucleation centers may be impurities (eg, residual gypsum particles), particles of gypsum added as seeds to accelerate setting, or strained areas on undissolved hemihydrate particles. The consequent depletion of calcium and sulfate ions in the aqueous phase allows more hemihydrate to go into solution and, in turn, to precipitate out as gypsum. The setting process is therefore one of heterogeneously nucleated recrystallization, characterized by a continuous solution of hemihydrate, diffusion of calcium and sulfate ions to nucleation centers, and the precipitation of microscopic gypsum crystals. The setting reaction is the reverse of the first stage of dehydration and so is exothermic. It is represented by the following equation:

$$2CaSO_4 \cdot \frac{1}{2}H_2O + 3H_2O \rightarrow 2CaSO_4 \cdot 2H_2O$$

Water requirement

The differing **water requirements** of plaster, stone, and high-strength stone are mainly the result of differences in the apparent density of the powder. The factors that promote adhesiveness of the particles in the dry powder persist when they are suspended in water.[10] For this reason, dry-calcined plaster, with its low apparent density, produces a flocculated suspension and needs a relatively high proportion of mixing water to give a mix of workable viscosity. **Water/powder (W/P) ratios** of 0.5 to 0.6 are usual. Hemihydrate powders produced by wet calcination, because of their higher apparent densities, require less water; typical W/P ratios are 0.30 to 0.33 for ordinary dental stones and 0.18 to 0.23 for high-strength stones.

In setting, 100 g of hemihydrate combines with 18.6 g of water. Therefore, at the completion of the reaction in normal mixes, there is always some excess of unreacted water (as a saturated solution of calcium sulfate) remaining in the set mass, and this residual water weakens the cast. It can be removed by low-temperature drying but leaves microscopic porosity that weakens the dry cast. Both wet and dry strengths of the set material depend on the relative amount of unreacted water remaining after setting, and also on the W/P ratio of the original mix. The relative amount of residual water is least in high-strength stone, which therefore has the strongest set mass.

Stages in setting

The setting process is continuous from the beginning of mixing until the setting reaction is complete, by which time the material has reached its full wet strength. However, important physical changes can be recognized during this process. Initially, the mix is a viscous liquid, exhibiting **pseudoplasticity** as it flows readily under vibration. In this stage the mix has a glossy surface with **specular** reflections. As the setting reaction proceeds, gypsum crystals continue to grow, and the viscosity of the mix increases. When the clumps of growing gypsum crystals interact, the mix becomes plastic; it will not flow under vibration but can readily be molded. At this time the glossy surface disappears as the fluid portion is drawn into pores formed when the growing gypsum crystals thrust apart. Continued crystal growth converts the plastic mass into a rigid solid, weak and friable at first but gaining strength as the relative amount of solid phase increases. These four stages may be designated (1) fluid, (2) plastic, (3) friable, and (4) carvable.

Volume changes during setting

The setting reaction causes a decrease in the true volume of the reactants, and under suitable conditions this contraction can be observed early in the setting process when the mix is still fluid. However, once the mix begins to attain rigidity (marked by the loss of surface gloss), an **isotropic** expansion is observed, resulting from growth pressure of the gypsum crystals that are forming. There is therefore a decrease in apparent density of the mix during the latter stages of setting, accompanied by the

formation of microscopic voids separating individual crystals in the aggregate.

The initial contraction is unlikely to affect the important dimensions of a gypsum cast, because in the still-fluid mix, it will occur mainly in a vertical direction. Gravity will keep the mix adapted to the anatomic portion of an impression. The expansion observed after the mix attains rigidity takes place in all directions and will affect the dimensions of the cast. The point at which the initial contraction ceases is used as zero in laboratory measurements of effective setting expansion.

Rate of the setting reaction

Within wide limits, the rate of hydration during setting is independent of the W/P ratio.[11] However, the rate at which the associated physical changes described earlier occur is highly dependent on the W/P ratio of the mix, because these changes result from the interaction of clumps of gypsum crystals growing from nucleation centers in the slurry. Thick mixes (low W/P ratios) harden more quickly because available nucleation centers are concentrated in a smaller volume; interaction of the growing solid phase occurs earlier and is more effective in promoting expansion.

The effect of additives

Many salts and colloids are known to alter the setting characteristics of hemihydrate plasters by affecting the rate of the setting reaction. They have been used in the formulation of dental plasters and stones for many years, mainly on an empirical basis, because their modes of action are not always completely understood.

Finely powdered gypsum is an efficient accelerator, which acts by providing seeds for heterogeneous nucleation. In low concentrations, soluble sulfates and chlorides are accelerators, apparently increasing the rate of solution of the hemihydrate. However, salts of relatively low solubility, such as sodium chloride and sodium sulfate, act as retarders in higher concentrations because, as setting proceeds, the amount of free water in the mix decreases and the concentration of the additive increases. When its limit of solubility is exceeded, the salt precipitates on nuclei of crystallization, thus poisoning them. Acetates, borates, citrates, and tartrates are retarders, which may act by **nuclei poisoning**, by reducing the rate of solution of hemihydrate, or by inhibiting the growth of dihydrate crystals. Reaction of some additives with hemihydrate can occur; soluble tartrates and citrates

Fig 4-5 Fracture surface of cast gypsum. *(a)* Plaster, W/P = 0.50; *(b)* high-strength stone, W/P = 0.25. (Scanning electron micrographs, original magnification ×3,000.) (Reprinted from Bever[14] with permission.)

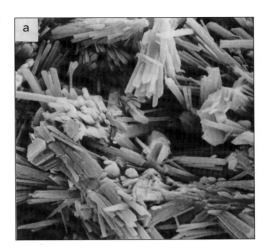
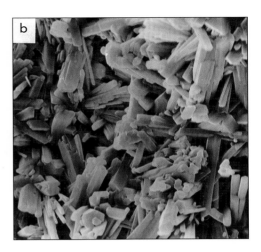

precipitate calcium tartrate and citrate, respectively. Colloids are effective retarders, presumably acting by nuclei poisoning.

Many accelerators and retarders reduce the setting expansion, sometimes by changing the crystal habit of growing gypsum crystals from acicular to a more compact form and inhibiting spherulite formation[12]; both factors reduce the effect of the crystals' growth pressure and thus the strength of the set material as well.

◼ The Microstructure of Cast Gypsum

The set material consists of a tangled aggregate of monoclinic gypsum crystals, usually acicular in shape, with lengths in the range of 5 to 20 μm. The aggregate exhibits two distinct types of inherent porosity on a microscopic scale:

1. Microporosity caused by the presence of residual unreacted water. These voids are roughly spheric and occur between clumps of gypsum crystals.
2. Microporosity resulting from growth of gypsum crystals. These voids are associated with setting expansion and are smaller than the first type; they appear as angular spaces between individual crystals in the aggregate.

The effect of W/P ratio

The relative amounts of both types of porosity are affected by the W/P ratio of the mix, but in opposite ways:
1. A low W/P ratio (thick mix) leaves less residual water in the set mass and so decreases the amount of the first type of porosity.
2. A low W/P ratio increases the effect of crystal growth during setting, because available nucleation centers are concentrated in a smaller total volume of mix. The interaction of growing gypsum crystals occurs earlier and is more effective, so the amount of the second type of porosity is increased.
3. At any W/P ratio, the total proportion of inherent porosity in the set mass is the sum of these two types. The effect of the first type predominates, so for any given plaster or stone there is always a decrease in the total inherent porosity of the set mass (ie, an increase in apparent density) as the W/P ratio of the mix is reduced. Inherent porosity represents about 40% of the total cast volume at a W/P ratio of 0.50 and about 20% at a W/P ratio of 0.25.[13]

Typical microstructures of casts made from plaster mixed in a W/P ratio of 0.50 and high-strength stone mixed in a W/P ratio of 0.25 are shown in Fig 4-5. The microporosity resulting from residual water can be seen clearly in Fig 4-5a, where the voids occur between spherulitic clumps of gypsum crystals. Both micrographs reveal the microporosity that results from crystal growth. The higher apparent density of the set high-strength stone is obvious.

Table 4-2 Linear setting expansions of typical dental gypsum products (setting in air)

TYPE	W/P RATIO	SETTING EXPANSION (%)
Impression plaster	0.60	0.13
Plaster	0.50	0.30
Stone	0.30	0.15
Stone, high-strength, low-expansion	0.20	0.10
Stone, high-strength, high-expansion	0.19	0.26

◉ Properties

Rate of setting

Manipulation time

Recognition of the physical changes occurring in the mix during setting is important in the manipulation of plaster and stone.

1. When casting (eg, pouring casts or dies), manipulation must be completed before the mix loses fluidity. The change is marked by the disappearance of the glossy surface from the mix.
2. When molding (eg, taking impressions or jaw registrations, articulating casts, flasking wax pattern dentures), manipulation must be completed before the mix loses plasticity and enters the friable stage. There is no recognized objective method of measuring this time.

Setting time

An arbitrary setting time (initial set) can be determined by using suitable penetrometers (eg, Gillmore or Vicat initial needles; both give approximately the same initial setting time). Measured in this way, the initial set is a guide to the time when the rigid material is strong enough to handle and, in particular, when it can be carved or trimmed to the final shape.

If a dental manufacturer specifies a setting time, it will be a Gillmore or Vicat initial set. Both the setting reaction and the increase in strength continue for some time after this initial set. Gillmore and Vicat final needles may be used to establish a final setting time, but this is not usual in dental technology.

Control of rate of setting

1. *The use of additives.* In formulating dental products, manufacturers adjust the rate of setting of raw hemihydrates by adding accelerators and retarders, often as a balanced mixture. Typical accelerators are potassium sulfate and potassium sodium tartrate (Rochelle salts), and typical retarders are sodium citrate and sodium tetraborate decahydrate (borax). The action of accelerators and retarders has already been discussed.
2. *W/P ratio.* It has already been pointed out that changing the W/P ratio has a marked effect on the rate at which the physical changes associated with setting of the mix occur. These changes take place more rapidly as the W/P ratio is reduced. Manipulation and setting times are thus directly proportional to W/P ratio.

Setting expansion

Typical values for the setting expansion in air of five types of widely used dental gypsum plaster are presented in Table 4-2.

When dental plaster or stone sets, the observed expansion is volumetric. In dental testing it may be assumed that linear setting expansion is isotropic; however, this assumption is not always justified. If restraint is imposed in some directions but not others (eg, by a rigid impression), setting expansion can be far from isotropic.

Effect of immersion

Gypsum products exposed to additional water while setting (eg, by immersion) show a greater expansion than when setting in air, a phenomenon commonly (but inaccurately) called *hygroscopic expansion*. When expansion begins, externally available water is drawn into pores forming in the setting mass, and this maintains a continuous aqueous phase in which crystal growth takes place freely. Under dry conditions, this additional water is not available, and as expansion occurs, the aqueous phase in the mix is reduced to a film over the growing gypsum crystals. Surface tension forces in this liquid film restrain further crystal growth, thereby reducing the observed setting expansion of the mix.[15] Thus, the so-called hygroscopic expansion is simply an enhanced setting expansion that occurs in the presence of additional water.

Control of setting expansion

1. *Use of additives.* A low setting expansion is desirable in applications where dimensional accuracy is important (eg, in impression taking and pouring working casts and dies). A balanced blend of accelerator and retarder, such as potassium sulfate–borax and potassium sodium tartrate–sodium citrate to the raw hemihydrate can reduce setting expansion and control setting time.

   The reduction in strength that these additives can cause is not a disadvantage in impression plasters, but, in stones, strength as well as dimensional accuracy is important. Formulation of the latter materials therefore involves striking a compromise between a desirable reduction in setting expansion and an undesirable reduction in strength.

   Normally, die stones in particular are formulated to have a low setting expansion. As their name indicates, they are used to make cast gypsum dies on which restorations such as inlays, crowns, and fixed partial dentures are constructed by the indirect method, and they are required to reproduce the prepared teeth with high dimensional accuracy. Such materials constitute the ISO type 4 high-strength, low-expansion stones, which have a setting expansion of less than 0.15%. These materials would be used where the investment expansion is sufficient to compensate completely for the casting shrinkage of the alloy. Another category of die stone has been introduced: ISO type 5, which is high-strength, high-expansion, with a setting expansion in the range of 0.16% to 0.30%. The higher expansion results from a lower concentration of modifying additives, so these materials also generally achieve higher strengths when set. They are intended for use in casting techniques when investment expansion alone may not be high enough to compensate fully for alloy shrinkage. Here the setting expansion of the die stone is intended to contribute to the total mold expansion by producing an oversized pattern,[16] but it is important that the impression be soft and flexible enough for isotropic setting expansion to occur. In an impression made from a stiff elastomeric material in a closely fitting rigid tray, setting expansion will likely occur in a vertical direction, producing a distorted die.

2. *W/P ratio.* For any given gypsum product, reducing the relative amount of aqueous phase in the process allows more effective interaction of growing gypsum crystals during setting, thus increasing the setting expansion. Setting expansion is therefore inversely proportional to the W/P ratio. Because of their lower water requirement, the raw hemihydrates used to produce stones and die stones have a higher inherent setting expansion in normal mixes than does plaster. This effect is masked, however, by the additives used in their formulation (Fig 4-6).

Strength

Cast gypsum is a brittle material and so is weaker in tension than in compression. Materials with the highest compressive strengths are the most brittle, and their tensile strengths are proportionally lower. For set plaster, the tensile strength is about 20% of the compressive strength; for set high-strength stone, it is about 10%. Since fracture of cast gypsum typically occurs in tension, tensile strength is a better guide to fracture resistance. However, compressive strength gives a better indication of surface hardness. Values for tensile and compressive strengths of five typical dental gypsum plasters are shown in Table 4-3.

1. *The effect of W/P ratio.* In general, strength properties are inversely related to W/P ratio and so to the total amount of inherent porosity (Fig 4-7). Therefore, when maximum strength is required, a given material should be mixed in as low a W/P ratio as practicable. The limiting factor is the viscosity of the mix, because it increases with decreasing W/P ratio and can become so high that the ability to pour sound casts is jeopardized.

   In high-strength stones mixed even in normal W/P ratios, there is little water present in excess of the theoretic W/P ratio (0.186) required for complete conversion of hemihydrate to dihydrate. Since the setting reaction depends on diffusion of ions, it may not proceed to completion in standard mixes. Donnison et al[18] showed that, in normal mixes, the hydration may

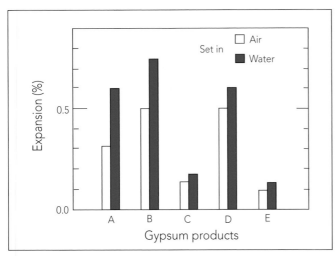

Fig 4-6 Linear setting expansion in air and in water of various types of gypsum products. (A) Plaster (W/P = 0.50); (B) unmodified stone (Hydrocal, W/P = 0.32); (C) commercial stone based on Hydrocal (W/P = 0.32); (D) unmodified high-strength stone (Densite K5, W/P = 0.24); (E) commercial high-strength stone based on Densite (W/P = 0.24).

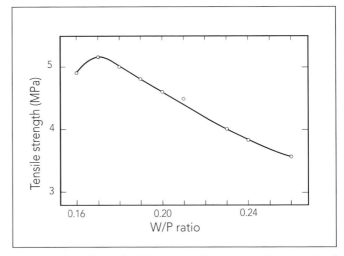

Fig 4-7 The effect of W/P ratio on the wet tensile strength of a high-strength stone. (Reprinted from Selby.[17])

Table 4-3 Strength properties of typical dental gypsum products*

TYPE	TENSILE STRENGTH (MPa)			COMPRESSIVE STRENGTH (MPa)	
	W/P RATIO	WET	DRY	WET	DRY
Impression plaster	0.60	1.3	—	5.9	—
Plaster	0.50	2.3	4.1	12.4	24.9
Stone	0.30	3.5	7.6	25.5	63.5
Stone, high-strength, low-expansion	0.20	6.1	10.6	58.4	126.4
Stone, high-strength, high-expansion	0.19	6.2	12.6	76.4	145.2

*The materials tested were the same as those in Table 4-2.

be up to 3% short of completion and that the proportion of residual hemihydrate increases as the W/P ratio decreases. Residual hemihydrate particles are often seen in micrographs of set high-strength stone. The content of unreacted hemihydrate becomes much greater in very thick mixes, but, as Fig 4-7 shows, this change does not adversely affect the strength until the W/P ratio is well below that theoretically needed for complete hydration. Such thick mixes would be impossible to manipulate successfully in most dental applications.

With any plaster or stone, using a low W/P ratio to obtain maximum strength properties also increases setting expansion, which must be accepted. But in applications where dimensional accuracy is more impor-

tant than strength (eg, impressions), higher W/P ratios can be used.

2. *The effect of drying.* Removal of all uncombined water from cast gypsum by low-temperature drying approximately doubles strength properties (see Table 4-3), but there is no strength increase until the last 2% of free water is removed. This strength increase on drying is reversible; soaking a dry cast in water reduces its strength to the original level.

Gypsum is stable only below about 40°C. Drying at higher temperatures must be carefully controlled; loss of water at crystallization occurs rapidly at 100°C or higher and causes shrinkage and a reduction in strength.

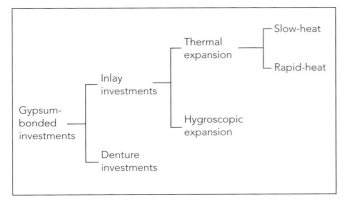

Fig 4-8 Classification of gypsum-bonded investments.

Table 4-4 Typical gypsum-bonded investments

TYPE	EXAMPLE
Inlay investment, thermal expansion (type 1)	Cristobalite Inlay (Kerr/Sybron)
Inlay investment, thermal expansion, rapid heat (type 1)	Cristoquick (GC International)
Inlay investment, hygroscopic expansion (type 1)	Beauty-Cast (Whip Mix)
Denture investment (type 2)	R&R Gray (Dentsply/ Ransom and Randolph)

Solubility

Because gypsum is sparingly soluble in water, long-term immersion is contraindicated. If dried gypsum casts have to be soaked, it is better to use a saturated solution of calcium sulfate.

Disinfection of Gypsum Casts

To prevent cross-infection, the practice of disinfecting impressions is becoming increasingly common. However, prolonged immersion in disinfectant solutions can cause unacceptably large dimensional changes in hydrocolloid[19,20] and polyether[21] impressions. Moreover, during subsequent clinical procedures, casts or dies can become reinfected with pathogenic organisms, which can then be transferred to technical staff. As an alternative, the addition of disinfectants to the mixing water when casts are poured has been investigated; 5% phenol[22] and 2% glutaraldehyde[23] have proved to be effective and to not adversely affect the properties of the set material. However, both are known tissue irritants. Alternatively, casts and dies may be treated by immersion in a disinfecting solution after each clinical stage. Dental stones that contain a disinfectant are also available.[24,25]

Autoclave sterilization of casts has been suggested.[26] Some loss of strength and surface hardness and an increase in dimensions occur, but it is claimed that under carefully controlled conditions, the casts retain adequate properties for ordinary laboratory use.

Gypsum-Bonded Investments

Gypsum-bonded investments are the mold materials most commonly used in the casting of dental gold alloys with liquidus temperatures no higher than 1,080°C. They are normally used for gold inlays, crowns, and fixed and removable partial dentures. Because of their tendency to decompose at high temperatures, these investments are not suitable for casting high-melting gold alloys, palladium alloys (used for copings in alloy-ceramic restorations), or most base-metal alloys, such as nickel-chromium and cobalt-chromium. Gypsum-bonded investments were classified by the ISO[27] as:

Type 1: For casting inlays and crowns
Type 2: For casting complete and partial denture bases

This classification is illustrated in Fig 4-8, and typical materials are listed in Table 4-4. Some materials, classified by their manufacturers as *universal*, are claimed to be suitable for casting all gold-alloy restorations.

Composition

All gypsum-bonded investment powders consist basically of a **refractory** filler and a binder. There may also be small amounts (less than 5%) of important modifying agents present.

Refractory

The refractory component is either cristobalite or quartz (or occasionally a mixture of the two), usually present in

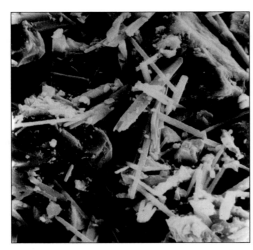

Fig 4-9 Scanning electron micrograph of fracture surface. Microstructure of a set gypsum-bonded investment (Cristobalite Inlay, Kerr Dental; W/P = 0.38). The large particles are cristobalite; the small acicular crystals are gypsum formed during setting (original magnification ×3,000).

the range of 55% to 75%. Both of these components are **polymorphs** of silica (SiO_2).

Binder

In the investment powder, the binder is calcium sulfate hemihydrate, either plaster or stone. When the investment sets, the silica is unaffected, and the hemihydrate binder combines with water to form dihydrate (gypsum) as occurs in the setting of other gypsum products. The setting reaction is therefore the same as that shown in the equation given previously. The set investment consists of fine particles of silica embedded in an interlocking aggregate of smaller acicular gypsum crystals (Fig 4-9). The continuous porosity characteristic of cast gypsum provides the necessary mold venting to assist in the production of sound castings.

Modifying agents

Small amounts of modifying agents are added to many commercial gypsum-bonded investments. These agents may be accelerators or retarders to control the rate of setting, reducing agents such as powdered graphite or copper to protect embedded gold-alloy components in "casting-on" techniques, or additives to increase the thermal expansion of the investment. Typical additives of

the last type are boric acid and soluble halide salts, particularly those of alkali or alkaline earth metals.

Effect of composition on setting and thermal behavior

Refractory

Although silica is referred to as the *refractory component*, cast gypsum itself is sufficiently heat resistant to be used as a mold material, because it can be heated to temperatures as high as 1,000°C without decomposing.[28] Adding silica reduces its heat resistance, because in such mixtures, at temperatures above 900°C, the following reaction occurs:

$$CaSO_4 + SiO_2 \rightarrow CaSiO_3 + SO_3$$

At high temperatures, the sulfur trioxide liberated by this reaction causes rapid corrosion of the casting.

Crystalline silica is used in dental investments to control dimensional changes on heating. When heated, cast gypsum shows a marked contraction, and because both quartz and cristobalite have high expansions when heated, they offset the shrinkage of the binder and provide a positive thermal expansion if needed.

Silica exists in 22 different condensed phases. Five of these are amorphous, and 17 are crystalline; the latter are the polymorphs of silica. Of this group, only one phase, low-temperature quartz, is thermodynamically stable at normal temperature and pressure. Two more, tridymite S-1 and low-temperature cristobalite, exist under normal atmospheric conditions as metastable (but actually long-lived) phases.

Only two polymorphs of silica are of importance in dental investments: quartz and cristobalite. Quartz is a common mineral; cristobalite occurs naturally as a rare mineral but is normally manufactured by prolonged heating of quartz at high temperatures to induce the appropriate slow inversion. Both quartz and cristobalite exist in low-temperature (α) and high-temperature (β) phases, and in both materials the change between low- and high-temperature phases is rapid and readily reversible on cooling. This change is known as the *high-low* **inversion**.

In both quartz and cristobalite, the high-temperature phase is less dense than the low-temperature phase, so the α → β inversion is accompanied by an isothermal expansion. This expansion is added to the normal thermal expansion to give a large overall expansion at high temperatures.

As in all crystalline materials, single crystals of quartz and cristobalite show anisotropy of physical properties, including their coefficients of thermal expansion. However, in dental investments, they are used as a fine powder with random orientation of individual particles. So in the aggregate, they behave isotropically, and properties such as the coefficient of thermal expansion have a uniform average value.

Typical linear thermal expansion curves for powdered quartz and cristobalite are shown in Fig 4-10. Specimens were made by densely compacting the powders into aggregates with a minimum amount of binder in the interstices, so the thermal expansion of the specimens was essentially that of the silica component in dental investments.

The temperature of the $\alpha \to \beta$ inversion of cristobalite varies according to the source of the sample and its previous thermal history; in the manufactured cristobalite used in dental investments it is about 250°C (see Fig 4-10, curve A). The inversion gives an isothermal expansion of about 1.3%, and the total expansion at 700°C is about 2.2%. Dental investments designed to have a high thermal expansion usually contain cristobalite as the refractory.

Quartz (Fig 4-10, curve B) undergoes its $\alpha \to \beta$ inversion at 573°C, producing an isothermal expansion of about 0.7%. The high-temperature form has a negative coefficient of thermal expansion, and the overall total expansion at 700°C is about 1.6%.

Binder

When the set investment is heated, the cast gypsum binder shows a marked contraction, which occurs in several stages. In the early stages of heating, a contraction accompanies loss of water of crystallization, as the dihydrate reverts to hemihydrate and then to hexagonal calcium sulfate. A large contraction then accompanies its $\gamma \to \beta$ transformation, which occurs in the approximate temperature range of 300°C to 400°C. A further large contraction begins at about 650°C, which is probably the result of densification by sintering. The total linear contraction of cast gypsum prepared from plaster (W/P = 0.50) and heated to 700°C can be as high as 3%; the corresponding shrinkage for cast gypsum prepared from a high-strength stone (W/P = 0.25) is about 1%. The latter is usually preferred as a binder in gypsum-bonded investments, not only because of its lower shrinkage on heating, but because its superior strength when set allows a higher concentration of silica to be used in the in-

vestment, thereby further reducing the effect of binder contraction.

Effects of varying composition

Within practical limits, increasing the proportion of silica in the investment powder increases the manipulation time (given by the time of loss of fluidity) and the initial setting time (Fig 4-11); the setting expansion, both in air and in water, and the thermal expansion (Fig 4-12); and reduces the compressive strength (Fig 4-13). The rate of the setting reaction itself is unchanged; the increases in observed manipulation and setting times occur because the particles of refractory filler interfere with the interlocking of growing gypsum crystals, making this less effective in developing a solid structure. The compressive strength of the set investment is reduced for the same reason. Setting expansion is increased when interlocking of growing gypsum crystals is inhibited by the refractory particles, because more of the crystal growth is directed outward. Thermal expansion is increased because, at any temperature, it is achieved by summing the binder contraction and the refractory expansion; thus, increasing the proportion of the expanding component increases the observed expansion.

Effects of modifying agents

Important modifying agents such as boric acid and soluble halide salts of alkali or alkaline earth metals are added to commercial investments to increase their thermal expansion. All of them act mainly by reducing the two large contractions of the gypsum binder that occur on heating to temperatures above 300°C.

Boric acid, when heated above 150°C, forms a viscous liquid with a composition intermediate between metaboric acid and boron oxide; this viscous liquid impedes the evaporation of the last traces of water, delaying the $\gamma \to \beta$ transformation of calcium sulfate.[29] The presence of the viscous liquid phase also reduces the high-temperature contraction that results from sintering, because it stabilizes the original contacts formed between the gypsum crystals and silica during setting.[30]

The presence of halide anions greatly reduces the first major shrinkage and completely eliminates the second, although the reason is not yet understood. If alkali metal or alkaline earth cations are also present (eg, as halide salts), the effect of the halide anion is nullified at temperatures above 650°C, and a rapid contraction occurs,

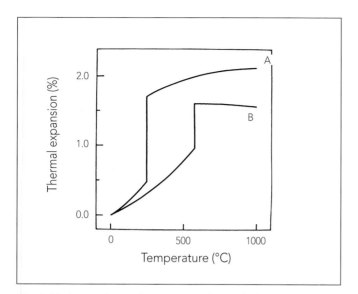

Fig 4-10 Linear thermal expansion of cristobalite (curve A) and quartz (curve B). The specimens were aggregates of fine powders, united with a minimum amount of binder; their thermal behavior was thus similar to that of the refractory component of dental casting investments. Cristobalite undergoes inversion at about 250°C, quartz at 573°C.

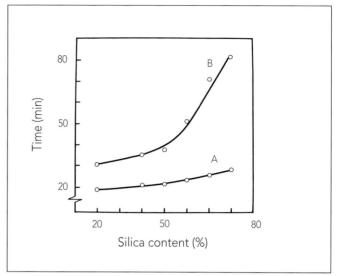

Fig 4-11 Effect of silica content on the manipulation time (curve A) and setting time (curve B) of experimental investments. Manipulation time was determined by the time of loss of gloss, which indicates loss of fluidity; setting time by the Vicat initial set. The investments were mixtures of cristobalite and a high-strength stone, and all specimens were mixed in a W/P ratio of 0.40.

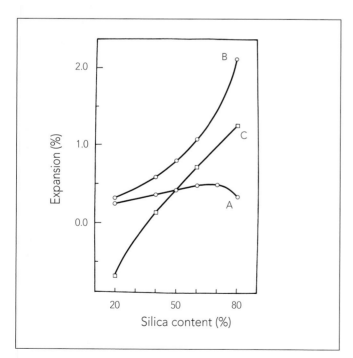

Fig 4-12 Effect of silica content on the setting expansion in air (curve A), the setting expansion in water (curve B), and the thermal expansion (curve C) of experimental investments (compositions and W/P ratio as in Fig 4-11). Setting expansions were recorded 2 hours after mixing, and thermal expansions after heating to 700°C.

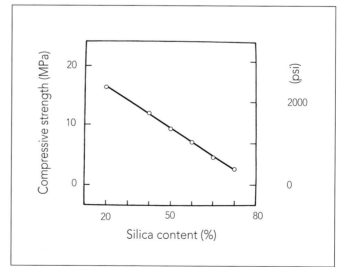

Fig 4-13 Effect of silica content on the compressive strength of experimental investments (compositions and W/P ratio as in Fig 4-11). Tests were made on wet specimens, 2 hours after mixing.

probably as the result of accelerated sintering. This large high-temperature shrinkage of the binder is not observed in gypsum-bonded investments containing alkali metal or alkaline earth halides, because at a concentration of 50% or more of silica, the silica particles in the set investment form a continuous "skeleton" that resists overall shrinkage.

The presence of modifiers added to increase the thermal expansion also affects the strength changes of the investment that occur on heating, again because of their effects on the calcium sulfate binder.

On heating, gypsum-bonded investments without these additives show a rapid increase in compressive strength of about 100% in the range of 100°C to 175°C; this is the result of drying and is analogous to that occurring in cast gypsum. Between 175°C and 225°C, there is an equally rapid decrease in compressive strength, attributable to the dehydration reaction dihydrate → hemihydrate, bringing the strength back to about that of the original wet specimens. Relatively minor strength fluctuations occur during subsequent heating to higher temperatures, attributable to (1) further phase changes in the binder, (2) the α → β inversion in the refractory, and (3) sintering of the binder.[31] Investments of this type, heated to temperatures in the range of 670°C to 700°C, show compressive strength changes ranging from +10% to −40%, compared with the wet strength at ambient temperatures.

Investments containing boric acid, when heated to the same temperatures, show increases in compressive strength ranging from +40% to +50%, probably the result of the effect of the viscous liquid phase stabilizing contacts between calcium sulfate and silica particles. Investments containing halides of alkali metals and alkaline earths (eg, sodium, barium, and strontium chlorides) show a marked strength decrease on heating to 700°C, ranging from −50% to −85%, which is probably the result of the increased sintering contraction of the binder at temperatures over 650°C. The silica skeleton resists shrinkage of the investment as a whole, so the high sintering contraction occurs independently in the binder, reducing the strength of its bond with the silica particles.

Properties

Particle size of the powder

The particle size affects the smoothness of the mold cavity surface (and thus of the casting) and also the inherent porosity of the mold (and thus the venting of the mold cavity). Only the particle size of the refractory filler is of practical importance, as it is the major constituent and remains unchanged in the set investment. The gypsum crystals formed during setting of the binder are much smaller than the silica particles (see Fig 4-9).

Excessive surface roughness of the casting can interfere with its fit; a refractory with a fine particle size ensures a smooth mold surface and a smooth casting. In gypsum-bonded investments, venting of the mold cavity is normally provided by the continuous porosity inherent in the set material. The porosity is greatest when packing of the silica particles is least dense, which in turn is achieved by ensuring that the particle size is uniform.

Therefore, the refractory powder used in making the investment should have a uniform, fine particle size. A particle size of no more than 75 mm is usual.

Rate of setting

The same physical changes that occur during the setting of gypsum plasters can also be recognized when gypsum-bonded investments set.

Manipulation time. Investing the wax pattern or pouring the investment cast must be completed while the mix is still fluid. As with gypsum plasters, loss of fluidity is indicated by the disappearance of the glossy surface.

Setting time. The initial setting time is usually determined using a Gillmore or Vicat needle. These measures indicate when the investment is strong enough for the sprue base and sprue former to be removed. Mold heating should be delayed until setting expansion is complete (usually between 1 and 2 hours from the start of mixing).

Expansion

The total expansions of currently available inlay investments are in the range of 1.5% to 2.5% (measured under laboratory conditions). The increased strength of denture investments is gained at the expense of the refractory component because of the higher content of hemihydrate binder, so the total expansions are less; the lower figure for the expansion range is about 1.3%. It is not certain, however, that such figures show the expansion of the mold cavity that can be expected under practical conditions.

Modern methods of casting small restorations can be classified into two groups:

1. In *hygroscopic expansion techniques*, all or most of the mold expansion is gained when the investment sets; the setting expansion is greatly increased by exposure to additional water. Thermal expansion of the investment is low.
2. In *thermal expansion techniques*, both setting and thermal expansion contribute importantly to mold expansion.

Setting expansion.
1. *Setting expansion in air.* Linear setting expansions of most inlay investments, measured under dry conditions, are in the range of 0.1% to 0.6%.
2. *Setting expansion in water (hygroscopic setting expansion).* Inlay investments show a much greater setting expansion if exposed to additional water during setting (eg, by immersion in a water bath). The phenomenon is the same as that described for gypsum plasters, but the effect on setting expansion is much greater because of the presence of the refractory particles (see Fig 4-12). If no constraint is imposed, the linear setting expansion of inlay investments can be as high as 4%.[32] But even a small restraining force causes a large reduction, and when measured under usual laboratory conditions, the hygroscopic setting expansion of most inlay investments is in the range of 0.3% to 2.0%. Investments specifically designed for use in hygroscopic expansion techniques have setting expansions, when immersed in water, of at least 1.3%.
3. *The effect of the casting ring liner.* In most casting techniques, the investment mold sets and is heated in a casting ring made of heat-resistant alloy, which has a much lower thermal expansion than the investment mold. The need for a soft ring liner to eliminate or at least reduce restraint to investment expansion was first recognized by Souder,[33] who advocated the use of asbestos tape to provide the necessary cushioning. Since asbestos readily absorbs water, the liner could be prewetted to prevent absorption of water from the unset investment mix.

The technique of lining a casting ring with wet asbestos was first described in 1930 by Taylor and coworkers,[34] and then until recent times, it has been a standard procedure. This technique made additional water available to the setting investment and allowed an increased setting expansion. Even when the investment mold set in air, some hygroscopic setting expansion occurred. Investments used with thermal expansion techniques had a relatively high silica content, so the increase in setting expansion produced by exposure to water was high (see Fig 4-12). Because this high setting expansion was uncontrollable and likely to be anisotropic, techniques were developed in which a dry, waterproofed asbestos ring liner was used[14,35] or the casting ring and liner were not used at all.[36]

In 1980, the potential dangerous effects of asbestos fibers in casting-ring liners, such as asbestosis or mesothelioma were detailed.[37] Another report claimed that the acceptable threshold limit for asbestos fibers in air can be considerably exceeded when castings are removed from asbestos-lined casting rings.[38] For this reason and because of the increasing unavailability of asbestos products, asbestos as a casting-ring liner has been almost completely replaced by alternative materials. Two types of materials currently used are *(1) cellulose*, which readily absorbs water and therefore must be prewetted, and *(2) ceramic materials*, which at atmospheric pressure will not absorb water and are normally used dry. The ceramic materials are made from fibers of an aluminosilicate glass derived from Kaolin, and are formed into sheets by means of standard paper-making techniques.[39] The major components of the glass are alumina (47% to 65%) and silica (38% to 50%), which makes the material highly heat resistant. The cellulose materials, on the other hand, will burn if heated in air and, at a burnout temperature of 700°C, they disappear completely from the casting ring. However, if liners are kept short of both ends of the ring, the investment mold is retained in place during casting.

Cellulose liners have a water uptake similar to asbestos and a similar effect on the setting expansion of the investment. Although ceramic liners absorb negligible amounts of water when immersed at atmospheric pressure, they absorb it readily under vacuum as evidenced during vacuum investing. Since the previously dry liners obtain the water from the investment mix, the W/P ratio of the unset investment is greatly reduced. The combination of a low W/P ratio and a wet liner considerably increases the investment's setting expansion; the total expansion is higher than when prewetted cellulose liners are used with normal W/P ratios.

Thermal expansion. After it has set, the investment mold is heated to the recommended temperature for casting. This preparation is necessary to dry the investment, to melt and burnout the wax pattern, to oxidize residual carbon from the mold, and to prevent premature freezing of thin sections when the alloy is cast. Heating also causes thermal expansion of the mold and therefore of the mold cavity.

1. *Hygroscopic expansion techniques.* With these techniques, the mold is heated to about 480°C, at which temperature its thermal expansion is relatively low (Fig 4-14). Investments for use in these techniques are based on a quartz refractory that does not undergo inversion until heated to 573°C (see Fig 4-10).

   A mold temperature as low as 480°C has the advantage of ensuring a fine grain structure in the solidified casting, though this is not an important consideration if the alloy contains grain-refining elements. It has the disadvantage that carbon remaining from burnout of the wax pattern is oxidized very slowly. Excessive carbon deposits interfere with venting of the mold cavity, so prolonged heating at the casting temperature (preferably 1 hour) is needed to ensure that casting defects caused by inadequate venting ("back-pressure porosity") do not occur.

2. *Thermal expansion techniques.* With thermal expansion techniques, the mold is usually heated to about 700°C to gain maximum mold expansion. A higher mold temperature should not be used or breakdown of the calcium sulfate binder can occur in the presence of carbon, thereby liberating sulfur dioxide. The carbon may be present as graphite added to the original investment powder as a reducing agent or may simply be carbon residue from burnout of the wax pattern. The reaction, which involves reduction of the calcium sulfate binder, takes place in two stages:

$$CaSO_4 + 4C \rightarrow CaS + 4CO$$
$$3CaSO_4 + CaS \rightarrow 4CaO + 4SO_2$$

   The sulfur dioxide formed by the second reaction causes sulfide formation on the gold-alloy casting, resulting in discoloration and embrittlement of the alloy, as first showed by O'Brien.[40]

   Investments for thermal expansion techniques may contain either cristobalite or quartz as the refractory; occasionally a mixture of both is used. Cristobalite investments have the advantage that thermal expansion is fairly constant over the temperature range of 400°C to 700°C, but have the disadvantage that the large ex-

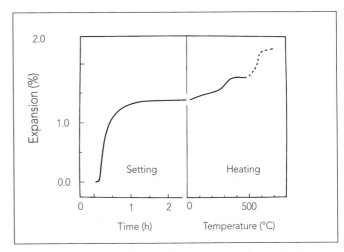

Fig 4-14 Setting and thermal expansion of a typical investment of the hygroscopic expansion type (Whip Mix Beauty-Cast, W/P = 0.30). The specimen was immersed in room-temperature water during setting and then heated to 480°C. This investment is based on quartz and contains a halide, which gives it a small positive thermal expansion, uniform over a range of about 150°C. The dashed continuation of the curve shows the effect of heating the investment to 700°C.

pansion at 250°C, resulting from the $\alpha \rightarrow \beta$ inversion of cristobalite, can cause mold cracking if heating is not carefully controlled (Fig 4-15, curve A). It should be slow in the temperature range of 230°C to 270°C while the inversion of cristobalite is occurring throughout the mold.

Quartz has a lower thermal expansion than cristobalite (see Fig 4-10), so most quartz investments for use in thermal expansion techniques contain additives to increase their thermal expansion. The expansion on heating is more gradual, so controlling the heating rate is not as important, but maximum expansion is available only in the temperature range of 600°C to 700°C (Fig 4-15, curve B).

At a burnout temperature of 700°C, residual carbon is oxidized rapidly, so venting of the mold cavity is not a problem.

3. *The effect of a wet liner.* In thermal expansion techniques, if a wet ring liner is used, not only the setting expansion but also the subsequent thermal expansion can be affected. Once the investment has set, the extra water it absorbed from the liner has the same effect as if it had been added during mixing (ie, an increased W/P ratio). Therefore, the thermal expansion may be reduced.

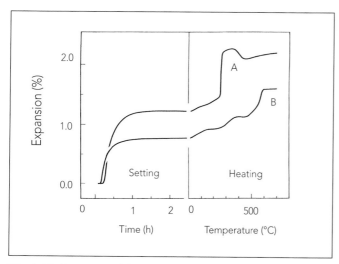

Fig 4-15 Setting and thermal expansion of two typical investments of the thermal expansion type (curve A: Kerr Cristobalite Inlay, W/P = 0.38; curve B: R&R Gray, W/P = 0.25). With both materials the specimens were surrounded by a wet ring liner while setting and were then heated to 700°C. The former material is an inlay investment based on cristobalite. The latter material is described as a universal investment but is most commonly used for casting dentures and is based on quartz, with the addition of sodium chloride to increase its thermal expansion.

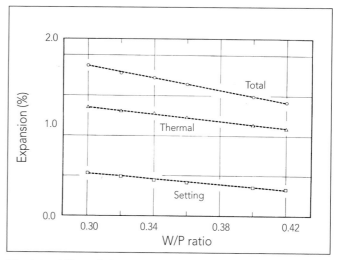

Fig 4-16 Effect of changing the W/P ratio on the setting, thermal, and total expansions of a typical investment of the thermal expansion type, set against a dry ceramic liner without vacuum investing, and then heated to 700°C.

The same considerations apply to denture investments. The investment cast forms part of the final mold, and its expansion is the major factor determining the accuracy of the casting. It sets in contact with a duplicating impression, usually an aqueous gel, which, like a wet ring liner, makes free water available to the setting investment with the same effects as those already described.

Control of expansion.

1. *Composition.* The manufacturer adjusts investment expansion by the choice of refractory and binder and sometimes by the use of suitable additives.
2. *W/P ratio.* Decreasing the W/P ratio increases both setting expansion (in air or water) and thermal expansion. The W/P ratio must be carefully controlled for reproducible mold expansion. Changes in expansion can most easily be effected by changing the W/P ratio (Fig 4-16).
3. *Period of exposure to water.* In hygroscopic expansion techniques, additional control can be obtained by varying the length of time the setting investment is exposed to an aqueous environment, such as by reducing the time for which the setting investment is immersed in a water bath, or by adding controlled amounts of water to the top of the investment mix in the ring instead of immersing it. In the latter case, if only a small volume of water is added, it will be completely absorbed by the investment before setting is complete, and subsequent expansion will be reduced. Varying the amount of added water varies the setting expansion proportionally.

Strength

The mold must be strong enough to withstand stresses at ambient temperatures (eg, during removal of the sprue former) and when heating to the recommended mold temperature for casting (eg, during rapid entry of molten alloy). Strength properties of investments are usually determined by testing in compression. Inlay investments have wet compressive strengths mostly in the range of 2 to 6 MPa. Because of the need to make a working cast, denture investments have higher compressive strengths when set, mostly in the range of 9 to 14 MPa. In both investment types, changes in the compressive strength on heating to the recommended casting temperature vary according to the presence of additives to control invest-ment thermal expansion. Unless it is known whether an additive is present in an investment, and if so what it is, it is impossible to predict strength at the casting tem-perature from measurements made at ordinary ambient temperatures. Little information is available on the com-pressive strength of gypsum-bonded investments at the casting temperature (hot strength). In one study on a lim-ited number of materials,[41] it was found that the hot strength of four investments without additives was in the range of 1.8 to 9.4 MPa. For three investments containing boric acid it was 6.3 to 13.3 MPa, and for three invest-ments containing sodium chloride it was 3.1 to 5.2 MPa.

Rapid-heat investments

Although it was stated earlier that investments based on a cristobalite refractory require slow heating while the $\alpha \rightarrow \beta$ inversion is occurring, some "rapid-heat" invest-ments have been introduced, which immediately after setting are placed into a furnace preheated to 700°C. At least some of these contain cristobalite as the refractory. The recommended technique is to place the mold, 30 minutes after the pattern is invested, into the preheated furnace for an additional 30 minutes. The casting is then made. A setting and thermal expansion curve for a typi-cal example is shown in Fig 4-17.

Little information is available on these materials. It can be seen in Fig 4-17 that setting expansion is still occur-ring rapidly at 30 minutes; measured under ordinary con-ditions, it is not complete until 2 hours after mixing and measures 1.1%. The rapid rate of expansion at 30 min-utes means that precise timing of placement of the mold in the furnace is critical if reproducible mold expansion is to occur.

Such a drastic heating program could be expected to cause severe thermal cracking in an ordinary cristobalite investment. Measurements on a mold in a lined inlay ring showed that the periphery of the investment mass reached 250°C within 6 minutes of entering the hot fur-nace, while the center was at only 110°C. The center of the mold did not reach 250°C until 4 minutes later. Both the periphery and center had reached a maximum of 690°C within the 30-minute heating period.

The indicated temperatures shown in Fig 4-17 were recorded by a thermocouple whose hot junction was em-bedded in the center of a specimen that had about the same thickness as an inlay mold. The expansion caused by the inversion of cristobalite, shown on the graph as

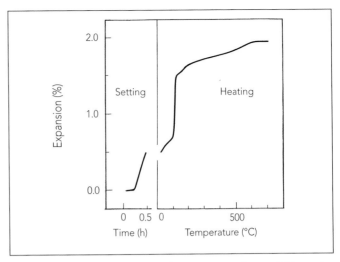

Fig 4-17 Setting and thermal expansion of a rapid-heat in-vestment of the thermal expansion type (GC Cristoquick, W/P = 0.33). As the manufacturer instructed, the investment was al-lowed to set against a dry ceramic liner for 30 minutes and was then immediately transferred to a furnace preheated to 700°C.

beginning at 110°C and finishing at 170°C, obviously took place when enough of the outer parts of the speci-men had reached 250°C to produce a volume change.

These rapid-heat investments save laboratory time and simplify the casting procedure, as the furnace is maintained at 700°C instead of being repeatedly heated and cooled. Despite the curtailed setting expansion, the investment's total expansion under these conditions was 1.95%, more than enough to compensate for the casting shrinkage of ordinary dental gold alloys.

Casting accuracy

In all casting procedures, after the molten metal or alloy has filled the mold, a volumetric contraction occurs in the liquid and then in the solid casting as it cools. In addi-tion, with almost all metals and alloys there is a volumet-ric contraction during solidification.

In dental casting, thermal contraction of the liquid alloy and its solidification contraction do not affect the dimensions of the casting because, under the influence of the casting force, continued feeding of liquid alloy oc-curs from the excess in the sprue and button. Interruption to the flow of liquid during solidification, which may be caused by premature freezing of an incorrectly designed sprue, will not cause an overall contraction of the casting but will lead to localized shrinkage porosity.

Table 4-5 Measured values for the linear casting shrinkage of pure gold

SPECIMENS (MM)	LINEAR CASTING SHRINKAGE (%)*
Cylindric rod[42] (5.6 × 25)	1.67 ± 0.02 (8)
Cylindric rod[43] (6.3 × 60)	1.74 ± 0.03 (6)
Rectangular prism[44] (3 × 5 × 20)	1.73 ± 0.04 (9)

*Values are shown as mean and standard deviation, with number of tests in parentheses.

Therefore, thermal contraction of the solidified casting, as it cools from solidus to ambient temperature, remains the sole cause of the observed casting shrinkage. Although this is a volumetric contraction, in dental technology, dimensional changes are usually studied on a linear basis. It is assumed that these changes occur isotropically—an assumption that is frequently unjustified.

The fact that the observed casting shrinkage is therma contraction of the solid alloy can be confirmed, at least for pure gold, by comparing measured values for its linear casting shrinkage with a value calculated from its coefficient of linear thermal expansion (α) and the temperature difference between its freezing temperature and ambient.

Results of direct measurements of the linear casting shrinkage of gold are shown in Table 4-5. A theoretic value can be calculated as follows:

$$\alpha_{(20°C-900°C)} = 16.7 \times 10^{-6}/K$$
$$\text{Melting temperature} = 1,064°C$$

If 20°C is taken as an average ambient temperature, the solidified gold cools through 1,044 K. Total linear contraction per unit length is given by $1,044 \times 16.7 \times 10^{-6}$ = 0.0174, which converts to 1.74%.

Alloying gold will alter the value for α and for solidus temperature. Calculations similar to that given previously have been made on a group of 12 high-noble-metal casting alloys, and the calculated linear casting shrinkages varied from 1.65% to 1.80%.[36] Thus, an average value of 1.7% would apply to gold and high-gold alloys.

It is conventionally assumed that compensation for this casting shrinkage is provided by mold expansion. Calculations of available compensation, however, must be based on measurements of investment expansion made under conditions that reproduce those obtained in the casting ring.[45]

Another factor that must be considered is the effect of the ring liner on investment expansion. Absorbent liners (asbestos and cellulose) vary in thickness, water uptake, and compressibility when wet. In thermal expansion techniques, some may not have sufficient compressibility to accommodate all of the increased setting expansion provided by the availability of extra water, so that restriction of expansion could occur in a diametral direction in the ring.[46] Thus they affect the available mold expansion to a varying degree.[47] Ceramic liners also vary in thickness and compressibility, and if vacuum investing is used, they vary in the amount of water they absorb from the investment mix.

The choice of casting-ring liner can therefore affect, often to a significant extent, the dimensional accuracy of the casting. Figures 4-18 and 4-19 show the great variation in casting inaccuracy produced when the same investment is used with different casting-ring liners. This variation in inaccuracy is often unpredictable; in these experiments, only when the ceramic liners were used with vacuum investing was there any correlation between measured liner properties and casting inaccuracy.

Although with gypsum-bonded investments mold expansion is the major factor affecting relative casting inaccuracy, mold strength at the casting temperature must also be considered. The average value of 1.7% for alloy thermal contraction represents the inherent casting shrinkage of the alloy—the shrinkage that would occur in a casting that was free to contract without constraint. Under practical conditions the casting is enclosed in a mold, and in all but the simplest castings its shape allows some interlocking between investment and mold. In the early stages of cooling, the mold has a lower rate of thermal contraction than the casting; the thermal contraction of a typical high-gold alloy, cooling from its solidus temperature to 500°C, would be 0.74%, while for a typical cristobalite inlay investment, cooling from 700°C to

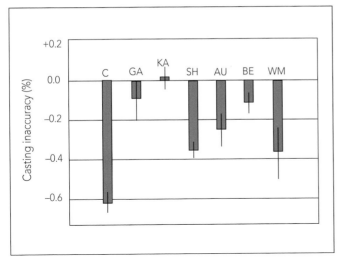

Fig 4-18 Effect of different prewetted ring liners on the relative inaccuracy of gold-alloy full-crown castings. The castings were made with a cristobalite inlay investment of the thermal expansion type used with vacuum investing. C = control castings made without a liner; GA, KA, and SH = castings made with asbestos liners; and AU, BE, and WM = castings made with cellulose liners. The height of each bar shows the mean of at least 10 castings, while the narrow superimposed bar shows the standard deviation.

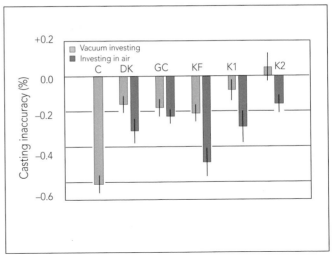

Fig 4-19 The effect of different dry ceramic ring liners on the relative inaccuracy of gold-alloy full-crown castings. Conditions were the same as in Fig 4-18, except that castings were made with and without vacuum investing. C = control castings made without a liner; DK, GC, and KF = castings made with ceramic liners supplied for dental use; and K1 and K2 = castings made with liners cut from commercial insulating material of the same type, supplied in sheets nominally 1 mm and 2 mm thick.

500°C, it would be 0.20%. If the investment has a high hot strength, alloy thermal contraction will be opposed by the mold; the degree of constraint will depend on the casting shape and is usually directional. At temperatures near its solidus, the alloy is weak and plastic, and mold constraint can cause anisotropic thermal contraction. When the alloy has cooled enough to attain rigidity, a strong mold can cause plastic deformation by hot-working the alloy. Both factors cause anisotropic contraction and distortion of the casting.

A constant pattern of distortion of gold-alloy mesio-occluso-distal inlays has been reported[48] and can be attributed to directional restraint of alloy shrinkage by the mold.[41] The gypsum-bonded investment used in Teteruck and Mumford's experiments had a compressive strength at 700°C in the range of 4 to 6 MPa.[48]

Therefore, although with gypsum-bonded investments the total investment expansion that occurs in the casting ring is the major factor affecting the casting inaccuracy, the hot strength of the mold must be considered. For the casting to accurately reproduce the size and shape of the original pattern, the investment expansion must compensate fully for the thermal contraction of the solid alloy,

the ring and ring liner must allow the potential expansion of the investment to be achieved isotropically, and the investment at the burnout temperature must not be so strong that it restricts the shrinkage of the alloy in any direction. On the other hand, it should not be so weak that it may fracture during casting. A safe minimum compressive strength at 700°C is 1.8 MPa, and this strength allows substantially isotropic alloy contraction.[49]

◉ Storage of Gypsum Products

When hemihydrate powders are exposed to the atmosphere, water vapor is adsorbed; the extent to which this occurs depends on the prevailing water vapor pressure.[8] If sufficient water is adsorbed to form a liquid film, and if this film becomes thick enough to function as a solvent, the setting reaction begins on the surface of the powder particles, causing deterioration of the material. Newly formed gypsum crystals act as nucleation centers when the powder is mixed with water and accelerate the setting rate. But if exposure of the powder continues, surface hydration will form a layer of gypsum on each particle, hindering the access of water to the hemihydrate, and the subsequent setting rate is retarded. If exposure continues over a long period, eventually the material will not set properly because insufficient unreacted hemihydrate remains to form a coherent set mass. This situation is equally likely to occur in gypsum-bonded investments and will have the same effects.

A long-standing recommendation[50] to store gypsum products at relative humidities less than 70% appears satisfactory only at temperatures of 25°C or lower, but of uncertain validity at higher temperatures. To avoid deterioration, especially at high temperatures and high relative humidities, bulk gypsum products should be stored in closed bins, in a cool dry area of the laboratory. "Topping up" of bins should not be done over old stock. Packaging of small quantities of powder in waterproof containers is a preferable method of storage in the laboratory; many die stones and gypsum-bonded investments are now packaged in this way by their manufacturers.

◖ Glossary

acicular (of a crystal) Slender, needle like.

apparent density (of a powder) The mass of a sample divided by the volume it occupies, measured at a specified degree of compaction. The measured volume includes all interstitial spaces and porosities, so powders with a poor packing ability show a low apparent density.

calcination Prolonged heating of a substance at some temperature below its melting temperature.

crystal habit (crystalline form) The external geometric shape of a crystal.

crystal structure The regular three-dimensional arrangement of atoms within a crystal. This internal atomic arrangement is characteristic of a particular crystalline solid, but may or may not be the same as the external shape of individual crystals.

inversion A temperature-dependent change from one polymorphic form to another. **Rapid (high-low) inversions** involve only an alteration in bond angles within the crystal structure (shear or displacive transformation). **Slow inversions** involve breaking of interatomic bonds and atomic diffusion to form a new crystal structure (reconstructive transformation).

isotropic Occurring equally in all directions.

nucleation center In an aqueous solution, a region where spontaneous, orderly deposition of ions or molecules forms nuclei that continue to grow, beginning the process of crystallization.

nuclei poisoning The inactivation of nuclei of crystallization by the deposition of foreign material on their surfaces.

polymorphism The existence of an element or chemical compound in more than two different crystalline forms.

pseudomorphic A crystalline material whose crystal habit differs from the normal shape that would be dictated by its crystal structure.

pseudoplasticity The behavior of non-Newtonian fluids in which the rate of shear increases more than in proportion to the shearing stress (shear-thinning liquids). Thick mixes of plaster or stone are typical examples; they appear to be very viscous when at rest but flow readily when subjected to a shear stress (eg, stirring or vibration).

refractory Capable of resisting high temperatures.

relative surface area (of a powder) The total surface area of a given mass.

specular (of reflections) Mirror like.

spherulite A spheric aggregation of needle-shaped crystals radiating out from a common center.

water/powder (W/P) ratio The mixing proportions of plaster or stone, expressed as a decimal fraction. If 100 g of plaster is to be mixed with 50 g of water, the W/P ratio is 0.50.

water requirement The amount of water that must be added to a given mass of plaster or stone to produce a mix of suitable viscosity.

◖ Discussion Questions

1. How many different applications do gypsum products have in dentistry, as well as other fields?

2. Why are storage conditions and shelf life important considerations in the use of gypsum products? Why do these present special problems for the dental services of large organizations such as the armed forces?

3. Why is it essential to follow directions to achieve the higher strengths possible with improved die stones?

4. What are the main methods of reducing bubbles in gypsum casts and molds?

Study Questions

(See appendix E for answers.)

1. What differences in chemical composition are there in the powders of plaster, stone, and die stone?

2. What physical differences are there in the powders of plaster, stone, and die stone? How are these differences related to the methods of manufacture of the powders?

3. Give typical W/P ratios for plaster, stone, and die stone. Why are these different? For each type, assuming that the setting reaction goes to completion, what percentage of the mass of the set material would consist of free water?

4. What chemical and physical changes accompany the setting of gypsum products?

5. What is the difference between the microstructures of gypsum casts made from plaster and stone? What is the cause of this difference, and what is its effect on strength properties?

6. What is meant by the setting time of gypsum products? What is the practical significance of *(a)* the loss of surface gloss, *(b)* the Gillmore initial set, and *(c)* the Vicat initial set?

7. Explain how the manufacturer of a dental gypsum product adjusts its rate of setting.

8. For a given gypsum product, what is the effect of increasing the W/P ratio on the rate of setting? Explain.

9. Theoretically, the setting of gypsum products should be accompanied by a volumetric contraction. Why is a setting expansion observed in practice?

10. Why do gypsum products show a greater setting expansion in water than in air?

11. What is the practical significance of the setting expansion of dental gypsum products?

12. Give typical values for the linear setting expansion in air of impression plaster, plaster, stone, and low-expansion and high-expansion die stones.

13. Explain how the manufacturer of a gypsum product controls its setting expansion.

14. What practical limits are placed on the extent of this control?

15. For a given gypsum product, what is the effect of increasing the W/P ratio on setting expansion? Explain.

16. What is the practical significance of the tensile strength and the compressive strength of dental gypsum products?

17. For a given gypsum product, what is the effect of increasing the W/P ratio on tensile strength and compressive strength? Explain.

18. What is the effect of drying on the tensile strength and the compressive strength of cast gypsum? Explain.

19. What constituents are likely to be present in a gypsum-bonded investment powder? Give the function of each.

20. Within normal limits, what effect does increasing the proportion of refractory filler in an investment have on *(a)* rate of setting, *(b)* setting expansion in air, *(c)* setting expansion in water, *(d)* thermal expansion, and *(e)* compressive strength?

21. How does the investment set?

22. What is the practical significance of microscopic porosity formed in the investment mass during setting?

23. What are the requirements for the particle size of an investment powder? Give reasons.

24. Why is the particle size of the refractory filler more important than that of the binder?

25. What is the most important property of an investment? Why?

26. What is a hygroscopic expansion technique?

27. What is a thermal expansion technique?

28. In hygroscopic expansion techniques, why is prolonged heating of the mold at the burnout temperature necessary?

29. How can the user of a dental investment discover whether it contains cristobalite or quartz as a refractory? What is the practical importance of this information?

30. Why is control of the heating rate more important with a cristobalite investment than with a quartz investment?

31. Why is an accurate furnace pyrometer more important with a quartz investment than with a cristobalite investment?

32. Why should gypsum-bonded investments not be heated above 700°C?

33. In thermal expansion techniques, what is the effect of a wet liner on the investment's setting expansion?

34. What is the effect of increasing the W/P ratio on (a) the investment's setting expansion in air, (b) its setting expansion in water, and (c) its thermal expansion?

35. In hygroscopic expansion techniques, how can mold expansion be controlled by the user?

36. In thermal expansion techniques, how can mold expansion be controlled by the user?

37. What is the practical significance of the compressive strength of the investment at the casting temperature?

38. How should gypsum products be stored in a dental laboratory? How can incorrect storage conditions affect these materials?

■ References

1. International Organization for Standardization. ISO 6873:1998. Dental Gypsum Products, ed 2. Geneva: International Organization for Standardization, 1998.
2. Andrews H. The Production, Properties and Uses of Calcium Sulphate Plasters. London: Building Research Congress, Division 2, Part F, 135, 1951.
3. Khalil AA, Hussein AT, Gad GM. On the thermochemistry of gypsum. J Appl Chem Biotechnol 1971;21:314.
4. Weiser HB, Milligan WD, Eckholm WC. The mechanism of dehydration of calcium sulfate hemihydrate. J Am Chem Soc 1936;58:1261.
5. Gay P. Some crystallographic studies in the system COMP: see p 4-5 for format $CaSO_4 – CaSO_4 \cdot 2H_2O$. I. The polymorphism of anhydrous $CaSO_4$. Mineral Mag 1965;35:347.
6. Gay P. Some crystallographic studies in the system $CaSO_4 – CaSO_4 \cdot 2H_2O$ COMP: see p 4-5 for format. II. The hydrous forms. Mineral Mag 1965;35:354.
7. Earnshaw R, Mori T. Contraction of cast gypsum between 200°C and 500°C. J Dent Res 1985;64:658.
8. Torrance A, Darvell BW. Effect of humidity on calcium sulphate hemihydrate. Aust Dent J 1990;35:230.
9. Gregg SJ. The Surface Chemistry of Solids, ed 2. London: Chapman and Hall, 1965:232.
10. Ridge MJ. Factors determining the water requirement of gypsum plaster. J Appl Chem 1961;11:287.
11. Lautenschlager EP, Harcourt JK, Ploszaj LC. Setting reactions of gypsum materials investigated by X-ray diffraction. J Dent Res 1969;48:43.
12. Koslowski T, Ludwig U. Retardation of gypsum plasters with citric acid: mechanism and properties. In: Kuntze RA (ed). The Chemistry and Technology of Gypsum ASTM STP861. Philadelphia: American Society for Testing and Materials, 1984:97–104.
13. Lautenschlager EP, Corbin F. Investigation on the expansion of dental stone. J Dent Res 1969;48:206.
14. Bever MB (ed). Encyclopedia of Materials Science and Engineering. Elmsford, NY: Pergamon Press, 1986:1098.
15. Mahler DB, Ady AB. An explanation for the hygroscopic setting expansion of dental gypsum products. J Dent Res 1960;39:578.
16. Fusayama T. Synthetic study on precision casting. Bull Tokyo Med Dent Univ 1964;11:165.
17. Selby A. The Relationship Between the Viscosity of the Mix and the Tensile Strength of Cast Gypsum [thesis]. Sydney: University of Sydney, 1979.
18. Donnison JA, Chong MP, Docking AR. Calorimetric study of the hygroscopic setting of calcined gypsum. Aust Dent J 1960;5:269.
19. Bergman B, Bergman M, Olsson S. Alginate impression materials, dimensional stability and surface detail sharpness following treatment with disinfectant solutions. Swed Dent J 1985;9:255.
20. Olsson S, Bergman B, Bergman M. Agar impression materials, dimensional stability and surface detail sharpness following treatment with disinfectant solutions. Swed Dent J 1987;11:169.
21. Johnson GH, Drennon DG, Powell GL. Accuracy of elastomeric impressions disinfected by immersion. J Am Dent Assoc 1988;116:525.
22. McGill S, Narea EM, Suchak AJ, Stanford JW. The effect of disinfecting solutions on alginate and gypsum materials. J Dent Res 1988;67:281.
23. Ivanovski S, Savage NW, Brockhurst PJ, Bird P. Disinfection of dental stone casts: antimicrobial effects and physical property alterations. Dent Mater 1995;11:19.
24. Donovan T, Chee WWL. Preliminary investigation of a disinfected gypsum die stone. Int J Prosthodont 1989;2:245.
25. Schutt RW. Bactericidal effect of a disinfectant dental stone on irreversible hydrocolloid impressions and stone casts. J Prosthet Dent 1989;62:605.
26. Whyte MP, Brockhurst PJ. The effect of steam sterilisation on the properties of set dental gypsum models. Aust Dent J 1996;41:128.
27. International Organization for Standardization. ISO 7490:2000. Dental Gypsum-Bonded Casting Investments, ed 2. Geneva: International Organization for Standardization, 2000.
28. Gutt WH, Smith MA. The a form of calcium sulphate. Trans Br Ceram Soc 1967;66:337.
29. Mori T. Thermal behavior of the gypsum binder in dental casting investments. J Dent Res 1986;65:877.
30. Mori T. The effect of boric acid on the thermal behavior of cast gypsum. Dent Mater J 1982;1:73.
31. Ohno H, Nakano S, Miyakawa O, Watanabe K, Shiokawa N. Effects of phase transformations of silicas and calcium sulfates on the compressive strength of gypsum-bonded investments at high temperatures. J Dent Res 1982;61:1077.
32. Earnshaw R. The effect of restrictive stress on the hygroscopic setting expansion of gypsum-bonded investments. Aust Dent J 1969;14:22.
33. Hollenback GM. A brief history of the cast restoration. J South Calif State Dent Assoc 1962;30:8.
34. Taylor NO, Paffenbarger GC, Sweeney WT. Dental inlay casting investments: physical properties and a specification. J Am Dent Assoc 1930;17:2266.
35. Fusayama T. Factors and technique of precision casting. J Prosthet Dent 1959;9:468, 486.
36. Finger W, Jørgensen KD. An improved dental casting investment. Scand J Dent Res 1980;88:278.
37. Priest G, Horner, JA. Fibrous ceramic aluminium silicate as an alternative to asbestos liners. J Prosthet Dent 1980;44:51.
38. Yli-Urpo A, Øilo G, Syverud M. The effect of asbestos-alternatives on the accuracy of cast veneer crowns. Swed Dent J 1982;6:127.
39. Barnard G. Recent developments in using ceramic fibres in reducing atmospheres. Metals Australasia 1981;13:10–11.
40. O'Brien WJ, Nielsen JP. Decomposition of gypsum investment in the presence of carbon. J Dent Res 1959;38:541.
41. Earnshaw R. The compressive strength of gypsum-bonded investments at high temperatures. Aust Dent J 1969;14:264.
42. Hollenback GM, Skinner EW. Shrinkage during casting of gold and gold alloys. J Am Dent Assoc 1946;33:1391.
43. Earnshaw R. Further measurements of the casting shrinkage of dental cobalt-chromium alloys. Br Dent J 1960;109:238.
44. Nakai A, Nakamura Y, Seki S-I, Kakuta K, Kawashima J-I. Measurement of casting shrinkage with U-type tungsten die. J Jap Dent Apparat Mat 1980;21:122.
45. Earnshaw R. The effect of casting ring liners on the potential expansion of a gypsum-bonded investment. J Dent Res 1988;67:1366.
46. Morey EF, Earnshaw R. The fit of gold-alloy full-crown castings made with pre-wetted casting ring liners. J Dent Res 1992;71:1858.

47. Earnshaw R, Morey EF. The fit of gold-alloy full-crown castings made with ceramic casting ring liners. J Dent Res 1992;71:1865.
48. Teteruck WR, Mumford G. The fit of certain dental casting alloys using different investing materials and techniques. J Prosthet Dent 1966;16:910.
49. Morey EF, Earnshaw R. The effect of potential investment expansion and hot strength on the fit of full-crown castings made with a gypsum-bonded investment. Dent Mater 1995;11:312.
50. Farmer GJ, Skinner EW. Effect of relative humidity on the setting time of plaster of Paris. Northwestern Univ Bull 1942;43:12.

◼ Recommended Reading

Anusavice K. Phillips' Science of Dental Materials, ed 10. Philadelphia: Saunders, 1996,196–198.

Asgar K. Casting alloys in dentistry. In: Dickson G, Cassel JM (eds). Dental Materials Research. Washington, DC: National Bureau of Standards, SP, 1972:354, 363.

Asgar K, Mahler DB, Peyton FA. Hygroscopic technique for inlay casting using controlled water additions. J Prosthet Dent 1955;5:711–724.

Beretka J, Crook DN, King GA, Middleton LW. Applications of by-Product Gypsum in the Plaster Industry. Presented at the Eighth Australian Chemical Engineering Conference, Melbourne, August 1980.

Buchanan AS, Worner HK. Changes in the composition and setting characteristics of plaster of Paris on exposure to high humidity atmosphere. J Dent Res 1945;24:65.

Collins PF, inventor. Dental Investment Composition and Process. US Patent: 2,006,733; 1935.

Collins PF, inventor. Dental Investment Composition. US Patent: 2,247,571; 1941.

Collins PF, inventor. Dental Investment Composition. US Patent: 2,247,572; 1941.

Collins PF, inventor. Dental Investment Composition. US Patent: 2,247,573; 1941.

Combe EC. Recent developments in model and die materials. In: von Fraunhofer JA (ed). Scientific Aspects of Dental Materials. London: Butterworths, 1974:402–415.

Combe EC, Smith DC. The effects of some organic acids and salts on the setting of gypsum plaster. II. Tartrates. J Appl Chem 1965;15:367.

Combe EC, Smith DC. The effects of some organic acids and salts on the setting of gypsum plaster. III. Citrates. J Appl Chem 1966;16:73.

Combe EC, Smith DC. Studies on the preparation of calcium sulphate hemihydrate by an autoclave process. J Appl Chem 1968;18:307.

Craig RG (ed). Restorative Dental Materials, ed 10. St Louis: Mosby, 1997:347.

Dootz ER, Craig RG, Peyton FA. Influence of investments and duplicating procedures on the accuracy of partial denture castings. J Prosthet Dent 1965;15:679.

Earnshaw R. The effect of restrictive stress on the setting expansion of gypsum-bonded investments. Aust Dent J 1964;9:169.

Earnshaw R. Effects of additives on the thermal expansion of cast gypsum. J Dent Res 1976;55:518.

Earnshaw R, Marks BI. The measurement of setting time of gypsum products. Aust Dent J 1964;9:17.

Eberl JJ, Ingram AR. Process for making high-strength plaster of Paris. Ind Eng Chem 1949;41:1061–1065.

Fairhurst CW. Compressive properties of dental gypsum. J Dent Res 1960;39:812–824.

Finger W, Jørgensen KD, Ono T. Strength properties of some gypsum-bonded investments. Scand J Dent Res 1980;88:155.

Gibson CS, Johnson RN. Investigations of the setting of plaster of Paris. J Soc Chem Ind (Transactions) 1932;51:25.

Greener EH, Harcourt JK, Lautenschlager EP. Materials Science in Dentistry. Baltimore: Williams & Wilkins, 1972:276.

Haddon CL. Gypsum plaster products. Chem Ind 1944;22:190.

Haddon CL, Cafferata BJ, inventors. Improvements in the manufacture of plaster of Paris. British Patent 563,019; 1944.

Harcourt JK, Lautenschlager EP. Accelerated and retarded dental plaster setting investigated by X-ray diffraction. J Dent Res 1970;49:502.

Hoggatt GA, inventor. Method of producing gypsum plaster. US Patent:2,616,789, 1952.

Jastrzebski ZD. The Nature and Properties of Engineering Materials, ed 2. New York: John Wiley & Sons, 1976:59.

Jørgensen KD, Posner AS. Study of the setting of plaster. J Dent Res 1959;38:491.

Kingery WD, Bower HK, Uhlmann DR. Introduction to Ceramics, ed 2. New York: John Wiley & Sons, 1976:81–87.

Lager GA, Armbruster T, Rotella FJ, Jørgensen JD, Flinks DG. A crystallographic study of the low-temperature dehydration products of gypsum. Am Mineral 1984;69:910.

Matsuya S, Yamane M. Decomposition of gypsum-bonded investments. J Dent Res 1981;60:1418.

Moore TE, inventor. Method of making dental castings and composition employed in said method. US Patent:1,924,874; 1933.

Mori T. Transformation of CaSO4(III) to CaSO4(II) in gypsum-bonded investments. J Dent Res 1985;64:658.

Mori T, Yamane M. Fractography of cast gypsum. Aust Dent J 1982; 27:30.

Neiman R, inventor. Investment. US Patent: 2,247,395; 1941.

Neiman R, Ernst RC, Steinbock EA, inventors. Investment composition. US Patent: 2,313,085; 1943.

Neiman R, Ernst RC, Steinbock EA, inventors. Investment composition. US Patent: 2,313,086.

Offutt JS, Lambe CM. Plasters and gypsum cements for the ceramic industry. Am Ceram Soc Bull 1947;26:29.

Pomés CD, Slack GL, Wise MW. Surface roughness of dental castings. J Am Dent Assoc 1950;41:545.

Randel WS, Dailey MC. High strength calcined gypsum and process of manufacture of same. US Patent: 1,901,051; 1933.

Ridge MJ. Acceleration of the set of gypsum plaster. Aust J Appl Sci 1959;10:218.

Ridge MJ. Mechanism of setting of gypsum plaster. Rev Pure Appl Chem 1960;10:243.

Ridge MJ. The hydration of calcium sulphate hemihydrate. Proc Royal Austral Chem Inst 1972;39:55.

Ridge MJ, Beretka J. Calcium sulphate hemihydrate and its hydration. Rev Pure Appl Chem 1969;19:17.

Russell JJ. The effect of moisture content on the compressive strength of small cubes of some cast gypsum plasters. Zement-Kalk-Gips 1960;13:345.

Sodeau WH, Gibson CS. The use of plaster of Paris as an impression material. Br Dent J 1927;48:70.

Sosman RB. The Phases of Silica. New Brunswick: Rutgers University Press, 1965:32, 36–42. 4

Souder W, Paffenbarger GC. Physical Properties of Dental Materials. Washington, DC: National Bureau of Standards, C433, 1942:80–93.

Suffert LW, Mahler DB. Reproducibility of gold castings made by present day dental casting technics. J Am Dent Assoc 1955;50:1.

Sweeney WT, Taylor DB. Dimensional changes in dental stone and plaster. J Dent Res 1950;29:749.

Weinstein LJ. Composition for dental moulds. US Patent: 1,708,436; 1929.

Worner HK. Dental plasters. Part I. Aust J Dent 1942;46:1.

Surface Phenomena and Adhesion to Tooth Structure

Surface phenomena include surface energy, wetting, adsorption, capillary penetration, and adhesion. Applications include capillary penetration around restorations, dentures, and teeth, and adhesion to tooth structure by sealants and restorative materials.

● Surface Energy

Atoms and molecules at the surfaces of liquids and solids possess more energy (**surface energy**) than do those in the interior. In the case of liquids, this energy is called **surface tension**. As illustrated in Fig 5-1, the molecules at the surface are farther apart due to loss of molecules by evaporation. From Fig 5-2 it can be seen that this greater average separation leads to a higher net energy of attraction. This reaction results in a surface contractile force or surface tension, which causes the liquid to form drops and to exhibit a surface skin that resists extension or penetration.

The surface energies of oxides and metals are greater than those of liquids (Table 5-1). In general, the higher the bond strength of a substance, the greater the surface energy. Since metallic bonds are much stronger than the van der Waals bonds of liquids, metals have higher surface energies. The units of surface energy are ergs/cm^2, but the surface tension of liquids is often expressed in the equivalent units of dynes/cm. The total surface energy of a system is the product of the surface energy of the material and the total area. Therefore, a high total surface energy exists if a material is finely divided (powder or **colloid**) to provide a large surface area, especially if the material has a high surface energy per unit area (eg, metals or ionic crystals).

Sintering

The firing of porcelain is a **sintering** process used for forming denture teeth and porcelain-fused-to-metal crowns. *Sintering* is a densification process in which finely divided particles are heated in contact. The driving force for this method is the reduction of total surface area and, thus, total surface energy.

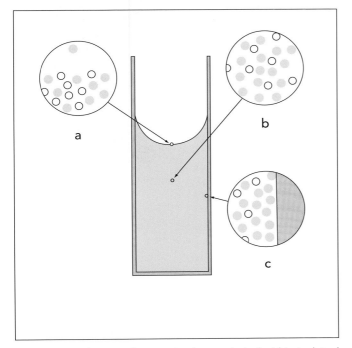

Fig 5-1 Distribution of vacancies (*open circles*) within isolated capillary liquid. More vacancies are present at (a) the surface as compared to (b) the bulk. Fewer vacancies are found at (c) the liquid-solid interface. (Modified with permission from O'Brien.[1])

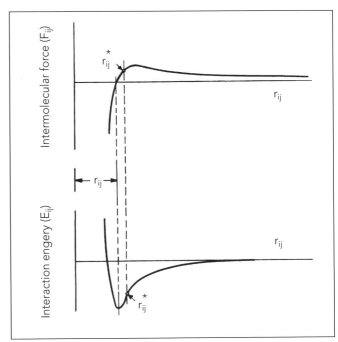

Fig 5-2 Relations between intermolecular forces, intermolecular energies, and distance as affected by distance (r_{ij}) between molecules. Departure from equilibrium distance r_{ij} causes repulsion or attraction. (Reprinted with permission from O'Brien.[1])

Table 5-1 Surface energies of various substances

SUBSTANCE	SURFACE ENERGY (ERG/CM²)	TEMPERATURE (°C)
Water	72	20
Benzene	29	20
Olive oil	36	20
Saliva	56	23
NaCl crystal	300	25
Dental porcelain	365	1,000
Copper, solid	1,430	1,080
Silver, solid	1,140	750

Table 5-2 Contact angles of liquids on solids

SOLID	LIQUID	CONTACT ANGLE (DEGREES)
Amalgam alloy	Water	80
Silicate cement	Water	10
Acrylic resin	Water	75
Teflon	Water	110
Ag₃Sn	Mercury	140
Gold alloys	Porcelain enamel	40–50
Nickel alloys	Porcelain enamel	80–100
Hydron	Water	0
Etched enamel	Pit and fissure sealants	0

▣ Wetting

The degree of spreading of a liquid drop on a solid surface is called **wetting**. The **contact angle** (θ), formed by the liquid surface and the interface separating the liquid and solid, is used as a measure of the degree of wetting (Fig 5-3). A 0-degree contact angle indicates complete wetting, and low values correspond to good wetting. Values above 90 degrees indicate poor wetting. Table 5-2 lists contact angles for several systems. Good wetting promotes **capillary penetration** and **adhesion**

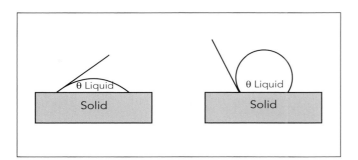

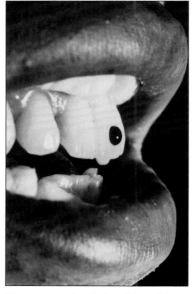

Fig 5-3 Wetting. Low contact angle indicates good wetting *(left)*; high contact angle indicates poor wetting *(right)*. (Reprinted with permission from O'Brien and Ryge.[2])

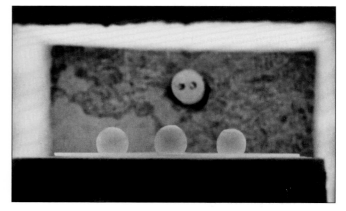

Fig 5-4 Hydrophobic film of fluorinated polymer on enamel giving high contact angle. (Reprinted with permission from O'Brien.[3])

Fig 5-5 Poor wetting shown by porcelain enamel drops on nongold alloy at 1,040°C. The furnace thermocouple is seen above the drops. (Reprinted with permission from O'Brien and Ryge.[4])

and indicates strong attraction between the liquid and solid surface molecules. Good wetting is important in soldering and is a factor in better denture retention. A more natural appearance is achieved if restorative materials are wetted by a thin film of saliva. **Hydrophobic** substances are those that exhibit high contact angles with water (eg, Teflon, silicone coatings) (Figs 5-4 and 5-5).

■ Adsorption

To reduce surface energy, atoms and molecules that are mobile will concentrate at high-energy surfaces. For ex-

ample, finely divided charcoal will adsorb quantities of several gases, and detergent (or soap) molecules will concentrate at the surface of water, leading to a large reduction in surface energy. Adsorption is strongest when there is large energy saving (high surface energy and large surface area) and slows down as the surface is covered.

Adsorption occurs only at the surface, whereas *absorption* involves penetration and uptake by the interior of the material (as in swelling of hydrocolloid impression materials in water). Gold foil adsorbs gases readily and must be degassed before use.

Colloids

Colloids contain material that is present in particles larger than ordinary atoms or molecules but still invisible to the unaided eye (ie, 10 to 10,000 Å). There are three types of colloidal systems.

Insoluble dispersed particles

Lyophobic is the term used to describe materials that are insoluble in a liquid medium (eg, sulfur in water) (Table 5-3). These fine particles acquire electric charges that keep them in suspension. Colloidal gold, for example, is used to form a gold coating on alloys to be bonded to porcelain. Although lyophobic systems may last for many years, they are unstable and can be precipitated by electric methods (smokes) or gravity (emulsions).

Large molecules

These systems are solutions in which the dispersed molecules are of colloidal dimension. They are stable but the large size of the macromolecules gives the solutions properties similar to those of lyophobic systems.

Dental materials consisting of such solutions include agar and alginate hydrocolloid impression materials. These materials aggregate to form gels through van der Waals bonding between the long chain molecules, and the gels undergo imbibition and syneresis (absorption and exudation of solvent) with resulting swelling and shrinkage, respectively. This behavior is responsible for the dimensional instability of these impression materials. As with other colloidal systems, the liquid state is called the *sol state*.

Association colloids

Surface active agents, such as soaps and detergents, are examples of association colloids, which are aggregates of smaller molecules that achieve colloidal size. Each molecule consists of a long-chain hydrocarbon with a small charged polar group at one end (eg, sodium palmitate). The aggregates formed by these molecules, called **micelles**, often are spheric; in aqueous systems, the hydrocarbon ends gather in the center of the micelle, and the polar groups are exposed on the outside. This system is useful in cleaning because grease and other organic films are dissolved in the interior of the micelles and held in suspension.

Table 5-3 Classification of lyophobic colloids

DISPERSED PHASE	CONTINUOUS PHASE	TYPE
Solid	Liquid	Sol
Solid	Gas	Aerosol (smoke)
Liquid	Liquid	Emulsion
Liquid	Gas	Aerosol (fog)
Gas	Liquid	Foam
Gas	Solid	Foam

Capillary Penetration

The surface energy of a liquid creates pressure that drives the liquid into crevices, narrow spaces, and thin tubes. Saliva penetration around restorations (leakage) and around teeth are important examples. Capillary penetration of saliva is also partially responsible for denture retention.

Capillary rise

If a glass tube is immersed in a liquid (Fig 5-6a), the capillary rise, h, is given by the formula:

$$h = 2\gamma \cos \theta / rdg$$

where γ is the surface tension, θ is the contact angle, r is the tube radius, d is the liquid's density, and g is the gravitational constant of 980 dynes/g. If the contact angle is less than 90 degrees, as in water-glass and saliva-enamel systems, elevation of the liquid occurs. However, if the contact angle exceeds 90 degrees (eg, mercury on glass or water on Teflon), depression takes place and pressure must be applied to force the liquid into the space (Fig 5-6b). If the capillary liquid is not connected with a reservoir of liquid, isolated capillaries (**isocaps**) are formed (Fig 5-7). The liquids in isocaps exert adhesive force on the walls of the capillary, which can be strong for thin layers. This capillary adhesion is a factor in denture retention.

To increase the penetration of saliva around acrylic dentures, surface coatings of silica are applied to reduce the contact angle. The main factor here, however, is

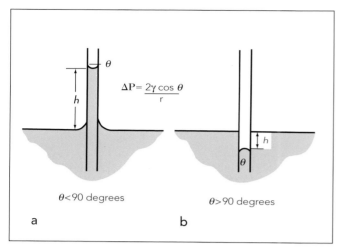

Fig 5-6 Effect of contact angle on capillary penetration. *(a)* Capillary elevation with concave meniscus (low contact angle). *(b)* Capillary depression with convex meniscus (high contact angle). ∆P is the capillary pressure. (Modified with permission from O'Brien et al.[5])

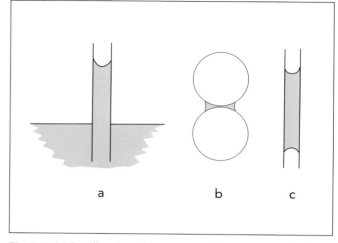

Fig 5-7 *(a)* Capillary liquid in contact with a reservoir. *(b, c)* Isolated capillaries. (Modified with permission from O'Brien and Fan.[6])

Fig 5-8 Capillary space between denture and mucosa.

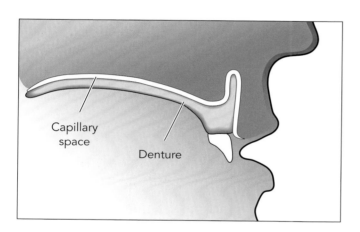

maintenance of a small gap distance (ie, close adaptation between denture and mucosa), as shown in Fig 5-8.

Penetration coefficient

The rate of movement of a liquid into a capillary space is related to the surface tension (γ), contact angle (θ), and viscosity (η), as given by the **penetration coefficient** (PC):

$$PC = \gamma \cos \theta / 2\eta$$

Therefore, a liquid with low viscosity, high surface tension, and low contact angle (ie, good wetting) will penetrate faster than one with the opposite combination of properties. These properties are important in adhesives such as pit and fissure sealants, which must penetrate

into surface roughness and crevices quickly for good bonding.

■ Adhesion

Adhesion is the attachment of materials in contact that resists the forces of separation. It is critical when using different types of dental restorative materials to understand the properties of adhesion, such as when bonding porcelains to metals and the adhesion of resins to tooth structure. Several types of adhesive bonds may be identified according to the classification (Fig 5-9). *Mechanical adhesion* depends on mechanical interlocking of the two phases and may include microscopic attachments, as in the case of resin bonding to etched enamel or

Fig 5-9 Classification of bonding mechanisms.

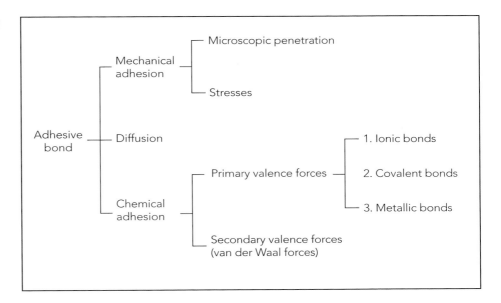

hoop stresses of a porcelain around a metal core. *Chemical adhesion* relies on chemical bonding between two phases. *Diffusion bonding* results when one phase penetrates by diffusion into the surface of a second phase and forms a hybrid layer, which is a composite of the two materials.

Several factors affect the strength of an adhesive bond:

1. *Cleanliness.* The surfaces to be attached should be free of debris and contamination.
2. *Penetration of surface.* Liquid adhesives (eg, sealants and bonding agents) must penetrate into crevices created by acid etching of enamel and dentin.
3. *Chemical reactions.* The formation of strong chemical bonds across an interface will increase the number of attachment sites. This is believed to occur between porcelain enamels and the oxides of tin, indium, and iron formed on the surfaces of alloys containing high proportions of precious metals. On the other hand, a weak compound may be formed by a chemical reaction, resulting in a weak boundary layer (eg, certain oxides) rather than attachment sites.
4. *Shrinkage of adhesive.* When liquid adhesives solidify by processes such as solvent evaporation and polymerization, shrinkage results. The adhesive may then pull away from the substrate, or stresses may be created that weaken the bond. Shrinkage is toward the center of the adhesive mass (Fig 5-10). However, shrinkage in light-cured systems occurs toward the light source.

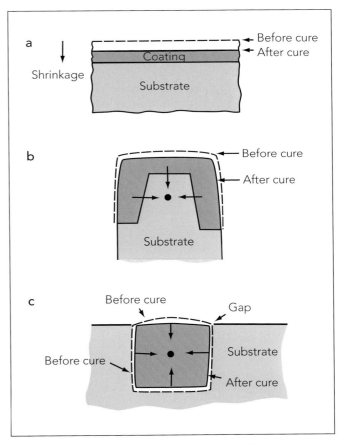

Fig 5-10 Shrinkage of adhesive (*grey*) toward center of mass during curing: (*a*) film, (*b*) crowns, (*c*) filling. (Modified from Lee.[7])

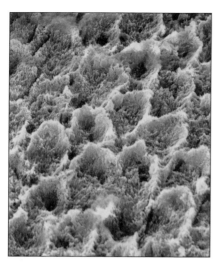

Fig 5-11 Microstructure of enamel etched with phosphoric acid (original magnification ×4,100).

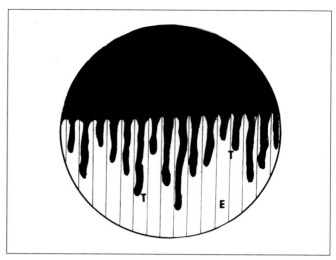

Fig 5-12 Attachment sites of polymer tags (T) in etched enamel (E).

5. *Thermal stresses.* If the adhesive and substrate have different thermal expansion coefficients, changes in temperature will produce stresses in the bond. For example, porcelain enamels are bonded to alloys at high temperatures and then cooled to room temperature. Close matching of the thermal expansion coefficients of porcelain enamel and alloy is required to minimize stresses.

6. *Corrosive environment.* The presence of water or corrosive liquid or vapor will often lead to deterioration of an adhesive bond. For example, acrylic resins will initially adhere to clean unetched tooth enamel, but the bond deteriorates when immersed in water.

Adhesion to enamel

Enamel is highly mineralized tissue composed of hydroxyapatite (about 95%), water (about 4%), and collagen (about 1%). Treatment with 35% to 50% phosphoric acid results in selective demineralization of exposed enamel rod ends, leaving a surface with increased area and high energy (Fig 5-11). High surface energy permits efficient wetting by the hydrophobic resin, which penetrates to form tags (Fig 5-12) and provides bond strength through mechanical interlocking. Contamination of the dry, etched surface by saliva or water, or incomplete removal of the etching agent or dissolved minerals, adversely affects the long-term stability of the bond. The **acid-etch technique** produces shear bond strengths during laboratory testing of 20 to 22 MPa, on

average above those produced at the composite-enamel interface by shrinkage due to polymerization (~18 MPa).

Acid etching of enamel is a widely accepted clinical procedure and has increased the life of resin composite restorations by decreasing the possibility of marginal staining, secondary caries, and postoperative sensitivity due to sealing of the enamel margins. The acid-etch technique allows the use of a more conservative cavity preparation and, to a certain extent, restores fracture resistance to the bonded structure.

Adhesion to dentin

Human dentin is composed of hydroxyapatite (45%), water (25%), and organic matrix (30%). Bonding to dentin is routinely achieved by etching and the diffusion of hydrophilic primers, followed by application of bonding resins. Composite restorative materials are then bonded to the resin layer; the resin-dentin interface has laboratory bond strengths of 22 to 35 MPa.

The stages of conditioning and resin impregnation are illustrated in Fig 5-13. In the first stage, the conditioning dissolves the smear layer of debris on the dentinal surface and in tubules, partially decalcifies the dentin to an optimum depth of around 5 μm, and opens dentinal tubules. In the second stage, hydrophilic primer coupling agents such as 2-hydroxyethyl methacrylate (2-HEMA), 4-methacryloxyethyl trimellitate anhydride (4-META), and glutaraldehyde are applied, penetrating

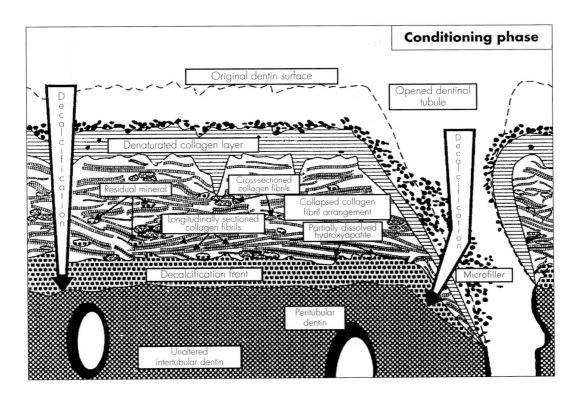

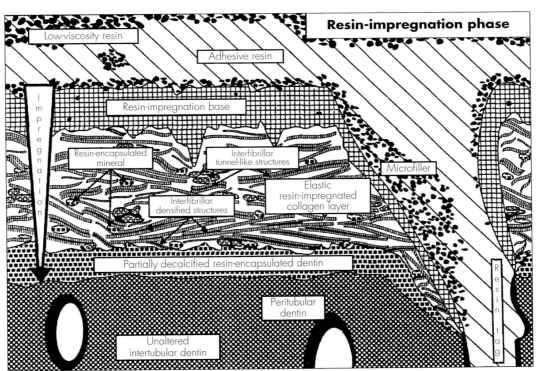

Fig 5-13 Schematic of the resin-dentin interdiffusion zone at *(top)* the conditioning phase and *(bottom)* the resin-impregnation phase. (Reprinted with permission from Van Meerbeek.[8])

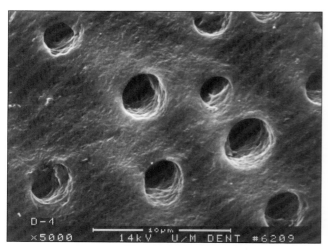

Fig 5-14 Dentin after deep etching with 20% phosphoric acid for 2 minutes (original magnification ×5,000).

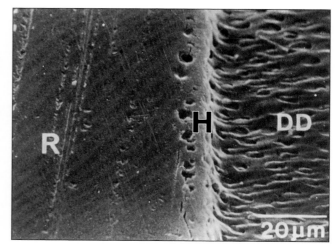

Fig 5-15 Cross-section of resin-etched bovine dentin interface showing resin (R), the hybrid zone (H), and demineralized dentin (DD). (Reprinted with permission from Wang and Nakabayashi.[9])

Fig 5-16 Scanning electron micrograph of a fractured resin-dentin interface showing resin tags plucked from tubules. DD = demineralized dentin. (Reprinted with permission from Wang and Nakabayashi.[9])

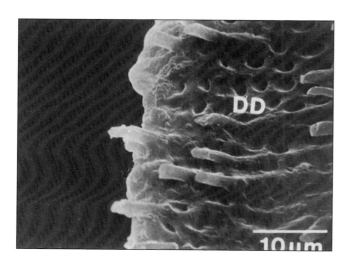

into both the tubules and the decalcified intertubular dentin. The primer stabilizes collagen and facilitates the penetration of the bonding resins, which are bisphenol A glycidyl methacrylate (bis-GMA) or urethane dimethacrylate (UDMA) monomers.

There are two main types of conditioner components in current use. The strong acids (eg, phosphoric and citric acids) nonselectively attack the dentin and the smear layer and expose the tubules (Fig 5-14). Other acids (eg, 10% maleic acid) are used to dissolve both inorganic and organic tissues, but they are less aggressive. The weak acids (eg, polyacrylic acid) are used to dissolve only the smear layer without demineralizing dentin.

The layer of resin penetration is known as the **hybrid zone** and may extend from 1 to 5 μm deep (Fig 5-15).

A layer of decalcified dentin below the hybrid zone will weaken the bond unless the depth of etching is limited, etching times are decreased, or less concentrated acids are used. Excessive drying of the dentin layer before primer application will lead to collapse of the surface collagen layer and reduce primer diffusion. Lateral penetration of resin into peritubular dentin may also occur if the resin has first penetrated the tubules. Figure 5-16 shows a scanning electron micrograph of a fractured hybrid layer with tags that have been plucked from the tubules during bond testing. Resin tags in tubules are not strongly anchored due to polymerization shrinkage and dentinal fluid.

Bond-strength values of materials to enamel and dentin are given in Table 5-4. The laboratory bond-strength values to dentin vary significantly more than

Table 5-4 Tensile bond strengths obtained between various restorative materials and tooth substance[10]

BONDING COUPLE	BOND STRENGTH (MPa)
Acid-etched enamel + resin (eg, bis-GMA)	16–20
Enamel + glass ionomer	5
Dentin + glass ionomer	1–3
Dentin + glass ionomer (light cured)	3–11
Enamel + NPG-GMA	2–5
Dentin + 4-META	2
Dentin + mordant ion + 4-META	18
Dentin + phosphate esters of bis-GMA	3–5
Acid-etched enamel + phosphate esters of bis-GMA	20
Dentin + maleic acid/HEMA + HEMA/bis-GMA	18
Acid-etched enamel + HEMA/bis-GMA	23
Dentin + isocyanate	4
Dentin + glutaraldehyde/HEMA	18

NPG-GMA = N-phenylglycine and glycidyl methacrylate.

those reported for enamel. Therefore, bonding to dentin is less reliable.

A major difference among commercial products is the number of components that need to be applied in sequence. Several multicomponent products contain an etchant (conditioning agent), a primer, and a bonding resin. Currently available materials may be divided into two general types, etch-and-rinse and self-etch, with four subtypes as shown in Fig 5-17. They may also be classified in terms of generations of products. A short description of these products and examples follow:

Etch and rinse

The three-step fourth-generation method is still widely used and involves etching, rinsing, and separately applying the primer and adhesive, such as Scotchbond Multipurpose (3M ESPE). A fifth-generation etch-and-rinse method involves two steps: etching and rinsing to remove the smear layer, followed by application of both primer and adhesive in a single solution (eg, Optibond Solo Plus, Kerr Dental; and Prime & Bond NT, Dentsply International). The main advantages of the three-step etch-and-rinse adhesives are consistent results supported by laboratory and clinical studies, and lower technique sensitivity. However, the procedures are time consuming, and there is a higher risk of overetching from the concentrated acid, which may lead to more postoperative sensitivity. The two-step systems are simpler to use, with fewer bottles and less complicated procedures. However, the time savings is minimal because of the need for multiple-layer applications, and there is a risk of overetching with these systems as well.

Self-etch systems

These products do not need a separate etch-and-rinse step; thus, there are fewer bottles and steps. Two- and one-step types are available. The two-step products use two bottles, one containing a self-etching primer with acidic monomers having carboxylic or phosphate groups that reduce the pH to between 1.0 and 4.7, and the second containing the resin adhesive. The one-step self-etching products have one bottle, which contains the etchant, primer, and adhesive resin together (eg, Adper Prompt L-Pop, 3M ESPE; Optibond, Kerr; and i-Bond, Heraeus Kulzer) (Figs 5-18 and 5-19). Both types of self-etch adhesive systems have the advantages of being simpler and time efficient compared with the etch-and-rinse systems. Also, both self-etching types appear to

71

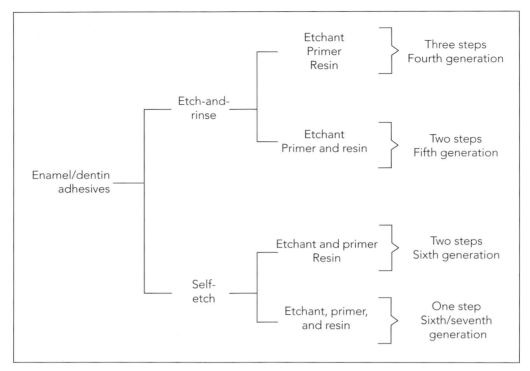

Fig 5-17 Classification of dental bonding agents.

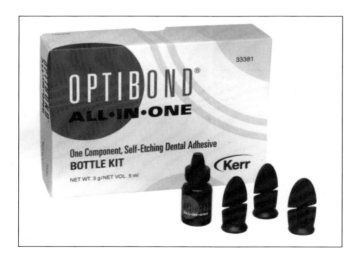

Fig 5-18 Optibond one component, self-etching dental adhesive. (Courtesy of Kerr.)

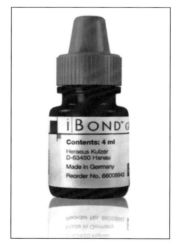

Fig 5-19 i-Bond one-step dental adhesive. (Courtesy of Heraeus Kulzer.)

be less sensitive to variations in dentin wetness. On the negative side, many self-etch products contain water, which can interfere with polymerization of the resin. Also, there are many conflicting data on bond strength values with self-etch systems, especially for mild-etch adhesives on enamel. Generally, strongly acidic products (pH between 0.4 and 1.0) yield stronger bonds with enamel but lower dentin bond strengths. The milder acidic products (pH 2 to 2.2) yield the opposite results, with poorer enamel bonding and stronger dentin bonding. Clearly, the self-etch products are still in a state of development, with less laboratory and clinical data available compared with the etch-and-rinse products.

Glossary

acid-etch technique The method of etching enamel with an acid to produce a roughened surface for resin bonding.

adhesion Surface attachment of two materials (as opposed to cohesion, which is the bonding within a single material).

capillary penetration Movement of a liquid into a crevice or tube because of capillary pressure.

colloid Material in which a constituent in a finely divided state that is invisible to the eye but capable of scattering light is suspended. Although colloids are not true solutions, many have long-term stability.

contact angle Angle formed between the surface of a liquid drop and the solid surface on which it rests. Usually designated by the Greek letter θ and used as a measure of wetting.

hybrid zone A layer of dentin that contains resin. Produced by etching and resin diffusion.

hydrophobic Water-repellent; showing a high contact angle.

isocaps Isolated capillary bridges formed between solid surfaces.

lyophobic colloid An unstable colloid made from insoluble dispersed material in fine suspension.

micelles Aggregated molecules formed in association colloids.

penetration coefficient Combination of the properties of viscosity, surface tension, and contact angle that promotes rapid capillary penetration.

sintering Densification process in which solid particles are fused together, usually at high temperatures.

surface energy Extra energy that atoms or molecules on the surface of a substance have over those in the interior. The units are erg/cm^2.

surface tension The surface energy of a liquid.

wetting The spreading of a liquid drop on the surface of a solid.

Discussion Questions

1. Why is wetting by an adhesive so important for bonding to tooth structure or any other material?

2. Why is the strength of enamel and dentin a limiting factor in the adhesive bond strength?

3. What is the essential role that hydrophilic primer coupling agents play in the formation of the hybrid layer?

4. How could the geometry of a restoration affect the final bond strength to tooth structure?

Study Questions

(See appendix E for answers.)

1. Why does surface tension exist in liquids?

2. How does wetting affect capillary penetration of a liquid?

3. How do *absorption* and *adsorption* differ?

4. Name three colloidal systems of importance to dental materials.

5. Which properties affect the penetration rate of liquids into capillaries?

6. In terms of innovation, would the bonding of restorative materials to dentin by etching and forming a hybrid layer be classified as a major, medium, or minor product improvement?

References

1. O'Brien WJ. Surface energy of liquid isolated in narrow capillaries. Surface Sci 1970;19:387.
2. O'Brien WJ, Ryge G. Wettability of poly(methyl methacrylate) treated with silicone tetrachloride. J Prosthet Dent 1965;15:304–308.
3. O'Brien WJ. Capillary effects on adhesion. In: Moskowitz H (ed). Symposium Proceedings on Adhesive Dental Materials. New York: New York Univ, 1973.
4. O'Brien WJ, Ryge G. Contact angles of drops of enamel on metals. J Prosthet Dent 1965;15:1094–1100.
5. O'Brien WJ, Craig RG, Peyton FA. Capillary penetration around a hydrophobic filling material. J Prosthet Dent 1968;19:399–405.
6. O'Brien WJ, Fan PL. Capillary adhesion. In: Lee LH (ed). Adhesion Science and Technology. Part B. New York: Plenum Press, 1975: 621–633.
7. Lee H. Adhesion of polymeric materials to tooth structure. In: Moskowitz H (ed). Symposium Proceedings on Adhesive Dental Materials. New York: New York Univ, 1973.
8. Van Meerbeek B, Dhem A, Goret-Nicaise M, Braem M, Lambrechts P, VanHerle G. Comparative SEM and TEM examination of the ultrastructure of the resin-dentin interdiffusion zone. J Dent Res 1993;72:495.
9. Wang T, Nakabayashi N. Effect of 2-(Methacryloxy) ethyl phenyl hydrogen phosphate on adhesion to dentin. J Dent Res 1991; 70(1):59–66.
10. McCabe JF. Applied Dental Materials. London: Blackwell, 1990.

◼ Recommended Reading

Adamson AW. Physical Chemistry of Surfaces. New York: Interscience Publishers, 1960.

Asmussen E. Clinical relevance of physical, chemical and bonding properties of composite resins. Oper Dent 1985;10:61–73.

Asmussen E, Antonucci JM, Bowen RL. Adhesion to dentin by means of Gluma resin. Scand J Dent Res 1988;96:584–589.

Asmussen E, Munksgaard EC. Bonding of restorative resins to dentine: Status of dentine adhesives and impact on cavity design and filling techniques. Int Dent J 1988;38:97–104.

Baran G, O'Brien WJ. The wetting of silver-tin phases by mercury in air. J Am Dent Assoc 1977;94:898–900.

Bayne SC, Heymann HO, Sturdevant JR, Wilder AD, Sluder TB. Contributing co-variables in clinical trials. Am J Dent 1991;4:247–250.

Berry EA III, von der Lehr WN, Herring HK. Dentin surface treatments for the removal of the smear layer: An SEM study. J Am Dent Assoc 1987;115:65–67.

Bowen RL. Bonding agents and adhesives: Reactor response. Adv Dent Res 1988;2:155–157.

Bowen RL, Cobb EN, Rapson JE. Adhesive bonding of various materials to hard tooth tissues: Improvement in bond strength to dentin. J Dent Res 1982;61:1070–1076.

Bowen RL, Eichmiller FC, Marjenhof WA. Glass-ceramic inserts anticipated for megafilled composite restorations. J Am Dent Assoc 1991;122:71–75.

Brannstrom M. Smear layer: Pathological and treatment considerations. Oper Dent Suppl 1984;3:35–42.

Bryant RW, Mahler DB. Modulus of elasticity in bonding of composite and amalgams. J Prosthet Dent 1986;56:243–248.

Clinical Research Associates. CRA Newsletter. November 2000.

Douglas WH. Clinical status of dentine bonding agents. J Dent 1989;17:209–215.

Duke ES, Lindemuth J. Polymeric adhesion to dentin: Contrasting substrates. Am J Dent 1990;3:264–270.

Duke ES, Lindemuth J. Variability of clinical dentin substrates. Am J Dent 1991;4:241–246.

Duncanson MG Jr, Miranda FJ, Probst RT. Resin dentin bonding agents—Rationale and results. Quintessence Int 1986;17:625–629.

el-Kalla IH, Garcia-Godoy F. Saliva contamination and bond strength of single-bottle adhesives to enamel and dentin. Am J Dent 1997;10:83–87.

Fan PI. Dentin bonding systems: An update. J Am Dent Assoc 1987;114:91–95.

Fan PI, O'Brien WJ. Penetrativity of sealants. J Dent Res 1974;54:262–264.

Fan PI, O'Brien WJ. Strain resulting from adhesive action of water in capillary bridges. Nature 1975;256:717–718.

Gaberolglio R, Brannstrom M. Scanning electron microscopic investigation of human dentinal tubules. Arch Oral Biol 1976;21:355–362.

Glantz PO. On wettability and adhesiveness. Odontol Revy 1969;20(suppl 17):1–132.

Heymann HO, Sturdevant JR, Bayne S, Wilder AD, Sluder TB, Brunson WD. Examining tooth flexure effects of dentinal adhesives in class V cervical lesions. J Am Dent Assoc 1991;122:179–183.

Jörgensen KD, Asmussen E, Shimokobe H. Enamel damage caused by contracting restorative resins. Scand J Dent Res 1975;83:120–122.

Jörgensen KD, Matono R, Shimokobe H. Deformation of cavities and resin fillings in loaded teeth. J Dent Res 1976;84:46–50.

Lambrechts P, Braem M, Vanherle G. Buonocore memorial lecture. Evaluation of clinical performance for posterior composite resins and dentine adhesives. Oper Dent 1987;12:53–78.

Lewis AF, Natarajan RT. The attachment site theory of adhesive joint strength. In: Lee LH (ed). Adhesion Science and Technology. Part B. New York: Plenum Press, 1975:563–575.

McGuckin RS, Tao L, Thompson WO, Pashley DH. Shear bond strength of Scotchbond in vivo. Dent Mater 1991;7(1):50–53.

Morin DL, DeLong R, Douglas WH. Cusp reinforcement by the acid-etch technique. J Dent Res 1984;63:1075–1078.

Morin DL, Douglas WH, Cross M, DeLong R. Biophysical stress analysis of restored teeth: Experimental strain measurement. Dent Mater 1988;4:41–48.

Nakabayashi N, Pashley DH. Hybridization of Dental Hard Tissue. Chicago: Quintessence, 1998.

O'Brien WJ. Capillary Penetration of Liquids Between Solids [dissertation]. Ann Arbor: Univ of Michigan, 1967.

O'Brien WJ. Capillary action around dental structures. J Dent Res 1973;52:533–549.

O'Brien WJ. Effects of capillary penetration and negative pressure at sites of caries susceptibility. In: Stiles HM, Loesche WJ, O'Brien TC (eds). Microbial Aspects of Dental Caries. Washington, DC: Information Retrieval, 1976.

Pashley DH. Smear layer: Physiological consideration. Oper Dent Suppl 1984;3:13–29.

Pashley DH. Dentin bonding: Overview of the substrate with respect to the adhesive material. J Esthet Dent 1991;3(2):46–50.

Pashley DH. In vitro simulations of in vivo bonding conditions. Am J Dent 1991;4:237–240.

Pashley DH, Livingston MJ, Greenhill JD. Regional resistances to fluid flow in human dentine in vitro. Arch Oral Biol 1978;23:807–810.

Pashley DH, Carvalho RM, Sano H, et al. The microtensile bond test: A review. J Adhes Dent 1999;1:299–309.

Perdigão J. An Ultra-Morphological Study of Human Dentin Exposed to Adhesive Systems [thesis]. Leuven, Belgium: Univ of Leuven, 1995.

Selna LG, Shillingburg HT Jr, Kerr PA. Finite element analysis of dental structures: Axisymmetric and plane stress idealizations. J Biomed Mater Res 1975;9:237–244.

Shahverdi S, Canay S, Sahin E, Bilge A. Effects of different surface treatment methods on the bond strength of composite resin to porcelain. J Oral Rehabil 1998;25:699–705.

Tao L, Pashely DH, Boyd L. Effect of different types of smear layers on dentin and enamel shear bond strengths. Dent Mater 1988;4:208–216.

Tate WH, You C, Powers JM. Bond strengths of compomers to dentin using acidic primers. Am J Dent 1999;12:235–242.

Thresher RW, Saito GE. The stress analysis of human teeth. J Biomech 1973;6:443–449.

Van Meerbeek B, Lambrechts P, Inokoshi S, Braem M, Vanherle G. Factors affecting adhesion to mineralized tissues. Oper Dent Suppl 1992;5:111–124.

Yettram AL, Wright KW, Pickard HM. Finite element stress analysis of the crowns of normal and restored teeth. J Dent Res 1976;55:1004–1011.

Yoshii E. Cytotoxic effects of acrylates and methacrylates: Relationships of monomer structures and cytotoxicity. J Biomed Mater Res 1997;37:517–524.

Ziemiecki TL, Dennison JB, Charbeneau GT. Clinical evaluation of cervical composite resin restorations placed without retention. Oper Dent 1987;12:27–33.

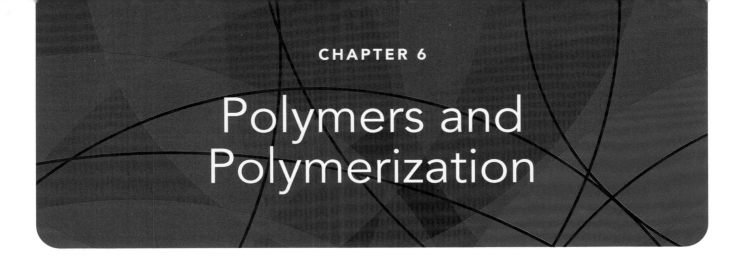

CHAPTER 6

Polymers and Polymerization

The distinctive properties of polymers allow a range of clinical applications not possible with other types of materials. The most widely used impression materials (alginates, polyethers, polysulfides, and silicones) are either synthetic or natural polymers. A polymeric matrix with a particulate ceramic filler is the most common material used in anterior esthetic restorations. Additional applications include denture teeth, cements, dies, provisional crowns, endodontic fillings, tissue conditioners, and pit and fissure sealants. However, the primary use of polymers in terms of quantity is in the construction of complete dentures and the tissue-bearing portions of partial dentures. This chapter introduces concepts related to polymer composition and properties and concludes with a discussion of those polymers currently used in the construction of complete and partial dentures, liners, and tissue conditioners.

◼ Polymers

Composition

A **polymer** is a molecule made up of many units (poly = many; mer = unit). An **oligomer** is a short polymer composed of two, three, four, or more but usually fewer than 10 mer units. A *mer* is the simplest repeating chemical unit of a polymer, and is often the basis for naming the material. Thus, *polystyrene* is a polymer composed of styrene units.

Monomers (mono = single) are the molecules that unite to form a polymer, and the process by which this occurs is termed **polymerization**. If monomers of two

or more different types are joined, **copolymers** are formed. Copolymers may be either *random* (mers do not appear in specific order) or *block* (large numbers of one type of mer appear arranged in sequence). Atoms along the length of any polymer are joined through strong, primary covalent bonds.

Molecular weight

The **degree of polymerization** is defined as the total number of mers in a polymer molecule. The **molecular weight** (molar mass) of a polymer molecule is the mass of one polymer molecule and is often calculated approximately from the sum of the molecular weights of the mers of which it is made. Typical polymer molecules may be composed of thousands to millions of mers. Often, a distribution of molecular sizes is present in a material, and the reported molecular weight is the average molecular weight. The particular distribution is the result of conditions present during polymerization. Variations in conditions have a pronounced effect on the properties of the final material.

Spatial structure

There are three basic spatial structures of polymers: linear, branched, and cross-linked (Fig 6-1). Linear and branched molecules are discrete but are bonded to one another through weak physical bonds. On heating, the mobility of the chains increases and the weak bonds break. The ability of the chains to then slide past one another results in a softened material. On cooling, the chain mobility decreases, the physical bonds reform, and hardening occurs. Materials that are able to undergo this process are termed **thermoplastic**, and ex-

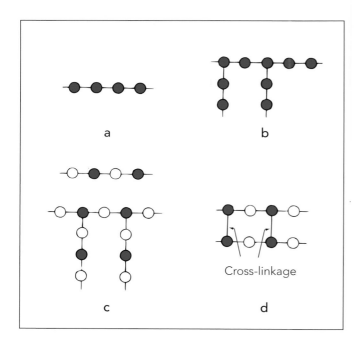

Fig 6-1 Polymer chains. *(a)* Linear chain; *(b)* branched chain; *(c)* copolymer chains, linear *(upper)* and branched *(lower)*; *(d)* cross-linking chains.

amples include polystyrene, polyvinyl acrylics, and poly(methyl methacrylate) (PMMA).

Cross-linking results in the formation of a network structure of covalently bonded atoms; primary linkages occur between chains, and the polymer actually becomes a single giant macromolecule. The spatial structure that allows chain sliding on heating is not present in cross-linked materials; therefore, cross-linked polymers do not undergo softening on heating and are termed **thermosets**. These crosslinked polymers may swell but do not dissolve in solvents. Typical examples are cross-linked PMMA, cis-polyisoprene, bisphenol A-diacrylate, and silicones.

Properties

Many factors affect the properties of polymers, including the chemical composition of the chain, its degree of polymerization, and the number of branches and/or cross-links between polymer chains. In general, longer chains and a higher molecular weight result in the polymer's increased strength, hardness, stiffness, and resistance to creep along with increased brittleness (Fig 6-2). Resin composites, for example, have a highly cross-linked matrix, in which a large number of strong covalent linkages between chains transforms the molecules into a rigid, very-high-molecular-weight material. The resulting increased strength and stiffness contribute to

the ability of this material to withstand occlusal stresses during function.

In contrast, elastomeric impression materials are composed primarily of individual coiled chains with just a few cross-links. This type of molecular structure permits the large-scale uncoiling and recoiling of chains that give these materials high flexibility.

The amount of crystallinity present in a polymer affects its properties. Materials that are highly crystalline have atoms with a very regular arrangement in space and are stronger, stiffer, and absorb less water than do noncrystalline materials. Few dental polymers are crystalline. Most are *amorphous*, meaning that the atoms of which they are composed have irregular arrangements in space. Amorphous polymers are often called **glassy polymers**.

Small **plasticizer** molecules, when added to a stiff un–cross-linked polymer, reduce its rigidity. When small molecules surround large ones, the large molecules are able to move more easily. A plasticizer therefore lowers the **glass-transition temperature** (T_g) of the polymer, so a material that is normally rigid at a particular temperature may become more flexible. The *glass-transition temperature* is the temperature at which a polymer ceases to be glassy and brittle and becomes rubberlike. The temperature of a polymer, as shown in Fig 6-3, has a strong effect on its strength properties.

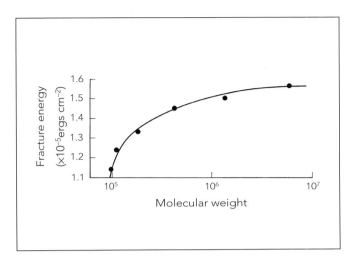

Fig 6-2 Relationship between strength and polymer molecular weight. (Reprinted with permission from Mark.[1])

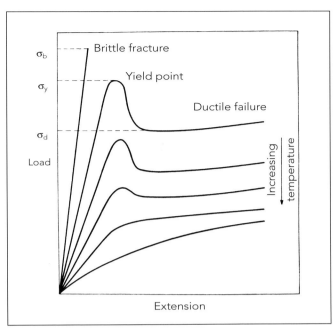

Fig 6-3 Effect of temperature on the tensile properties of a polymer. The temperature below which brittle failure occurs is called the *glass-transition temperature*. (Reprinted with permission from Berry and Bueche.[2])

Finally, during polymerization a volumetric decrease occurs, resulting in shrinkage (up to 21% for unfilled acrylic resins, 6% for denture resins, and 1% to 3% for resin composites) and the production of internal stresses. A change in shape, often called *warpage*, may occur when the polymer is reheated. Additionally, polymers have varying abilities to absorb water. A small amount of expansion may occur during this process.

Polymerization

Most polymerization reactions are of two types: **addition polymerization**, in which no by-product is formed, and **condensation polymerization**, in which a low-molecular-weight by-product such as water or alcohol is formed. Materials that set by addition polymerization include PMMA, used in the construction of dentures, and bisphenol A glycidyl methacrylate (bis-GMA), a common component of the matrix of resin composites. Materials that set by the condensation mechanism include polysulfide rubber and some silicone rubber impression materials.

The three stages in the free-radical addition polymerization reaction are described in the following subsections. They may be accelerated by heat, light, or small amounts of peroxides.

Initiation

The initiation step involves the production of free radicals, which initiate the growth of polymer chains (Fig 6-4). Free-radical molecules have chemical groups with unshared electrons and are usually formed by thermal decomposition of molecules, photodissociation of molecules, or redox reactions. The most common initiators are thermal initiators, which have one weak bond that breaks at a significant rate at a moderate temperature to yield free radicals. This weak bond is usually peroxide (-O-O-) or azo (-N=N-). Various initiators are used at different temperatures depending on their rates of decomposition. The differences in the decomposition rates of initiators are conveniently expressed in terms of the initiator half-life, $t\frac{1}{2}$, which is defined as the time for the concentration of initiator to decrease its original value by one half. Table 6-1 lists the initiator half-lives for several common initiators at different temperatures.

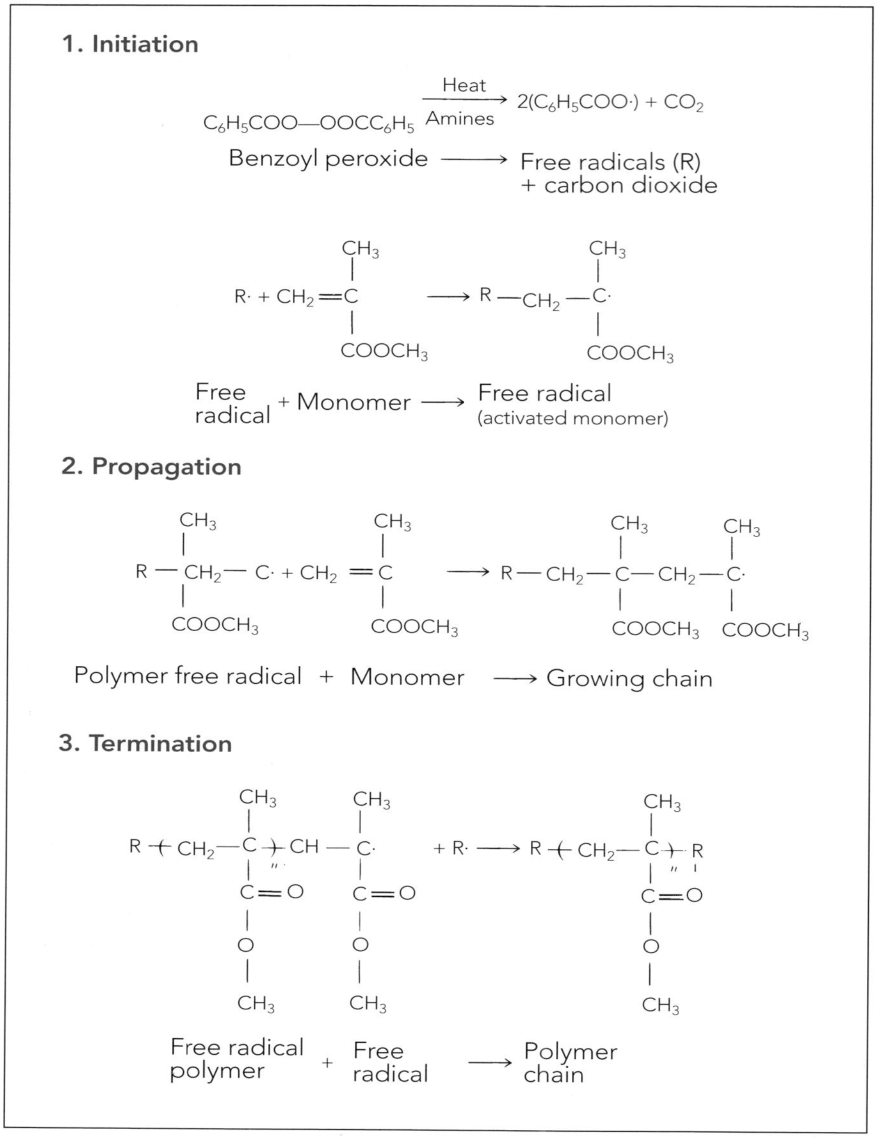

1. Initiation

$$C_6H_5COO{-}OOCC_6H_5 \xrightarrow[\text{Amines}]{\text{Heat}} 2(C_6H_5COO\cdot) + CO_2$$

Benzoyl peroxide $\longrightarrow$ Free radicals (R)
+ carbon dioxide

$$R\cdot + CH_2{=}\underset{\underset{COOCH_3}{|}}{\overset{\overset{CH_3}{|}}{C}} \longrightarrow R{-}CH_2{-}\underset{\underset{COOCH_3}{|}}{\overset{\overset{CH_3}{|}}{C}}\cdot$$

$$\underset{\text{radical}}{\text{Free}} + \text{Monomer} \longrightarrow \underset{\text{(activated monomer)}}{\text{Free radical}}$$

2. Propagation

$$R{-}CH_2{-}\underset{\underset{COOCH_3}{|}}{\overset{\overset{CH_3}{|}}{C}}\cdot + CH_2{=}\underset{\underset{COOCH_3}{|}}{\overset{\overset{CH_3}{|}}{C}} \longrightarrow R{-}CH_2{-}\underset{\underset{COOCH_3}{|}}{\overset{\overset{CH_3}{|}}{C}}{-}CH_2{-}\underset{\underset{COOCH_3}{|}}{\overset{\overset{CH_3}{|}}{C}}\cdot$$

Polymer free radical + Monomer $\longrightarrow$ Growing chain

3. Termination

$$R{-}(CH_2{-}\underset{\underset{\underset{\underset{CH_3}{|}}{O}}{\overset{C=O}{|}}}{\overset{\overset{CH_3}{|}}{C}}){-}CH{-}\underset{\underset{\underset{\underset{CH_3}{|}}{O}}{\overset{C=O}{|}}}{\overset{\overset{CH_3}{|}}{C}}\cdot + R\cdot \longrightarrow R{-}(CH_2{-}\underset{\underset{\underset{\underset{CH_3}{|}}{O}}{\overset{C=O}{|}}}{\overset{\overset{CH_3}{|}}{C}}){-}R$$

$$\underset{\text{polymer}}{\text{Free radical}} + \underset{\text{radical}}{\text{Free}} \longrightarrow \underset{\text{chain}}{\text{Polymer}}$$

Fig 6-4 Three stages of addition polymerization of methyl methacrylate.

Photodissociation occurs when light is absorbed by a molecule and causes one of its bonds to break to form free radicals. A *redox reaction* involves the transfer of one (or more) electron(s) from one species to another to generate free radicals. Whatever the means of production, the free radicals attack the double bonds of available monomer molecules, resulting in the shift of the unshared electron to the end of the monomer and the formation of activated monomer molecules.

Propagation

Activated monomers attack the double bonds of additional available monomers, resulting in the rapid addition of monomer molecules to the free radical. This second stage, *propagation*, continues as the chain grows in length.

Termination

Termination of the growing free radical may occur by several mechanisms and can result in the formation of branches and cross-links. Small amounts of inhibitors, such as hydroquinone, may be added to the monomer to increase storage life. Hydroquinones react with free radicals, thereby decreasing the rate of initiation.

Table 6-1 Half-lives of initiators

INITIATOR	HALF-LIFE*			
Azobisisobutyronitrile	74 h (50°C)	4.8 h (70°C)	7.2 min (100°C)	
Benzoyl peroxide	7.3 h (70°C)	1.4 h (85°C)	19.8 min (100°C)	
Acetyl peroxide	158 h (50°C)	8.1 h (70°C)	1.1 h (85°C)	
Lauryl peroxide	47.7 h (50°C)	12.8 h (60°C)	3.5 h (70°C)	31 min (85°C)
t-Butyl peracetate	88 h (85°C)	12.5 h (100°C)	1.9 h (115°C)	18 min (130°C)
Cumyl peroxide	13 h (115°C)	1.7 h (130°C)	16.8 min (145°C)	
t-Butyl peroxide	218 h (100°C)	34 h (115°C)	6.4 h (130°C)	1.38 h (145°C)
t-Butyl hydroperoxide	338 h (100°C)	44.9 h (155°C)	4.81 h (175°C)	

*The half-life values are for benzene or toluene solutions of the initiators.

▣ Denture Base Polymers

The polymeric **denture base** can consist of either a simple stiff base on which the teeth are arranged, or a sandwich of stiff base and a resilient liner to provide greater retention and comfort. When the tissue underlying a loose denture is traumatized due to the constant motion of the hard plastic over the mucosa, a viscoelastic gel known as a **tissue conditioner** can be molded onto the fitting surface of the denture in situ so the tissue can heal and an accurate impression of the untraumatized fitting surface can be taken before making a new, better-fitting denture. A classification is shown in Fig 6-5.

Advances in denture design have been mediated by the materials available at the time. In the 1800s, the art of hand carving ivory and wooden denture bases resulted in dentures retained by mechanical devices such as springs. Goodyear's invention of vulcanized rubber vulcanite in 1839 provided not only a thermoplastic material that could be molded accurately but also one that did not biodegrade and was strong enough to withstand masticatory forces for many years. Vulcanite's intrinsic dark color and opacity meant that the translucency and reflectivity of living mucosa was impossible to mimic.

With the commercial availability of man-made polymers in the early 1930s came an opportunity to apply some of the optically brilliant polymers to dentistry. It was the need for custom fit that delayed their use, however, since polymerization of the free monomer, with its inherent massive volume shrinkage, did not lend itself easily to the vulcanizing techniques used at the time. It was the adoption of the *dough technique*, first described in the mid-thirties, that made the use of acrylics in dentistry possible. In the dough technique, a liquid component (monomer) is mixed with a powder component (polymer) to achieve a dough-like consistency, which is packed into the mold before polymerization.

Adoption of the new denture bases was rapid in America. However, in Europe, rubber shortages during World War II forced the profession to use alternative materials. By the end of the war, the use of vulcanite for dentures had almost ceased. After the war, resins developed for aircraft production and the burgeoning plastics industry were offered for use as denture base materials, but the simplicity of the dough technique and the lifelike results have sustained acrylics as the market leader to the present day. Table 6-2 compares current denture base materials.

Composition and manufacture
Heat-cured acrylic
The bulk of denture base acrylic is supplied in the form of a free-running powder and a liquid. Originally, the powder was produced by grinding blocks of PMMA. However, it was soon found that smoother, more consistent doughs resulted from the use of a spheric bead polymer. By suspending a monomer liquid in water with the aid of either a surfactant or water-soluble polymer,

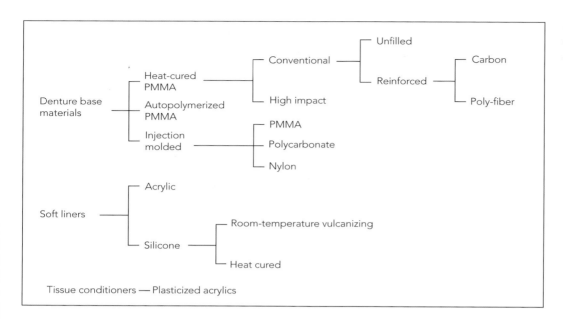

Fig 6-5 A classification of denture bases, liners, and tissue conditioners.

Table 6-2 A comparison of denture base materials

MATERIAL	ADVANTAGES	DISADVANTAGES	IDEAL PROPERTIES
Heat-cured	Good appearance High glass-transition temperature Ease of fabrication Low capital costs Good surface finish	Free-monomer content or formaldehyde can cause sensitization Low impact strength Flexural strength low enough to penalize poor denture design Fatigue life too short Radiolucency	Good appearance High flexural strength High impact resistance High stiffness Long fatigue life High craze resistance High creep resistance High radiopacity
Heat-cured, rubber-reinforced	Improved impact strength	Reduced stiffness	Low free-monomer content Good adhesion with teeth and liners

Heat-cured, fiber-reinforced	High stiffness
	Very high impact strength
	Good fatigue life
	Polypropylene fibers:
	  Good translucency
	  Good surface finish
		Carbon and Kevlar fibers:
		  Poor color
		  Poor surface
			Low solubility
			Low water uptake
			Dimensional stability
			Dimensional accuracy

Autocured	Easy to deflask Dimensional accuracy Capable of higher flexural strength than heat cured	No cheaper over long term Increased creep Increased free-monomer content Color instability Reduced stiffness Tooth adhesion failure	———
Injection-molded	Dimensional accuracy Low free-monomer content Polycarbonate and nylon Good impact strength	High capital costs Difficult mold design problems Less craze resistance Less creep resistance	———
Light-activated	No methacrylate monomer Decreased polymerization shrinkage Possible improved fit compared to conventional material Requires little equipment Time-saving	Decreased elastic modulus	———

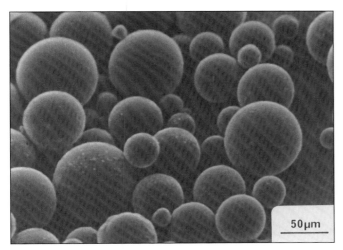

Fig 6-6 Scanning electron micrograph of PMMA beads.

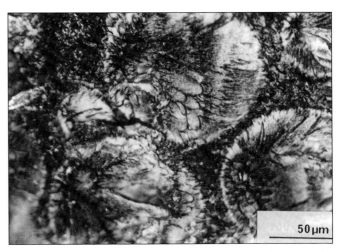

Fig 6-7 Fracture surface of heat-cured denture base acrylic resin. Note that the bead structure remains and that cracks pass through, rather than around, beads during fracture.

the rate of polymerization can be well controlled by the cooling action of the surrounding water. The additives required for the beads to easily achieve a dough-like consistency are fortunately very soluble in monomer globules and relatively insoluble in water. The globules can be thermally polymerized without a catalyst; however, benzoyl peroxide is usually added, partly to act as a catalyst in the polymerization of the beads, and partly so the beads become the source of the peroxy free radical during the polymerization of the dough in the dental flask (Fig 6-6).

To assist dough formation, a plasticizer is also incorporated into the bead polymer. For many years this was an *external plasticizer*, that is, one that resided between the polymer chains rather than being chemically attached to them. Any inert, nontoxic organic molecule would suffice; dibutylphthalate was used for many years. Today, internal plasticizers are used instead, containing various methacrylate or acrylate monomers. They locally soften the bead and allow the monomer to diffuse more rapidly into the bead during the dough stage. Pigment can be added to the bead either during polymerization or after, by *ball milling*. This method enables the manufacturer to produce a PMMA bead mixture having a fairly wide molecular weight distribution, with an average molecular weight of 1 million. The all-important doughing characteristics of the bead are governed by particle size distribution, molecular weight distribution, and plasticizer content. The highest molecular weight and lowest plasticizer content are favored, be-

cause they result in better physical and mechanical properties in the cured denture base.

The monomer used to form the dough is largely the same as that used to make the methyl methacrylate beads. Methyl methacrylate quickly diffuses into the polymer beads on contact, causing them to swell and extracting some low-molecular-weight polymer into the monomer trapped in the interstices between the beads. As the beads swell, entanglements occur between the juxtaposed beads, and the bead-monomer mixture becomes a cohesive gel. The beads never dissolve completely (Fig 6-7), although the monomer infiltrates well into the core of each bead. In the swollen state, benzoyl peroxide can diffuse from the bead into the interstices, where later it will initiate the curing of the dough.

Cross-linking agent molecules, which are capable of diffusing into the beads, are also present in this monomer phase. The cross-linking agent confers two useful properties on the cured gel. It reduces the denture base's solubility to organic solvents, and it reduces the tendency of the denture base to **crazing** (forming precracks) under stress. From a practical point of view, cross-linking agents help to simplify the denture-making apparatus. For a monomer to be converted to a solid polymer, the polymer chain produced must achieve a certain minimal length. Polymers with molecular weights below 5,000 are liquid and viscous; resilient polymers need to achieve a minimum molecular weight of about 150,000. Without a cross-linking agent, the flask would have to be airtight and the monomer flushed with nitrogen to achieve the molecular weight required without being inhibited by air. Free-monomer levels would then be unacceptably high, and the denture would have a lower stiffness level and a greater tendency to creep. The cross-linking agent accelerates the increase in the curing system's molecular weight and combats the effects of oxygen inhibition. However, excessive levels of cross-linking agent in the monomer result in denture bases that are brittle. The most common cross-linking agents are dimethacrylates, either ethylene glycol dimethacrylate or 1,4-butylene glycol dimethacrylate.

High-impact acrylic

The heat-cured dough method is also used for high-impact acrylic denture bases. Impact resistance is ensured by the incorporation of a rubber phase into the beads during their suspension polymerization. Certain rubbers will dissolve in methyl methacrylate monomer, notably copolymers of butadiene with styrene and/or methyl methacrylate. The rubber remains soluble in the monomer globule until the polymer content of the globule becomes too high and the rubber begins to precipitate out. During precipitation, some of the growing chains of PMMA may become grafted to the butadiene rubber. This event results in what is known as a **phase inversion**, which causes the dispersion throughout the bead of tiny islands of rubber containing small inclusions of rubber/PMMA graft copolymer (Fig 6-8). Why these inclusions improve the impact strength of the cured denture base will be discussed later. There are, however, many patents that describe the formation of the beads. In dentistry, beads have either uniformly distributed rubber inclusions or a core of rubber-included polymer covered by an outer shell of conventional polymer to give a more conventional dough formation. Beads that have no shell often gel very quickly and may entrap air as a result. The monomer used to get high-impact beads differs from conventional monomers in that it contains either very little or no cross-linking agent. Fortunately, the inclusion of rubber does have a craze-inhibiting effect, as will be explained later.

Autopolymerizing denture base

The autopolymerizing, or pour-type, denture base is chemically similar to the heat-cured denture base except that a reducing agent is added to the monomer. The reducing agent is usually a tertiary aromatic amine, although barbituric acid derivatives also have been used. The reducing agent reacts with the benzoyl peroxide at room temperature to produce peroxy free radicals, which initiate the polymerization of the monomer in the denture base. There is wide variation among manufacturers in the molecular weights of the polymers in the beads. Some have average molecular weights as low as 190,000. Also, cross-linker concentrations vary greatly in the monomer liquid, from 0% to 9%; interestingly, excess cross-linker is associated with high creep. The size, molecular weight, and plasticizer content should be balanced for high penetration of monomer into the bead at a low viscosity to allow pouring of the acrylic into the mold and good wetting of the plastic teeth. This compromise is difficult to achieve and often results in high residual free-monomer contents and low cross-link densities. Manufacturers' attempts to achieve the best compromise have led to the wide ranges of molecular weights and cross-linker concentrations found in materials, which inevitably result in large differences in physical and mechanical properties between various products, especially where creep is concerned.

Injection-molded plastic

Injection-molded plastics have the advantage of consistent molecular weight but the disadvantages of capital equipment costs, low craze resistance, and difficulties associated with attachment of teeth to the denture base. The plastics still used as injection-molded denture base acrylic are polycarbonate and nylon. Although they represent a very small fraction of the market, polycarbonate and nylon offer an alternative to metal dentures for patients sensitized to conventional methacrylate, nickel, or cobalt.

Acrylic.

Acrylic is supplied as granules of low-molecular-weight (MW = 150,000) linear PMMA with a narrow molecular weight range and a small amount of residual free monomer. Note that there is no cross-linking, as this would increase the melt viscosity during molding. Plasticization is low and often results in stiffness slightly in excess of conventional heat-cured denture bases despite the low molecular weight.

Polycarbonate.

This tough plastic is supplied as granules but is not suited to injection into damp molds. It has a high melt viscosity and may depolymerize explosively if overheated in the presence of water. Again, the absence of cross-linking results in poor solvent resistance and craze resistance. Furthermore, the high melt viscosity exacerbates problems in tooth attachment.

Nylon or polyamides.

This family of condensation polymers results from the reaction of a diacid with a diamine. The physical and mechanical properties of the resulting polyamides depend on the linking groups between the acid or amine groups. The first dental use of nylon was not a success because of the excessive water absorption of the type chosen, which resulted in excessive creep and some biodegradation. More recent work on glass-reinforced nylons with much lower water absorptions (eg, nylon 66) has produced more encouraging results. These nylons are either filled with specially coated glass beads or chopped glass fibers. The glass fibers increase the stiffness of the nylon to about that of a conventional heat-cured denture base from a stiffness of half that when only glass-bead reinforcement is used. Glass-fiber reinforcement should be used with care, and patients should be warned not to abrade the fitting surface so as to avoid exposing irritation-causing fibers.

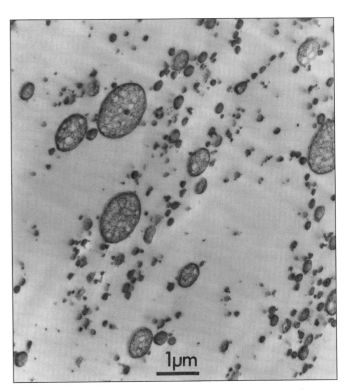

Fig 6-8 Scanning electron micrograph of high-impact denture base showing the size and shape of the polystyrene-butadiene rubber inversion phase.

Light-activated materials

In recent years, a light-activated system has come on the market and is now used for many prosthetic applications. This material consists of a urethane dimethacrylate matrix with an acrylic copolymer and a microfine silica filler. It is supplied in premixed sheet or rope form. A baseplate is made by adapting the material to a cast and polymerizing in a light chamber at 400 to 500 nm. Teeth are then added to the base with additional material followed by a second period of light exposure. The system eliminates the need for flasks, wax, boil-out tanks, packing presses, and heat-processing units required for the construction of conventional dentures. The manufacturer claims a significant time savings in both the dental office and the laboratory.

Fabrication and its effect on physical and mechanical properties

When fabricating a denture base from polymers—by whatever means—certain physical and mechanical properties of the final polymer are important. The cured polymer should be stiff enough to hold the teeth in oc-clusion during mastication and to minimize uneven loading of the mucosa underlying the denture. The polymer should not creep under masticatory loads if good occlusion is to be maintained, and it must have sufficient strength and resilience to withstand not only normal masticatory forces but sudden high stress caused by impact forces. It should not deteriorate in the aqueous oral environment nor craze as the result of solvents in food, drinks, or medicaments. The cured polymer should be biologically inert and slow to foul when in contact with oral flora.

During fabrication of a denture, the physical and mechanical properties can be influenced by cure conditions and choice of materials. Each cure cycle or fabrication technique is a compromise that attempts to optimize the important properties for a given application and patient. In a patient with allergies, low free-monomer content may be more important than stiffness. In a patient requiring a soft lining, stiffness is important to avoid problems with stability or loading due to the reduced cross-sectional area.

Heat-cured denture base

When manipulating the dough before packing, the stages of gelation need to be recognized: the initial melting of the beads with the monomer; the sandy stage; the formation of first entanglements as the outer layers of the bead swell; and, when the dough is pulled, the formation of stringy threads that can be drawn out as low-molecular-weight components dissolve into and thicken the interstitial monomer. In the last stage, the dough becomes elastic as monomer penetration reaches the core of the beads, plasticizing them and lowering their glass-transition temperature from an initial 125°C to well below room temperature. At this point, the beads have become rubber. Curing the dough before the monomer has diffused to the core of the beads may result in reduced flexural strength and a tendency for cracks to propagate along lines of weakness between the cross-linked interstitial phase and the linear, more pliable beads. Allowing the monomer and cross-linker to diffuse to the center of the beads results in a more homogeneous distribution of stress and the formation of a tough, three-dimensional network within the existing amorphous bead polymer to form what is known as an **interpenetrating polymer network** (IPN) (see Fig 6-7).

The curing cycle is designed to raise the temperature to a point at which (1) sufficient benzoyl peroxy radicals are produced to overcome the scavenging effect of oxygen, and (2) polymer chains form by free-radical addition polymerization. Too rapid a rise in temperature produces large numbers of radicals—a radical avalanche—and, as a result, many growing polymer chains. These chains collide either with other radicals or with polymer chains and increase branching and cross-linking of the interstitial polymer, thus reducing toughness. The polymerization reaction itself is exothermic; if the rate of reaction is too high, heat builds up in the dough until the boiling point of the monomer is exceeded. Porosity of the final denture base results, with a subsequent loss of strength and esthetics and an increase in the possibility of fouling.

Slow cures result in much tougher denture bases, producing fewer cross-links and branches and a higher overall molecular weight between cross-links due to fewer polymer chains growing at any one time. Free-monomer content is often lower, also, because the steadier rise in internal viscosity of the curing polymer allows the monomer easier access to the growing free radicals. The cross-linker is more completely polymer-ized in heat-cured systems, resulting in significantly lower creep values due to removal of the plasticizing effect of unreacted pendant cross-linker groups.

The shrinkage that occurs when a liquid monomer is converted to a solid polymer can be largely compensated for by keeping the curing dough under compression. There are, however, hybrid systems that deliberately start the polymerization of the dough on one side of the mold, while forcing uncured dough into the mold on the opposite side. As curing progresses across the mold, the mold space is kept filled, resulting in an improvement in dimensional accuracy. The advantage of this system is that there is less tendency to raise the bite by overpacking the mold with dough, which can occur with conventional flasks.

Heat-cured systems have one great advantage over autopolymerized and injection-molding methods: an increased rate of monomer diffusion at the higher temperature. This factor is most beneficial when acrylic teeth are used, because it leads to better wetting of the teeth by the dough and the formation of chemical welds between the teeth and denture base. Conversely, an increased temperature of cure can also result in the annealing of stresses that build up in the structure due to polymerization shrinkage. If this stress is not released, it can act as the foci for crazes or distortions caused by overzealous cleaning regimes.

Autopolymerizing acrylic

The pour technique for dentures, originally developed during the 1960s, has lost much of its popularity because of problems that stem from incorrect processing. In this technique, the acrylic is mixed to a liquid consistency and poured into a sprued mold that consists largely of reversible hydrocolloid. The fitting surface of the mold consists of the plaster cast itself; the acrylic teeth occupy their positions in the agar mold in the same way they do in a conventional plaster mold.

The pour-type mold has design weaknesses. The gelatinous agar cannot grip the teeth as easily as rock-hard plaster, and hence there is a greater tendency for the teeth to be displaced during the pouring of acrylic. In addition, before being placed in the mold, any wax remaining on the teeth from the waxing will prevent the monomer from wetting the surfaces. This problem is far less common when solution and diffusion of the wax can occur at the elevated temperatures of the heat-curing process.

The use of a hydroflask to increase the atmospheric pressure around the mold has two main advantages: *(1)* porosity caused by monomer boiling is prevented by raising its boiling point; and *(2)* air included during mixing is compressed, raising the density of the cured resin and improving its transverse strength. However, the technician can do little to reduce free-monomer content to achieve high toughness, because this factor is built into the formulation when the manufacturer chooses the powder/liquid ratio, the cross-linker content, and the accelerator/catalyst ratio. In general, the creep of these products is greater than that of heat-cured acrylics.

Injection molding

The technician has little leeway when using injection-molded plastics. The mold should be dry to prevent the generation of steam during molding. Patience is required to ensure that the melt has reached the right temperature and cools sufficiently after molding. Inadequate spruing will lead to underfilled molds, as can underheating the melt; overheating the melt can cause explosions, especially when polycarbonate is injected into moist molds. Depolymerization or oxidation from overheating the melt can result in porosity, loss of strength, color changes, and increased fouling.

Injection moldings rely almost completely on mechanical forces to retain the teeth. Low melt temperatures will cause strong forces to be put on the teeth during the injection phase and may dislodge some molars, even from plaster molds.

Light-activated materials

Light-activated materials compare well with conventional heat-cured materials in terms of impact strength and hardness but have a considerably lower elastic modulus.[3] A denture constructed of light-cured material would therefore be expected to deform elastically to a greater extent than a heat-cured denture under the forces of mastication. However, *transverse strength*—a measure of the load required to fracture a thin strip of material in the transverse direction—is just slightly lower than that of the conventional material.

As a consequence of the higher-molecular-weight oligomers used in light-cured systems, polymerization shrinkage is smaller, about 3%, rather than the 6% shrinkage found in conventional systems. A lack of polymerization shrinkage would allow the best fit.

Since light-activated materials contain no methyl methacrylate monomer, they may be considered for use in those patients who have demonstrated a sensitivity. The formulation of light-activated denture bases contains a copolymer of urethane dimethacrylate and an acrylic resin along with silica fillers. Blue light is used to polymerize thin sheets of the plastic raw material in a light chamber.

Future improvements in polymeric denture bases

Radiopacity, impact strength, and stiffness are projected to be improved features of polymeric denture bases products.

Denture wearers, be they motorists, members of the security forces, or athletes, can endure serious complications if their denture fractures and a portion of it is either inhaled or ingested or, in more serious incidents, is driven through the skull into the brain. Fragments of radiolucent denture base are difficult to find even when sophisticated ultrasound techniques are used, and their presence is often suspected only after a secondary infection sets in.

The use of radiopaque salts and fillers often reduces esthetic properties and strength, and organometallic components have often proved too toxic for use. Bromine-containing organics can give good esthetics but often lack the heat stability necessary for heat processing or have to be added in such high quantities that the bulky bromine groups overplasticize the resulting acrylic denture base, causing creep, water adsorption, and stiffness problems. However, by phase-separating a bromo-polymer additive within the bead phase, it has been shown that sufficiently high glass-transition temperatures of 110°C and stiffnesses of 2.0 GPa (290,000 psi) can be achieved, while at the same time preserving esthetic properties and achieving high levels of radiopacity.

High-impact denture base materials can be prepared using inversion-phase–separated polymer beads. However, a 50% improvement in impact strength (2.1 J/m) could be achieved, in combination with good esthetics and radiopacity, by the formation of a three-phase bead consisting of *(1)* PMMA, *(2)* styrene/butadiene rubber, and *(3)* poly(2,3-dibromopropyl methacrylate). Processing conditions must be well controlled.

The availability and quality of high-modulus fibers is improving quickly, as is the variety of materials from which the fibers are made. Early experiments with glass fibers resulted in failure because of the irritating nature of the fibers that protruded from the finished surfaces. Carbon fibers had no such irritant effects and greatly increased impact strength and flexural stiffness of the denture base for little material expense. However, carbon fibers are black, so their use must be restricted to the lingual aspects of a denture. Kevlar fibers (poly-*p*-phenylene terephthalamide) have stiffnesses of 90 GPa (13 million psi), are straw-colored, and are not easy to pack. They can, however, greatly enhance the mechanical properties of the denture. As with carbon fibers, they need to be restricted to lingual aspects of the denture for esthetic reasons, although they can be extended to the midline of the teeth without being noticeable. If this were done with carbon fibers, it would create a black shadow beneath the teeth in the plastic gum work.

Incorporation of the fibers into dentures produces conventional dentures that can withstand uncommonly rigorous treatment. When the fibers are combined with bis-GMA, the flexural strength is such that they do not break in the conventional three-point flexural test apparatus, yet they have the Young moduli of 30 GPa (4 million psi), a figure comparable with that of ceramics. Lingual bars for partial dentures could be made using such materials, and, perhaps, with some changes in partial denture design, much less obtrusive polymeric partial dentures could be fabricated with only the clasps being made of metal.

◖ Permanent Soft Lining Materials

Permanent **soft lining materials** are resilient polymers used to replace the fitting surface of a hard plastic denture because the patient cannot tolerate a hard fitting surface or to improve retention of the denture. Because the lining is soft, its dimensional stability is important, as are its durability and resistance to fouling. However, because soft lining materials are above their glass-transition temperature when in the mouth, such physical phenomena as water absorption, osmotic presence of soluble components, and biodegradability play a greater role in the clinical success of a liner than they do in the glassy polymers used as denture bases.

Acrylics and silicones are the two main families of polymers used commercially as soft liners, although other rubbers have been used in limited clinical experiments. Table 6-3 presents a comparison of soft lining materials.

Acrylic soft liners

The acrylics consist of either highly plasticized intrinsically glassy polymers or soft acrylics that have a natural glass-transition temperature at least 25°C less than that of the mouth. The plasticizer used to soften acrylic can either be unbound to the acrylic and hence free to diffuse out during use, resulting in a loss of resilience, or it can be reacted into the cured matrix of the acrylic. The latter method is preferred because it should increase the clinical life of the soft liner; unfortunately, in practice, such acrylics are hard to formulate.

The reactive plasticizer often has a much lower rate of polymerization than the acrylic monomer. The result is a form of phase separation that leads to an uneven uptake of water by the soft liner. Water accumulates in the plasticizer-rich phase, and soluble impurities in the polymer create an osmotic pressure that causes it to swell and distort. Therefore, although such internally plasticized acrylics have been produced commercially, they have often been withdrawn after distortion problems have been noted in practice, often due to insufficient curing of very finely balanced formulations.

The plasticized acrylics are based on copolymer beads consisting mainly of ethyl methacrylate; both *n*- and isobutyl methacrylate can be used, as can 2-ethoxyethyl methacrylate. However, the latter monomer is used mainly in the liquid component. The beads are copolymerized with acrylates, which, in general, have much lower glass-transition temperatures than their methacrylate homologues but unfortunately have very unpleasant odors. So that the beads are free-flowing, the bead polymers have glass-transition temperatures slightly above room temperature. The monomer usually contains the plasticizer, which is a large phthalate ester. The monomer must swell sufficiently for the plasticizer to enter the beads. The plasticizer is then trapped inside the beads as the monomer polymerizes and the mean free path between the polymer chains decreases. The monomer can be methyl methacrylate, although its T_g, even when plasticized, is rather high; *n*- or isobutyl methacrylate is preferred because it has a much lower

Table 6-3 A comparison of soft liners and tissue conditioners

MATERIAL	ADVANTAGES	DISADVANTAGES	IDEAL PROPERTIES
Soft liners			
Acrylic	High peel strength to acrylic denture base High rupture strength Some can be polished if cooled Reasonable resistance to damage by denture cleansers	Poor resilience Loses plasticizer in time Some buckle in water	High resilience Unaffected by aqueous environment and cleansers Good bond to denture base Good abrasion resistance
Silicone (RTV)	Resilience	Low tear strength Low bond strength to dentures Attacked by cleansers Buckle in water Poor abrasion resistance	Biocompatible Antifouling properties Good dimensional stability
Silicone (heat-cured)	Resilience Adequate bond strength to acrylic More resistant to aqueous environment and cleansers than RTV	Low tear strength Poor abrasion resistance	———
Tissue conditioners	Rheologic and viscoelastic properties almost ideal Can be applied chairside Dentures fit well Can record freeway space	Low cohesive strength Affected by cleansers Alcohol can sting inflamed mucosa	Flow under constant force Resilient at high rates of deformation Remain viscous for several days Have a high tack to aid retention to denture base

T_g when polymerized. Some manufacturers use isobutyl methacrylate to produce a balance of properties such that in ice water the liner can be polished like denture base acrylic, while the liner remains resilient in the mouth.

Water can, of course, be used as the plasticizer in **hydrophilic liners**. This was the principle behind the hydroxyethyl methacrylate soft liners. However, the water is not present when the denture is fabricated, and its uptake leads to a swelling of the liner, which must be compensated for. Water-swollen liners also allow ions into their matrices, which can subsequently crystallize and thus harden the lining as well as cause osmotic pressure effects, as in the polymerizable plasticizers.

Silicone soft liners

The silicones used as soft liners can be divided into two types: room-temperature vulcanizing (RTV) and heat curing. The resilience of silicones makes them seem ideal as soft lining materials. However, silicones have poor tear strength, no intrinsic adhesion to acrylic denture base, and, if not properly cured, a tendency to osmotic pressure effects. The RTV silicones' greatest drawback is their lack of adhesion, which is especially a problem around the edges of the attachment between acrylic and silicone. Heat-cured silicones contain a siloxane methacrylate that can polymerize into the curing denture base. The RTV silicones use a condensation cross-linking system based on organotin derivatives such as those used in impression rubbers. Their degree of cross-linking is lower, and their serviceability is low as a result, with frequent reports in the literature of swelling and buckling during use and excessive sensitivity to denture cleansers.[4,5] The rupture strength of some RTV silicones is known to deteriorate considerably when exposed to water for long periods. The heat-cured silicones achieve a greater degree of cross-linking and have much longer clinical lifetimes.

■ Temporary Soft Liners and Functional Impression Materials

Temporary soft liners, or *tissue conditioners*, need only survive in the mouth for a few weeks—although some are so well formulated as to remain resilient and in place for many months. However, it is their viscoelastic properties that are important, specifically their ability to flow under masticatory and linguistic forces, spreading the load on the mucosa evenly. When first mixed, they flow easily, recording such voids as mean freespace. They soon become highly viscous, however, and thereafter only respond to persistent forces, such as changes in the shape of the mucosa beneath the denture. In this way swollen mucosa traumatized by ill-fitting dentures can recover while the denture, with its tissue conditioner lining, adapts to any fitting difficulties caused by masticatory forces.

Many materials were used for the temporary soft liners when the technique was first developed and included many nontoxic, puttylike materials, such as plasticine and chewing gum. Modern materials are exclusively acrylic gels. An acrylic gel can be made by mixing swellable acrylic beads with alcohol. PMMA is unsuitable for this purpose, although poly(ethyl methacrylate) or its copolymers with acrylates have proved most popular. To maintain the softness of the gel in the mouth, plasticizer is added to the alcohol, which diffuses into the polymer beads and lowers their glass-transition temperature to well below that of the mouth. The beads are made of low-molecular-weight polymer and have a high tack when swollen. This characteristic has the advantage of increasing the cohesive strength of the gel and causing it to be well retained by the denture base acrylic.

There is no polymerization or curing reaction involved in the setting of the gel, just the entanglement of outer polymer chains of juxtaposed beads. The rate of gelling is increased by lowering the molecular weight of the bead, reducing its size, or increasing the amount of acrylate in its copolymers. The alcohol content of the liquid also can be used to control the rate of gelling, as can the size of the plasticizer molecule; the more alcohol used, the faster the rate of gelling. However, because the alcohol diffuses out of the gel and is only partially replaced by water, high-alcohol-content gels tend to harden much faster than others. Practitioners should be aware of the alcohol content of these products, first because they sting when initially inserted, and second because they give false-positive results if the patient is given a breathalyzer test.

■ Glossary

addition polymerization A polymerization process (such as a free radical-initiated one) in which no by-product is formed as the chain grows.

condensation polymerization A polymerization process in which a by-product, such as water or alcohol, is formed as the chain grows.

copolymer A polymer consisting of two or more types of mers, or units, joined together.

crazing Minute surface cracks on polymers; precursors to crack growth and subsequent failure of the material.

cross-linking agent A monomer having two or more groups per molecule capable of polymerization. When polymerized, each active group is capable of incorporation in a growing polymer chain, causing either a loop in the chain or a cross-link between two chains.

degree of polymerization The total number of mers in one polymer molecule.

denture base Materials used to contact the oral tissues and support artificial teeth.

glass-transition temperature (T_g) The temperature at which the polymer ceases to be glass-like (ie, fractures in a brittle manner) and becomes rubber-like or leather-like (ie, tends to permanently deform under a load too small to cause fracture). Also called *softening temperature*.

glassy polymer An amorphous polymer that behaves as a brittle solid.

hydrophilic liner A soft liner that is readily wet by water.

interpenetrating polymer network (IPN) A combination of two polymers in network form, at least one of which is synthesized and/or polymerized in the immediate presence of the other. An IPN can be distinguished from simple polymer blends, blocks, and grafts in two ways: (1) An IPN swells but does not dissolve in solvents, and (2) creep and flow are suppressed.

molecular weight The mass of one polymer molecule, which is often calculated approximately as the sum of the molecular weights of the mers of which the polymer is made.

monomer A molecule that becomes a repeating chemical unit of a polymer (eg, ethylene is the monomer of a long chain polyethylene).

oligomer A polymer made up of two, three, four, or more but usually fewer than ten monomer units.

phase inversion The inversion of the internal and external phases in an emulsion, eg, the change of an oil-in-water emulsion to a water-in-oil emulsion.

plasticizer A small molecule that, when added to a polymer, lowers its glass-transition temperature and increases the rate at which solvents penetrate the polymer.

polymer A molecule made up of thousands or millions of repeating units. Polymers may be linear, branched, or cross-linked.

polymerization The process by which monomers unite to form a polymer.

soft lining material A soft polymer used as a thin layer on the tissue-bearing surface of a denture; also called a *soft liner*.

thermoplastic A polymer that softens upon heating and rehardens upon cooling.

thermoset A polymer that is not able to undergo softening upon heating.

tissue conditioner A soft liner used to treat traumatized mucosa.

▪ Discussion Questions

1. Why is higher impact strength an important advantage for denture base materials?

2. How does the heat-curing rate affect the porosity and strength of acrylic denture bases?

3. Although cross-linking can improve mechanical properties, how can it lead to problems in the bonding between acrylic teeth and the denture base?

4. Why do acrylic polymers still dominate the denture base market?

▪ Study Questions

(See appendix E for answers.)

1. What are the main types of denture base materials used?

2. What are the ideal properties of a denture base material?

3. What are the advantages and disadvantages of heat-cured acrylic denture base materials?

4. What are the advantages and disadvantages of autocured denture base materials?

5. What are the advantages and disadvantages of rubber-reinforced denture base materials?

6. What are the advantages and disadvantages of fiber-reinforced denture base materials?

7. What are the advantages and disadvantages of injection-molded denture bases?

8. What are the advantages and disadvantages of light-activated denture base materials?

9. What are the materials currently being used as soft liners?

10. What are the advantages and disadvantages of RTV silicones?

11. What are the advantages and disadvantages of heat-cured silicones?

12. What are the advantages and disadvantages of acrylic soft liners?

13. What are the ideal properties of tissue conditioners?

▪ References

1. Mark FF. Future trends for improvement of cohesive and adhesive strength of polymers. In: Weiss P (ed). Adhesion and Cohesion. Amsterdam: Elsevier, 1962:241.

2. Berry JP, Bueche AM. Ultimate strength of polymers. In: Weiss P (ed). Adhesion and Cohesion. Amsterdam: Elsevier, 1962:20.

3. Smith LT, Powers JM, Ladd D. Mechanical properties of new denture resins polymerized by visible light, heat and microwave energy. Int J Prosthodont 1992;5:315–320.

4. Kawano F, Dootz ER, Koran A 3rd, Craig RG. Sorption and solubility of 12 soft denture liners. J Prosthet Dent 1994;72:393–398.

5. Kimoto S, Kitamura M, Kodaira M, et al. Randomized controlled clinical trial on satisfaction with resilient denture liners among edentulous patients. Int J Prosthodont 2004;17:236–240.

■ Recommended Reading

Anderson GC, Schulte JK, Arnold TG. Dimensional stability of injection and conventional processing of denture base acrylic resin. J Prosthet Dent 1988;60(3):394–398.

Bafile M, Graser GN, Myers ML, Li EKH. Porosity of denture resin cured by microwave energy. J Prosthet Dent 1991;66:269–274.

Cunningham JL, Benington IC. An investigation of the variables which may affect the bond between plastic teeth and denture base resin. J Dent 1999;27:129–135.

Davy KWM, Causton BE. Radio-opaque denture base: A new acrylic copolymer. J Dent 1982;10:253–264.

Eichold WA, Woefel JB. Denture base acrylic resins: Friend or foe? Compend Contin Educ Dent 1990;11:720–725.

Goll G, Smith DE, Plein JB. The effect of denture cleansers on temporary soft liners. J Prosthet Dent 1983;50:466–472.

Khan Z, von Fraunhofer JA, Razavi R. The staining characteristics, transverse strength, and microhardness of a visible light-cured denture base material. J Prosthet Dent 1987;57:384–386.

MacGregor AR, Graham J, Stafford GD, Huggett B. Recent experience with denture polymers. J Dent 1984;12:146–157.

Mack PJ. Denture soft linings: Materials available. Aust Dent J 1989;34:517–521.

Qudah S, Harrison A, Huggett R. Soft lining materials in prosthetic dentistry: A review. Int J Prosthodont 1990;3:477–483.

Ruyter IE. Methacrylate-based polymeric dental materials: Conversion and related properties. Acta Odontol Scand 1982;40:359–376.

Ruyter IE, Svendsen SA. Flexural properties of denture base polymers. J Prosthet Dent 1980;43:95–104.

Schmidt WF, Smith DE. A six-year retrospective study of Molloplast-B-lined dentures. Part 1. Patient response. J Prosthet Dent 1983;50(3):308–313.

Smith LT, Powers JM. Relative fit of new denture resins polymerized by heat, light and microwave energy. Am J Dent 1992;5(3):140–142.

Takamata T, Setcos JC. Resin denture bases: Review of accuracy and methods of polymerization. Int J Prosthodont 1989;2:555–562.

Wright PS. Soft lining materials: Their status and prospects. J Dent 1976;4:247–256.

CHAPTER 7

Impression Materials

To replicate the structures of the oral cavity, impression materials are converted from a liquid state into either elastic or nonelastic (ie, plastic or brittle) negative replicas of the soft and/or hard tissues of the mouth by physical change, chemical reaction, or polymerization. A **cast material** (eg, high-strength stone) is then poured into the impression and, on setting, produces a positive impression of the tissues. Nonelastic materials include impression plaster, impression compound, and zinc oxide–eugenol. Agar hydrocolloid, alginate, polysulfide, condensation silicone, addition silicone, and polyether are examples of elastic materials currently used. A classification is shown in Fig 7-1.

The American Dental Association's (ADA's) Council on Dental Materials, Instruments, and Equipment is responsible for developing and disseminating specifications for dental materials, instruments, and equipment. The American National Standards Institute (ANSI) has made the Council the Administrative Secretariat of the American National Standards Committee MD156 for Dental Materials, Instruments, and Equipment. Specifications are available for several dental impression materials: dental agar impression material[1]; alginate impression material[2]; nonaqueous, elastomeric impression material[3]; and dental duplicating material.[4]

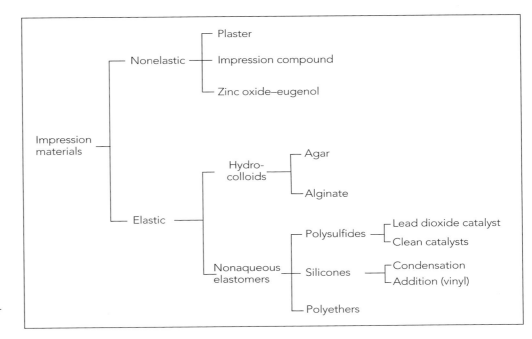

Fig 7-1 A classification for impression materials.

■ Nonelastic Materials

Impression plaster

Plaster of Paris is seldom used as an impression material now that elastomeric materials are available, but it can be used as a *wash impression* material (a thin lining material placed over a stiffer base material or tray) for edentulous impressions. The main component of impression plaster is calcium sulfate hemihydrate, which reacts with water to form calcium sulfate dihydrate. Manufacturers incorporate additives to adjust the setting time and setting expansion. The water/powder (W/P) ratio recommended by the manufacturer should be measured out carefully. The powder should be sprinkled into the water, allowed to sit for 30 seconds to wet the powder, and then mixed for the minimum time necessary to obtain a homogeneous mix. Impression plaster is rigid and will break rather than bend. The plaster must be stored in an airtight container, because it will absorb water from the air which may adversely affect its setting time.

Dental impression compound (types I and II)

Although dental compound has fallen into disuse, it can be used for full-crown impressions (type I), impressions of partially or completely edentulous jaws (type I), and impression trays in which a final impression is taken with another material (type II). Dental compound cannot be used to record undercuts because it is not elastic. Impression compound is available in either cakes or sticks in various colors from a number of manufacturers.

Composition
Natural resins give the compound its **thermoplastic** character and make up about 40% of the formulation. Shellac is often used. Waxes (about 7%) also have thermoplastic properties, and stearic acid (about 3%) acts as a lubricant and plasticizer. Fillers (eg, diatomaceous earth, soapstone, and talc) and inorganic pigments account for the remaining 50% of the formulation.

Thermal and mechanical properties
Dental compound's thermoplastic property allows it to be used warm (45°C) and then cooled to oral temperature (37°C), at which it is fairly rigid. The setting mechanism is therefore a reversible physical process rather than a chemical reaction. Dental compound is limited by its thermal properties. Type I materials have a **flow** of at least 85% at 45°C and less than 6% at 37°C. Type II materials flow about 70% at 45°C but less than 2% at 37°C. Both types become quite plastic with only an 8°C rise in temperature. The **thermal conductivity** of dental impression compounds is very low. These materials require heat soaking to attain a uniform temperature throughout the mass. When heated or cooled, they soften or harden quickly on the outside, but time is needed for the temperature to become uniform throughout the entire mass. If the impression is removed from the mouth before it has cooled completely, severe distortion may occur. Since these materials contain resins and waxes, they have high thermal expansion and contraction coefficients. Contraction from oral temperature to room temperature may be as high as 0.3%. Therefore, the dimensions of the resulting impression could be significantly different from those of the mouth. Since the compound has such a high viscosity, it is difficult to record details.

Manipulation
Impression compound is softened by heating over a flame or in a water bath. Care must be taken to prevent volatilizing ingredients over a direct flame. Kneading in water also may cause changes in composition and flow properties. The aim, therefore, is thorough heating without excessive temperatures or long periods of storage in water. A room-temperature water spray is used to cool the impression in the mouth. Cooling must be continued until the entire mass is rigid to reduce plastic flow. Care must also be taken to prevent overheating and burning of the tissues being replicated. Also, cooling water should not be too cold, to prevent thermal shock.

To ease separation of the die stone, the impression should first be softened by immersion in warm water.

Advantages
Dental impression compound is compatible with die and cast materials and is easily **electroplated** to form accurate and abrasion-resistant dies.

Disadvantages
The handling of dental impression compound is very technique sensitive. If it is not prepared properly, volatiles can be lost on heating or low-molecular-weight ingredients can be lost during immersion in a water bath.

Also, excessive wet kneading can incorporate water into the mix and change the flow properties of the compound. Due to a high coefficient of thermal expansion, the dimensions of the impression are not likely to be the same as the dimensions in the mouth. These materials are nonelastic and may distort on removal from the mouth. The casts should be poured within 1 hour.

Troubleshooting

1. *Distortion.* If the material is not completely cooled, the inner portions of the impression will still be soft when the impression is removed, resulting in distortion. Also, if water has been incorporated as the result of wet kneading, the material could have excessive flow at mouth temperature, producing distortion during removal from the mouth. If the tray used to carry the compound to the mouth is too flexible, distortion can result. It is important to select a tray that is strong and rigid. A delay in preparing the stone cast also may cause distortion. The cast should be poured as soon as possible after the impression has been removed from the mouth.

2. *Compound is too brittle or grainy.* Prolonged immersion in the water bath will cause low-molecular-weight components to leach out.

Disinfection

Dental impression compound can be disinfected by immersion in sodium hypochlorite, iodophors, or phenolic glutaraldehydes. The manufacturer's recommendations for proper disinfection should be followed.

Zinc oxide–eugenol

The main use of zinc oxide–eugenol is for dentures on edentulous ridges with minor or no undercuts. It can also be used as a wash impression over the compound in a tray or in a custom acrylic tray. Zinc oxide–eugenol is also used as a bite registration material.

Composition

This material is commercially available in a powder and liquid form and as two pastes. One paste, called the *base* or *catalyst paste*, contains zinc oxide (ZnO), oil, and hydrogenated rosin. The second paste, the *accelerator*, contains about 12% to 15% **eugenol**, oils, rosin, and a filler such as talc or Kaolin. These two pastes have contrasting colors so it can be determined when the pastes are thoroughly mixed.

These materials are supplied as a soft- or hard-set type. Equal lengths of the two pastes, or properly proportioned amounts of the powder and liquid, are mixed with a stiff spatula on a special oil-resistant paper pad or a glass slab. The mixed material is placed in a preliminary impression made from tray compound or tray acrylic. The setting time is shortened by increases in temperature and/or humidity. The set material does not adhere to set dental plaster or stone.

Eugenol

Zinc oxide, in the presence of moisture, reacts with eugenol to form zinc eugenolate, which acts as a matrix holding together the unreacted zinc oxide:

$$\text{ZnO (excess)} + \text{eugenol} \xrightarrow{\text{H}_2\text{O}} \text{Zn eugenolate}$$
$$\text{(powder)} \quad \text{(liquid)} \qquad + \text{ZnO (unreacted)}$$
$$\text{(solid)}$$

The setting reaction is accelerated by the presence of water, high humidity, or heat. A dimensional change of only about 0.1% shrinkage accompanies the setting.

These impression materials are classified as *hard-* and *soft-set*. The hard-set material sets faster (in about 10 minutes, compared with 15 minutes for the soft-set material), although the hard- and soft-set materials both begin to set in about 5 minutes. The hard-set material is more fluid before setting than the soft-set material; after setting, it is harder and more brittle.

Noneugenol pastes containing carboxylic acids (eg, lauric or ortho-ethoxybenzoic acid) in place of eugenol are available to avoid the stinging and burning sensation experienced by some patients.

Mechanical properties

The hardness of zinc oxide–eugenol impression materials is determined using a Krebs penetrometer with a load of 100 g for 10 seconds. The hardness for type I (hard-set) materials should be no greater than 0.5 mm, and the hardness for type II (soft-set) materials should be between 0.8 and 1.5 mm. The shrinkage of these materials during the hardening process is approximately 0.1%. Subsequently, no additional dimensional change should occur.

Manipulation

These materials are usually mixed on a mixing pad with a spatula. Equal lengths of base and catalyst are extruded on the mixing pad. The components are mixed thoroughly with a stiff stainless steel spatula. Adequate mixing time is 45 to 60 seconds, after which the mix should appear streak free. The pastes have an initial set time of 3 to 5 minutes, with the setting time decreasing as the temperature and/or humidity increases. The cast should only be made from gypsum-type plaster or stone. After the stone has set, the impression is immersed in warm water (60°C) to ease its removal from the cast. The spatula may be cleaned by warming or by wiping with available solvents.

Advantages

Zinc oxide–eugenol gives high accuracy of soft tissue impressions due to its low viscosity. The material is stable after setting, has good surface detail reproduction, and is inexpensive. It also adheres well to dental impression compound.

Disadvantages

This material is messy and has a variable setting time due to temperature and humidity. Eugenol is irritating to soft tissues. This material is nonelastic and may fracture if undercuts are present.

Troubleshooting

1. *Inadequate working or setting time.* An increase in humidity and/or temperature results in decreased working and setting time. It is important to select a material that provides the required setting time.
2. *Distortion.* If the tray warps on standing, the impression will also become distorted. It is important to select a stable tray material.
3. *Loss of detail.* If there is loss of detail, the impression material may not be compatible with the stone used to prepare the cast, and/or there may be adhesion between the impression and the stone.

Disinfection

Zinc oxide–eugenol impressions can be disinfected by immersion in 2% glutaraldehyde or 1:213 iodophor solutions at room temperature. The manufacturer's recommendations for proper disinfection should be followed.

■ Elastic Materials

Agar (reversible) hydrocolloid

Agar hydrocolloids have been largely replaced by rubber impression materials but are still used for full-mouth impressions without deep undercuts, quadrant impressions without deep undercuts, and single impressions (less frequently). Because of their high accuracy, they can be used for fixed partial denture impressions.

Composition

Agar hydrocolloids are available in both tray and syringe consistencies. The material is supplied as a **gel** in plastic tubes and contains agar (12% to 15%) as a gelling agent, borax (0.2%) to improve strength, potassium sulfate (1% to 2%) to provide good surfaces on gypsum models or dies, alkylbenzoates (0.1%) as preservatives, and coloring and flavoring agents (traces) for ease of "reading" the impression and esthetics. The balance of the formulation (~85%) is water. The syringe consistency is prepared by increasing the water content and decreasing the agar content.

The gel material can be converted to a **sol** (liquid) by heating; cooling the sol will return the material to the gel state:

$$\text{agar hydrocolloid (hot)} \underset{\substack{\text{heat to}\\100°C}}{\overset{\substack{\text{cool to}\\43°C}}{\rightleftarrows}} \text{agar hydrocolloid (cold)}$$
$$\text{(sol)} \qquad\qquad\qquad \text{(gel)}$$

The gel-to-sol and sol-to-gel transformations depend on time and temperature. The liquefaction and gelation temperatures are different (the latter being lower), and the effect is called **hysteresis**. A typical value of the gelation temperature is 43°C (109°F).

Mechanical properties

The mechanical properties of agar **hydrocolloids** are presented in Table 7-1. They are highly elastic (98.8%)

and sufficiently flexible (11%) to give accurate impressions of teeth with undercuts. They are stronger when stressed quickly; therefore, rapid removal is recommended.

Manipulation

Agar requires a special water bath with three chambers for heating and water-cooled trays. The following sequence is used:

1. Heat in water at 100°C (212°F) for 8 to 12 minutes.
2. Store in water at 65°C (149°F).
3. Place in a tray (containing cooling coils) at 65°C (149°F).
4. Temper in 46°C (115°F) water for 2 minutes before taking the impression.
5. After seating the tray, cool it with water at no less than 13°C (55°F) until gelation occurs.
6. After the impression is removed from the mouth, wash it to remove saliva, which will interfere with the setting of the gypsum.
7. Shake off excess water and lightly blow off remaining excess with air.
8. Disinfect the impression.
9. Pour mixed dental stone into the impression. If the impression is stored for a short time in 100% relative humidity, it should be washed as described in steps 6 and 7 to remove any exudate on the surface caused by **syneresis** (the exudation of water, accompanied by contraction) before pouring the cast.
10. After the initial setting of the stone, store the gypsum cast and impression in a humidor.

Agar impressions become less accurate during storage, so prompt pouring of gypsum casts is necessary. Table 7-2 lists the dimensional changes that occur during storage under different conditions. If agar impressions must be stored, the minimum changes in dimensions occur in 100% relative humidity for no longer than 1 hour. However, the gel structure can absorb water, a process called **imbibition**, which is usually accompanied by expansion.

As the values in Table 7-3 indicate, agar materials have a long **working time**. Handling, however, offsets this convenience because of the need for storage tanks. Gelation, produced by circulating cool water through the special trays, also requires special equipment. Thermal shock produced by suddenly cooling the warm colloid may be painful to patients who have metallic restorations.

Contact with agar retards the setting of gypsum, resulting in dies and casts with poor surface finish. With older products, soaking the impression in a 2% potassium sulfate solution was necessary to achieve a smooth surface finish. Most agar products now contain potassium sulfate, which acts as an accelerator for the gypsum setting reaction, and soaking is no longer necessary.

Advantages

Agar impression materials are inexpensive, have no unpleasant odors, and are nontoxic and nonstaining. They do not require a custom tray or adhesives, and the components do not require mixing. These materials are **hydrophilic** and can be used in the presence of moisture and are able to displace blood and body fluids. In addition, they are easily poured in stone, and the stone casts are easily removed from the hydrocolloid impressions.

Disadvantages

These materials require the use of expensive equipment and must be prepared in advance. They tear easily, must be poured immediately, are dimensionally unstable, can only be used for single casts, and cannot be electroplated. The surface of stone casts will be weakened by compositions containing borax.

Troubleshooting

Sometimes problems of distorted impressions or loss of detail may be encountered when using agar hydrocolloids. The following are factors that could lead to distortion:

1. *Slow removal from the mouth.* To avoid permanent deformation, the impression should be removed with a quick jerk.
2. *Removal from the mouth before the gel reaches a temperature of 37°C (98.6°F) or less.* Above this temperature the impression material will still be plastic. The cooling rate of hydrocolloid depends on the temperature of water circulating through the tray.
3. *Cooling water that is too cold (< 13°C).* Rapid cooling of the impression may cause a concentration of internal stresses that may be subsequently released.
4. *Application of force on the tray during gelation.* After the load is removed, relaxation of stresses will occur.

Table 7-1 Properties of elastomeric impression materials*

	AGAR	ALGINATE	POLYSULFIDE	CONDENSATION SILICONE	ADDITION SILICONE	POLYETHER
Elastic recovery (%)	98.8	97.3	96.9–94.5	99.6–98.2	99.9–99.0	99.0–98.3
Flexibility (%)	11	12	8.5–20	3.5–7.8	1.3–5.6	1.9–3.3
Flow (%)	—	—	0.4–1.9	< 0.10	< 0.05	< 0.05
Reproduction limit (μm)	25	75	25	25	25	25
Shrinkage, 24 hours (%)	—	—	0.4–0.5	0.2–1.0	0.01–0.2	0.2–0.3
Tear strength (g/cm)	700	380–700	2,240–7,410	2,280–4,370	1,640–5,260	1,700–4,800

*See glossary for definitions of terms.

Table 7-2 Dimensional change of hydrocolloid impressions

STORAGE CONDITIONS	DIMENSIONAL CHANGE	CAUSES
Air	Shrinkage	Evaporation of water from gel
H_2O	Expansion	Imbibition and absorption of water
100% relative humidity	Shrinkage	Syneresis
Inorganic salt solutions	Expansion or shrinkage	Depends on relationship of electrolyte in gel and in solution

Table 7-3 Handling properties of elastomeric impression materials*

	AGAR	ALGINATE	POLYSULFIDE	CONDENSATION SILICONE	ADDITION SILICONE	POLYETHER
Preparation	Boil, temper, store	Powder, water	2 pastes	2 pastes or paste-liquid	2 pastes	2 pastes
Handling	Complicated	Simple	Simple	Simple	Simple	Simple
Ease of use	Technique sensitive	Good	Fair	Fair	Good	Good
Patient reaction	Tedious, thermal shock	Pleasant, clean	Unpleasant, stains	Pleasant, clean	Pleasant	Unpleasant, clean
Ease of removal	Very easy	Very easy	Easy	Moderate	Moderate	Moderate to difficult
Working time (min)	7–15	2.5	5–7	3	2–4.5	2.5
Setting time (min)	5	3.5	8–12	6–8	3–7	4.5
Stability	1 h at 100% RH	Immediate pour	1 h	Immediate pour	1 w	1 w kept dry
Wetting and ease of pouring	Excellent	Excellent	Excellent	Fair	Fair to good	Good
Die material	Stone	Stone	Stone	Stone	Stone	Stone
Electroplating	No	No	Yes	Yes	Yes	Yes
Disinfection	Poor	Poor	Fair	Excellent	Excellent	Fair
Comparative	Low	Very low	Low	Moderate	High to very high	Very high

*See glossary for definitions of terms.

5. *Delay in pouring the cast*. Waiting any length of time to pour the cast will result in shrinkage of the impression due to the loss of water.

6. *Instability of tray*. If there is loss of detail, it may be caused by movement of the tray before gelation is complete. Failure to keep the impression stabilized will result in a multiple impression of the oral structures.

Disinfection

Agar hydrocolloids can be disinfected by immersion in sodium hypochlorite, iodophors, or phenolic glutaraldehydes. The manufacturer's recommendations for proper disinfection should be followed.

Alginate (irreversible) hydrocolloid

Alginates are the most widely used impression materials in dentistry. They are used for making impressions for removable partial dentures with clasps, preliminary impressions for complete dentures, and orthodontic and study casts. They are not accurate enough for fixed partial denture impressions.

Composition

Alginates are supplied as a powder containing sodium or potassium alginate (12% to 15%) and calcium sulfate dihydrate (8% to 12%) as reactants; sodium phosphate (2%) as a retarder; a reinforcing filler (70%), such as diatomaceous earth, to control the stiffness of the set gel; potassium sulfate or alkali zinc fluorides (~10%) to provide good surfaces on gypsum dies; and coloring and flavoring agents (traces) for esthetics. The sodium phosphate content is adjusted by the manufacturer to produce either *regular-* or *fast-set* alginates.

The powder is mixed with water to obtain a paste. Two main reactions occur when the powder reacts with water during setting. First, the sodium phosphate reacts with the calcium sulfate to provide adequate working time:

$$2Na_3PO_4 + 3CaSO_4 \rightarrow Ca_3(PO_4)_2 + 3Na_2SO_4$$

Second, after the sodium phosphate has reacted, the remaining calcium sulfate reacts with the sodium alginate to form an insoluble calcium alginate, which forms a gel with the water:

$$\begin{array}{c} H_2O \\ \text{Na alginate} + CaSO_4 \xrightarrow{\hspace{1cm}} \text{Ca alginate} + Na_2SO_4 \\ \text{(powder)} \hspace{3cm} \text{(gel)} \end{array}$$

To avoid the inhalation of alginate dust, some materials have been introduced in a dustless version in which the powder is coated with a glycol (eg, Identic Dust Free, Cadco; Jeltrate Plus, Dentsply Caulk).

Some products contain a chemical disinfectant in the alginate powder to control infection (eg, Coe Hydrophilic Gel, GC America; Identic Dust Free). Two examples of these disinfectants are didecyl-dimethyl ammonium chloride and chlorhexidine acetate. When the quaternary ammonium compound is used, the detail reproduction and gypsum compatibility of the alginate improve. However, the impressions made from these materials should still be disinfected on removal from the mouth.

Mechanical properties

Table 7-1 gives an **elastic recovery** value of 97.3% for alginates, which indicates less elasticity and therefore less accuracy than agar hydrocolloids and silicone and polyether impression materials. The compressive and tear strengths increase with increasing rates of deformation. The limit of reproduction is also lower, thus, less fine detail will be obtained. Figure 7-2 compares the elasticity of alginates with the more accurate agar materials. Alginates have a higher permanent deformation on stretching to pass over undercuts.

Manipulation

Although easy to use, care is required in handling alginate hydrocolloids. The powder, supplied in a can, should be shaken up for aeration, and one scoop of powder should be used for one measure of water. A powder scoop and a graduated cylinder for water are usually supplied with the product. With predispensed powder products, one packet of powder is used with the amount of water specified by the manufacturer. A lower W/P ratio increases strength, tear resistance, and consistency, and decreases working and setting times and **flexibility**. Also, cooling the water increases the working and setting times. Insufficient mixing results in a grainy mix and poor recording of detail. Adequate spatulation gives a smooth, creamy mix with a minimum of voids.

One minute of thorough mixing for the regular-set material and 45 seconds for the fast-set material are generally recommended. Alginates have a relatively short working time of about 2.5 minutes (see Table 7-3) and set about 3.5 minutes after mixing. They are as un-

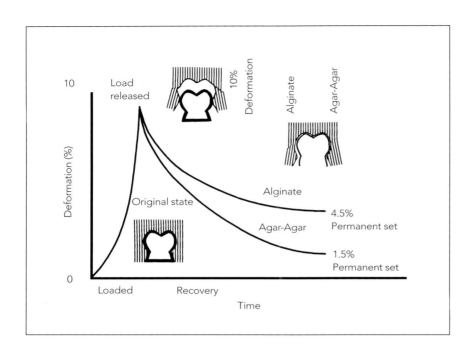

Fig 7-2 The greater accuracy of agar hydrocolloids is due to their greater degree of recovery after deformation around undercuts. (Reprinted with permission from Roydhouse.[5])

stable as agar hydrocolloids because both are gels, and they undergo shrinkage or expansion when water is lost or gained. Storage in either air or water results in significant dimensional change; however, storage at 100% humidity results in the least dimensional change. Therefore, the cast should be poured soon after removal of the impression and cleaning (see Table 7-3). Alginates, like agar, retard the setting of the gypsum cast and die materials when in contact. Potassium sulfate is added by the manufacturer to accelerate the setting of the gypsum and to obtain smooth cast and die surfaces.

An alginate tray material can be combined with an agar syringe material to prepare impressions. These impressions take advantage of the agar hydrocolloid's detail reproduction and compatibility with gypsum qualities and at the same time minimize equipment needs. A simple heater can be used to prepare the syringe material, and the water-cooled trays are no longer necessary. The alginate is placed in a tray, the agar is dispensed around the preparation, and then the alginate is seated on top of the agar. Care must be taken to select an agar-alginate impression pair with suitable bond strengths. It is best to select combinations recommended by the manufacturers. Best results are obtained when single-unit impressions are made by this technique.

Advantages

Alginate impression materials are inexpensive, easy to manipulate, pleasant tasting, able to displace blood and body fluids, hydrophilic, and easily poured in stone. They can be used with stock trays.

Disadvantages

Alginates tear easily, must be poured immediately after removal from the mouth, have limited detail reproduction, are dimensionally unstable, and can only be used for single casts. The gypsum compatibility varies with the brands of alginates and dental stones used. They are incompatible with many epoxy resin die materials.

Troubleshooting

Problems may sometimes be encountered when using alginate hydrocolloids. The following should serve as a guide for troubleshooting problems with these materials:

1. *Inadequate working or setting time.* The temperature of the mixing water may be too high. Generally, the temperature of the water should range between 18°C and 24°C (65°F and 75°F). If the mixture is incompletely spatulated, it may be inhomogeneous and may set prematurely. Under normal conditions, ade-

quate spatulation requires 45 to 60 seconds. If the W/P ratio is too low as the result of incorrect dispensing, the setting time could be too fast. Improper storage of the alginate powder can result in deterioration of the material and shorter setting times.

2. *Distortion.* If the tray moves during gelation or if the impression is removed prematurely, the result will be a distorted impression. The amount and duration of compression should be considered. It is important, therefore, to remove the impression from the mouth rapidly. Since the weight of the tray can compress or distort the alginate, the impression should not be placed face down on the bench surface. If the impression is not poured immediately, distortion could occur.

3. *Tearing.* If the impression tears, it is possible that it was removed from the mouth before it was adequately set. Wait 2 to 3 minutes after loss of tackiness to remove the impression for development of adequate tear strength. Also, the rate of removal from the mouth may be a factor. Because the tear strength of alginate increases with the rate at which a stress is applied, it is desirable to rapidly remove the impression from the mouth. In addition, thin mixes are more prone to tearing than those with lower W/P ratios. The presence of undercuts also can produce tearing. Blocking out these areas will place less stress on the impression material during removal. It is also possible that there is not enough impression material; there should always be at least 3 mm of material between the tray and the oral tissues.

4. *Loss of detail.* If there is loss of detail, the impression may have been removed from the mouth prematurely. Multiple impressions of the oral structure will result if the material is still in the plastic state when removed.

5. *Consistency.* If the preset mix does not have the proper consistency (either too thick or too thin), the W/P ratio is incorrect. Care must be taken to fluff the powder before measuring and not to overfill the powder dispenser. Vigorous spatulation and mixing for the full recommended time is required to avoid consistency problems caused by inadequate mixing. If hot water is used, the mix may become grainy and prematurely thick.

6. *Dimensional change.* If dimensional change is a problem, a delay in pouring the impression might be the cause. Such delays will result in a cast that is distorted as well as undersized, because alginate impressions lose water when stored in air.

7. *Porosity.* Whipping air into the mix during spatulation can cause the impression to be porous. After the powder has been wetted, the alginate should be mixed so as to squeeze the material between the spatula blade and the side of the rubber bowl.

8. *Poor stone surface.* If the set gypsum remains in contact with the alginate for too long, the quality of the stone surface will suffer.

Disinfection

Alginate hydrocolloids can be disinfected by immersion in sodium hypochlorite or iodophors. The manufacturer's recommendations for proper disinfection should be followed.

Polysulfide rubber (mercaptan)

Due to their high accuracy and relatively low cost, **polysulfide** rubbers are widely used for fixed partial denture application. These materials are useful for multiple impressions when extra time is needed. Polysulfides are supplied in tubes of base paste and catalyst paste, which are mixed together. They are available in low, medium, and high viscosities.

Composition

The base paste contains the polysulfide polymer, fillers, and plasticizers. Low-molecular-weight (~4,000 MW) polysulfide polymer, having both terminal and pendant (near the center of the polymer) mercaptan groups (-SH), is used:

$$HS - R_n - S - S - \overset{\displaystyle \overset{C_2H_5}{|}}{C} \underset{\displaystyle \underset{SH}{|}}{} - S - S - R_n - SH$$

Mercaptan

The content of the reinforcing fillers (eg, zinc oxide, titanium dioxide, zinc sulfide, and silica) varies from 12% to 50% depending on the consistency (ie, low, medium or high viscosity). The accelerator or catalyst paste contains lead dioxide (30%), hydrated copper oxide or organic peroxide as a catalyst, sulfur (1% to 4%) as a promoter, and dibutyl phthalate or other nonreactive oils (17%) to form the paste. The balance of the catalyst paste is made up of inorganic fillers used to adjust the consistency and reactivity. Those materials containing an organic peroxide may have decreased dimensional stability due to evaporation of the peroxide.

The lead dioxide catalyzes the condensation of the terminal and pendant -SH with -SH groups on other molecules, resulting in chain lengthening and cross-linking. In the process, the material changes from a paste to a rubber. The reaction is accelerated by increases in temperature and by the presence of moisture.

mercaptan + lead dioxide → polysulfide rubber + lead oxide + water
(base paste) (catalyst)   (impression)

Note that this is a **condensation** polymerization with water as a by-product.

Mechanical properties

The values for the mechanical properties of these materials are summarized in Table 7-1. For elastic recovery, the polysulfides have values of about 96%, slightly lower than those for the other rubber impression materials (eg, silicone and polyether). Values for flow range from 0.4% to 1.9%, indicating a tendency to distort when in storage. The flow tends to be highest for the light-bodied and least for the heavy-bodied materials. Light-bodied polysulfides have flexibilities of about 16%; regular-bodied polysulfides, about 14%; and heavy-bodied polysulfides, about 10%. Removal from undercut areas is therefore easier than with the stiffer addition silicones and polyethers. Polysulfides have the highest tear strength of the rubber materials, which allows their use in deep subgingival areas where removal is difficult.

Manipulation

Equal lengths of base and catalyst are extruded on a disposable mixing pad, and the components are mixed thoroughly with a stiff tapered spatula. The catalyst is dark and the base is white, so thorough mixing is readily observed by lack of streaks in the mix. Adequate mixing time is 45 to 60 seconds, and the working time is about 5 to 7 minutes (see Table 7-3). Both working and

setting times are shortened by higher temperatures and humidity. A value of 0.45% is given for shrinkage after 24 hours. Although this period is less than that of the condensation silicones, the cast or die should be poured within 1 hour of taking the impression. Since polysulfides take longer to set than silicones, they require more chair time. They can be electroplated, and some products can be silverplated, but copperplating is not recommended.

Advantages

These materials have a long working time, good tear strength, good flow before setting, good reproduction of surface detail, high flexibility for easier removal around undercuts, and lower cost compared with silicones and polyethers.

Disadvantages

Polysulfides have an unpleasant odor and a tendency to run down the patient's throat due to lower viscosity and will stain clothing permanently. Also, custom-made rather than stock trays are needed because of the greater chance of distortion. Further, polysulfides must be poured within 1 hour and cannot be repoured.

Troubleshooting

Sometimes problems may be encountered when using polysulfide rubber impression materials:

1. *Inadequate working time.* An increase in humidity and/or temperature results in decreased working and setting times. An improper base-to-catalyst ratio could also produce inadequate working time (too much catalyst will reduce working time).
2. *Distortion.* A number of factors cause distortion, one of which is too much load. Because recovery after deformation is dependent on the amount and duration of loading, the impression should not be placed face down on the laboratory bench. Improper removal from the mouth could also cause distortion of the impression; removal should be rapid because permanent deformation is a function of duration of stress. If a bubble is located just below the surface adjacent to a preparation (internal porosity), the impression may distort.
3. *Loss of detail.* Removal before sufficient polymerization or before the material is sufficiently elastic will result in inaccurate registration of detail. Also, failure

to incorporate all of the catalyst into the base will result in incomplete polymerization of portions of the surface. Movement of the tray before removal could also cause loss of detail. The impression tray should be held firmly until the elastic stage is attained.

4. *Surface bubbles or voids.* The incorporation of air into the mix may cause surface bubbles. The impression material should always be mixed carefully with only the flat surface of the blade. If the material is partially polymerized before insertion into the mouth, voids may occur in the impression.

Disinfection

Polysulfide impressions can be disinfected by immersion in sodium hypochlorite, iodophors, complex phenolics, glutaraldehydes, or phenolic glutaraldehydes. The manufacturer's recommendations for proper disinfection should be followed.

Condensation silicone rubber

Condensation silicone rubber impression materials are used mainly for fixed partial denture impressions and are ideal for single-unit inlays. These materials are supplied either as two-paste or paste-liquid catalyst systems. Condensation silicones are available in low, medium, high, and very high (putty) viscosities.

Composition

The base paste usually contains a moderately high-molecular-weight poly(dimethylsiloxane) with terminal hydroxy groups (-OH), an orthoalkylsilicate for cross-linking, and inorganic filler. A paste will contain 30% to 40% filler, whereas a putty will contain as much as 75%. The catalyst paste or liquid usually contains a metal organic ester, such as tin octoate or dibutyl tin dilaurate, and an oily diluent. A thickening agent is also used when making catalyst pastes. Sometimes a catalyst will contain both the orthoalkylsilicate and the metal organic ester:

hydroxy terminated poly(dimethyl-siloxane)   orthoalkylsilicate   tin octoate

The metal organic ester catalyzes the reaction. One part of the polymerization involves chain extension by condensation of the terminal -OH group in a siloxane. The other part consists of cross-linking between chains by the orthoalkylsilicate molecules:

hydroxy terminated poly(dimethyl-siloxane) (base paste)   orthoalkyl-silicate   tin octoate   silicone rubber   alcohol

(catalyst paste or liquid)   (impression)

A volatile alcohol is formed as a by-product.

Mechanical properties

Accepted values for the mechanical properties of these materials are given in Table 7-1. The average value of 99% for elastic recovery is excellent. The flow of silicones is low; most values are less than 0.1%, indicating that less distortion is likely to be caused by light pressure on standing. The silicones are stiffer than polysulfides, as indicated by lower flexibility values in Table 7-1. The shrinkage in 24 hours ranges from 0.2% to 1.0%. About half the shrinkage takes place in the first hour, and it is greater than for polysulfides or polyethers. Polymerization and evaporation of the alcohol formed in the reaction are responsible for this high shrinkage. Accuracy is greatly improved by first taking an impression with a highly filled silicone putty and, after setting, taking a second impression with a light-bodied silicone. Thus, the final total shrinkage is lower.

Manipulation

The manipulation of condensation silicones is the same as for polysulfides, except that the silicone material may be supplied as a base paste plus a liquid catalyst. When it is supplied in this form, one drop per inch of extruded base paste is usually recommended. The setting time (6 to 8 minutes) is less than that of the polysulfides, which saves some chair time. Electroplating is an option. Because of the high polymerization shrinkage, the cast or die must be poured as soon as possible. Higher temperatures and humidity shorten the setting time.

Advantages

Condensation silicones are clean, favorable materials for the patient. They are highly elastic, and the setting time can be controlled with the amount of accelerator. The use of a putty-wash method improves accuracy and eliminates the need for a custom tray.

Disadvantages

These materials tend to be inaccurate due to shrinkage on standing and should be poured within 1 hour. They are very **hydrophobic**, require a very dry field, and are difficult to pour in stone.

Troubleshooting

1. *Inadequate working time.* Although not as critical as polysulfide rubber, the setting times of silicone impression materials are influenced by temperature and humidity. Increases in these conditions tend to shorten both working and setting times. An improper base-to-catalyst ratio could also produce inadequate working time; insufficient catalyst will result in prolonged setting times. Failure to polymerize in the predicted time may result from deterioration during storage.

2. *Distortion.* Failure to remove the impression in a rapid, jerking motion may cause the impression to become permanently deformed. An impression can also become distorted if there is inadequate support of the impression after removal from the mouth. It may undergo permanent deformation if allowed to rest face down on the bench. Excessive delay in pouring the cast (30 minutes or more) also may result in dimensional changes. Possible shrinkage may result from continued polymerization and vaporization of volatiles in the **silicone rubber**. This shrinkage can be compensated for by the double impression technique in which a preliminary impression is made with a very high-viscosity material (putty), providing space for the final impression, which is made with a low-viscosity material using the preliminary impression as the tray.

3. *Loss of detail.* Premature removal of the impression from the mouth could cause loss of detail or plastic deformation. Loss of detail also can be caused by incomplete mixing. Failure to adequately incorporate all of the catalyst into the base will result in incomplete polymerization. Loss of detail can also result from movement of the tray after the impression has been seated; a blurred impression will result if the tray is not stable.

Disinfection

Condensation silicone impressions can be disinfected by immersion in sodium hypochlorite, iodophors, complex phenolics, glutaraldehydes, or phenolic glutaraldehydes. The manufacturer's recommendations for proper disinfection should be followed.

Addition (vinyl) silicones

The accuracy of **addition silicones** is due to a change in polymerization reactions to an addition type and the elimination of an alcohol by-product that evaporates, causing shrinkage. These materials are available as two-paste systems in four viscosities—light, medium, heavy, and putty—and a range of colors, allowing monitoring of the degree of mixing. Addition silicones are rigid after setting. Due to their high accuracy, these materials are suitable for fixed and removable partial denture impressions. They are expensive, however, and therefore are not used for routine study casts. Hydrophilic materials have been introduced that reportedly contain surfactants to improve the wetting characteristics compared with those of unmodified silicones (Fig 7-3). Monophase materials have been formulated with sufficient shear thinning to be used as both low-viscosity and high-viscosity materials.

Composition

These materials are based on silicone prepolymers with vinyl and hydrogen side groups, which can polymerize by addition polymerization. They are therefore called *vinyl* or *addition* silicones. The setting reaction is produced by mixing one paste containing the vinyl-poly(dimethylsiloxane) prepolymer with a second paste that contains a siloxane prepolymer with hydrogen side groups. One of the pastes contains a platinum catalyst, chloroplatinic acid, which starts the addition polymerization reaction as follows:

$$\underset{\substack{\text{vinyl terminated}\\\text{siloxane}}}{\overset{\displaystyle \begin{array}{c} CH_3 \\ | \\ -Si-\\ | \\ CH_3 \end{array}}{}} \overset{\substack{\text{silane}}}{\underset{}{\begin{array}{c} | \\ CH=CH_2 + H-Si-CH_3 \\ | \end{array}}} \xrightarrow{\substack{H_2PtCl_6 \\ \text{chloroplatinic}\\ \text{acid}}} \underset{\substack{\text{silicone rubber}}}{\begin{array}{c} | \quad\quad | \\ CH_3-Si-CH_2-CH_2-Si-CH_3 \\ | \quad\quad | \end{array}}$$

Other reactions may release hydrogen gas, which on rare occasion can produce porosity. Some manufacturers include hydrogen absorbers in their formulations to eliminate this problem. Since no volatile by-products are produced in the reaction, addition silicones have a much greater dimensional stability than condensation silicones.

Mechanical properties

The working and setting times of addition silicones are faster than polysulfides; a retarder is often supplied to extend the working and setting times. Addition silicones have excellent elasticity and show very low dimensional shrinkage when stored (see Table 7-1). Therefore, addition silicones can be safely poured later or sent to a dental laboratory. Addition silicones do have greater rigidity, however, and therefore it is difficult to remove the impression around undercuts, as indicated by the lower flexibility value. The tear strength of addition silicones is similar to that of condensation silicones but less than that of polysulfides.

Manipulation

Addition silicones are as easy to handle as condensation silicones. Because there is the possibility of hydrogen release on setting, finely divided palladium is added to some products to absorb the hydrogen and prevent bubbles from forming on stone die surfaces. If a product does not contain a hydrogen absorber, an hour should pass before pouring dies, and the impression should stand overnight before epoxy dies are poured. Automatic mixers that provide quick, bubble-free mixes are available with several products. Addition silicones can be electroplated with both copper and silver.

Advantages

Addition silicones are highly accurate and have high dimensional stability after setting. Recovery from deformation on removal is excellent. The material stays in the tray of reclined patients, does not stain clothing, is available in pleasant colors and scents, may be used with stock or custom trays, and can be copper- or silver-plated. The materials may be poured 1 week after taking the impression, and multiple pours are possible.

Disadvantages

The material is expensive—twice the cost of polysulfides; it is more rigid than condensation silicones and is difficult to remove around undercuts; it has a moderate tear strength, making removal from gingival retraction areas somewhat risky; and it may release hydrogen gas on setting, producing bubbles on die surfaces if the material does not contain a hydrogen absorber. Hydro-

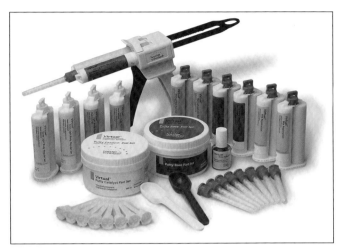

Fig 7-3 A current hydrophilic impression material. (Courtesy of Ivoclar Vivadent.)

phobic materials are difficult to electroplate and to pour in stone. Also, sulfur in latex gloves and rubber dam can inhibit polymerization.

Troubleshooting

1. *Inadequate working time.* As the temperature increases, the working and setting times decrease. If the impression material does not set, the catalyst may have been contaminated. The platinum-containing catalyst becomes inactive after contacting certain substances, such as tin or sulfur compounds. If addition silicones are combined with condensation silicones, the material will not set. Components from these two systems are not compatible and cannot be mixed together.

2. *Loss of detail.* The use of unmodified addition silicones could result in loss of detail. These hydrophobic materials cannot displace any moisture or hemorrhage that is not removed before placement of the impression material.

3. *Porosity.* The stone surface may appear porous if hydrogen gas is evolved, and so it is recommended that the pouring of dies be delayed for at least 1 hour.

4. *Distortion.* If the polysiloxane adhesive does not provide adequate retention, distortion may occur. Mechanical retention may be required in combination with the adhesive.

Disinfection

Addition silicone impressions can be disinfected by immersion in sodium hypochlorite, iodophors, complex phenolics, glutaraldehydes, or phenolic glutaraldehydes. The manufacturer's recommendations for proper disinfection should be followed.

Polyether rubber

The high stiffness and short working time of **polyether** rubbers restricts their use to impressions of a few teeth. They give accurate impressions without severe undercuts. Polyethers are available in low-, medium-, and high-viscosity materials.

Composition

These materials are supplied as two-paste systems. The base paste contains low-molecular-weight polyether with ethyleneimine **terminal groups**:

$$-N \begin{cases} CH_2 \\ | \\ CH_2 \end{cases}$$

along with fillers, such as colloidal silica, and plasticizers:

$$CH_3 - \overset{\overset{\displaystyle H}{|}}{C} - CH_2 - \overset{\overset{\displaystyle O}{||}}{C} - O - R - O - \overset{\overset{\displaystyle O}{||}}{C} - CH_2 - \overset{\overset{\displaystyle H}{|}}{C} - CH_3$$

$$\begin{matrix} N \\ | \\ CH_2 - CH_2 \end{matrix} \qquad \begin{matrix} N \\ | \\ CH_2 - CH_2 \end{matrix}$$

Polyether

The catalyst paste contains an aromatic sulfonic acid ester plus a thickening agent and fillers:

$$SO_3CH_2CH_3$$

Sulfonic ester

When the base paste is mixed with the catalyst paste, ionic polymerization occurs by ring opening of the ethyleneimine group and chain extension. The reaction converts the paste to a rubber as follows:

polyether + sulfonic ester → polyether rubber
(base paste)   (catalyst)   (impression)

Mechanical properties

Polyethers are similar to addition silicones. The early polyethers had short working and setting times and low flexibilities. Thinners were available to increase the working time and flexibility without any significant loss of other physical or mechanical properties. However, more recent formulations have a working time of 2.5 minutes and a setting time of 4.5 minutes (see Table 7-3). Shrinkage values of 0.3% in 24 hours place the polyethers at the upper end of the range for accuracy, but they are inferior to some addition silicones. Because this rubber absorbs water and changes dimensions, storage in water is not recommended. Elastic recovery values average 98.5%, between those for polysulfides and addition silicones (see Table 7-1). The flow of polyethers is very low and contributes to accuracy. The flexibility also is low (ie, the stiffness is high). This quality causes some problems on removal of the impression from the mouth or the die from the impression. More rubber between the tray and the impression area is recommended to relieve this problem. Polyethers have low tear strength values.

Manipulation

The manipulation of polyethers is similar to that of polysulfides and silicones. Equal lengths of base and catalyst paste are mixed vigorously and rapidly (30 to 45 seconds), because the working time is short. They are easy to mix. The impressions can be readily silverplated to produce accurate dies. Precautions should be taken to mix the material thoroughly and to avoid contact of the catalyst with the skin or mucosa because tissue reactions have been observed.

A handheld gun-type mixer that provides quick, bubble-free mixes is available for Permadyne Garant (3M ESPE). Also, an automatic mixing device (Pentamix, 3M ESPE) (Fig 7-4) is available for use with a polyether packaged in polybags (Impregum Penta).

Advantages

Polyethers are easy to handle and to mix. These materials are more accurate than polysulfide or condensation silicone impression materials. They have good surface detail reproduction and are easily poured in stone. If kept dry, they will be dimensionally stable for up to 1 week.

Disadvantages

The cost of these materials is high, working and setting times are short, and there is high stiffness after setting,

Fig 7-4 The Pentamix 2 is used for mixing a variety of impression materials (3M ESPE).

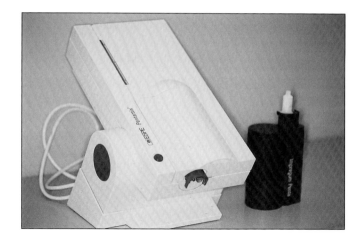

which limit their use. Their bitter taste is objectionable to some patients. Storage of polyether impressions is critical, as they will distort if stored in water or high humidity. They cannot be left in disinfectant solutions for long periods.

Troubleshooting

1. *Inadequate working time.* An increase in temperature will decrease the working and setting times. An improper base-to-catalyst ratio (too much catalyst) will also decrease the working time.
2. *Tearing.* The rigidity of this material may result in tearing on removal of the impression from the mouth or of the die from the impression. Tearing may occur if the rubber thickness is inadequate (at least 4 mm).
3. *Distortion.* The impression may distort due to moisture absorption and/or plasticizer extraction. These phenomena may result in dimensional change when impressions are stored in high-humidity environments or are exposed to water. The use of the thinner may increase water absorption. Delay in impression placement also may cause distortion. The onset of setting will result in the formation of elastic properties, which will cause deformation on removal from the mouth.
4. *Loss of detail.* Failure to obtain a homogeneous mix will result in incomplete polymerization. If problems are encountered with multiple dies, it may be the result of gingival tearing and/or swelling. The rigidity and the relatively low tear strength of the polyethers

may result in progressive deterioration at the gingival margin of the impression. The impression may absorb enough moisture from the gypsum that multiple pours could produce swelling.

Disinfection

Polyether impressions can be disinfected by immersion in sodium hypochlorite. The manufacturer's recommendations for proper disinfection should be followed.

Dental Duplicating Materials

Dental duplicating materials are used to prepare duplicate casts for prosthetic appliances and orthodontic casts. These materials are used to make an impression of the original dental cast. Agar hydrocolloid duplicating materials are used most frequently. Their composition has a higher water content than agar hydrocolloid impression materials, and subsequently, a lower agar content. Therefore, the compressive strengths for duplicating materials are generally lower than those of impression materials. Advantages of the reversible materials are that they can be reused a number of times and may be stored in the liquid state for use as needed. Disadvantages include the necessity for immediate pours as well as accelerated degradation of the material by contamination. A classification is shown in Fig 7-5.

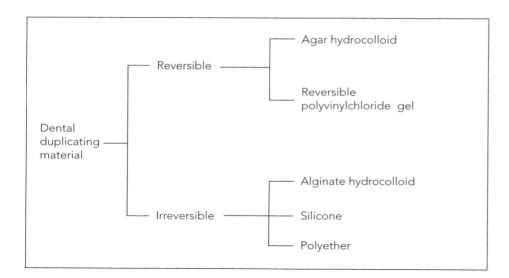

Fig 7-5 A classification for dental duplicating materials.

■ Clinical Decision Scenarios for Dental Impression Materials

This section presents one approach for choosing impression materials for specific situations based on consideration of the advantages and disadvantages of each material and taking into account the different practitioner requirements, such as skill level, cost factors, among others, as applicable.

Each scenario includes *(1)* a description of the situation; *(2)* a list of the critical factors; *(3)* a list of the advantages and disadvantages of each material prioritized using the following codes: • of minor importance, •• important, ••• very important; and *(4)* an analysis of the situation and the decision reached.

■ Glossary

addition silicone A silicone polymer resulting from the free-radical polymerization of vinyl groups by a platinum catalyst.

agar An ingredient in agar impression material. It is usually extracted from seaweed as a polysaccharide.

alginate Alginate impression material containing salts of alginic acid.

cast material Material used to form casts or dies from impressions.

condensation (in polymerization) In a condensation polymerization (eg, to form silicone impression materials), two molecules unite and one small molecule (eg, H_2O, ROH) is released as a by-product.

$$\sim\text{Si-OH} + \text{R-O-Si}\sim \rightarrow \text{ROH} + \sim\text{Si-O-Si}\sim$$

Materials Polysulfides vs addition silicones in a dental school clinic

Situation An instructor at a dental school has been asked to determine which impression material will be used in the undergraduate crown-and-bridge clinics. There is a fixed budget that, typical of universities, dictates the use of inexpensive materials. The students are slow and unskilled at their stage of training, so a material allowing long working time is desirable. In addition, the students have not yet developed their gingival retraction techniques to the point that they have a wide sulcus into which to inject their syringe material. Therefore, a material with a high tear strength is desirable so the gingival area will not tear off from the main part of the impression and remain in the sulcus on removal of the tray. After review of the materials available, all are rejected except for the polysulfides (mercaptans) and the addition silicones (polyvinyl siloxanes).

Critical Factors Low cost, long working time, high tear strength

POLYSULFIDES	ADDITION SILICONES
ADVANTAGES	ADVANTAGES
••• Longer working time ••• Lower cost ••• Good tear resistance • High flexibility (easy to remove from undercuts) ••• Good accuracy	• Good dimensional stability (can be mailed unpoured) • Short setting time ••• Very accurate • Easy to mix and clean up • No disagreeable odor or taste • Rigid material
DISADVANTAGES	DISADVANTAGES
• Disagreeable odor and taste • Can stain clothing • Low dimensional stability (should be poured within 1 hour) • Longer setting time	••• High cost • Low flexibility (harder to remove from undercuts) ••• Shorter working time ••• Lower tear resistance (may tear off in deep subgingival areas) • Some emit hydrogen gas (pouring must be delayed)

Analysis/Decision Since the factors identified as important were low cost, high tear strength, and long working time, all these properties are marked ••• under advantages or disadvantages, as is the property of good accuracy. This trait is essential in any impression material used for crown-and-bridge procedures. Because accuracy is an advantage of both materials, it cancels out and is not a deciding factor.

In this example, the factors the dentist is interested in are advantages for the polysulfides but not for the addition silicones. The choice is easy—polysulfides are selected.

The next step is to conduct a trial of the chosen material to see if this decision is well founded. For example, one-half of the class takes impressions with polysulfide, and the other half uses the material previously used. If the polysulfide works well in the hands of students and is less expensive than the addition silicone, the trial confirms the decision.

Materials Polysulfides vs addition silicones in a busy practice

Situation An experienced clinician in a busy practice has been using agar hydrocolloid in water-cooled trays but has heard that the new elastomeric impression materials have become more dimensionally stable than they were originally. She is interested in trying either a polysulfide or an addition silicone. She has always obtained very good impressions with the agar hydrocolloid material but has never liked having to interrupt her busy schedule to pour the impressions right away. She feels that her time could be better used if a technician could set the dowel pins and pour the impression, but she has not felt that her practice is large enough to justify an in-office laboratory technician. She has likewise been unable to send the agar hydrocolloid impressions to a laboratory for pouring because of the material's properties.

The clinician realizes that to use a polysulfide material, she should use custom trays due to the lack of dimensional stability of the material. However, she does not like to take the dental assistant away from chairside for the time required to make a tray because productivity is decreased. She would prefer a material with sufficient dimensional stability that it could be used in a disposable stock plastic tray. She is also looking for a material that will set much faster than the agar so she can decrease chair time for a crown impression.

Critical Factors Low cost, short setting time, good dimensional stability

POLYSULFIDES	ADDITION SILICONES
ADVANTAGES	ADVANTAGES
• Longer working time ••• Lower cost • Good tear resistance • High flexibility (easy to remove from undercuts) ••• Good accuracy	••• Good dimensional stability (can be mailed unpoured) ••• Short setting time ••• Very accurate • Easy to mix and clean up • No disagreeable odor or taste • Rigid material
DISADVANTAGES	DISADVANTAGES
• Disagreeable odor and taste • Can stain clothing ••• Low dimensional stability (should be poured within 1 hour) ••• Longer setting time	••• High cost • Low flexibility (harder to remove from undercuts) •• Shorter working time • Lower tear resistance (may tear off in deep subgingival areas) • Some emit hydrogen gas (pouring must be delayed)

Analysis/Decision Here the decision is less obvious than in the previous example. The addition silicone seems to offer much of what the dentist desires, but it costs twice as much as the polysulfide. In this case, the decision might be in favor of the polysulfide due to the significant cost difference. After the trial period, however, the dentist confirmed her suspicion that the polysulfide was not stable enough to use stock trays, and it took 15 to 30 minutes for either her or her assistant to fabricate the custom trays. She also found that that use of "putty" material to line the stock tray greatly reduced the cost of the addition silicone. Furthermore, she found that placing dowel pins and pouring up the polysulfide took another 15 to 30 minutes of someone's time. The amount of time lost from chairside production more than offset the higher cost of the addition silicones, whose properties allowed her to use stock trays and to mail the impressions to her laboratory. Seeing this in her trial, the dentist reconsidered and changed to the addition silicone, which satisfied her needs.

Materials Polysulfides vs addition silicones for "triple tray"

Situation The dentist has been using the polysulfides and is quite content but wishes to try a new impression technique that is gaining great favor among his peers. This method uses what is known as a triple tray and has the advantage for the single crown of obtaining the working impression, the opposing impression, and the bite relation all at the same time. A significant amount of time could be saved for each patient. The dentist finds, however, that the sides of the flimsy plastic trays sometimes spread apart when the dental arches impinge on them as the patient bites into position. The tray then attempts to spring back from this distortion when it is removed from the mouth. The recovery from the spreading requires that he use a material with sufficient rigidity that it can maintain its shape against this elastic recovery of the tray. If not, the tray recovery may distort the impression and result in a nonfitting crown.

Critical Factors Low flexibility, good dimensional stability

POLYSULFIDES	ADDITION SILICONES
ADVANTAGES	ADVANTAGES
• Longer working time • Lower cost • Good tear resistance ••• Good accuracy	••• Good dimensional stability (can be mailed unpoured) • Short setting time ••• Very accurate • Easy to mix and clean up • No disagreeable odor or taste ••• Rigid material
DISADVANTAGES	DISADVANTAGES
••• High flexibility (easy to remove from undercuts) • Disagreeable odor and taste • Can stain clothing ••• Low dimensional stability (should be poured within 1 hour) • Longer setting time	• High cost ••• Low flexibility (hard to remove from undercuts) • Shorter working time • Lower tear resistance (may tear off in deep subgingival areas) • Some emit hydrogen gas (pouring must be delayed)

Analysis/Decision In this case, the trial period showed that the addition silicone was the only feasible choice. The need for rigidity in the impression material for the triple tray is important enough that it becomes the deciding factor. Although other factors, such as accuracy, are important, unless the material is rigid enough to hold its shape, these other properties are meaningless.

Materials   Polysulfides vs addition silicones for full-arch impression

Situation   In this situation, the dentist is a prosthodontist in an established specialty practice. He has a dental laboratory in his office and employs two laboratory technicians. He therefore has the capability of having custom trays made in his office and the impressions poured right away. Most of his patients have been referred from dentists who do the easier cases themselves. Consequently, his patients usually already have multiple crowns or fixed partial dentures in different areas of the mouth. He feels that full-arch impressions are better because, in the more extensive cases, he needs the accuracy in bite relations that can only come from full-arch registration. He has heard that addition silicones are very accurate and that they have better dimensional stability than the material he has been using. This appeals to him for "pickup" impressions where a rigid material and better dimensional stability greatly enhance the probability of success. On the other hand, he is concerned that the stiffness of the addition silicone will make the removal of full-arch impressions from the mouth much more difficult. He is also concerned that the stiffness may pose a greater risk of inadvertently removing crowns or fixed partial dentures that his patients already have in other areas of the mouth.

Critical Factors   Good accuracy, high flexibility, good dimensional stability

POLYSULFIDES	ADDITION SILICONES
ADVANTAGES	ADVANTAGES
<ul><li>Longer working time</li><li>Lower cost</li><li>Good tear resistance</li><li>••• High flexibility (easy to remove from undercuts)</li><li>••• Good accuracy</li></ul>	<ul><li>••• Good dimensional stability</li><li>Short setting time</li><li>••• Very accurate</li><li>Easy to mix and clean up</li><li>No disagreeable odor or taste</li><li>Rigid material</li></ul>
DISADVANTAGES	DISADVANTAGES
<ul><li>Disagreeable odor and taste</li><li>Can stain clothing</li><li>••• Low dimensional stability (should be poured within 1 hour)</li><li>Longer setting time</li></ul>	<ul><li>High cost</li><li>••• Low flexibility (harder to remove from undercuts)</li><li>Shorter working time</li><li>Lower tear resistance (may tear off in deep subgingival areas)</li><li>Some emit hydrogen gas (pouring must be delayed)</li></ul>

Analysis/Decision   The high flexibility listed under the advantages of polysulfides is offset by the rigidity listed as an advantage under addition silicones. He found that the rigidity was desirable for pickup impressions, but the flexibility was desirable for regular impressions. He decided to try the addition silicone and found that it did, indeed, give very accurate and dimensionally stable impressions. His pickup impressions were better than they had ever been. However, in normal situations the rigidity of the material made removal of the full-arch impressions much more difficult. Some crowns and fixed partial dentures on which he was not working came off in the impression material because of its rigidity. He found, however, that he could compensate for this rigidity by filling the impression tray only partially full in the areas where he only needed the occlusal registration and filling it full in the area of the preparations.

condensation silicone A silicone polymer resulting from the condensation of terminal -OH groups by ortho-alkylsilicates and releasing alcohol as a by-product.

elastic recovery The amount of rebound after a cylinder of material is strained 10% for 30 seconds.

electroplate The process of depositing metal from solution onto the surface of an impression using an electric current.

eugenol Oil of cloves. As a derivative of phenol, eugenol reacts as an acid with zinc oxide.

flexibility The amount of strain produced when a sample is stressed between 100 and 1,000 g/cm². A flexible material shows a higher value of flexibility than a stiff material.

flow The amount of shortening of a cylinder when placed under a light load for 15 minutes.

gel A colloid system in which the solid (eg, agar) and liquid (eg, water) are continuous phases. A gel is usually flexible.

hydrocolloid A colloid system in which the liquid phase is water. Agar impression material is a hydrocolloid (agar + water).

hydrophilic Having a strong affinity for water; can be readily wetted by water.

hydrophobic Resistant to wetting by water.

hysteresis The phenomenon of a gel's having a liquefaction temperature different from the solidification temperature of the sol.

imbibition The taking up of fluid by a colloidal system, resulting in swelling.

plasticizer A material that is added to increase flow.

polyether The polymer resulting from the ionic polymerization with ring opening of the ethyleneimine group and chain extension.

polysulfide The polymer resulting from the condensation of terminal mercaptan groups catalyzed by lead dioxide or other catalysts.

silicone rubber A polymer resulting from the formation of silicon-oxygen-silicon bonds (-Si-O-Si-). Silicone impression material is a silicone rubber.

sol A colloid system in which the solid phase is dispersed in the liquid phase. A sol usually has fluid properties.

syneresis The exudation of a liquid film on the surface of a gel.

terminal group A chemical group at the end of a molecule (eg, -SH).

thermal conductivity The quantity of heat passing through a body 1 cm thick with a cross section of 1 cm² when the temperature difference between the hot and cold sides of the body is 1°C.

thermoplastic The property of softening on heating and hardening on cooling.

working time Duration from the start of mixing to the time when a test rod leaves a permanent indentation in the material on withdrawal.

Discussion Questions

1. Why are there so many impression materials in dentistry?

2. How could the movement of soft tissues during impression taking affect the accuracy of the final impression?

3. Since elastic impression materials are viscoelastic, wouldn't immediate pouring of a gypsum cast result in inaccuracy?

4. Why is it essential to sterilize an impression before sending it to a laboratory, and how is this done?

5. Why is the impression tray an important factor in obtaining a good impression?

Study Questions

(See appendix E for answers.)

1. What are the components of dental compound, and what is the purpose of each?

2. What term describes the quality of dental compound that allows it to be repeatedly softened on heating and hardened on cooling?

3. What is the principal difference between the properties of impression and tray-type compounds?

4. What precautions should be taken when heating dental compound?

5. What importance does low thermal conductivity have on the clinical handling of dental impression compound?

6. What factors affect the flow of impression compound?

7. What are the reactive ingredients in a zinc oxide–eugenol material?

8. What is responsible for the setting of zinc oxide–eugenol impression paste?

9. What factors affect the setting time of zinc oxide–eugenol?

10. What are the functions of the various components in agar hydrocolloid?

11. What is meant by *hysteresis* in agar hydrocolloid?

12. What kinds of dimensional changes occur when an agar impression is stored in air, water, 100% relative humidity, or potassium sulfate solution?

13. What is the function of each of the components in alginate powder?

14. What factors affect the setting time of alginates?

15. What reaction is responsible for providing the working time of alginate, and what other reaction is responsible for the setting of alginate?

16. Why are alginate impression materials called *irreversible hydrocolloids*?

17. What effect does the W/P ratio of alginates have on their properties?

18. What effect does spatulation of alginates have on their properties?

19. What effect does water temperature have on the working and setting times of alginates?

20. How do the properties of alginate impression materials compare with those of agar impression materials?

21 Describe the setting reactions for polysulfide, silicone, and polyether rubber impression materials.

22. What effect do proportioning and temperature have on the working and setting times of the three rubber impression materials?

23. What impression material may be used if you wish to use either a gypsum die, a silverplated die, or a copperplated die?

24. Compare the elastic recoveries of polysulfide, silicone, and polyether impression materials. How does elastic recovery affect clinical usage?

25. Compare the flexibilities of polysulfide, silicone, and polyether impression materials.

26. How would you disinfect your impression before sending it to the laboratory?

27. List the advantages of each of the following recent advances in impression materials: *(a)* addition silicones with hydrophilic properties; *(b)* single-viscosity or monophase, addition silicones; *(c)* automatic mixers for addition silicones and polyethers.

■ References

1. American National Standards Institute/American Dental Association. ANSI/ADA Specification No. 11-1997. Dental Agar Impression Material. Chicago: American Dental Association, 1997.
2. American Dental Association. ADA Specification No. 18-1992. Dental Alginate Impression Material. Chicago: American Dental Association, 1992.
3. American National Standards Institute/American Dental Association. ANSI/ADA Specification No. 19-2003. Dental Elastomeric Impression Materials. Chicago: American Dental Association, 2003.
4. American National Standards Institute/American Dental Association. ANSI/ADA Specification No. 20-1972. Dental Duplicating Material. Chicago: American Dental Association, 1972.
5. Roydhouse RH. Materials in Dentistry. Chicago: Year Book Medical Publishers, 1962.

■ Recommended Reading

Albers HF. Impressions: A Text for Selection of Materials and Techniques. Santa Rosa, CA: Alto Books, 1990.

Allen EP, Bayne SC, Donovan TE, et al. Annual review of selected dental literature. J Prosthet Dent 1996;76:75.

Anderson JN. Flow and elasticity in alginates. Dent Progr 1960;1:63–74.

Anusavice KJ. Dental impression materials: Reactor response. Adv Dent Res 1988;2:65–70.

Boening KW, Walter MH, Schuette U. Clinical significance of surface activation of silicone impression materials. J Dent 1998;26:447.

Braden M. Characterization of the setting process in dental polysulfide rubbers. J Dent Res 1966;45:1065–1071.

Braden M, Causton B, Clarke RL. A polyether impression rubber. J Dent Res 1972;51:889–896.

Braden M, Elliot JC. Characterization of the setting process of silicone dental rubbers. J Dent Res 1966;45:1016–1023.

Buchan S, Peggie RW. Role of ingredients in alginate impression compounds. J Dent Res 1966;45:1120–1129.

Chee WW, Donovan TE. Polyvinyl siloxane impression materials: A review of properties and techniques. J Prosthet Dent 1992;68:728–732.

Chen SY, Liang WM, Chen FN. Factors affecting the accuracy of elastoometic impression materials. J Dent 2004;32:603.

Chong JA, Chong MP, Docking AR. The surface of gypsum cast in alginate impressions. Dent Pract 1965;16:107–109.

Council on Dental Materials and Devices. Status report on polyether impression materials. J Am Dent Assoc 1977;95:126–130.

Council on Dental Materials, Instruments, and Devices. Vinyl polysiloxane impression materials: A status report. J Am Dent Assoc 1990;120:595–596, 598, 600.

Council on Dental Materials, Instruments, and Devices. Disinfection of impressions. J Am Dent Assoc 1991;122(8):110.

Council on Dental Materials, Instruments, and Devices. Retarding the setting of vinyl polysiloxane impressions. J Am Dent Assoc 1991;122(8):114.

Council on Dental Materials, Instruments, and Devices; Council on Dental Therapeutics; Council on Dental Research; Council on Dental Practice. Infection control recommendations for the dental office and the dental laboratory. J Am Dent Assoc 1992;123 (suppl):1–8.

Council on Dental Materials, Instruments and Equipment; Council on Dental Therapeutics. Clinical Products in Dentistry: A Desktop Reference. Chicago: American Dental Association, 1993.

Craig RG. A review of properties of rubber impression materials. J Mich Dent Assoc 1977;59:254–261.

Craig RG. Evaluation of an automatic mixing system for an addition silicone impression material. J Am Dent Assoc 1985;110:213–215.

Craig RG. Review of dental impression materials. Adv Dent Res 1988; 2:51–64.

Craig RG, O'Brien WJ, Powers JM. Dental Materials—Properties and Manipulation, ed 6. St Louis: Mosby, 1996.

Craig RG, Sun Z. Trends in elastomeric impression materials. Oper Dent 1994;19:138–145.

Craig RG, Urquiola NJ, Liu CC. Comparison of commercial elastomeric impression materials. Oper Dent 1990;15:94–104.

Farah JM, Powers JM. Impressions and accessories. The Dental Advisor 1992;9(4):1–8.

Donovan TE, Chee WW. A review of contemporary impression materials and techniques. Dent Clin North Am 2004;48:445.

Fish SF, Braden M. Characterization of the setting process in alginate impression materials. J Dent Res 1964;43:107–117.

Harris WT Jr. Water temperature and accuracy of alginate impressions. J Prosthet Dent 1969;21:613–617.

Johnson GH, Craig RG. Accuracy and bond strength of combination agar/alginate hydrocolloid impression materials. J Prosthet Dent 1986;55:1–6.

Kahn RL, Donovan TE, Chee WW. Interaction of gloves and rubber dam with a poly(vinyl siloxane) impression material: A screening test. Int J Prosthodont 1989;2:342–346.

Kim K-N, Craig RG, Koran A III. Viscosity of monophase addition silicones as a function of shear rate. J Prosthet Dent 1992;67:794–798.

Lautenschlager EP, Miyamoto P, Hilton R. Elastic recovery of polysulfide base impressions. J Dent Res 1972;51:773–779.

MacPherson GW, Craig RG, Peyton FA. Mechanical properties of hydrocolloid and rubber impression materials. J Dent Res 1967; 46:714–721.

Marker VA. Dental impression materials. In: Okabe T, Takahashi S (eds). Transactions of the First International Congress on Dental Materials. Honolulu, HI: Univ of Hawaii, 1989:114–138.

Merchant VA. Update on disinfection of impressions, prostheses, and casts. J Calif Dent Assoc 1992;20:31–35.

McCabe JF, Wilson HJ. Addition curing silicone rubber impression materials: An appraisal of the physical properties. Br Dent J 1978; 145:17–20.

McLean JW. Physical properties influencing the accuracy of silicone and thiokol impression materials. Br Dent J 1961;110:85–91.

Myers GE, Peyton FA. Clinical and physical studies of the silicone rubber impression materials. J Prosthet Dent 1959;9:315–324.

Myers GE, Peyton FA. Physical properties of the zinc oxide–eugenol impression pastes. J Dent Res 1961;40:39–48.

Myers GE, Stockman DG. Factors that affect the accuracy and dimensional stability of the mercaptan rubber base impression materials. J Prosthet Dent 1960;10:525–535.

Naylor WP, Evans DB. An overview of impression materials and techniques for fixed prosthodontics. In: Hardin JF (ed). Clark's Clinical Dentistry, vol 4. Hagerstown, MD: Harper and Row, 1991.

Pratten DH, Craig RG. Wettability of a hydrophilic addition silicone impression material. J Prosthet Dent 1989;61:197–202.

Pratten DH, Novetsky M. Detail reproduction of soft tissue: A comparison of impression materials. J Prosthet Dent 1991;65:188–191.

Rosenblum MA, Asgar K, Leinfelder KF. Dental prosthetic materials. In: Reese JA, Valega TM (eds). Restorative Dental Materials, vol I. London: Quintessence, 1985:158–168.

Smith DC, Wilson HJ. Further studies on alginate impression materials. Dent Pract 1965;15:380–382.

Stackhouse JA Jr. The accuracy of stone dies made from rubber impression materials. J Prosthet Dent 1970;24:377–386.

Stackhouse JA Jr. Electrodeposition in dentistry: A review of the literature. J Prosthet Dent 1980;44:259–263.

Stackhouse JA Jr. Impression materials and electrodeposits. Part I. Impression materials. J Prosthet Dent 1981;45:44–48.

Stackhouse JA Jr. Impression materials and electrodeposits. Part II. Electrodeposits. J Prosthet Dent 1981;45:146–151.

Stannard JG, Sadighi-Nouri M. Retarders for polyvinylsiloxane impression materials: Evaluation and recommendations. J Prosthet Dent 1986;55:7–10.

Wilson HJ. Some properties of alginate impression materials relevant to clinical practice. Br Dent J 1966;121:463–467.

Wilson HJ. Elastomeric impression materials. I. The setting material. Br Dent J 1966;121:277–283.

Wilson HJ, Smith DC. Alginate impression materials. Br Dent J 1963;114:20–26.

CHAPTER 8

Polymeric Restorative Materials

The first material developed for use as a direct esthetic restorative was silicate cement, which was prepared from an alumina-silica glass and a phosphoric acid liquid. Introduced in the late 1800s, the cement remained the favored material until the early 1950s. Its main advantage was the slow release of fluoride from the glass phase, but silicate is highly soluble in oral fluids and deteriorates rapidly. Dissolution, discoloration, loss of translucency, and lack of adequate mechanical properties contributed to its eventual replacement.

Self-curing unfilled acrylic resins were introduced around 1945 as a substitute for silicate cement and were in moderate use in the 1950s. These materials were related to denture base resins and were much less soluble and more color stable than silicates. In addition, they were easy to use and polishable and provided good initial esthetics. Their main problems were high shrinkage during polymerization, large thermal dimensional change, eventual discoloration, and a high wear rate.

A *composite* is a material composed of two or more distinct phases. **Resin composites** for dental use were formulated to combine the esthetics and ease of use of a polymerizable resin base with the improved properties to be gained from the addition of a ceramic filler. This combination of hard, inorganic filler particles bonded to soft dimethacrylate polymer was introduced in the 1960s, originally intended for use in anterior Class 3, 4, and 5 restorations where esthetics are important. As a consequence of the bonded filler phase, these materials had much better mechanical properties than did unfilled resins, approaching the properties of dentin and enamel.

Improvements have included light curing, bonding to tooth structure, and reduced wear. Continued development in wear resistance, dentin bonding, and reduced polymerization shrinkage has led to their increased use in posterior restorations.

Composition and Reaction

Polymer matrix

The organic polymer matrix in currently available composites is most commonly an aromatic or urethane diacrylate **oligomer** such as bisphenol A glycidyl methacrylate (bis-GMA) or urethane dimethacrylate, represented by the simplified formula:

$$CH_2 = C - R - C = CH_2$$
$$\;\;\;\;\;\;\;\; | \;\;\;\;\;\;\;\; |$$
$$\;\;\;\;\;\;CH_3 \;\;\;\; CH_3$$

where R may be any of a number of organic groups, such as methyl-, hydroxyl-, phenyl-, carboxyl-, and amide-.

Oligomers have reactive double bonds at each end of the molecule that are able to undergo addition polymerization in the presence of free radicals. The oligomer molecules are highly viscous and require the addition of low-molecular-weight diluent **monomers**, usually triethylene glycol dimethacrylate, so a clinically workable consistency may be maintained when the filler is incorporated.

Coupling agents

A bond between filler particle and matrix in the set composite is achieved by use of an organic silicon compound, or silane **coupling agent**. The silane molecule has reactive groups at both ends and is coated on the filler particle surface by the manufacturer before mixing with the oligomer. During polymerization, double bonds on the silane molecule also react with the polymer matrix. A bond between filler and matrix allows the distribution of stresses generated under function. The net result is a material with strength properties greater than those of the particulate filler or the matrix separately or the filler combined with the unsilanated matrix. Bonding also enhances the retention of the filler particle during abrasive action at the composite surface, greatly improving the wear resistance of the material. Effective silane coupling of each filler particle to the organic resin matrix also reduces the absorption of water from the oral environment. Decreased water sorption will result in better dimensional and color stability of the material over time.

Initiators and accelerators

Polymerization of composites may be initiated by chemical means (self cure) or by visible-light activation. Dual cure is a combination of light and chemical curing. In chemically activated systems, an organic peroxide **initiator** (or catalyst) reacts with a tertiary **amine accelerator**, producing **free radicals** that attack the double bonds of oligomer molecules and initiate addition polymerization.

Initiation of polymerization in light-activated systems depends on generation of free radicals with a diketone (camphorquinone) and aliphatic amine when irradiated with blue light. For both systems, the following general reaction occurs:

Dimethacrylate + Initiator (benzoyl-peroxide or diketone with blue light) + Accelerator (aromatic amine or aliphatic amine)

+ Silane-treated filler particles → Dental composite

Because **dimethacrylate** oligomers as well as dimethacrylate diluent monomers have reactive double bonds at each end of the molecules, polymerization results in a highly **cross-linked polymer**.

Other ingredients

Inorganic oxide pigments are added to composites in small amounts to provide a range of standard shades. Most often, four shades, ranging from yellow to gray, are supplied. In response to consumer interest, manufacturers now offer an extended range of 16 to 25 shades, matched to the Vita ceramic shade guide. Most manufacturers offer modifiers such as highly pigmented tints for characterizing standard shades and creating opaque layers to block out tooth discolorations. There are also highly translucent incisal shades, extra-white bleach shades, and surface glazes to customize esthetic procedures. Polymerization inhibitors and stabilizers are added to the composite to lengthen shelf life.

Filler composition

Filler particles are of inorganic composition. In addition to quartz, fine-sized particles may be composed of barium or lithium aluminum silicate glasses; borosilicate glass; or barium, strontium, or zinc glasses. Colloidal silica particles make up microfilled composites, and radiopaque composites are made by incorporating elements of high atomic weight, such as barium, strontium, zirconium, or ytterbium, into the glass filler particles. Resin composites are often classified according to the size of the ceramic filler particle (Fig 8-1 and Tables 8-1 and 8-2).

Fine-particle resin composites contain ground glass or quartz particles 0.5 to 3.0 μm in diameter, which occupy 60% to 77% of the composite by volume. Since the filler has a density greater than that of the **polymer** matrix, the fraction of the filler by weight is higher, about 70% to 90%. Particles may be of uniform diameter or have a distribution of diameters, in which case smaller particles fit in the spaces between larger particles, and packing is more efficient.

Microfilled resin composites contain spheric colloidal silica particles 0.01 to 0.12 μm in diameter. Colloidal silica is produced by vapor-phase hydrolysis of silicon compounds, resulting in an average surface area of 200 m²/g, which greatly increases the viscosity of the polymer matrix on incorporation. Filler loading in these composites is therefore limited to about 30% to 55% by volume or 35% to 60% by weight, and low-molecular-weight organic diluents of low viscosity are often added to give the composite a workable clinical consistency. Filler content may be increased and properties improved by grinding a polymerized microfilled composite into particles 10

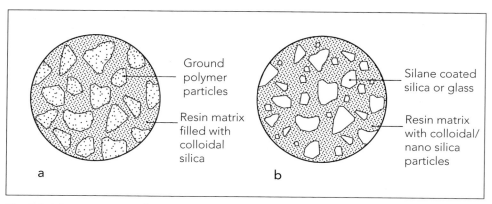

Fig 8-1 Microstructures of resin composite materials: *(a)* microfilled, *(b)* microhybrid.

Table 8-1 Average properties of resin composites

PROPERTY	MICROFILLED	MICROHYBRID
Inorganic filler content (vol %)	30–55	60–70
Thermal conductivity	Insulator	Insulator
Coefficient of thermal expansion (/°C $\times$ 10^{-6})	50–68	20–40
Hardness (Knoop)	22–36	50–80
Water sorption (mg/cm²)	1.2–2.2	0.5–0.7
Compressive strength (MPa)	225–300	200–350
Tensile strength (MPa)	25–35	35–60
Young modulus (GPa)	3–5	7–14
Polymerization shrinkage (%)	2–3	1–1.7

Table 8-2 Clinical characteristics and selection of resin composites

	MICROFILLED	MICROHYBRID
Filler size	0.01–0.12 µm	0.01–3.0 µm
Appearance	Optical properties similar to enamel	Good gloss, luster, and smoothness
Polishability	Highly polishable	Polishable
Usage	Non-stress-bearing esthetic restorations*	Anterior and posterior restorations

*Only heavily filled microfilled materials may be used for posterior restorations.

to 20 µm in diameter and subsequently using these reinforced particles as filler along with colloidal silica. Heavily filled microfilled composites have a filler content of 32% to 66% by volume or about 40% to 80% by weight (Fig 8-2).

Hybrid resin composites have a combination of colloidal and fine particles as filler. The colloidal particles fill the matrix between fine particles, resulting in a filler content of around 60% to 65% by volume. Hybrids (Fig 8-3a) have dominated the market over the past decade.

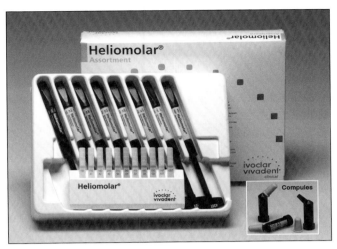

Fig 8-2 A microfilled light-cured composite restorative material in compules. (Courtesy of Ivoclar Vivadent.)

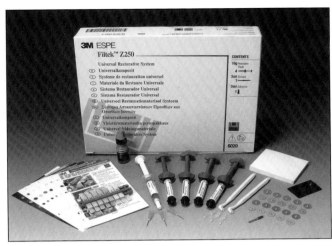

Fig 8-3a A well-established hybrid composite. (Courtesy of 3M ESPE.)

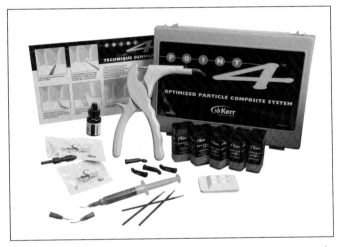

Fig 8-3b A microhybrid composite with low average particle size (0.4 μm). (Courtesy of Kerr.)

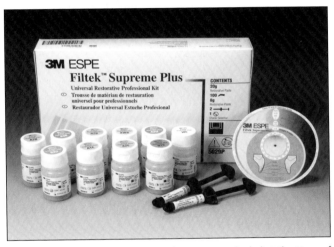

Fig 8-3c A nanocomposite with an extended distribution of filler particle sizes. (Courtesy of 3M ESPE.)

Microhybrid resin composites contain a combination of microfillers and ultrafine glass particles and are so called because of their reduced filler particle size range (0.04 to 1.0 μm). They are marketed as all-purpose "universal" composites, offering both esthetics and enhanced wear resistance for use in both anterior and posterior applications (Fig 8-3b).

Nanofilled composites are microhybrid composites with even smaller sized particles prepared using nanotechnology. Nanometer-sized particles range from 20 nm to 75 nm, depending on the desired shade and translucency. They can be partially fused or sintered into small nanoclusters that act as silanated fillers. These materials tend to have a smoother surface texture after finishing

and also after clinical wear. They blend shades better with natural tooth structure and create more esthetic restorations in critical anterior areas. With these characteristics comes no decrease in the physical properties. Nanofilled composites are recommended for both anterior and posterior restorations (Fig 8-3c).

Composite Product Systems

Chemically cured composites supplied as two pastes are typically used as resin cements or for core applications. Each jar contains dimethacrylate and filler; one jar also contains the peroxide initiator, and the other contains the

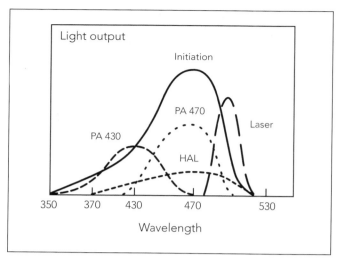

Fig 8-4 Spectra of curing lights including halogen (HAL), plasma arc (PA), and argon laser, along with the absorption spectrum needed for initiation with camphorquinone.

amine accelerator. The initiator and the accelerator are kept separate until mixing. A few composites are offered as two-paste, dual-cure systems. Setting begins after the catalyst and base are mixed and can be accelerated by light curing.

Composites designed for restorative applications are supplied as single pastes in opaque, disposable syringes or in color-coded compules to be used with a syringe. Light-activated composites are currently the most widely used systems available.

Commercially available curing units transmit light from a halogen lamp to the tooth surface by way of a curved quartz rod, a liquid-filled transmission tube, or a bundle of flexible quartz fibers attached to a fiber-optic handpiece. Ultraviolet light is generally filtered out at the light source.

The initiator present in most photocuring monomers is camphorquinone, which is sensitive to light with the spectrum shown in Fig 8-4. To initiate polymerization, curing lights must emit light within this spectrum, which is in the blue range. Filtered halogen lights produce a broad range of wavelengths within the camphorquinone spectrum and are the standard.

Other lights that have higher intensities for faster polymerization have been introduced. These include plasma arc lamps (PAC) and argon laser lights (see Fig 8-4). Although more intense, not all PAC and laser lights have the broad spectrum of the halogen lamps. It is important to match the spectrum of any light to the ab-

sorption characteristic of the initiator in the product being used. Lasers are expensive, and the quality and dimensional change of the composite material cured at such fast speeds is still in question.

Halogen curing lights are available with continuous operation and programmed cycles. One program is called a *stepping function*, which raises the light intensity from about 25% to 100% in specified steps over the curing period. Another program is the *ramped function*, which has a similar action but works on a continuously increasing light intensity over the set curing period. These curing variables reduce polymerization shrinkage during the curing process by having some of the initial shrinkage take place while the material is still in a plastic stage. Figure 8-5a shows a halogen curing light for composite materials.

The latest advancement in light technology to enter the dental marketplace is the light-emitting diode (LED) curing lights. They are usually portable and rechargeable instruments that are very conducive to clinical applications (Fig 8-5b). However, the light source is emitted from a stimulated blue chip or an array of chips that can produce high-power densities but over more restricted spectral ranges. The first and second generations of these lights were somewhat underpowered because the higher intensities generated internal heat sufficient to melt the chip and external heat that could affect the dental pulp in the prepared tooth. In a newer generation of the LED lights, a pulsed intensity (micropulsing) and an array of smaller chips with variations in frequencies produce a more controlled heat.

In selecting a light source, every effort must be made to have the spectral distribution of the light match the absorption of the initiator in the material. In general, it is most desirable to use a light with the highest power density level that is consistent with minimal biologic response from the heat generated. From a material standpoint, the most important factor is to obtain sufficient depth of cure. The external surface will cure with most available light sources, but the internal aspects of the material may be insufficiently activated and result in a restoration with inferior physical properties. The best measure of the effectiveness of a light/resin composite combination is the depth of cure that can be obtained within the specific material.

As with ultraviolet light used in early curing units, blue light has the potential to cause retinal damage if observed directly. Protective eyewear during operation of

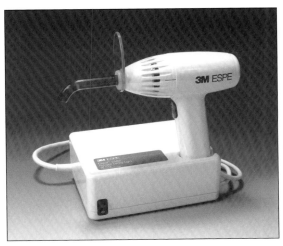

Fig 8-5a A halogen blue curing light. (Courtesy of 3M ESPE.)

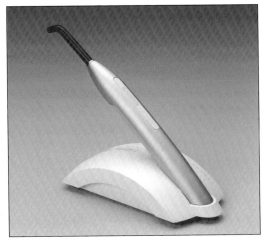

Fig 8-5b An LED blue curing light. (Courtesy of 3M ESPE.)

curing units is highly recommended; however, the glasses or shields used should be wavelength specific to absorb between 450 and 500 nm. Normal sunglasses will not provide adequate protection.

Properties

Setting time

Composite systems that are chemically activated have setting times ranging from 3 to 5 minutes from the start of mixing. The setting time is determined at the time of manufacture by control of the concentrations of initiator and accelerator. However, studies show that even after a curing time of 24 hours, polymerization is incomplete, and 25% to 45% of double bonds remain unreacted.

The setting time and the depth of cure of light-initiated materials depend on the intensity and penetration of the light beam. Polymerization is approximately 75% complete at 10 minutes after exposure to blue light, and curing continues for a period of at least 24 hours. At 24 hours, up to 30% of double bonds still remain unreacted.

Polymerization shrinkage

The occurrence of shrinkage during polymerization creates stresses (~18 MPa) at the tooth-composite interface that may exceed the strength of any bond between composite and enamel or dentin. Bond failure at the interface allows an influx of oral fluids and greatly contributes

to the possibility of postoperative sensitivity, marginal staining, and secondary caries. In addition, stresses at the tooth-composite interface may exceed the tensile strength of enamel perpendicular to the enamel rods, resulting in fractures through the enamel along the interface.

Shrinkage is a direct function of the volume fraction of polymer matrix in the composite, and thus occurs to a larger degree in microfilled composites than in fine-particle composites or hybrids. Microfilled composites typically show setting contractions of 2% to 4% as compared with 1.0% to 1.7% for fine-particle composites (see Table 8-1).

The shrinkage problem can be partially overcome in three ways. First, incremental addition and polymerization of thin layers of a light-initiated material will result in decreased total setting contraction as opposed to bulk curing a single thick layer. However, although this method does result in lower stresses at the tooth-composite interface, studies show that marginal gaps may still occur.

A second method is to use a graduated curing process by varying the light intensity during the curing exposure. The initial polymerization is done at a low intensity and then the final aspect is cured at full light intensity. This stepped sequence allows some of the initial shrinkage that takes place when the reaction kinetics are at the highest rate to be accommodated for while the material is still in the flow state. As a result, the absolute shrinkage is reduced and the stresses on the adhesive bonds are reduced.

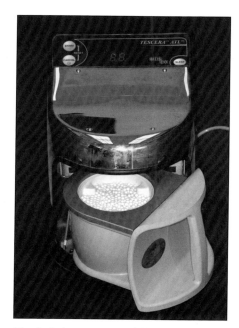

Fig 8-6 A composite laboratory curing unit.

The third approach involves the preparation of a composite inlay either directly in the mouth or indirectly as a laboratory procedure. In the latter procedure the inlay is heat processed (Fig 8-6), allowing the degree of polymerization to approach 100%, and then cemented in the mouth with a thin layer of resin cement. The bulk of the resin composite cement layer needed is small, producing a very small amount of shrinkage and low interfacial stresses. Composite inlays produced in this way are expected to show improved durability and increased wear resistance due to enhanced physical properties. The major drawback of this procedure is that a more extensive cavity preparation is required, and the procedure is significantly more expensive.

Thermal properties

The organic polymer matrix has low thermal conductivity, and composites therefore provide good thermal insulation for the dental pulp. The thermal conductivity of all composites closely matches those of enamel and dentin and is much lower than that of dental amalgam.

As a consequence of the weak physical bonds by which individual polymer molecules are held together, polymers have a marked tendency to expand and contract in response to temperature changes. In contrast, the highly inorganic content of tooth structure is affected to a much smaller degree. Dimensional changes in the resin composite resulting from thermal cycling in the mouth (approximately between 5°C and 55°C) produce further strain on the bond at the tooth-composite interface, increasing the possibility of marginal percolation. This effect occurs to a larger extent with resin-rich microfilled composites than with the more highly filled hybrid materials. The normal thermal cycling of resin materials over extended periods of time also produces a thermal fatigue effect within the material that can be manifested in surface, bulk, or adhesive failure.

Water sorption and solubility

The polymer matrix is able to absorb water; thus, there is some swelling of the composite but not enough to counteract polymerization shrinkage. The uptake of water by composites has been correlated with decreases in surface hardness and wear resistance. As a result of their larger volume fraction of matrix, microfilled composites have higher water sorption values and therefore a greater potential for discoloration by water-soluble stains.

The solubility of resin composites ranges from 1.5% to 2.0% of the original material weight. The major component found to leach in water is residual oligomer or monomer, revealing that incomplete polymerization of the composite results in markedly increased solubility. Additional leachable molecules include degradation products of various composite components and may include formaldehyde, benzoic acid, and methacrylic acid. The largest part of the dissolution occurs within the first few hours of placement.

Elements from filler particles dissolve in water to varying degrees and are detected in quantities as high as 180 μmol/g. Boron and silicon are the main elements, but barium, strontium, and lead—other additives to glass particles—also leach out. The presence of silicon in solution may indicate degradation of the surface treatment of the filler.

Alcohol, a solvent of bis-GMA, and acidulated fluoride gels increase the rate of dissolution of filler particles. Therefore, alcohol-free rinses and neutral fluoride products should be used.

Color stability

Darkening and a color shift to yellow or gray has often been noted in self-curing systems, and has been attributed to the tertiary amine accelerator, which produces color on oxidation. Photo-initiated systems do not con-

Table 8-3 Mechanical properties of enamel and dentin

	COMPRESSIVE STRENGTH (MPa)	TENSILE STRENGTH (MPa)	YOUNG MODULUS (GPa)	HARDNESS NUMBER KNOOP (VICKERS)
Enamel	384	10.3	84.1	343 (408)
Dentin	297	51.7	18.5	68 (60)

tain a tertiary amine and have shown considerable improvement in color stability over long periods of time.

Under accelerated aging conditions in a weathering chamber, erosion of the resin matrix and exposure of filler particles of microfilled composites resulted in lightening of color. The color stability of microfilled composites, however, was affected by erosion only to a small degree.

Radiopacity

A degree of radiopacity slightly exceeding that of enamel may be useful in diagnosis. Radiopacity may be conferred by incorporating elements of high atomic number, such as barium, strontium, and zirconium, into the filler. The relative number of these atoms is still small, however, and the materials are much less radiopaque than is amalgam. Almost all composites currently available have some degree of radiopacity. The international standard[1] for the radiopacity of resin composites used in posterior restorations requires it to be equal or greater than that of enamel.[2] This property is judged by comparing the radiograph of the material with that of an aluminum stepped wedge with graded radiopacities.

Mechanical properties

The higher compressive and tensile strengths of fine-particle and hybrid composites, as compared with microfilled composites, reflect the higher volume fraction of the high-strength filler component. Note that for all materials, compressive strengths are several times higher than tensile strengths, reflecting the somewhat brittle behavior of composites. More highly filled composites have tensile strengths near that of dentin and compressive strengths similar to or higher than that of dentin (Table 8-3). Some highly filled composites have compressive strengths greater than that of enamel.

The Young modulus, also called the *elastic modulus*, is a measure of a material's stiffness. A material with low elastic modulus deflects under stress. As a group, composites have elastic moduli that are only a fraction of that of enamel. Fine-particle materials, however, have moduli similar to that of dentin. Under high loads, such as those that occur in posterior teeth during mastication, deflection of the restoration strains the tooth-composite bond. Deflection additionally places considerable tensile stresses on adjacent cusps.

The lower filler content of microfilled composites results in elastic moduli of one quarter to one half that of the more highly filled composites. They are therefore recommended for cervical (Class 5) restorations, since some deflection within the material could reduce stresses at the tooth-composite interface.

Microindentation hardness of composites is directly related to volume fraction of the hard, inorganic filler component. Hardness is also related to the degree of polymerization. In laboratory experiments, composites that underwent a secondary heat treatment to increase the degree of polymerization showed higher Knoop hardness values than did composites that were light cured only.

As a group, the hardness of composites is a fraction of that of enamel but is similar to or higher than that of dentin.

Wear

Wear in composites is a complex phenomenon that depends on several intrinsic and extrinsic factors. The large amount of data collected for various available composites is confusing, at least in part because measuring techniques have not been standardized. In vivo, wear has not been shown to correlate well with any single material property. In addition, the appearance of wear patterns (Fig 8-7) in restorations of long duration is complicated by the presence of *erosion*, a degradative uniform loss of material across the composite surface. Nevertheless, a number of factors that contribute to wear have been identified.

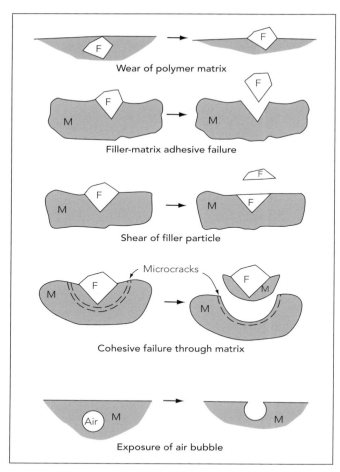

Fig 8-7 Several possible wear mechanisms for dental composites (F = filler particle; M = matrix). (Modified with permission from O'Brien and Yee.[3])

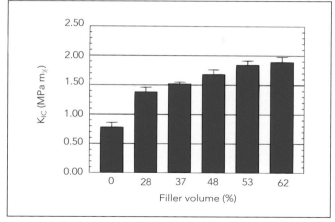

Fig 8-8 The effect of filler volume fraction on fracture toughness, K_{IC}. (Courtesy of J. Ferracane.)

than 1.0 µm is greatest in the year after placement, declining thereafter.

The incorporation of softer filler particles with hardness characteristics similar to that of enamel appears to result in decreased wear. It is thought that soft particles are more capable than hard particles of absorbing energy generated during the masticatory process, thereby transmitting lower stresses to the matrix. Scanning electron micrographs of a material with hard quartz particles and another with soft glass particles are shown in Figs 8-9 and 8-10, respectively, illustrating the difference in the shapes of the particles that project from the occlusal surface.

It is notable that the presence of filler particles with hardness values greater than that of enamel has been shown to increase the roughness of opposing enamel over time.

Tooth position in the arch

In general, the more distally located the restoration, the higher the rate of wear. Under normal functioning occlusion, molars will show much greater wear than premolars.

Porosity

Internal porosity, particularly in stress-bearing areas, increases wear. It has been proposed that porosities concentrate stresses in the matrix and, under loading, contribute to the formation of microcracks. In addition, voids, produced during the spatulation process or during incorporation of filler at the time of manufacture, are air-filled. An air-inhibited layer of incompletely polymerized matrix may exist at the void surface. Light-initiated sys-

Filler content, particle size, and hardness

Increased filler volume results in decreased wear. Laboratory studies demonstrate a greater loss of material volume during abrasive action for microfilled as compared with more highly filled composites. A higher filler volume results in a higher fracture toughness, as shown in Fig 8-8.

Keeping volume fraction constant, wear resistance is increased by decreasing the size of the filler particle. Large, hard particles transmit considerable stress to the matrix, possibly resulting in microcracking and subsequent loss of material (Fig 8-9). By contrast, a reduced load per particle results when a large number of small particles is present per unit volume.

It has been reported that wear of composites with filler particles smaller than 1.0 µm occurs at a constant rate with time. Wear of composites with particles larger

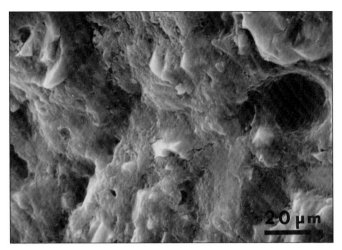

Fig 8-9 Worn surface of a composite restoration showing a protruding hard quartz filler particle with an adjacent microcrack (scanning electron microscope; original magnification ×1,000). (Reprinted with permission from O'Brien and Yee.[3])

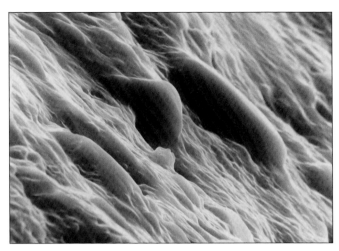

Fig 8-10 Worn surface of a composite with a soft glass filler (scanning electron microscope; original magnification ×2,500).

tems requiring no spatulation have demonstrated higher wear resistance than self-curing systems.

Degree of polymerization

Strength properties of polymers are directly related to molecular size. During polymerization, molecular size increases enormously. The enhanced wear resistance found in some studies of heat-processed composite inlays is thought to be related to their higher degree of polymerization.

Coupling agent

The absence of a silane coupling agent at the matrix-filler interface reduces wear resistance by about half.

Depth of cure

Polymerization in both chemically and light-activated composites is incomplete. Degrees of conversion are reported to be in the range of 60% to 75%. The number of unreacted double bonds at 24 hours is higher in light-activated than in chemically activated systems and results from several factors affecting depth of cure.

Light intensity at the surface and time of exposure are critical. The tip of the light source should be held within 1 to 2 mm of the surface to cure a light shade of material to a depth of 2.0 to 2.5 mm using a standard exposure time of 40 seconds. A longer exposure time will increase the degree of polymerization at all depths and is necessary when using darker shades or more opaque materials.

A reduction in thickness of the increment to be cured is a more reliable way of achieving polymerization than is an increase in exposure time. In addition, the hardness of the top surface of a cured restoration is not a good indication of the extent of polymerization at the bottom surface.

Depth of cure can be measured in the dental office by taking an opaque straw, cutting it to a length of 6 to 8 mm, and placing it on the white background of a mixing pad. The straw should be filled flush with the test material and then light cured with a normal exposure from the light to be evaluated (usually 40 seconds for a quartz-halogen source). The straw can then be cut open from the side and the specimen removed. The soft material should be scraped away with a dull-bladed instrument. A rough estimate of effective depth of cure is obtained by dividing the length of the remaining specimen in millimeters in half. For most material/light combinations, 2 to 2.5 mm is the optimum depth of cure that should be expected, and each increment of new material added to a restoration should not exceed that thickness.

Depth of cure is also influenced by the wavelength of light and the concentration of the activator-initiator system. The refractive indices of the resin and filler, as well as the size, shape, and number of filler particles, are important to the dispersion of the light beam. The small, highly numerous colloidal-sized particles of microfilled composites scatter incident light very efficiently, necessitating a longer exposure time to obtain adequate polymerization.

Chemically activated systems are considered to have an infinite depth of cure, and polymerization should be uniform at all levels of the cured restoration.

Biocompatibility

Histologic studies of the effect of residual monomer molecules on pulp tissue have shown a moderate degree of cytotoxicity, even in low concentrations. Recent in vivo biocompatibility studies, however, show that resin composites, whether completely or incompletely cured, cause little irritation to the pulp if an adequate marginal seal is present. It has been proposed that a significant degree of sensitivity after the placement of a restoration is a consequence of microbial invasion from the oral environment and not of toxicity of the material itself. Postoperative sensitivity also may be a consequence of debonding between dentin and the composite at the cavity floor, causing a pumping action of dentinal fluid during chewing (percolation), possibly expressing irritants or bacterial toxins into dentinal tubules.

Until the precise mechanisms involved are understood, pulpal protection is recommended at the depths of extensive cavity preparations.

● Manipulation

Placement

Eugenol inhibits the polymerization of resin composites. Therefore, liners, bases, and interim restorations containing eugenol are not recommended. The use of cavity varnish is not recommended under composite restorations, because monomers in the composite may solubilize and disrupt the integrity of the varnish film. Also, varnish will prevent bonding.

Following cavity preparation and before placement of the composite, a sealing procedure of some type should be done. Once a **dentin bonding agent** is applied, the use of rubber dam or similar isolation procedure is indicated because moisture will interfere with bonding. The dentin is first conditioned according to the manufacturer's directions. Deep preparations may require the placement of a glass-ionomer or hybrid ionomer liner or base over the dentin. Very deep cavities also require a thin layer of a calcium hydroxide product on the dentin over the pulp before placing a liner or base.

Enamel and dentin are treated strictly according to manufacturer's directions depending on the bonding agent used. Generally, enamel and dentin are **acid etched** for 15 seconds using a 35% to 50% phosphoric acid solution or acid gel. High-viscosity gel etchants have the advantage of ease of control of the application to enamel walls. The preparation is thoroughly washed with water for at least 15 seconds to remove all residue. The surface is then gently air-dried, at which point the enamel should have an opaque, white appearance. Any contamination by saliva after this step requires re-etching to clean the surface thoroughly.

A dentin bonding agent is applied to the clean enamel and dentin according to the manufacturer's directions. The bonding resin should be blotted or air-blown gently to ensure a thin film application. Dentin bonding agents also work on enamel by penetrating into the etched surface and producing retentive resin tags. While components of bonding systems should not be interchanged, any composite can be used with most bonding agents.

A transparent mylar matrix band is placed when indicated to establish the restoration contour.

Two-paste system (autopolymerized)

To ensure uniform distribution of filler particles in the matrix, each paste should be stirred periodically with disposable plastic mixing sticks, taking care to avoid cross-contamination that will cause polymerization in the jars. Less particle settling and an increase in shelf life will result if the pastes are refrigerated.

Equal amounts of the two pastes are dispensed onto a mixing pad with a disposable two-bladed plastic spatula. One blade of the spatula should be used to dispense one paste, and the other blade, the second paste. When needed, the two pastes are mixed thoroughly, requiring 20 to 30 seconds. Care should be taken to avoid the incorporation of air during mixing. Metal spatulas are not recommended for mixing, because filler particles are capable of abrading metal and small amounts of metal may be incorporated into the composite, resulting in discoloration.

Two-paste composites have a working time from the start of mixing of 1 to 1.5 minutes and a setting time of 3 to 5 minutes. Viscous material is best placed with plastic instruments that do not adhere to the unset material. A small amount of bonding resin on the tip of the plastic instrument will prevent sticking. If the viscosity of the mixed material is low enough, it may be injected into the cavity preparation from a syringe. Syringe placement tends to minimize the incorporation of voids into the restoration.

The cavity preparation should be slightly overfilled. At 3.5 to 4 minutes after the start of mixing, the matrix band, if used, is removed. After an additional 2 to 6 minutes, the composite surface is sufficiently hard for finishing to begin.

Single-paste system (photo-activated)

The shelf life of composites supplied as single pastes and stored in a cool, dry environment is about 1 year.

The composite is best placed in small layers to minimize polymerization shrinkage, and each layer should be light cured for at least 40 seconds. After curing, there should be a tacky, air-inhibited layer, to which the subsequent layer bonds.

Microfilled composites require longer exposure times than do hybrid composites because their colloidal-sized and more numerous filler particles scatter blue light more efficiently.

Finishing

Composites are finished and polished to establish a functional occlusal relationship and a contour that is physiologically in harmony with supporting tissues. In addition, proper contour and high gloss give the restoration the appearance of a natural tooth structure. Early composites had large, hard quartz particles. Polishing preferentially removed the resin matrix, leaving filler particles exposed and giving the surface a dull appearance. In addition, quartz has a hardness about 2.5 times that of enamel and is difficult to polish compared with glasses, which have hardness characteristics similar to that of enamel.

Particles smaller than about 0.05 μm cannot be detected visually and allow polishing to a high luster. Fine-particle composites have no microfilled particles, are considered to be only semipolishable, and tend to have a rather opaque appearance. The colloidal-sized filler particles of microfilled materials scatter light efficiently, giving these restorations a pleasing esthetic appearance. Hybrid composites are polishable but are not as translucent as microfilled composites.

The composite surface may be contoured with a plastic matrix strip, but some gross reduction is often required. Finishing begins with coarse abrasives, such as 9- and 12-blade finishing burs and fine diamonds, and progresses to 16- and 30-blade finishing burs, ultrafine diamonds, and medium-grit abrasive points, disks, and strips. Polishing is accomplished with aluminum oxide or diamond polishing pastes on a rubber cup at low speed.

Wear resistance decreases with the use of carbide or diamond finishing burs. Their use is thought to weaken the surface through the formation of microcracks or to degrade the matrix through the generation of heat. Pitting has also been observed on the surface of microfilled-particle–reinforced composites after polishing. The pits are thought to occur at the junction of the new resin and the prepolymerized resin/filler, resulting in an increased susceptibility to chipping. Voids can also occur as a result of excessive manipulation during the placement of resin increments or plucking of filler clusters during polishing. A postocclusal adjustment cure of 40 seconds further hardens the surface. It is recommended that finishing or adjustment be followed by re-etching and the application and curing of a low-viscosity filled or unfilled resin glaze coating. The resin penetrates microcracks and voids on the finished surface, limiting crack propagation and further reducing wear.

Wear resistance of composites developed for posterior use has improved steadily over recent years, although it is still a major disadvantage in restorations with extensive occlusal surface exposure.

A properly placed anterior composite restoration has an expected clinical life of 7 to 10 years. Posterior restorations are generally serviceable for less than that. The major reasons for replacing any composite include deterioration of esthetics, interfacial staining, wear, microleakage, bulk fracture, and secondary caries.

Material Selection

A variety of materials is available for use as direct esthetic dental restorations: resin composites, compomers, hybrid ionomers, and glass ionomers. Each has a resin component, except the traditional glass ionomer. The unique characteristics of each of these materials make them desirable for a range of applications. Choosing the most suitable material requires matching a material's desired properties and manipulation to the application for use. The continuum of resin composite to glass-ionomer esthetic restorative materials is illustrated in Fig 8-11, and their uses are presented in Table 8-4.

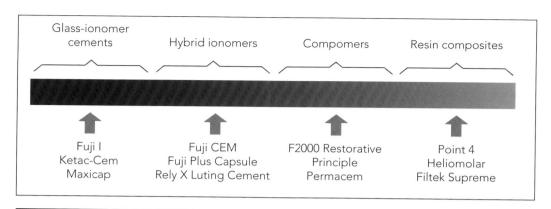

Fig 8-11 Continuum of glass-ionomer and composite restorative materials.[4]

Table 8-4 Direct esthetic materials and their uses

RESTORATIVE MATERIAL	APPLICATION
Flowable resin composite	Preventive resin restorations Small Class 5 restorations Liner/base under posterior composite
Hybrid, microhybrid, and nanofilled resin composite	Anterior restorations Posterior restorations
Microfilled resin composite	Areas of esthetic concern Anterior restorations
Packable resin composite	Class 1 and 2 restorations
Polyacid-modified resin composite (compomer)	Class 3 and 5 restorations Cervical erosion or abrasion lesions Class 1 and 2 restorations in pediatric patients Sandwich technique for Class 2 restorations
Glass ionomer	High caries–risk patients Cervical erosion or abrasion lesions Class 5 restorations where esthetics is not a concern Atraumatic restorative treatment restorations
Hybrid ionomer	Class 3 and 5 restorations Cervical erosion or abrasion lesions Class 1 restorations in pediatric patients Sandwich technique for Class 2 restorations Liners, bases, and luting cements Temporary restorations

Resin composites

The most commonly used direct esthetic restorative materials are resin composites. They offer excellent esthetics, strength, and wear resistance but have little or no fluoride release. Microfilled composites are used for anterior applications, and hybrid composites are recommended for posterior applications; however, the difference between posterior and anterior composites has become less distinct due to the development of the microhybrid and nanofilled composites.

Composites can also be selected based on their handling characteristics. **Packable composites** have been used as an alternative to amalgam (Fig 8-12). They differ from anterior and posterior composites in that they have higher filler loading (greater than 80% by weight and 66% to 70% by volume) with either fibers, porous filler particles, irregular filler particles, or viscosity modifiers. They are recommended for use in Class 1 and 2 cavity preparations. Because of the high depth of cure and lower polymerization shrinkage of packable composites, a bulk-fill technique may be possible. A low-viscosity (flowable) material (Fig 8-13) can be used as a liner to fill irregular internal surfaces and proximal boxes before placing the packable composite. Flowable composites or compomers will wet and adapt to the tooth surface, sealing it and possibly reducing postoperative sensitivity.

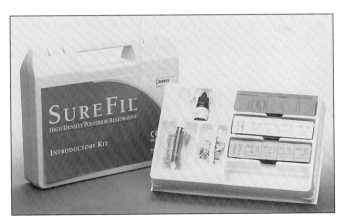

Fig 8-12 A packable composite material. An interlocking particle network allows the packable handling properties. (Courtesy of Dentsply Caulk.)

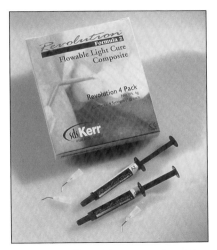

Fig 8-13 A flowable composite with a filler load of about 60% by weight and average particle size of 0.6 μm. (Courtesy of Kerr.)

Compomers

Compomers, or *polyacid-modified composites* (Fig 8-14), contain monomers modified by polyacid groups with fluoride-releasing silicate glasses. The properties and clinical characteristics of compomers are directly related to their composition of composite and glass ionomer. Compomers release fluoride by a mechanism similar to glass and hybrid ionomers, but the amount of release and its duration are lower. In addition, compomers do not recharge from fluoride treatments or brushing with fluoride dentifrices as much as do glass and hybrid ionomers. Like composites, compomers require a bonding agent to bond to tooth structure. Single-bottle bonding agents that contain acidic primers have been used with some compomers. Acidic primers will bond to both enamel and dentin without the need for phosphoric acid etching. However, studies have shown that the bond strength of compomers to teeth is improved with additional etching with phosphoric acid. Compomers set by light-activated polymerization and by an acid-base reaction with water absorbed from the tooth. They are packaged as single-paste formulations in compules and syringes. Compomers are recommended for low-stress-bearing areas and cementations.

Hybrid ionomers

Hybrid ionomers (or *resin-modified glass ionomers*) contain fluoride-releasing glass and polyacid monomers. They set by an acid-base reaction and both chemical and

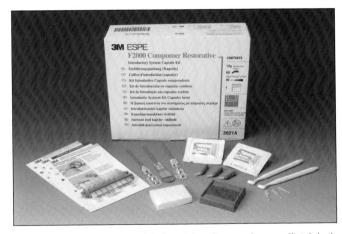

Fig 8-14 A compomer with fluoride-silicate glass, colloidal silica, dimethacrylate resin, and hydrophilic polymer. (Courtesy of 3M ESPE.)

light-cured free-radical reactions. They are recommended for cervical lesions, Class 3 and 5 restorations in adults, primary teeth, Class 1 restorations in children, the sandwich technique for Class 2 restorations, temporary restorations, and with high-caries-risk patients. Because of the resin content, these restorations are more esthetic and stronger than glass ionomers. Hybrid ionomers are packaged in powder-liquid form or are preencapsulated to be mixed in an amalgamator. The use of a bonding agent before placement is not recommended because it decreases fluoride release. Hybrid ionomers naturally bond to tooth structure once the tooth is conditioned

Table 8-5 Mechanical properties of glass ionomer and resin composite combinations*

MATERIALS CLASS	FLEXURAL STRENGTH (MPa)	FLEXURAL MODULUS (GPa)	COMPRESSIVE STRENGTH (MPa)	DIAMETRAL TENSILE STRENGTH (MPa)	SHEAR BOND STRENGTH (MPa)	SHRINKAGE (% VOL)
Conventional glass ionomer	25	8	180–200	22–25	3–5	3
Hybrid ionomer	35–70	4	170–200	35–40	8–14	3.5
Compomer	97	6–8	210–245	45–47	14	4.5
Fluoride-releasing resin composite	85	8	—	40	24	3
Flowable resin composite	111–167	4–8	—	—	20–22	5
Resin composite	140	18	350	65–75	24–28	3

*Used with permission from Burgess et al.[5]

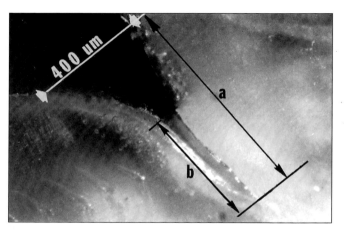

Fig 8-15 Penetration of a sealant into a fissure: (a) depth of sealant penetration, (b) total depth.

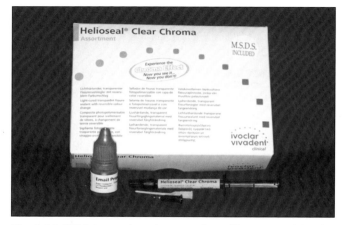

Fig 8-16 Widely used sealant product. (Courtesy of Ivoclar Vivadent.)

with polyacrylic acid or a primer. See chapter 9 for the use of hybrid ionomers as cements. A comparison of the properties of several of these materials is presented in Table 8-5.

● Pit and Fissure Sealants

Sealants are mainly fluid resins that are applied to posterior occlusal surfaces of caries-prone teeth to seal pits and fissures from bacterial action. The principal monomer used is bis-GMA, which may be lightly filled with ceramic filler particles to improve wear resistance. Before application of the fluid monomer, the tooth enamel is etched with phosphoric acid. When the fluid resin is applied, it penetrates the pits and fissures by capillary action (Fig

8-15). It also penetrates the microstructure of the etched enamel to form "tags" that lead to micromechanical action. Deep penetration is promoted by a high penetration coefficient, which results from low viscosity, high surface tension, and low contact angle, that is, good wetting (see chapter 5).

Sealants have been found to be effective in many clinical studies. Long-term studies have shown around 50% decay reduction in sealed teeth compared with controls. About 70% to 90% of sealants are at least partially present at 5 years. Also, partial loss or wear of a sealant does not limit its preventive action in deep fissures. One difficulty in selecting sealant treatment for a patient is that the diagnosis of caries in pits and fissures is a challenging decision. Often the fissure can look and feel noncarious, but there can be initial demineralization at the depth of the fissure and even bacterial penetration to the dentinoenamel junction. If incipient enamel caries or viable bacteria are trapped beneath a well-placed sealant, studies have shown that the bacteria become dormant and the caries can be arrested.[6,7] Sealants are particularly indicated for patients who are at more than minimal risk for caries activity and are primarily applied in the early eruption stages for optimum effectiveness. Fluoride-containing sealants are also available, but the clinical effectiveness of the fluoride release is not well documented. Due to the high probability of debonding and resulting microleakage under the sealant, patients with sealants should be under consistent recall for early failure detection and retreatment or repair. See Fig 8-16 for a widely used sealant product.

Clinical Decision Scenarios for Restorative Materials

This section presents a formal approach to choosing restorative materials for specific situations. Each scenario uses the same format as that presented in chapter 7. Advantages and disadvantages of each material are prioritized using the following codes: • of minor importance, •• important, ••• very important.

Materials Light-cured vs chemically cured composite materials for anterior Class 3 restorations

Situation A patient has a small proximal caries lesion on the mesial surface of a maxillary permanent central incisor and would like an esthetic restoration. The clinician has both visible light–cured composite material and chemically cured material in his armamentarium.

Critical Factor Esthetics

LIGHT CURE	CHEMICAL CURE
ADVANTAGES	ADVANTAGES
••• Good esthetics • Better color stability Less porosity More working time	••• Good esthetics • More complete cure Curing light not needed
DISADVANTAGES	DISADVANTAGES
Less complete cure Curing light needed	More porosity ••• Poorer color stability Less working time

Analysis/Decision Although either material would be satisfactory, the greater color stability provides the determining factor in this instance and leads to selection of the light-cured material. The greater working time of light-cured material is convenient but not necessary to a clinician experienced in the use of the chemically cured material. The higher porosity of the chemically cured material—induced by the need to mix the paste and catalyst—as well as the activators and accelerators needed in the chemical cure, probably contribute to the lower color stability.

Materials Resin composite vs amalgam for cores

Situation A patient comes to the office complaining of a broken tooth. On examination, the clinician finds that the lingual cusps of the mandibular right permanent first molar have fractured at the gingival line. The tooth already has a large mesio-occlusodistal amalgam in it, and the facial cusps are not sturdy. The patient is leaving for a winter vacation to Florida in 10 days and hopes to have the tooth repaired before then. The treatment plan is to prepare a pin-retained core buildup and then a full gold crown. The clinician has both amalgam and a composite core material available.

Critical Factor Time

AMALGAM	RESIN COMPOSITE
ADVANTAGES	ADVANTAGES
Greater strength Long clinical history	••• Immediate set Bonds to tooth Can be prepared immediately
DISADVANTAGES	DISADVANTAGES
••• 24-hour set No bond to tooth	Lesser strength

Analysis/Decision The seemingly abbreviated list represents the main considerations. While the strength of the amalgam is thought to be greater in these applications, composites have served well if properly done. The deciding factor is often that the composite can be placed and prepared for the crown immediately, whereas it is recommended that the amalgam be allowed to set 24 hours before preparation. Thus, the composite may be placed and the tooth prepared in one appointment. Amalgam would have required a second appointment for the crown preparation.

◉ Glossary

accelerator A chemical added to speed up a reaction. For example, amines are added to accelerate free radical polymerization; also called an *activator*.

acid etch Selective etching of portions of the enamel rods with phosphoric acid, resulting in both high surface area and increased surface energy. Resin is able to flow into the enamel substructure and, on polymerization, provides a mechanical bond to the enamel.

amine An organic compound containing nitrogen that is used as an accelerator in polymerization reactions. Tertiary amines are used in chemically activated composite materials, and aliphatic amines are use in light-activated materials.

compomer A blend of resin composite and glass ionomer; requires a bonding agent to bond to tooth; also known as *polyacid-modified resin composite*.

coupling agent A chemical attached to the filler surface to create a bond with the resin matrix on polymerization. The presence of a coupling agent improves several properties of the composite, including strength and wear resistance.

cross-linked polymer A polymer with a three-dimensional network structure.

dentin bonding agent Low-viscosity resin used for adhesion to enamel and/or dentin.

dimethacrylate A methacrylate monomer with reactive, or polymerizable, groups at each end.

Materials Microfilled resin composite vs hybrid composite for direct veneer

Situation A recent college graduate requests an improvement in the appearance of her maxillary lateral incisors, which are slightly crowded, and she wants it done before a job interview in 2 weeks. She is advised that orthodontic treatment would be a more permanent solution, but it would take 1 or 2 years. Due to urgency, the clinician agrees to place direct veneers using either a microfilled or hybrid composite material.

Critical Factors Appearance, strong bond to enamel, strength

HYBRID COMPOSITE	MICROFILLED COMPOSITE
ADVANTAGES	ADVANTAGES
Ease of placement • Stronger than microfilled composite •• More wear resistance Lower expansion and contraction ••• Strong bond to enamel	Ease of placement ••• More natural appearance • Smoother finish ••• Strong bond to enamel
DISADVANTAGES	DISADVANTAGES
••• Less natural appearance • Less smooth finish	•• Less wear resistance • Weaker than hybrid Higher expansion and contraction

Analysis/Decision Given that the microfilled composite material has a smoother and more natural appearance, the clinician chose to use this material. No tooth removal was necessary. The lateral incisors were isolated, cleaned with pumice, and enamel etched. Then natural-looking restorations were created. The patient was delighted with the results. The clinician explained to the patient that these restorations may need to be resurfaced/polished on a regular basis and replaced every 4 or 5 years due to wear.

fine-particle resin composite A composite containing fine-sized filler particles (0.5 to 3.0 μm); it is less polishable than a microfilled composite.

free radical A highly active chemical group that results from having an unpaired electron.

hybrid ionomer An ionomer that sets by an acid-base reaction and resin polymerization. The powder is similar to glass ionomer and the liquid contains monomers, polyacids, and water; also known as *resin-modified glass ionomer*.

hybrid (blend) resin composite A composite containing colloidal silica (0.01 to 0.12 μm) in addition to fine-sized particles.

initiator A chemical that starts a reaction. Benzoyl peroxide is used as an initiator in free radical polymerization of acrylic resins.

microfilled resin composite A composite containing colloidal silica as filler; it is the most polishable and translucent resin composite.

microhybrid resin composite A composite containing filler particles in the range of 0.4 to 1.0 μm; a blend of hybrid and microfilled composites.

monomer A single molecule with double or triple bonds that are capable of uniting the monomers into oligomers or polymers.

oligomer A short polymer made up of two to four monomer units.

packable composites A composite with a higher filler content than traditional resin composite with either fibers, porous filler particles, irregular filler particles, or viscosity modifiers.

polymer A macromolecule formed by the linkage of monomers or oligomers.

polymerization The process by which a polymer is formed from monomers or oligomers.

resin composite A physical mixture of silicate glass particles (filler) with an acrylic monomer (matrix phase) that is polymerized during application. A material having two or more distinct components and with properties different from those of the individual components.

■ Discussion Questions

1. Why are these materials called polymeric restorative materials when they usually contain mostly ceramic phases?

2. How have composites overcome many of the problems of unfilled resin restorative materials?

3. How well are composite materials competing against dental amalgam?

4. Although microfilled composite materials have inferior mechanical properties, they continue to be widely used. Why?

■ Study Questions

(See appendix E for answers.)

1. What is the general composition of resin composite restorative materials?

2. What are the applications for resin composite restorative materials?

3. How long do composite restorations last?

4. What are the advantages of fine-particle composites?

5. What are the advantages of microfilled composites?

6. What is a hybrid, or blend, composite?

7. What is polymerization shrinkage, and why is it a problem?

8. Which restorative materials release fluoride? List them in order of amount released.

9. What is the material of choice for cervical restorations?

■ References

1. International Organization for Standardization. ISO 4049:2000. Dentistry—Polymer-based filling, restorative and luting materials, ed 3. Geneva: International Organization for Standardization, 2000.
2. Turgut MD, Attar N, Onen A. Radiopacity of direct esthetic restorative materials. Oper Dent 2003;28:508–514.
3. O'Brien WJ, Yee JJ. Microstructure of posterior restorations of composite resins after clinical wear. Oper Dent 1980;5(3):90–94.
4. Albers HF. Tooth-Colored Restoratives, ed 8. Santa Rosa: Alto Books, 1996.
5. Burgess JO, Norling BK, Rawls HR, Ong JL. Directly placed esthetic restorative materials. Compend Contin Educ Dent 1996; 17(8):731–748.
6. Jensen OE, Handelman SL. Effect of an autopolymerizing sealant on viability of microflora in occlusal dental caries. Scand J Dent Rest 1980;88:382–388.
7. Handelman SL, Buonocore MG, Heseck DJ. A preliminary report on the effect of fissure sealant on bacteria in dental caries. J Prosthet Dent 1972;27:390–392.

■ Recommended Reading

al-Dawood A, Wennberg A. Biocompatibility of dentin bonding agents. Endod Dent Traumatol 1993;9:1–7.

Armstrong SR, Seol J, Boyer DB. Fracture toughness of direct tooth-colored restorative materials [abstract 811]. J Dent Res 1999;78: 207.

Asmussen E. Factors affecting the quantity of remaining double bonds in restorative resin polymers. Scand J Dent Res 1982;90: 490–496.

Attin T, Vataschki M, Hellwig E. Properties of resin-modified glass-ionomer restorative materials and two polyacid-modified resin composite materials. Quintessence Int 1996;27:203–209.

Barkmeier WW, Blake SM, Wilwerding TM, Latta MA. In-vitro wear assessment of compomer restoratives [abstract 1652]. J Dent Res 1999;78:312.

Bayne SC, Thompson JY, Swift EJ Jr, Stamatiades P, Wilkerson M. A characterization of first-generation flowable composites. J Am Dent Assoc 1998;129:567–577.

Braga RR, Ferracane JL. Alternatives in polymerization contraction stress management. Crit Rev Oral Biol Med 2004;15:176.

Albers HF. Tooth-Colored Restoratives, ed 8. Santa Rosa: Alto Books, 1996.

Burgess JO, et al. Directly placed esthetic restorative materials. Compend Contin Educ Dent 1996;17:8,731–748.

Choi KK, Condon JR, Ferracane JL. The effects of adhesive thickness on polymerization contraction stress of composites J Dent Res 2000;79:812.

Christensen GJ. Condensable restorative resins. Clin Res Associates Newsletter 1998;22(7):1.

Christensen GJ. Sorting out the confusing array of resin-based composites in dentistry. J Am Dent Assoc 1999;130:275–277.

Compoglass F. Physical properties [product information sheet]. Amherst, NY: Ivoclar Vivadent, 2007.

Condon JR, Ferracane JL. Reduction of composite contraction stress through non-bonded microfiller particles. Dent Mater 1998;14–256.

Craig RG. Restorative Dental Materials, ed 9. St Louis: Mosby, 1993.

Czerner A, Weller M, Lohbauer U, Ebert J, Frankenberger J. Wear resistance of flowable composites as pit and fissure sealants [abstract 1087]. J Dent Res 2000;79:279.

Dauvillier BS, Feilzer AJ, de Gee AJ, et al. Visco-elastic parameters of dental restorative materials during setting. J Dent Res 2000; 79:818.

Dhuru V, Benhamuerlaine M. Water sorption of selected tooth color materials [abstract 1100]. J Dent Res 2000;79:281.

Eick JD, Robinson SJ, Byerley TJ, Chappelow CC. Adhesives and nonshrinking dental resins of the future. Quintessence Int 1993; 24:632–640.

Eliades G, Palaghias G, Vougiouklakis G. Surface reactions of adhesives on dentin. Dent Mater 1990;6:208–216.

El-Kalla IH, Garcia-Godoy F. Mechanical properties of compomer restorative materials. Oper Dent 1999;24:2–8.

Farah JW, Powers JM. Anterior and posterior composites. Dental Advisor 1991;8(4):1–8.

Farah JW, Powers JM. Fluoride-releasing restorative materials. Dental Advisor 1999;15:1.

Ferracane JL. Current trends in dental composites. Crit Rev Oral Biol 1995;6:302.

Fortin D, Vargas MA. The spectrum of composites: New techniques and materials. J Am Dent Assoc 2000;131(suppl):26S–30S.

Iazetti G, Burgess JO, Tavares C. Mechanical properties of fluoride-releasing materials [abstract 417]. J Dent Res 1999;78:158.

Kelsey WP, Latta MA, Barkmeier WW. Physical properties of high density, composite restorative materials [abstract 810]. J Dent Res 1999;78:207.

Kerby R, Berlin J, Knobloch L. Fracture toughness of posterior condensable composites [abstract 415]. J Dent Res 1999;78:157.

Kerby R, Lee J, Knobloch L, Seghi R. Hardness and degree of conversion of posterior condensable composite resin [abstract 414]. J Dent Res 1999;78:157.

Latta MA, Randall CJ. Physical properties of compomer restorative materials [abstract 412]. J Dent Res 1999;78:157.

Lohbauer U, Schoch M, Frankenburger R, Braem MJA, Kramer N. Flexural strength characterization of resin composites by Weibull analysis [abstract 805]. J Dent Res 1999;78:206.

MacGregor KM, Cobb DS, Denehy GE. Physical properties of new packable composites vs. a conventional hybrid [abstract 1777]. J Dent Res 2000;79:366.

MacGregor KM, Cobb DS, Vargas MA. Physical properties of condensable versus conventional composites [abstract 411]. J Dent Res 1999;78:157.

Manhart J, Chen HY, Draegert U, Kunzelmann KH, Hickel R. Vickers hardness and depth of cure of light-cured packable composite resins [abstract 1807]. J Dent Res 2000;79:369.

McKinney JE, Wu W. Chemical softening and wear of dental composites. J Dent Res 1985;64:1326–1331.

Minato D, Ruse ND, Feduik D. Fracture toughness of a hybrid, a microfill, and a compomer using NTP test [abstract 2343]. J Dent Res 1999;78:398.

Musa A, Pearson GJ, Gelbier M. In vitro investigation of fluoride ion release from four resin-modified glass polyalkenoate cements. Biomaterials 1996;17:1019–1023.

Nguyen D, Angeletakis C, Shellard E. A new high polish retention microhybrid composite [abstract 1081]. J Dent Res 2000;79:279.

Pearson GJ, Longman CM. Water sorption and solubility of resin-based materials following inadequate polymerization by a visible-light curing system. J Oral Rehabil 1989;16:57–61.

Powers JM, Fan PL, Raptis CN. Color stability of new composite restorative materials under accelerated aging. J Dent Res 1980;59:2071–2074.

Price RB, Felix CA, Andreou P. Knoop hardness of ten resin composites irradiated with high power LED and quartz-tungsten-halogen lights. Biomaterials 2005;26:2631.

Roeder LB, Tate WH, Powers JM. Surface roughness of polished condensable composites [abstract 3024]. J Dent Res 1999;78:483.

Ruddle DE, Thompson JY, Stamatiades PJ, et al. Mechanical properties and wear behavior of condensable composites [abstract 407]. J Dent Res 1999;78:156.

Ruse ND. What is a compomer? J Can Dent Assoc 1999;65:500–504.

Ruyter IE, Øysæd H. Composites for use in posterior teeth: composition and conversion. J Biomed Mater Res 1987;21:11–23.

Sideridou I, Tserki V, Papanastasiou G. Study of water sorption, solubility and modulus of light cured dimethacrylate-based dental resins. Biomaterials 2003;24:655.

Transactions of the Academy of Dental Materials, vol 12. [Proceedings of Conference on Critical Reviews of Restorative Quandaries, 1–3 Oct 1998, Banff, Canada]. Lake Oswego, OR: Academy of Dental Materials, 1998.

Van Meerbeek B, Braem M, Lambrechts P, Vanherle G. Two-year clinical valuation of two dentine-adhesive systems in cervical lesions. J Dent 1993;21(4):195–202.

Van Meerbeek B, Lambrechts P, Inokoshi S, Braem M, Vanherle G. Factors affecting adhesion to mineralized tissues. Oper Dent 1992;5 (suppl):111–124.

Wendt SL Jr, Leinfelder KF. Clinical evaluation of a heat-treated resin composite inlay: 3-year results. Am J Dent 1992;5:258–262.

Willems G, Lambrechts P, Braem M, Vanherle G. Composite resins in the 21st century. Quintessence Int 1993;24:641–658.

Willems G, Lambrechts P, Braem M, Vanherle G. Three-year follow-up of five posterior composites; in vivo wear. J Dent 1993;21:74–78.

Winkler MM, Xu X, Burgess JO. In vitro contact wear of 8 posterior resin composites [abstract 1082]. J Dent Res 2000;79:279.

Zidan O, Gomez-Marin O, Tsuchiya T. A comparative study of the effects of dentinal bonding agents and application techniques on marginal gaps in Class V cavities. J Dent Res 1987;66:716–721.

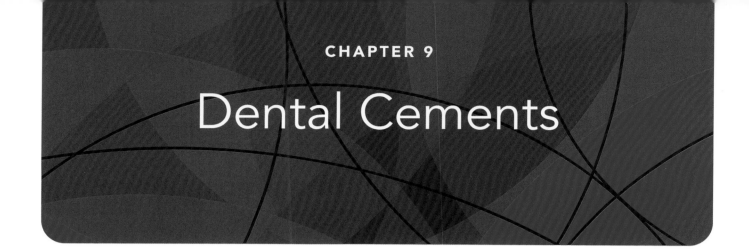

CHAPTER 9

Dental Cements

Although dental cements are used only in small quantities, they are perhaps the most important materials in clinical dentistry. These materials act as (1) luting agents to bond preformed restorations and orthodontic attachments in or on the tooth, (2) cavity liners and bases to protect the pulp and foundations and anchors for restorations, and (3) restorative materials. This multiplicity of applications requires more than one type of cement, because no one material has yet been developed that can fulfill the varying requirements.

Over the last two decades, there has been an emphasis on materials for **luting** in view of the increased use of fixed partial dentures. With the advent of glass-ionomer cements, interest in restorative applications has been revived, and most recent developments have introduced dual-cured multipurpose resin cements with self-curing and self-etching primers. Because different applications require different physical properties and clinical manipulative characteristics, new international standards are being developed (International Organization for Standards [ISO]), as are various national standards (American National Standards Institute/American Dental Association [ANSI/ADA]) based on performance criteria rather than specific composition.[1–3]

For acceptable performance in luting and restorative applications, the cement must have adequate resistance to dissolution in the oral environment and be biocompatible. It must also develop an adequately strong bond through mechanical interlocking and adhesion. High strength in tension, shear, and compression is required, as is good fracture toughness to resist stresses at the restoration-tooth interface. Good manipulation properties, such as adequate working and setting times, are necessary for successful use. The manipulation, including dispensation of the ingredients, should allow for some margin of error in practice.

Most cements are powder/liquid materials that may be dispensed and mixed manually or predispensed in capsules that are mixed mechanically. Some recent materials are composed of two pastes. Cements set by chemical reaction between the ingredients (often an acid-base reaction) or by polymerization of a monomeric component. In the early 20th century, zinc oxide–phosphoric acid, zinc oxide–eugenol (clove oil 85%), and silicate glass–phosphoric acid cements were discovered. These cements were widely used until the 1970s, when new cements began to be developed.

The introduction of new types of cements was prompted by the desire for improved biocompatibility and bonding to the tooth as well as esthetic demands that began to develop 30 years ago. New information on pulpal histopathologic changes due to particular clinical techniques and materials, as well as the demonstration of marginal leakage involving penetration of bacteria into the dentin interface and a reduction in retention of restorations, led to the realization that new materials with good wetting and bonding to enamel and dentin and low toxicity were needed.

These concepts prompted the development of cements based on polyacrylic acid: first the zinc polyacrylate (polycarboxylate) cements, then the glass-ionomer cements, and more recently the resin cements and hybrid ionomer cements. The newer cements have gradually become established as alternatives to zinc phosphate cement because of their minimal effects on pulp, similar strength and solubility characteristics, and adhesive properties.

The advent of the acrylic resins led to the development of poly(methyl methacrylate) (PMMA) in the mid-1950s, but limitations such as lack of adhesion, leakage, and toxicity terminated their use for routine cementation. In the last 20 years, polymerizable bisphenol-A diglycidyl-

Fig 9-1 Classification of dental cements according to bonding mechanism. EBA = ethoxybenzoic acid.

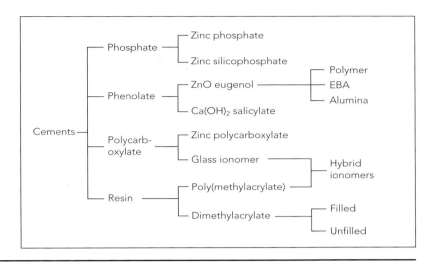

Table 9-1 Classification of dental cements

TYPE (MATRIX BOND)	CLASS OF CEMENT	FORMULATIONS
Phosphate	Zinc phosphate	Zinc phosphate Zinc phosphate fluoride Zinc phosphate copper oxide/salts Zinc phosphate silver salts
	Zinc silicophosphate	Zinc silicophosphate Zinc silicophosphate mercury salts
Phenolate	Zinc oxide–eugenol	Zinc oxide–eugenol Zinc oxide–eugenol polymer Zinc oxide–eugenol EBA/alumina
	Calcium hydroxide salicylate	Calcium hydroxide salicylate
Polycarboxylate	Zinc polycarboxylate	Zinc polycarboxylate Zinc polycarboxylate fluoride
	Glass ionomer	Calcium aluminum polyalkenoate Calcium aluminum polyalkenoate-polymethacrylate
Resin	Acrylic	PMMA
	Dimethacrylate	Dimethacrylate unfilled Dimethacrylate filled
	Adhesive	4-META
Resin-modified glass ionomers	Hybrid ionomers	Self-cured Light-cured

ether-dimethacrylate (bis-GMA) and other dimethacrylate monomer cements have become available in various forms for attachment of cast restorations and orthodontic brackets to enamel. More recently, similar systems containing (potentially) adhesive monomers have been marketed for fixed partial denture cementation.

The cements based on the reaction between calcium hydroxide and a liquid salicylate also originated 35 years ago. They were primarily fluid, two-paste materials intended for the lining of deep cavities that had actual or potential exposure, thus providing an antibacterial seal-

ing to facilitate the formation of reparative dentin. The susceptibility to acid erosion of the original formulations, both through marginal leakage of restorations and exposure to phosphoric acid during acid-etch techniques, has resulted in more resistant compositions and, recently, to a light-cured, resin-based material.

As a result of the research of the last 20 years, five basic types of cements are available, classified according to the matrix-forming species, as shown in Fig 9-1 and Table 9-1:

Table 9-2 "Permanent" luting cements

PRODUCT	TYPE	MANUFACTURER
Multilink Automix	Dual-cured resin	Ivoclar Vivadent
Panavia F 2.0	Dual-cured resin with Fl	Kuraray Dental
Maxcem	Dual-cured resin cement	Kerr Dental
Fuji Plus	Hybrid ionomer	GC America
Vitremer Luting	Hybrid ionomer	3M ESPE
Fleck's Extraordinary	Zinc phosphate	Mizzy
Fuji I	Glass ionomer	GC America
Fynal	Zinc oxide–eugenol	Dentsply Caulk
Hy-Bond Polycarboxylate Cement	Zinc carboxylate	Shofu Dental
Hy-Bond Zinc Phosphate Cement	Zinc phosphate	Shofu Dental
Ketac-Cem	Glass ionomer	3M ESPE
Rely X	Hybrid ionomer	3M ESPE
Modern Tenacin	Zinc phosphate	Dentsply Caulk
Super EBA	Zinc oxide–eugenol	Bosworth
Tylok Plus	Zinc carboxylate	Dentsply Caulk
Zinc Cement Improved	Zinc phosphate	Mission White Dental

Table 9-3 Selection of dental cements

APPLICATION	CEMENT TYPE
Luting inlays, crown posts, multiretainers, fixed partial denture in or on:	Glass-ionomer cement, hybrid ionomers, dual-cure resin
Nonvital teeth or teeth with advanced pulpal recession and average retention	Zinc phosphate
Vital teeth with average retention, average pulpal recession, thin dentin, especially for single units and small-span fixed partial dentures	Zinc polycarboxylate
Multiretainer splints on vital teeth with above-average retention, minimal dentin thickness; hypersensitive patients	Zinc oxide–eugenol polymer
Provisional cementation	Zinc oxide–eugenol polymer Zinc polycarboxylate (thin mix)
Provisional cementation and stabilization of old, loose restorations; fixation of facings and acid-etched cast restorations	Dimethacrylate resin composite
Base/liner in:	
Cavity with remaining dentin greater than about 0.5 mm	Glass-ionomer cement, resin ionomer Zinc polycarboxylate Zinc phosphate (low-acid type)
Cavity with minimal dentin or exposure	Calcium hydroxide salicylate Zinc oxide–eugenol polymer

Table 9-4 Properties of dental luting cements

MATERIAL	FILM THICKNESS (MM)	SETTING TIME (MIN)	SOLUBILITY (WT%)	STRENGTH (MPa) COMPRESSIVE	TENSILE	MODULUS OF ELASTICITY (GPa)
Zinc phosphate	25–35	5–14	0.2 max	80–100	5–7	13
Zinc oxide–eugenol						
Unmodified	25–35	2–10	1.5	2–25	1–2	—
Polymer reinforced	35–45	7–9	1	35–55	5–8	2–3
EBA-alumina	40–60	7–13	1	55–70	3–6	3–6
Zinc polycarboxylate	20–25	6–9	0.06	55–85	8–12	5–6
Glass ionomer	25–35	6–9	1	90–140	6–7	7–8
Polymer based	20–60	3–7	0.05	70–200	25–40	4–6

1. Phosphate bonded
2. Phenolate bonded
3. Polycarboxylate bonded
4. Dimethylacrylate bonded
5. Polycarboxylate and dimethylacrylate combinations

Numerous brands of each type are available, and there is some overlap between properties. Examples of current widely used brands of permanent luting cements are presented in Table 9-2. Since clinical and in vivo evaluation of cements is still very limited, the predictive value of laboratory data for assessment of clinical performance requires knowledgeable interpretation, especially because generalizations about specific types of cement cannot be made based on the behavior of one or two brands. The applications of the different types of cements are presented in Table 9-3. Typical properties of luting cements are presented in Table 9-4.

◼ Phosphate-Based Cements

Zinc phosphate cement

Applications

Because of their long history, these materials have the widest range of applications, from the cementation (luting) of fixed cast alloy and porcelain restorations and orthodontic bands (see Table 9-2) to their use as a cavity liner or base to protect pulp from mechanical, thermal, or electric stimuli.

Composition and setting

The powder is mainly zinc oxide with up to 10% magnesium oxide and small amounts of pigments. It is fired at high temperature (> 1,000°C) for several hours to reduce its reactivity. The liquid is an aqueous solution of phosphoric acid containing 45% to 64% H_3PO_4 and 30% to 55% water. The liquid also contains 2% to 3% aluminum and 0% to 9% zinc. Aluminum is essential to the cement-forming reaction, whereas zinc is a moderator of the reaction between powder and liquid, allowing adequate **working time** and permitting a sufficient quantity of powder to be added for optimum properties in the cement.

Some zinc phosphate cements have modified compositions. One material, widely used as a cavity liner, has 8% aluminum and only 25% H_3PO_4 in the liquid and a powder that contains calcium hydroxide. Others may contain fluoride and have as much as 10% stannous fluoride.

The amorphous zinc phosphate formed binds together the unreacted zinc oxide and other components of the cement. The set cement consists of a **cored structure** of residual zinc oxide particles in a phosphate matrix:

$$\text{zinc oxide} + \text{phosphoric acid} \rightarrow \text{amorphous zinc phosphate}$$

Manipulation

The mixing slab must be thoroughly dried before use. A chilled (5°C) thick glass slab will slow the initial reaction and allow incorporation of more powder, giving superior properties in the set cement.

The measurement of the components and the timing of mixing are necessary. The powder is added to the liquid in small portions to achieve the desired consistency. Increasing the powder/liquid ratio gives a more viscous mix, shorter setting time, higher strength, lower solubility, and less free acidity. Dissipation of the heat of reaction by mixing over a large area on a cooled slab will allow a greater incorporation of powder in a given amount of liquid. The cement must be undisturbed until the end of the **setting time**. It is kept sealed with a stopper to prevent changes in the water content. Cloudy liquid should be discarded.

Properties

Zinc phosphates have been used in clinical practice for many years. Under routine conditions, they can be easily manipulated, and they set sharply to a relatively strong mass from a fluid consistency. Although the properties are far from ideal, they are usually regarded as a standard against which to compare newer cements (see Table 9-4).

For a given brand, the properties are a function of the powder/liquid ratio. For a given cementing consistency, the higher the powder/liquid ratio, the better the strength properties and the lower the solubility and free acidity. At room temperature (21°C to 23°C) the working time for most brands at luting consistency is 3 to 6 minutes, and the setting time is 5 to 14 minutes. Extended working times and shorter setting times can be achieved by use of a cold mixing slab, which permits up to an approximate 50% increase in the amount of powder, improving both strength and resistance to dissolution.

The cement must have the ability to wet the tooth and restoration, flow into the irregularities on the joining surfaces, and fill in and seal the gaps between the restoration and the tooth. The minimum value of film thickness is a function of powder particle size, powder/liquid ratio, and mix viscosity. As measured by ISO and ANSI/ADA specifications,[1–3] acceptable cements give film thicknesses of less than 25 µm. In practice, the cement fills in the inaccuracies between the restoration and the tooth and allows most castings to seat satisfactorily. Unless escapeways or vents are provided with full crowns, separation of powder and liquid may occur, with marginal defects in the cement film.

At the recommended powder/liquid ratio (2.5 to 3.5 g/mL), the compressive strength of the set zinc phosphate cement is 80 to 110 MPa (11,000 to 16,000 psi) after 24 hours. The minimum strength for adequate re- tention of restorations is about 60 MPa (8,500 psi). The strength is strongly and almost linearly dependent on powder/liquid ratio. The tensile strength is much lower than the compressive strength, 5 to 7 MPa (700 to 900 psi), and the cement shows brittle characteristics. The modulus of elasticity (stiffness) is about 13 GPa (1.8×10^6 psi).

According to the standard method, the solubility and disintegration in distilled water after 23 hours may range from 0.04% to 3.3% for inferior material. The standard limit is 0.2%. The solubility in fluoride-containing cements is about 0.7% to 1.0% because of the leaching of fluoride. The solubility in organic acid solutions, such as lactic or citric acid, is 20 to 30 times higher. These data are only a rough guide to solubility under oral conditions. The comparative evaluation of cement solubility under clinical conditions has shown significant loss but conflicting results. Dissolution contributes to marginal leakage around restorations and bacterial penetration. This occurrence may be facilitated by dimensional change. The cement has been found to contract about 0.5% linearly, giving rise to slits at the tooth-cement and cement-restoration interfaces.

Biologic effects

The freshly mixed zinc phosphate is highly acidic, with a pH between 1 and 2 after mixing, and, even after setting 1 hour, the pH may still be below 4. After 24 hours, the pH is usually between 6 and 7. Pain on cementation is due not only to the free acidity of the mix but also to osmotic movement of fluid through the dentinal tubules. Hydraulic pressure developed during seating of the restoration may also contribute to pulpal damage. Prolonged pulpal irritation, especially in deep cavities that necessitate some form of pulpal protection, may be associated with prolongation of the low pH. Irritation is minimized by a high powder/liquid ratio and rapid setting. A material that has a low acid content and incorporates calcium hydroxide has little effect on pulp when used as a liner. Very thin mixes will also lead to etching of the enamel.

Advantages and disadvantages

The main advantages of zinc phosphate cements are that they can be mixed easily and that they set sharply to a relatively strong mass from a fluid consistency. Unless the mix is extremely thin (for instance, with a very low powder/liquid ratio), the set cement has a strength that is adequate for clinical service, so manipulation is less critical than with other cements.

However, zinc phosphates' distinct disadvantages include pulpal irritation, lack of antibacterial action, brittleness, lack of adhesion, and solubility in oral fluids.

Modified zinc phosphate cements

Copper and silver cements

Black copper cements contain cupric oxide (CuO), and red copper cements contain cuprous oxide (Cu_2O). Others may contain cuprous iodide or silicate. Because a much lower powder/liquid ratio is necessary to obtain satisfactory manipulation characteristics with these cements, the mix is highly acidic, resulting in much greater pulpal irritation. Their solubility is higher and their strength is lower than zinc phosphate cements. Their bacteriostatic or anticariogenic properties seem to be slight. Silver cements generally contain a small percentage of a salt such as silver phosphate. Their advantages over zinc phosphate cement have not been substantiated.

Fluoride cements

Stannous fluoride (1% to 3%) is present in some orthodontic cements. These materials have a higher solubility and lower strength than zinc phosphate cement due to dissolution of the fluoride-containing material. Fluoride uptake by enamel from such cements results in reduced enamel solubility and potentially anticariogenic effects. Fluoride is found in some hybrid iononomer and dual-cured resin cements.

Silicophosphate cements

These materials have been available for many years as a combination of zinc phosphate and silicate cements. The presence of the silicate glass provides a degree of translucency, improved strength, and fluoride release.

Applications

Their principal applications have been for the cementation of fixed restorations and orthodontic bands (type I), as a provisional posterior restorative material (type II), and as a dual-purpose material (type III).

Composition and setting

The powder in these materials consists of a blend of 10% to 20% zinc oxide (zinc phosphate cement powder) and silicate glass (silicate cement powder) mechanically mixed or fused and reground. The silicate glass usually contains 12% to 25% fluoride. Some materials have been labeled "germicidal" because of the presence of small amounts of mercury or silver compounds. The liquid is a concentrated orthophosphoric acid solution containing about 45% water and 2% to 5% aluminum and zinc salts.

The setting reaction has not been fully investigated, but may be represented as follows:

$$\text{zinc oxide/aluminosilicate glass + phosphoric acid} \rightarrow \text{zinc aluminosilicate phosphate gel}$$

The set cement consists of unreacted glass and zinc oxide particles bonded together by the aluminosilicophosphate gel matrix.

Manipulation

The mixing is analogous to that for a phosphate cement; a nonabradable spatula and a cooled mixing slab should be used. The filling mix should be glossy, with putty-like consistency.

Properties

At cementing consistency, the setting time is 5 to 7 minutes; working time is about 4 minutes and may be increased by using a cold mixing slab. These cements generally have shorter working times and a coarser grain size, leading to a higher film thickness than with zinc phosphate cements. One material is improved in these respects, and film thickness is adequate for cementation of cast gold and porcelain restorations.

The compressive strength of the set cement ranges from 140 to 170 MPa (20,000 to 25,000 psi); the tensile strength is considerably lower at 7 MPa (1,000 psi) (see Table 9-4). The toughness and abrasion resistance are higher than those of phosphate cements. The durability in bonding orthodontic bands to teeth is greater, and less decalcification is observed.

The solubility in distilled water after 7 days is about 1% by weight. Solubility in organic acids and in the mouth is less than for phosphate cements. In the presence of oral fluids, fluoride will leach out

The glass content gives considerably greater translucency than phosphate cements, making silicophosphate cements useful for cementation of porcelain restorations.

Biologic effects

Because of the acidity of the mix and the prolonged low pH (4 to 5) after setting, pulpal protection is necessary on all vital teeth. Fluoride and other ions are leached out from the set cement by oral fluids, resulting in increased enamel fluoride and probable anticariogenic action.

Advantages and disadvantages

Silicophosphate cements have better strength, toughness, and abrasion-resistance properties than zinc phosphate cements and show considerable fluoride release, translucency, and, under clinical conditions, lower solubility and better bonding.

However, the initial pH and total acidity are greater than those for zinc phosphate cements; thus, pulpal sensitivity may be of longer duration. Manipulation with these cements is more critical than with zinc phosphate cements.

● Phenolate-Based Cements

The main types of phenolate-bonded cements are:

1. Simple zinc oxide–eugenol combination that may contain setting accelerators
2. Reinforced zinc oxide–eugenol
3. Ortho-ethoxybenzoic acid (EBA)

Cements have also been formulated using other phenolic liquids, but have seen little use except for those materials containing calcium hydroxide and a salicylate.

Zinc oxide–eugenol cements

Applications

The basic combination of zinc oxide and eugenol finds its principal applications in the provisional cementation of crowns and fixed partial dentures, in the provisional restoration of teeth, and as a cavity liner in deep cavity preparations.

Composition and setting

The powder is pure zinc oxide (United States Pharmacopeia or equivalent, arsenic-free). Commercial materials may contain small amounts of fillers, such as silica. About 1% of zinc salts, such as acetate or sulfate, may be present to accelerate the setting. The liquid is purified eugenol or, in some commercial materials, oil of cloves (85% eugenol). One percent or less of alcohol or acetic acid may be included to accelerate setting together with small amounts of water, which is necessary for the setting reaction.

A chemical reaction occurs between zinc oxide and eugenol, with the formation of zinc eugenolate (eugenate):

$$\text{zinc oxide} + \text{eugenol} \xrightarrow{\text{water}} \text{zinc eugenolate} \atop \text{(eugenate)}$$

The precise mechanism is not fully understood, but the set mass contains residual zinc oxide particles bonded by a matrix of zinc eugenolate and some free eugenol. Water is essential to the reaction, which is also accelerated by zinc ions. The reaction is reversible because the zinc eugenolate is easily hydrolyzed by moisture to eugenol and zinc hydroxide. Thus, the cement disintegrates rapidly when exposed to oral conditions. The rate of reaction between the zinc oxide and eugenol depends on the nature, source, reactivity, and moisture content of the zinc oxide and on the purity and moisture content of the eugenol.

Manipulation

The zinc oxide is slowly wetted by the eugenol; therefore, prolonged and vigorous spatulation is required, especially for a thick mix. A powder/liquid ratio of 3:1 or 4:1 must be used for maximum strength.

Properties

The working time is long because moisture is required for setting. Variable results are obtained with different samples of zinc oxide, depending on their mode of preparation and reactivity. For a given oxide, set time is controlled by moisture availability, **accelerators**, and the powder/liquid ratio. Mixes of cementing consistency set very slowly unless accelerators are used and/or a drop of water is added. Commercial materials set in 2 to 10 minutes, resulting in adequate strengths at 10 minutes for amalgam restorations to be placed (see Table 9-4).

The particle size of the zinc oxide and the viscosity of the mix govern the film thickness. Use of a fluid mix gives values of about 40 μm.

Because of the weak nature of the binding agent, the compressive strength is low, in the range of 7 to 40 MPa (1,000 to 6,000 psi). The tensile strength is very low also.

The solubility is high, about 1.5% by weight in distilled water after 24 hours. Eugenol is extracted from the set cement by the hydrolytic decomposition of the zinc eugenolate/eugenate. The cement disintegrates rapidly when exposed to oral conditions.

Biologic effect

The presence of eugenol in the set cement under clinical conditions appears to lead to an **anodyne** and **obtundent** effect on the pulp in deep cavities. At the same time, eugenol is a potential allergen. When exposed directly to oral conditions, the material maintains good sealing characteristics despite a volumetric shrinkage of 0.9% and a thermal expansion of $35 \times 10^{-6}/°C$. The sealing capacity and antibacterial action appear to facilitate pulpal healing; however, when in direct contact with connective tissue, the material is an irritant. Reparative dentin formation in exposed pulp is variable.

Advantages and disadvantages

The main advantage of these materials is their bland and obtundent effect on the pulpal tissues, together with their good sealing ability and resistance to marginal penetration.

Disadvantages include low strength and abrasion resistance, solubility and disintegration in oral fluids, and little anticariogenic action.

Reinforced zinc oxide–eugenol cements

Applications

These materials have been used as cementing agents for crowns and fixed partial dentures, cavity liners and base materials, and provisional restorative materials.

Composition and setting

The powder consists of zinc oxide with 10% to 40% finely divided natural or synthetic resins (eg, colophony [pine resin], PMMA, polystyrene, or polycarbonate) together with accelerators. The liquid is eugenol, which may also contain dissolved resins as mentioned earlier and accelerators such as acetic acid, as well as antimicrobial agents such as thymol or 8-hydroxyquinoline.

The setting reaction is similar to zinc oxide–eugenol cements. Acidic resins such as colophony (abietic acid) may react with the zinc oxide, strengthening the matrix.

Manipulation

More powder is required for a cementing mix than with other cements. Measures are provided for some commercial materials, and the proper ratio must be adhered to for adequate strength properties. The mixing pad or slab should be thoroughly dry. The powder is mixed into the liquid in small portions with vigorous spatulation until the correct amount has been incorporated. Adequate time should be allowed for setting without disturbance of the cement. Both powder and liquid containers should be kept closed and stored under dry conditions.

Properties

These cements may have a long working time because moisture is needed for setting. Some commercial materials contain moisture and, therefore, have working and setting times in the same range as zinc phosphate cements, that is, 7 to 9 minutes in oral conditions. Setting time is also lengthened by reducing the powder/liquid ratio.

At cementing consistency, values of film thickness from 35 to 75 µm have been obtained with commercial materials (see Table 9-4). Clinical trials have shown satisfactory performance in seating castings for cements with the lowest values.

These materials have compressive strengths in the range from 35 to 55 MPa (5,000 to 8,000 psi). The tensile strength is 5 to 8 MPa (700 to 1,000 psi) (see Table 9-4). The strength is adequate as a lining material and for luting single restorations and retainers with good retention form. The modulus of elasticity is 2 to 3 GPa (300,000 to 400,000 psi). The mechanical properties of these cements are reduced by immersion in water, which results in loss of eugenol, although this appears to be slower than with simple zinc oxide–eugenol materials. This tendency seems less pronounced with the polymer-reinforced materials.

Because of the presence of the resin, the solubility of these cements appears to be lower than that of zinc oxide–eugenol materials.

Biologic effects

Polymer-reinforced zinc oxide–eugenol cements have biologic effects similar to basic materials, although there is some variation in inflammatory reaction in connective tissue with the brand of material. There may be softening and discoloration of some resin restorative materials.

Advantages and disadvantages

The main advantages of these materials are the minimal biologic effects, good initial sealing properties, and adequate strength for final cementation of restorations. The principal disadvantages are the lower strength, higher solubility, and higher disintegration compared with zinc phosphate cements; hydrolytic instability; and the softening and discoloration of some resin restorative materials.

EBA and other chelate cements

To further improve on the basic zinc oxide–eugenol system, many researchers have investigated mixtures of zinc and other oxides with various liquid **chelating** agents. The only system that has received extensive commercial exploitation for luting and lining is that containing ortho-EBA. (Noneugenol cements have also been developed in which fatty acids or low-odor phenolic derivatives are used to overcome the smell and taste of eugenol.)

Applications

These materials have been used for the cementation of inlays, crowns, and fixed partial dentures; for provisional restorations; and as base or lining materials.

Composition and setting

In EBA materials, the powder is mainly zinc oxide containing 20% to 30% aluminum oxide or other mineral fillers. Polymeric reinforcing agents, such as PMMA, may also be present. The liquid consists of eugenol and 50% to 66% EBA.

The setting mechanism has not been fully elucidated, but it appears to involve chelate salt formation between EBA, eugenol, and zinc oxide. The setting is accelerated by the same factors that are operative for zinc oxide–eugenol cements.

Manipulation

In general, the manipulation is similar to that of reinforced zinc oxide–eugenol cements. The cement mixes readily to a very fluid consistency even at a high powder/liquid ratio. To obtain optimal properties, it is important to use as high a powder/liquid ratio as possible—about 3.5 g/mL for cementation and 5 to 6 g/mL for liners or bases. Vigorous spatulation is required for about 2 minutes to incorporate all of the powder. The correct mix flows readily under pressure because of the long working time. Adequate setting time in the mouth should be allowed. Several days may be required to reach maximum strength.

Properties

The working time at room temperature is long because of the dependence on moisture. The setting time ranges between 7 and 13 minutes under oral conditions (see Table 9-4).

The film thickness may be between 40 and 70 μm depending on the brand, but for permanent cementation of restorations, the lower level is preferable.

At cementing consistency, the compressive strength of these materials is in the range of 55 to 70 MPa (8,000 to 10,000 psi); higher values, similar to those of zinc phosphate cements, can be obtained by increasing the powder/liquid ratio. The tensile strength is considerably lower, about 3 to 6 MPa (500 to 900 psi), and the modulus of elasticity is about 5 GPa (700,000 psi). The viscoelastic properties of EBA cements show very low strength and slow rates of large plastic deformation (0.1 mm/min) at oral temperature (37°C). These characteristics may explain why the retention values for crowns and orthodontic bands are considerably below those for zinc phosphate cements.

The solubility is similar to that of the polymer-reinforced zinc oxide–eugenol materials in distilled water, although loss of eugenol also occurs. The resistance to solubility in organic acids appears to be greater than that of the zinc phosphate cements. When exposed to moisture, greater oral dissolution occurs than for other cements. However, a clinical survey by Silvey and Myers[4] of the performance of an EBA-alumina cement during 3 years showed only slightly worse results than for zinc phosphate and polycarboxylate cements. Oral breakdown may thus depend on the precise brand and manipulation.

Biologic effects

The biologic properties of these materials appear to be similar to those of zinc oxide–eugenol materials.

Advantages and disadvantages

EBA cements are very easy to mix and have a long working time, good flow characteristics, and low irritation to pulp. Strength and film thickness can be comparable with those of zinc phosphate cements (see Table 9-4).

The main disadvantages are the critical proportioning, hydrolytic breakdown in oral fluids, liability to plastic deformation, and poorer retention than zinc phosphate cements. These materials seem best suited for luting restorations with good fit and retention where there is no undue stress and as cavity bases.

Calcium hydroxide chelate cements

The value of calcium hydroxide as a pulp-capping material that facilitates the formation of reparative dentin has long been recognized. This action appears to be largely attributable to its alkaline pH and consequent antibacterial and protein-lyzing effect. Although a number of aqueous paste materials based on calcium hydroxide are available, they are not easy to manipulate, and the dried films tend to crack. In the early 1960s, phenolate-type cements based on the setting reaction between calcium hydroxide and other oxides and salicylate esters were introduced.

Applications

These cements are used as liners in deep cavity preparations.

Composition and setting

Usually, two pastes are used: One contains calcium hydroxide, zinc oxide, and zinc salts in ethylene toluene sulphonamide; and the other contains calcium sulfate, titanium dioxide, and calcium tungstate (a radiopacifying agent) in a liquid disalicylate ester of butane-1,3-diol. An intentional excess of calcium hydroxide produces an alkaline pH to effect an antibacterial and remineralization action. There is some variation among the materials in this respect. At least one material contains fluoride.

Calcium and zinc oxide react with the salicylate ester to form a chelate similar to the zinc oxide–eugenol reaction. Likewise, the reaction is greatly accelerated by moisture and accelerators.

Manipulation

Equal lengths of the two pastes are mixed to a uniform color.

Properties

Working time may be 3 to 5 minutes, depending on the availability of moisture. In the mouth, setting is rapid, about 1 or 2 minutes.

The compressive strength at 7 minutes is about 6 MPa (900 psi), and the tensile strength is 1.5 MPa (200 psi); at 1 hour the corresponding values are about 10 MPa (1,500 psi) and 1.5 MPa (200 psi); at 24 hours the values are 14 to 20 MPa (2,000 to 3,000 psi) and 1.7 to 2.0 MPa (250 to 300 psi). Thin films become resistant to an 8 MPa (1,100 psi) penetration force in 90 seconds. Plastic flow without fracture occurs at 37°C.

The solubility in 50% phosphoric acid during acid-etching procedures is significant. These cements seem to be subject to hydrolytic breakdown. When continued marginal leakage takes place, complete dissolution of the linings of these materials can occur.

Biologic effects

These cements appear to exert a strong antibacterial action when free calcium hydroxide is available and to assist in remineralization of carious dentin. They facilitate the formation of dentin bridges when used for pulp capping on exposures. Their effect on exposed pulp is superior to that of zinc oxide–eugenol materials. These materials can also exert a pulpal protective action by neutralizing and preventing the passage of acid and by acting as a barrier to the penetration of other agents, such as methyl methacrylate.

Advantages and disadvantages

These cements are easy to manipulate, they rapidly harden in thin layers, and they have good sealing characteristics and beneficial effects on carious dentin and exposed pulp.

However, they show low strength even when fully set, exhibit plastic deformation, are weakened by exposure to moisture, and will dissolve under acidic conditions and if marginal leakage occurs. The data on physical properties and clinical experience suggest that further improvements in these materials are required before they can be used as the sole liner in deep cavity preparations.

More recently, polymerizable resin compositions containing calcium hydroxide have been introduced as alternatives to these materials.

◉ Polycarboxylate (Carboxylate)-Based Cements

Zinc polycarboxylate cements

The polycarboxylate cements were developed in the late 1960s as adhesive dental cements that combined the strength properties of the phosphate system with the biologic acceptability of the zinc oxide–eugenol materials.

Applications

Zinc polycarboxylates are used for the cementation of cast alloy and porcelain restorations and orthodontic bands, as cavity liners or base materials, and as provisional restorative materials.

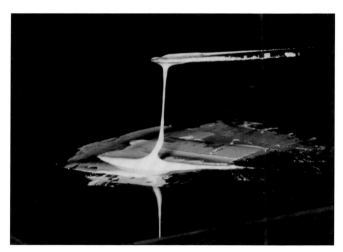

Fig 9-2 Typical consistency for water mix polycarboxylate and glass-ionomer cements. The mix is comparable with zinc phosphate cements.

Composition and setting

The powder in these cements is zinc oxide with, in some cases, 1% to 5% tin or magnesium oxide; 10% to 40% aluminum oxide or other reinforcing filler may be present in some brands. A small percentage of stannous or other fluoride may also be included to improve mechanical properties and provide leachable fluoride. The liquid is approximately a 40% aqueous solution of polyacrylic acid or an acrylic acid copolymer with other organic acids, such as itaconic acid. The molecular weight of the polymer is generally in the range of 30,000 to 50,000, which accounts for the viscous nature of the solution. In some brands, the polyacrylic acid component is dried and then added to the powder. In a brand that is encapsulated, the liquid is a weak solution of NaH_2PO_4, which both reduces the viscosity of the polyacrylic acid and retards the setting of the cement. In other brands, water is simply added to the powdered ingredients.

The zinc oxide reacts with the polyacrylic acid, forming a cross-linked structure of zinc polyacrylate. The set cement consists of the residual zinc oxide particles bonded together by this amorphous gel-like matrix:

zinc oxide + polyacrylic acid → zinc polyacrylate

Manipulation

The material should be carefully proportioned and the freshly dispensed components mixed rapidly in 30 to 40 seconds. The mix should be used while it is still glossy, before the onset of cobwebbing. The correct cementing mix is more viscous than a zinc phosphate mix, but because of its different **rheology** it flows adequately under pressure. The water mix materials are more fluid initially (Fig 9-2). The interior of restorations and tooth surfaces should be clean and free of saliva. The powder and liquid should be stored under cool conditions and kept sealed with a stopper. However, prolonged or cold storage may cause the liquid to gel. To reverse this effect, the gel must be warmed to 50°C. Loss of moisture from the liquid will lead to thickening.

Properties

The rate of setting is affected by the powder/liquid ratio, the reactivity of the zinc oxide, the particle size, the presence of additives, and the molecular weight and concentration of the polyacrylic acid. At luting consistency the recommended powder/liquid ratio for most materials is about 1.5:1.0 by weight. The working time is 2.5 to 3.5 minutes at room temperature, and the setting time is 6 to 9 minutes at 37°C; the water mix materials tend to give slightly longer setting times. As with other cements, working time can be substantially increased by mixing the material on a cold slab and by refrigerating the powder. The liquid should not be chilled, as this encourages gelation due to hydrogen bonding.

The freshly mixed cement shows shear thinning. Contrary to the subjective impression that the correct mix for a zinc polycarboxylate cement is much thicker than that of a luting zinc phosphate mix, under pressure they flow out to the same degree, to a film thickness of 25 to 35 μm. The zinc phosphate mix tends to thicken more quickly than the zinc polycarboxylate mix. One of the most common errors in preparing these cements is to make a mix that appears to be as fluid as a zinc phosphate mix, resulting in a low powder/liquid ratio and thus poor cement properties. Measuring devices for these materials will ensure correct proportions.

At cementing consistency, the compressive strength of these materials is in the range of 55 to 85 MPa (8,000 to 12,000 psi), and the tensile strength is 8 to 12 MPa (1,100 to 1,700 psi) (see Table 9-4). Strength increases with the powder/liquid ratio, reaching a maximum at about 2:1 by weight, and it is increased also by additives such as alumina and stannous fluoride. In general these cements have lower compressive strengths than zinc phosphate cements but are significantly stronger in tension. The cement gains strength rapidly after the initial setting period; the strength at 1 hour is about 80% of the

24-hour value. The modulus of elasticity is about 6 GPa (850,000 psi).

In distilled water, the solubility ranges from less than 0.1% to 0.6%. The latter high value relates particularly to cements that contain stannous fluoride. However, as in the zinc phosphate system, the solubility is appreciably higher in acids such as lactic and citric acid. In vivo solubility is similar to or less than that for zinc phosphate cements.

Bonding to clean enamel and dentin surfaces can occur through calcium complexation. In practice, adhesion to dentin may be limited because of debris and contamination. The material also sticks to clean stainless steel, amalgam, chromium-cobalt, and other alloys. Bond strength is related to the strength of the cement.

Biologic effects

The effect of zinc polycarboxylate cements on pulp is comparable with or less than that of zinc oxide–eugenol. The formation of reparative dentin in exposed pulp is variable. The generally good biocompatibility appears to be primarily due to the low intrinsic toxicity and also to (1) the rapid rise of the cement pH toward neutrality; (2) localization of the polyacrylic acid and limitation of diffusion by its molecular size and ion binding to dentinal fluid and proteins; and (3) the minimal movement of fluid in the dentinal tubules in response to the cement. The presence of stannous fluoride does not appear to affect the mild response. The fluoride-containing cements release fluoride, which is taken up by neighboring enamel and which presumably will exert anticariogenic effects.

Advantages and disadvantages

The main advantages of these materials are the low irritation, adhesion to tooth substance and alloys, easy manipulation, strength, solubility, and film thickness properties comparable with those of zinc phosphate cements.

The need for accurate proportioning for optimal properties and thus more critical manipulation, the lower compressive strength and greater viscoelasticity than zinc phosphate cements, the short working time of some materials, and the need for clean surfaces for adhesion are the disadvantages.

■ Polymer-Based Cements

Most of the materials in this group are polymethacrylates of two types: (1) materials based on methyl methacrylate and (2) materials based on aromatic dimethacrylates of the bis-GMA type. The closely related cyanoacrylate monomers, notably ethyl and isobutyl, have limited use for the attachment of facings and for pin cementation. The hydrolytic stability and biologic effects are questionable, however.

Acrylic resin cements

Applications

Acrylic resin cements are used for the cementation of restorations, facings, and provisional crowns.

Composition and setting

The powder in these materials is a finely divided methyl methacrylate polymer or copolymer containing benzoyl peroxide as the **initiator**. Mineral filler and pigments may also be present. The liquid is a methyl methacrylate monomer containing an amine accelerator.

The monomer dissolves and softens the polymer particles and concurrently polymerizes through the action of free radicals from the peroxide-amine interaction. The set mass consists of the new polymer matrix uniting the undissolved but swollen original polymer granules.

Manipulation

The liquid is added to the powder with minimal spatulation to avoid an incorporation of air. The mix must be used immediately because working time is short. Excess material must be removed at the final set, hard stage and not when the material is rubbery, otherwise marginal deficiencies will be created.

Properties

The properties of these materials are comparable with those of the cold-curing acrylic resin filling materials. They are stronger and less soluble than other types of cement but display low rigidity and viscoelastic properties. They have no effective bond to tooth structure in the presence of moisture; thus, they permit marginal leakage, although they may show better bonding than other cements to resin facings and polycarbonate crowns.

Biologic effects

As with acrylic resin filling materials, marked pulpal reaction may occur and pulpal protection is necessary.

Advantages and disadvantages

These materials have relatively high strength and toughness and low solubility, but they have a short working time, deleterious effects on pulp, and difficulty in removal of excess cement from margins.

Adhesive resin cements

Adhesive acrylic materials are formulated by adding an adhesion promoter, 4-methacryloxyethyl trimellitate anhydride (4-META), to the methyl methacrylate monomer as well as an additional polymerization initiator, tributyl boron, which is also believed to aid chemical bonding to dentin. Such materials have been developed as cements for metal fixed partial dentures, especially base metal (Super-Bond C&B, Sun Medical), and for bonding amalgam to dentin and composites (Amalgambond, Parkell). In vitro tests have shown high bond strengths for the luting cement to oxidized, etched, or silica-coated casting alloy surfaces. The shear bond strength to amalgam is significantly less than the bond strength to dentin (~20 MPa). Since these materials have only low filler content (<10%), the physical properties are typical of acrylic resins, that is, moderate strength with high deformation under load. Although the materials have been widely used for cementation of fixed partial dentures, there are little clinical data on longevity, and the cements are said to be *technique sensitive*.

Dimethacrylate cements

Cements of this type are usually based on the bis-GMA system: They are combinations of an aromatic dimethacrylate with other monomers containing various amounts of ceramic filler. They are basically similar to composite restorative materials.

Applications

Dimethacrylate cements are used for bonding crowns (usually porcelain), fixed partial dentures, inlays, veneers, and indirect resin restorations.

Composition and setting

Classification is by method of curing :

1. *Chemically (or auto-) cured:* Paste-paste systems used to cement metal and opaque ceramic core (eg, Procera, In-Ceram) restorations (Fig 9-3).
2. *Dual cured:* Cements that start curing with light and continue with chemical curing. The chemical cure will

polymerize more thoroughly than light curing alone (Fig 9-4). These products are used to cement translucent restorations (eg, porcelain, indirect resin restorations).

3. *Light cured/dual cured:* These products are used for both light-cure applications (eg, thin porcelain veneers) and dual-cure applications when dual-cure catalysts are added to the light-cure base (Fig 9-5).

In the powder/liquid materials, the powder is generally a finely divided borosilicate or silica glass together with fine polymer powder and an organic peroxide initiator. The liquid is a mixture of bis-GMA and/or other dimethacrylate monomers containing an amine promoter for polymerization. Some materials contain monomers with potentially adhesive groups, such as phosphate or carboxyl, similar to dentin bonding materials. The two-paste materials are of similar overall composition but with the monomers and fillers combined into two pastes. In light-cured and dual-cured materials, light-sensitive polymerization systems such as diketones (eg, camphorquinone) and amine promoters are present, respectively, in the two cement components in addition to the chemical-initiator systems.

On mixing the components, polymerization of the monomers occurs, leading to a highly cross-linked resin composite structure.

Manipulation

Correct proportioning of powder and liquid components using measures is important. Paste materials are usually proportioned 1:1 (equal lengths). Rapid, thorough mixing to minimize air inclusion until uniform is critical.

Properties

As with resin composite restorative materials, monomer conversion is incomplete, even under optimum cure conditions, and thus manipulation is critical to optimum physical properties. For light- and dual-cured materials, the maximum light exposure is desirable. Maximum properties are generally reached about 10 minutes after polymerization, and only small changes occur over the ensuing 24 hours.

Since polymerization systems vary and filler content ranges between 20% and 80% of the various products, physical properties vary widely (see Table 9-4) and the solubility of a specific material for a particular clinical application should be checked individually. Compressive strengths have been reported to range between 100 and

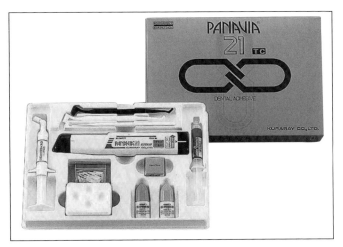

Fig 9-3 A chemically cured resin cement for use under opaque restorations. (Courtesy of Kuraray Dental.)

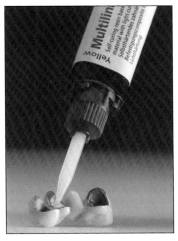

Fig 9-4 A dual-cured resin cement in mixing-syringe form for general use when light may not penetrate enough for complete curing. (Courtesy of Ivoclar Vivadent.)

200 MPa (14,000 and 28,000 psi), and diametral tensile strengths from 20 to 50 MPa (3,000 to 7,000 psi) with corresponding differences in microhardness. These values are considerably higher than traditional cements, and therefore high values can be obtained for retention of well-fitting crowns. However, optimum luting performance is dependent on fluidity, seating capability, and film thickness. Many resin cements tend to show unacceptably high values for film thickness. Recently, to improve wetting of the tooth, preparation, seating, and bond strength, some resin cements have been used with dentin bonding primers, thus increasing the clinical complexity of the system. Although these materials have been used widely in adhesive techniques, especially for ceramic restorations, there are comparatively few clinical reports of their longevity. Aside from failures induced by material and technique shortcomings during the critical clinical manipulation, studies indicate that resin cement bonds will most likely fail through cyclic fatigue stresses. Some studies on etched metal restorations cemented with chemically cured cements have indicated a median survival time of about 8 years.

Biologic effects

The materials themselves appear to pose few problems, although some patients experience objectionable odors. Cases of allergy among dental personnel have occurred, especially where reactive dentin bonding systems have been used. Skin contact should be avoided.

Pulpal pathology may be due to poor seating, polymerization contraction, and consequent microleakage.

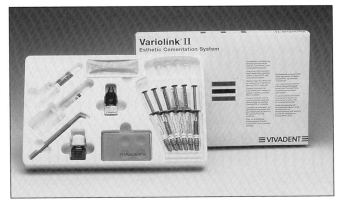

Fig 9-5 A light-cured/dual-cured cement may be cured with light or with addition of dual-cure catalyst, which will allow setting to continue after light is turned off. (Courtesy of Ivoclar Vivadent.)

All systems show some microleakage, which may contribute to tooth sensitivity and clinical failure. Microleakage appears to occur least with systems using dentin bonding agents, but there are no long-term studies on this aspect.

Advantages and disadvantages

These cements have high strength, low oral solubility, and high micromechanical (and possibly chemical) bonding to prepared enamel, dentin, alloys, and ceramic surfaces.

Disadvantages include the need for a meticulous and critical technique, more difficult sealing and higher film thickness than traditional cements, possible leakage and pulpal sensitivity, and difficulty in removal of excess cement.

■ Glass-Ionomer Cements

These materials were formulated in the 1970s by bringing together the silicate and polyacrylate systems. The use of an acid-reactive glass powder together with a polyacrylic acid solution leads to a translucent, stronger cement that can be used for luting and restorative materials.

Applications

Glass-ionomer cements are used for the cementation of cast-alloy and porcelain restorations and orthodontic bands, as cavity liners or base materials, and as restorative materials, especially for erosion lesions. They are being replaced, however, by hybrid ionomer cements, which allow better handling.

Composition and setting

The powder in these materials is finely ground calcium aluminum fluorosilicate glass with a particle size around 40 μm for the filling materials and less than 25 μm for the luting materials. One brand (Zionomer liner, Den-Mat) also contains zinc oxide. Silver powder is fused into the glass in Ketac-Silver (3M ESPE) for improved physical properties. The liquid is a 50% aqueous solution of a polyacrylic-itaconic acid or other polycarboxylic acid copolymer that contains about 5% tartaric acid. Some other materials contain 10% to 20% added silver, silver alloy, or stainless steel. In some materials the solid copolymer is added to the powder, and the solution contains tartaric acid; in others, all of the ingredients are in the powder, and the liquid is water.

On mixing, the polyacrylic and tartaric acids react with the glass, leaching calcium and aluminum ions from the surface, which cross-link the polyacid molecules into a gel. The tartaric acid serves to increase working time and gives a sharp setting by forming metal ion complexes.[5] Differences in composition between brands affect the hardening rate and properties.

Manipulation

The material should be carefully proportioned and the freshly dispensed components mixed rapidly in 30 to 40 seconds. Some brands are encapsulated, mechanically mixed, and injected. The powder/liquid ratio for luting is about 1.3:1 for the conventional types of glass-ionomer cement. This ratio appears to be critical with these cements to obtain optimal cementation properties. Best re-sults are obtained by mixing the chilled powder with the liquid on a chilled slab. The correct cementing mix is fluid, similar to zinc phosphate. The lining mix is more viscous, depending on the brand. The restorative mix should have a putty-like consistency and a glossy surface. Tooth surfaces should be clean and free from saliva but not dehydrated. Restoration surfaces should be free from debris and contamination. The cement hardens slowly and should be protected from loss or gain of moisture when set clinically. Restoration margins or filling surfaces should be protected with a varnish or a light-curing sealant. This is less important with light-cured materials.

Properties

For the luting materials, the setting time is in the range of 6 to 9 minutes. The lining materials set in 4 to 5 minutes, and the restorative materials set in 3 to 4 minutes. Materials that are light-cured set in approximately 30 seconds when exposed to a visible light source. The acid-base reaction continues slowly and properties improve over time.

Film thickness in the range of 25 to 35 μm is adequate to seat castings satisfactorily, although the flow properties are dependent on the powder/liquid ratio.

For the luting cements, the compressive strength increases over 24 hours to between 90 and 140 MPa (13,000 to 20,000 psi) depending on the brand, and the tensile strength increases to between 6 and 8 MPa (900 to 1,100 psi). The lining materials have compressive and tensile strengths in the same range with some light-cured materials at the higher end of the range, reaching 150 to 160 MPa (21,000 to 23,000 psi) in compression and 10 to 12 MPa (1,400 to 1,700 psi) in tension. The compressive modulus of elasticity is about 7 GPa (900,000 psi). The light-cured materials are significantly tougher in some brands, with a lower modulus of elasticity. The restorative materials range from 140 to 180 MPa (20,000 to 26,000 psi) in compression and 12 to 15 MPa (1,700 to 2,100 psi) in tension. The light-cured restorative materials may have strengths as high as 200 MPa in compression and 20 MPa in tension. Some silver-containing materials are in this range, and even higher strengths have been achieved in recent materials. In general, with light-cured materials, properties are dependent on the depth of cure.

The solubility of a luting material in water is about 1% and in lactic acid is higher. Good resistance to dissolution is observed under oral conditions. Resistance to dissolution and disintegration may be improved by varnish protection.

Acid phosphate fluoride solutions have been known to cause erosion of clinical restorations of conventional cements and therefore are contraindicated.

Glass-ionomer cements exhibit bonding to enamel, dentin, and alloys in a manner similar to zinc polycarboxylates. In vitro and in vivo, the adhesion is variable and is affected by surface conditions. Slight and variable marginal leakage has been observed. Bonding to dentin for conventional materials is not improved by pretreatment with polyacrylic acid solutions, whereas with light-cured materials it is dependent on the use of dentin primers.

Biologic effects

The pulpal response to the lining and restorative materials appears to be generally favorable. Postoperative sensitivity has been reported with various luting materials and is attributed to prolonged low pH coupled with the effects of the toxic ions in addition to dehydration of dentin and marginal leakage of bacteria. Leaching of fluoride and uptake by adjacent enamel also occurs with these cements and continues for at least a year, with potentially cariostatic effects. Antibacterial action has been attributed to low initial pH, leaching, release of silver and other ions, or a combination of these. Light-cured materials have been observed to show greater cytotoxicity.

Advantages and disadvantages

The advantages of glass-ionomer cement materials include easy mixing, high strength and stiffness, leachable fluoride, good resistance to acid dissolution, potentially adhesive characteristics, and translucency.

The disadvantages include initial slow setting and moisture sensitivity, variable adhesive characteristics, radiolucency, and possible pulpal sensitivity.

Hybrid ionomer cements

Applications

A recent addition to the spectrum of materials, these versatile cements (see Fig 8-11) have many uses: cavity liners, bases, core buildups, and luting cements. One hybrid ionomer (Fig 9-6) is used for permanent cementation of crowns, orthodontic appliances, and core buildups.

Composition and setting

In hybrid ionomers, the acid-base setting reaction in glass-ionomer cements has been modified by the introduction of water-soluble polymers and polymerizable monomers into the composition. The use of copolymers of acrylic acid and methacrylate monomers in the liquid gives these materials the capability to undergo the acid-base reaction on setting as well as to be light cured via the methacrylate groups. As a result, there is improved lining, and the restorative materials have an immediate command set and thus higher early strength and water resistance. Some commercial materials contain a preponderance of polymeric components with minimal acid-base reaction.

The classification of these materials as glass-ionomer cements is controversial. Some light-cured restorative glass-ionomer cements are used with a dentin primer similar to dentin-bonding resin composite systems and thus depend on surface infiltration for bonding in addition to chemical interaction.

Hybrid ionomers are available in hand-mixed and predosed capsules (Fig 9-7). The resin monomers in the liquid depend on the product and include bis-GMA, hydroxyethylmethacrylate, and methacrylate-modified polyacrylates along with photoinitiators.

Manipulation

For hand-mixed compositions, the powder should be fluffed before dispensing, and the powder and liquid should be mixed within 30 seconds on the pad. These cements have a working time of about 2.5 minutes. For luting, the cement is applied to the undesiccated tooth to avoid possible postoperative sensitivity.

Properties

Table 9-5 compares the properties of hybrid ionomers with those of glass ionomers. The strength properties of the two types of cements are similar but with considerable variations among brands. There is a major difference in flexibility, with the hybrid ionomers being twice as flexible as indicated by their lower modulus of elasticity. Also, many of the hybrid ionomers expand on setting, possibly due to the absorption of water, which is greater than for resin cements. Therefore, hybrid ionomers are not recommended for luting all-ceramic crowns, to avoid possible expansion stresses and crown fracture.

Biologic effects

Hybrid ionomers release fluoride from the glass component, which is favorable for caries prevention.[7]

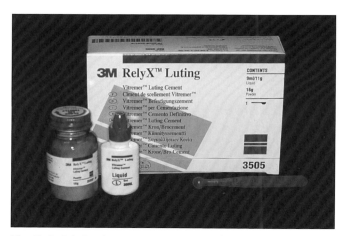

Fig 9-6 A hybrid ionomer. (Courtesy of 3M ESPE.)

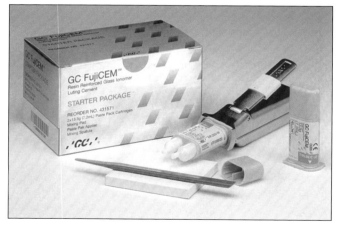

Fig 9-7 A hybrid ionomer luting cement. (Courtesy of GC America.)

Table 9-5 Mechanical properties of glass-ionomer and hybrid ionomer cements[6]

PROPERTIES	GLASS IONOMERS	HYBRID IONOMERS
Flexural strength (MPa)	25	35–70
Flexural modulus (GPa)	8	4
Compressive strength (MPa)	180–200	170–200
Diametral tensile strength (MPa)	22–25	35–40
Shrinkage (% vol)	3	3.5–expansion

Advantages and disadvantages

Among the advantages are dual cure, fluoride release, higher flexural strength than glass-ionomer cements, and ease of handling. Also, they are capable of bonding to composite materials.

One problem is a possible setting expansion that may lead to cracking of all-ceramic crowns. Therefore, resin cements, zinc phosphate, and glass-ionomer cements are still recommended for metal-free crowns.

◉ Selection and Use of Cements

None of the cements available is free from deficiencies in the required clinical characteristics, such as biocompatibility, ease of manipulation, satisfactory sealing, retentive properties, and long-term stability. A proportion of clini-

cal failures is inevitable, but this rate can be minimized by proper selection and manipulation of the cement. The following factors should be kept under review:

1. Rapid uniform and reproducible dispensing of the components
2. Rapid, thorough mixing
3. Moisture isolation where practical
4. An undisturbed setting
5. Careful removal of excess
6. Avoidance of excessive drying of dentin

Factors within the clinician's control, such as the design and execution of the preparation, adequate isolation, proper seating of the restoration, and finishing of the margins, are also important determinants of success as is the manipulation of the cement. These considerations may influence cement selection and use, but a governing factor is the biologic state of the tooth tissue. Thus, as indicated in Table 9-2, the selection of particular cements for specific clinical situations is limited both by the preparation and the properties of the cement.

Clinical Decision Scenarios for Dental Cements

This section presents one approach for choosing dental cements for specific situations. Each of the following scenarios uses the same format as that presented in chapter 7. Advantages and disadvantages of each material are prioritized using the following codes: • of minor importance, •• important, and ••• very important.

Materials Zinc phosphate vs resin cement for crown cementation

Situation A clinician has finished preparation of a full gold crown for a maxillary left permanent second molar and is ready to cement the crown. This is a routine crown cementation. The preparation is normal, the tooth is vital, and there is no known pulpal pathology. The clinician may choose between a resin cement and zinc phosphate cement.

Critical Factors Ease of use, cost-effectiveness

ZINC PHOSPHATE	RESIN
ADVANTAGES	ADVANTAGES
••• Low cost Long clinical history High rigidity Long working time ••• Easy to use	••• Bonds to tooth Fast setting time Higher strength ••• Easy to use
DISADVANTAGES	DISADVANTAGES
••• No bond to tooth Slow setting time Moisture sensitivity during mixing	••• High cost Short working time Film thickness varies widely among brands Difficult to remove excess

Analysis/Decision Comparing the properties of the two cements reveals that they are balanced in advantages and disadvantages for this situation. The choice finally rests in the personal preference of the clinician. Because this clinician had more experience with zinc phosphate, she chose to use that material.

Materials Glass ionomers vs zinc phosphate cement for crown cementation

Situation An older gentlemen with a history of periodontal surgery to correct bony defects has broken the cusps off a previously restored mandibular first molar. The patient's plaque control is only fair, and he is taking medications that could result in some degree of "dry mouth." He has had a slightly increased level of caries activity since the surgery and since beginning the medication. The clinician has elected to restore the tooth with a cast crown, which has now been returned from the laboratory and is ready for cementation. The clinician has both zinc phosphate and glass-ionomer luting cements available and must decide which to use.

Critical Factors Caries resistance, good seal

ZINC PHOSPHATE	GLASS IONOMER
ADVANTAGES	ADVANTAGES
••• Good seal •• Reasonable cost •• Adequate strength •• Little sensitivity	••• Good seal •• Fluoride release •• Adequate strength •• Reasonable cost
DISADVANTAGES	DISADVANTAGES
••• No fluoride release	•• Occasional sensitivity

Analysis/Decision Both cements have a good seal, but only the glass ionomer releases fluoride after cementation. Fluoride is generally accepted to reduce caries. For this reason, the glass ionomer was selected. Careful attention to instructions allowed cementation without the sensitivity sometimes experienced with glass-ionomer cements. The clinician was satisfied with this treatment choice.

Materials Glass ionomers vs zinc phosphate for bases under amalgam restorations

Situation A patient has a mandibular molar that exhibits extensive carious destruction. Due to the patient's financial situation, a large, pin-retained amalgam restoration is selected. Following caries removal and preparation, it is determined that the cavity needs a base prior to placement of the amalgam restoration. The clinician has zinc phosphate and glass-ionomer cements available and must choose between them for a base material.

Critical Factors Strength, modulus of elasticity

ZINC PHOSPHATE	GLASS IONOMER
ADVANTAGES	ADVANTAGES
••• Adequate modulus of elasticity ••• Adequate strength •• Ease of use •• No sensitivity	••• Adequate modulus of elasticity ••• Adequate strength •• Fluoride release •• Ease of use
DISADVANTAGES	DISADVANTAGES
•• No fluoride release	•• Occasional sensitivity

Analysis/Decision Since the advantages and disadvantages were balanced for this situation, neither cement had a clear advantage. The highly significant modulus of elasticity, essential for a good base, was roughly equivalent. In this case, the clinician chose glass ionomer because of the added advantage of fluoride release, which is thought to reduce recurrent decay. However, because that was not a problem with this patient, either cement would have been an acceptable choice.

Materials Zinc oxide–eugenol vs calcium hydroxide as liners under amalgam restorations

Situation A patient in need of a slightly deep mesio-occlusodistal amalgam on a mandibular left first molar was seen by the clinician. The patient reported that the last two amalgams the clinician placed had been sensitive for several weeks following placement. They had finally lost their sensitivity, but the patient felt they had hurt unusually long for new restorations. On preparation, the clinician decided that a base was indicated. Both calcium hydroxide and zinc oxide–eugenol base materials were available.

Critical Factors Strength, modulus of elasticity, reduction of sensitivity

ZINC OXIDE–EUGENOL	CALCIUM HYDROXIDE
ADVANTAGES	ADVANTAGES
•• Ease of use •• Decreased sensitivity •• Low cost	•• Ease of use •• Stimulates secondary dentin •• Low cost
DISADVANTAGES	DISADVANTAGES
••• Low strength ••• Low modulus of elasticity	••• Low strength ••• Low modulus of elasticity

Analysis/Decision In this situation, again, there is no clear advantage for either base. Both have low strength and low modulus of elasticity, necessitating that they be applied as very thin layers. The zinc oxide–eugenol has the advantage of the anodyne eugenol, which is known to reduce tooth sensitivity. The calcium hydroxide, on the other hand, will stimulate the formation of secondary dentin and thus is good if the restoration is near the pulp. This was true in the situation described, but the patient also had a history of sensitive teeth following placement of amalgam restorations. Therefore, the clinician selected the zinc oxide–eugenol as the liner of choice. Had the cavity preparation been deeper and the pulp visible through the dentin, calcium hydroxide would have been selected due to its ability to stimulate formation of secondary dentin.

Materials Flowable resin composite vs hybrid ionomer for Class 5 restorations in high-caries-risk patient

Situation An older patient has recurrent caries around the margins of a few old Class 5 amalgam restorations, probably due to poor hygiene and a mild xerostomia resulting from a cholesterol-lowering drug. The patient requested that the replacement restorations be more esthetic. The clinician considers flowable composites and hybrid ionomers.

Critical Factors Ease of placement, prevention of recurrent decay, reasonable esthetics

FLOWABLE COMPOSITE	HYBRID IONOMER
ADVANTAGES	ADVANTAGES
••• Very simple placement ••• Excellent esthetics • Less soluble	••• Ease of placement ••• Less recurrent decay ••• Reasonable esthetics •• Less sensitivity to moisture during placement
DISADVANTAGES	DISADVANTAGES
••• Higher incidence of recurrent decay •• Higher sensitivity to moisture contamination during placement	• More soluble than flowables

Analysis/Decision Due to the patient's high risk of recurrent decay, the clinician decided to use the hybrid ionomer restorative material. She chose a dual-cure hybrid ionomer for its ease of use and potential to be recharged with fluoride at future visits.

Materials All-purpose adhesives vs cavity varnish under amalgam restorations

Situation A patient is seen and diagnosed as needing numerous amalgam restorations, some large. After preparation, the cavities turn out to be normal in size and depth. There is little remarkable about the patient or the restorations. The clinician has both cavity varnish and new all-purpose adhesives to use under the amalgam restorations. The all-purpose adhesives are reported by the manufacturer to bond the amalgam to the teeth, but the clinician knows that such claims are as yet probably exaggerated.

Critical Factors Marginal leakage, bond to tooth, cost, time required for application

VARNISH	ADHESIVES
ADVANTAGES	ADVANTAGES
••• Low cost ••• Easy placement	••• Superior marginal seal ••• Bond to tooth
DISADVANTAGES	DISADVANTAGES
••• No bond to tooth ••• Mediocre seal	•• High cost ••• Complex placement

Analysis/Decision Since there is no evidence of excessively weakened cusps, the possible bonding of the new adhesives is not significant in this case. The superior seal makes them desirable, but their high cost and complex placement process complicates the choice. The clinician had been to a recent lecture on dental materials in which the speaker claimed the new materials should be a standard of practice, so he chose to place the adhesives. The patient reported a complete lack of postoperative sensitivity in the new restorations.

Materials Dentin adhesives vs glass-ionomer liners under composite restorations

Situation A patient has several Class 5 toothbrush-abrasion lesions on his maxillary and mandibular premolars. At first, they were no problem, but over the years they have become sensitive, and the patient wants the discomfort relieved. The lesions are not carious but are deep. The occlusal, mesial, and distal margins are on enamel, but the cervical margin is on cementum. The clinician decides against glass-ionomer restorations because she feels better esthetics can be obtained with a composite material. In addition, she feels the composite will better resist further toothbrush abrasion. She is uncertain whether to use a dentin bonding agent alone or a glass-ionomer lining cement under the cervical margin to prevent leakage. She has heard that composites often leak on margins that are on cementum.

Critical Factors Marginal seal, bond strength

DENTIN ADHESIVES	GLASS IONOMER
ADVANTAGES	ADVANTAGES
•• Good seal ••• Adequate bond strength •• Lower cost	••• Better marginal seal ••• Adequate bond strength
DISADVANTAGES	DISADVANTAGES
••• Poorer marginal seal	•• Additional cost •• Additional procedure

Analysis/Decision Although there are more advantages for the bonding agent, the most significant advantage—better marginal seal—favors the glass-ionomer liner. It adds to the cost and the time to do the procedure, but it provides a significantly better seal. The better seal results in a superior restoration that justifies the extra cost and time. The glass-ionomer liner was selected.

Materials Hybrid ionomer vs glass ionomer for treatment of recurrent caries at gold crown margins

Situation Patient examination reveals recurrent caries around the margins of a few gold crowns. Replacement of the crowns is not feasible due to the patient's lack of funds. Normally, the clinician would use a glass ionomer to restore the marginal areas after decay removal. However, he is considering the use of hybrid ionomers.

Critical Factors Prevention of recurrent caries, ease of placement, bond to tooth structure

HYBRID IONOMER	GLASS IONOMER
ADVANTAGES	ADVANTAGES
••• Easy to place ••• Tooth colored • Low cost ••• Fluoride release •• Bonds to tooth • Smoother finish •• Light/dual cure	••• Reasonably easy to place ••• Tooth colored • Low cost ••• Fluoride release ••• Bonds to tooth
DISADVANTAGES	DISADVANTAGES
• Less durable • Isolation is critical	• Less durable •• More plaque retentive • Isolation is critical •• Chemical cure only

Analysis/Decision Though the two materials have comparable fluoride release, the clinician chose a hybrid ionomer mainly for its greater ease of use. The hybrid ionomer can be placed and cured in less than 1 minute due to the dual-cure feature, while the traditional chemically cured glass ionomers require protection from oral fluids for 4 to 5 minutes during setting. The dual-curing hybrid ionomer may also release more fluoride because it contains more fluoride glass, which is the source of fluoride ions and aids in the chemical setting reaction.

Materials Glass-ionomer vs zinc phosphate cement

Situation A patient presents with a loose crown on the left side of the maxillary arch. Examination reveals a loose porcelain-fused-to-metal crown in the maxillary left second premolar, and a radiograph shows a cast post from a previous root canal treatment that seems to be of adequate length. A crown remover is used to remove the crown and the cast post, which are solidly attached together. There is little coronal tooth structure left, but no evidence of recurrent caries. The decision is made to recement the post and core (along with the attached crown) after properly cleaning the restoration and tooth.

Critical Factors Increased need for retention

ZINC PHOSPHATE	GLASS IONOMER
ADVANTAGES	ADVANTAGES
••• Low cost Long clinical history High rigidity Long working time ••• Easy to use	••• Reasonably easy to place Low cost ••• Fluoride release ••• Bonds to tooth
DISADVANTAGES	DISADVANTAGE
••• No bond to tooth Slow setting time Moisture sensitivity during mixing	Harder to clean excess

Analysis/Decision Even though either cement can be used, the clinician chose a glass-ionomer cement. His decision was influenced by the lack of adequate coronal structure on the premolar, which made the retention of the restoration dependent on the cast post. Use of a self-curing material that bonds to the tooth structure increases the chance of long-term success.

Materials Hybrid ionomer vs dual-cured resin cement

Situation An adult patient presents with a fractured mandibular left first molar. Examination reveals a large, old mesio-occlusodistal amalgam in the fractured molar with open margins and recurrent caries; the lingual wall of the molar fractured off about 2 mm supragingivally. A radiograph reveals no periapical pathology, and the patient relates no symptoms other than temperature sensitivity. Because the patient has no other metal restorations in her mouth, is very esthetically conscious, and does not want a new restoration with any metal in it, the tooth is restored with an Empress all-ceramic crown.

Critical Factors Adequate bond of crown to tooth structure

HYBRID IONOMER	DUAL-CURED RESIN
ADVANTAGES	ADVANTAGES
••• Easy to place ••• Tooth colored 　　Low cost ••• Fluoride release •• Bonds to tooth •• Light/dual cure	••• Bonds to tooth ••• Bonds to porcelain ••• Proper setting assured through dual-cure action 　　Higher strength ••• Proper marginal seal (composite closes any minor margin imperfections)
DISADVANTAGES	DISADVANTAGES
• Less durable • Isolation is critical ••• Expansion on setting can lead to fracture in porcelain	••• High cost •• Technique sensitive •• Time consuming to clean

Analysis/Decision Because all-ceramic restorations need to be bonded to the tooth, nonbonding luting agents are not indicated in these situations. Even though hybrid ionomers do bond to the tooth, they expand on setting, making them contraindicated for all-ceramic applications. The clinician chose the dual-cured resin, which bonds to the tooth and all-ceramic crown, increasing the strength and longevity of the restoration.

● Glossary

accelerator Substance that facilitates decomposition of an initiator; also called *promoter*.

anodyne Relieves pain.

chelating Ring structure reaction with metal ions.

cored structure A material consisting of at least two phases, for example, as residual particles of a component embedded in a matrix of reaction product.

initiator Substance capable of decomposing into free radicals that initiate polymerization.

lute A cement-like material that also fills and seals gaps.

obtundent A material that reduces irritation or has a soothing effect on tissue.

rheology Science of the deformation and flow of matter.

setting time Time from the beginning of mixing of the cement to the development of a hard and rigid (usually brittle) state in the mouth.

working time Time available, measured from the beginning of mixing at room temperature, for clinical manipulation of a cement before viscosity becomes too great for seating of the restoration.

◉ Discussion Questions

1. Why is fluoride release so important in a cement?

2. What is the source of fluoride in a glass-ionomer cement?

3. What is the difference in function between a cement liner and a cement base?

4. Why are polymer cements recommended for use with CAD/CAM inlays with poor marginal fits?

◉ Study Questions

(See appendix E for answers.)

1. What is the minimum compressive strength required of a dental cement for adequate retention of restorations?

2. What is the structure of set zinc phosphate cement?

3. How does the solubility of phosphate cements in citric or lactic acid compare with their solubility in water?

4. What are adhesive resin cements?

5. What are hybrid ionomers?

6. What agents accelerate the setting of zinc oxide–eugenol cements?

7. Why do zinc oxide–eugenol cements have a high solubility?

8. What materials can be added to zinc oxide–eugenol cements to improve their strength?

9. What effects do zinc oxide–eugenol cements have on resin restorative materials?

10. How does the composition of EBA cements differ from that of zinc oxide–eugenol cements?

11. What factors affect the setting reaction of polycarboxylate cements?

12. Give possible reasons for the minimal effect of polycarboxylate cements on pulp.

13. What are important considerations in manipulating polycarboxylate cements?

14. What are the advantages of light-curing glass-ionomer cements?

15. What are the major advantages of glass-ionomer cements?

16. Define the two types of polymer-based cement.

17. What are the principal disadvantages of polymer-based cement?

18. It has been reported that hybrid ionomers expand on setting, which could cause cracking of all-ceramic crowns. This was discovered years after the cements were marketed. Using the hierarchy of evidence, which type of study would have warned clinicians about this problem?

19. Although short-term pulpal studies on glass-ionomer cements gave a satisfactory overall biocompatibility, there were occasional signs of cytotoxicity with certain products. After many years of clinical use, it has been reported that, if the dentin has been dehydrated by excessive drying, there is a definite chance of postoperative sensitivity when these cements are used to cement crowns. Speculate on why this serious clinical problem was not clearly identified in the histologic analysis of treated tooth pulps that were used in the biocompatibility tests.

◉ References

1. American National Standards Institute/American Dental Association. ANSI/ADA Specification No. 96-2000. Dental Water-Based Cements. Chicago: American Dental Association, 2000.
2. International Organization for Standardization. ISO 9917-1:2007. Dental Water-Based Cements—Part 1: Powder/Liquid Acid-Base Cements, ed 2. Geneva: International Organization for Standardization, 2007.
3. International Organization for Standardization. ISO 9917-2:1998. Dental Water-Based Cements—Part 2: Light-Activated cements Cements. Geneva: International Organization for Standardization, 1998.
4. Silvey RG, Myers GE. Clinical studies of dental cements. VII. A study of bridge retainers luted with three different cements. J Dent Res 1978;57:703.
5. Nicholson JW. Chemistry of glass-ionomer cements: A review. Biomaterials 1998;19:485–494.
6. Burgess JO, Norling BK, Rawls HR, Ong JL. Directly placed esthetic restorative materials—the continuum. Compend Contin Educ Dent 1996;17:731–732, 734, 748.
7. Forss H. Release of fluoride and other elements from light-cured glass ionomers in neutral and acidic conditions. J Dent Res 1993;72:1257–1262.

◉ Recommended Reading

Albers HF. Tooth-Colored Restoratives, ed 8. Santa Rosa: Alto Books, 1996.

Antonucci JM, McKinney JE, Stansbury RW, inventors. Resin modified glass ionomer cement. US Patent: 160,856 1998.

Arfaci AH, Asgar K. Bond strength of selected cementing materials. Microfilmed Paper No. 549. Presented at the Annual Meeting of the International Association for Dental Research, Atlanta, GA, Mar 21–24, 1974.

Beagrie GS, Smith DC. Development of a germicidal polycarboxylate cement. J Can Dent Assoc 1978;44:409.

Berg JH Glass ionomer cements. Pediatr Dent 2003;24:430-436.

Boyer DB, Williams VD, Thayer KE, Denehy GE, Diaz-Arnold AM. Analysis of debond rates of resin-bonded prostheses. J Dent Res 1993;72:1244–1248.

Brännström M, Nyborg H. Bacterial growth and pulpal changes under inlays cemented with zinc phosphate cement and Epoxylite CBA 9080. J Prosthet Dent 1974;31:556.

Burgess JO, Barghi N, Chan DC, Hummert T. A comparative study of three glass ionomer base materials. Am J Dent 1993;6:137–141.

Burke FJ, McCaughey AD. Resin luting materials: The current status. Dent Update April 1993;20:109–110, 112–115.

Causton BE. Primers and mineralizing solutions. In: Smith DC, Williams DF (eds). Biocompatibility of Dental Materials, vol 2. Boca Raton, FL: CRC Press, 1982:125–144.

Croll TP, Nicholson. Glass ionomer cements in pediatric dentistry. Pediatr Dent 2002;24:423–426.

De Freitas JF. The long-term solubility of a stannous fluoride–zinc phosphate cement. Aust Dent J 1973;18:167.

Dennison JD, Powers JM. A review of dental cements used for permanent retention of restorations. Part I. Composition and manipulation. J Mich Dent Assoc 1974;56:116.

Eames WB, Hendri K, Mohler HC. Pulpal response in rhesus monkeys to cementation agents and cleaners. J Am Dent Assoc 1979;98:40.

Eames WB, O'Neal SJ, Miller CB. Cementation variables in the seating of castings. Microfilmed Paper No. 545. Presented at the Annual Meeting of the International Association for Dental Research, Atlanta, GA, Mar 21–24, 1974.

Eames WB, O'Neal SJ, Monteiro J, et al. Techniques to improve the seating of castings. J Am Dent Assoc 1978;96:432.

Friedl KH, Schmalz G, Hiller KA, Shams M. Resin-modified glass ionomer cements: Fluoride release and influence on *Streptococcus mutans* growth. Eur J Oral Sci 1997;105:81–85.

Glenn JF. Composition and properties of unfilled and composite resin restorative materials. In: Smith DC, Williams DF (eds). Biocompatibility of Dental Materials, vol 3. Boca Raton, FL: CRC Press, 1982;97–130.

Grieve AR. A study of dental cements. Br Dent J 1969;127:405–410.

Grieve AR, Jones JC. Marginal leakage associated with four inlay cementing materials. Br Dent J 1981;151:331.

Griffith JR, Cannon RWS. Cementation—materials and techniques. Aust J Dent 1974;19(2):92–99.

Grobler SR, Rossouw RJ, Van Wyk Kotze TJ. A comparison of fluoride release from various dental materials. J Dent 1998;26:259–265.

Hatton PV, Brook JM. Characterization of the ultrastructure of glass ionomer (poly-alkenoate) cement. Br Dent J 1993;173:275–277.

Hembree JH Jr, George TA, Hembree ME. Film thickness of cements beneath complete crowns. J Prosthet Dent 1978;39:533.

Hilton TJ. Cavity sealers, liners, and bases: Current philosophies and indications for use. Oper Dent 1996;21:134.

Hoard RJ, Caputo AA, Contino RM, et al. Intracoronal pressure during crown cementation. J Prosthet Dent 1978;40:520.

Hood JA, Childs WA, Evans DF. Bond strengths of glass ionomer and polycarboxylate cements to dentin. N Z Dent J 1981;77:141.

Jarzynka W. Effect of fluorine contained in the phosphate cement "Fluostable" on tooth pulp. Czas Stomatol 1978;31:1003.

Jendresen MD. New dental cements and fixed prosthodontics. J Prosthet Dent 1973;30:684.

Johnson GH, Herbert AJ, Powers JM. Properties of glass ionomer luting cements. Microfilmed Paper No. 189. Presented at the Annual Meeting of the American Association for Dental Research, Dental Materials Group, Cincinnati, OH, Mar 17–20, 1983.

Kent BE, Wilson AD. The properties of a glass ionomer cement. Br Dent J 1973;135:322.

Kidd EAM, McLean JW. The cavity sealing ability of cemented cast gold restorations. Br Dent J 1979;147:39.

Kohmura TT, Ida KA. A new type of hydraulic cement. J Dent Res 1979;58:1461.

Markowitz K, Moynihan M, Liu M, Kim S. Biologic properties of eugenol and zinc oxide–eugenol: A clinically-oriented review. Oral Surg Oral Med Oral Pathol 1992;73:729–737.

McCabe JF. Resin-modified glass-ionomers. Biomaterials 1998;19:521–527.

McComb D. Retention of castings with glass ionomer cement. J Prosthet Dent 1982;48:285.

McLean JW. The clinical use of glass ionomer cements. Dent Clin North Am 1992;36:693–711.

Meyer JM, Cattani-Lorente MA, Dupuis V. Compomers: Between glass-ionomer cements and composites. Biomaterials 1998;19:529–539.

Miller RA, Bussell NE, Richetts CK, et al. Analysis of purification of eugenol. J Dent Res 1979;58:1394.

Mitchem JC, Gronas DG. Clinical evaluation of cement solubility. J Prosthet Dent 1978;40:453.

Mitchem JC, Gronas DG. Continued evaluation of the clinical solubility of luting cements. J Prosthet Dent 1981;45:289.

Mount GO, Makinson OF. Clinical characteristics of a glass ionomer cement. Br Dent J 1978;145:67.

Myers CL, Drake JT, Brantley WA. A comparison of properties of zinc phosphate cements mixed on room temperature and frozen slabs. J Prosthet Dent 1978;40:409.

Norman RD, Swartz ML, Phillips RW, et al. A comparison of the intra-oral disintegration of three dental cements. J Am Dent Assoc 1969;78:777.

Øilo G. Adhesive bonding of dental luting cements: Influence of surface treatments. Acta Odontol Scand 1978;36:263.

Øilo G. Extent of slits at the interface between luting cements and enamel, dentin and alloy. Acta Odontol Scand 1978;36:257.

Øilo G, Espevik S. Stress/strain behavior of some dental luting cements. Acta Odontol Scand 1978;36:45.

Pameijer GH, Segal E, Richardson J. Pulpal response to a glass ionomer cement in primates. J Prosthet Dent 1981;46:36.

Peacocke LE, Jones DW, Sutow E, et al. Direct tensile strength of glass ionomer, polycarboxylate and phosphate cements. Microfilmed Paper No. 1212. Presented at the Annual Meeting of the International Association for Dental Research, Dental Materials Group, New Orleans, LA, Mar 29–Apr 1, 1979.

Peterson WG, Joos RW, Boyer LV, et al. Initial response of Ca(OH)$_2$ bases in simulated oral conditions. Microfilmed Paper No. 210. Presented at the Annual Meeting of the International Association for Dental Research, Dental Materials Group, Washington, DC, Mar 16–19, 1978.

Powers JM, Dennison JD. A review of dental cements used for permanent retention of restorations. Part II. Properties and criteria for selection. J Mich Dent Assoc 1974;56(7–8):218–225.

Reisbick MH. Working qualities of glass ionomer cements. J Prosthet Dent 1981;46:525.

Rueggeberg FA, Caughman WF. The influence of light exposure on polymerization of dual-cure resin cements. Oper Dent 1993;18:48–55.

Sidhu SK, Watson TF. Resin modified glass modified materials. Am J Dent 1994;8:59-67.

Smith DC. Dental cements. Dent Clin North Am 1971;15:3.

Smith DC. A review of the zinc polycarboxylate cements. J Can Dent Assoc 1974;37:22.

Smith DC. Past, present and future of dental cements. In: Craig RG (ed). Dental Materials Review. Ann Arbor: University of Michigan Press, 1977:52–77.

Smith DC. Glass ionomer contents. In: Kawahara H (ed). Implantology and Biomaterials in Stomatology. Tokyo: Ishikayn Publisher, 1980:26–54.

Smith DC. Composition and characteristics of dental cements. In: Smith DC, Williams DF (eds). Biocompatibility of Dental Materials, vol 2. Boca Raton, FL: CRC Press, 1982:143–199.

Smith DC. Dental cements. Current status and future prospects. Dent Clin North Am 1983;27:763–792.

Smith DC. Dental cements. Adv Dent Res 1988;2:131–141.

Smith DC. Dental cements. Curr Opin Dent 1991;1:228–234.

Suljak JP, Hatibovic-Kofman S. A fluoride release-adsorption-release system applied to fluoride-releasing restorative materials. Quintessence Int 1996;27:635–638.

Summitt JB, Robbins WJ, Hilton TJ, Schwartz RS (eds). Fundamentals of Operative Dentistry. Chicago: Quintessence, 2006:225–230.

Uno S, Finger WJ, Fritz U. Long term mechanical characteristics of resin-modified glass ionomer restorative materials. Dent Mater 1996;12:64–69.

Vougiouklakis G, Smith DC. The bonding of cervical restorative materials to dentin. J Oral Rehabil 1982;9:231.

White S, Yu Z. Compressive and diametral tensile strengths of current adhesive luting agents. J Prosthet Dent 1993;69:568–572.

White S, Yu Z. Physical properties of fixed prosthodontic resin composite luting agents. Int J Prosthodont 1993;6:384–389.

White SN, Yu Z, Kipmio V. Effect of seating force on film thickness of new adhesive luting agents. J Prosthet Dent 1992;68:476–481.

Wilder AD, Boghosian AA, Bayne SC, et al. Effect of powder/liquid ratio on the clinical and laboratory performance of resin-modified glass-ionomers. J Dent 1998;26:369–377.

Williams JA, Billington RW, Pearson GJ. The comparative strengths of commercial glass-ionomer cements with and without metal additions. Br Dent J 1993;172:279–282.

Wilson AD. The chemistry of dental cements. Chem Soc Rev 1978;7:265.

Wilson AD. Resin-modified glass-ionomer cements. Int J Prosthodont 1990;3:425.

Wilson AD, McLean JW. Glass Ionomer Cements. Chicago: Quintessence, 1988.

Wilson AD, Paddon JM, Crisp S. The hydration of dental cements. J Dent Res 1979;58:1065.

Wilson AD, Prosser HJ. Alumino silicate dental cements. In: Smith DC, Williams DF (eds). Biocompatibility of Dental Materials, vol 3. Boca Raton, FL: CRC Press, 1982;42–77.

Yoshida Y, Van Meerbee B, Nakayama Y, et al. Evidence of chemical bonding at biomaterial-hard tissue interfaces. J Dent Res 2000;79:709-714.

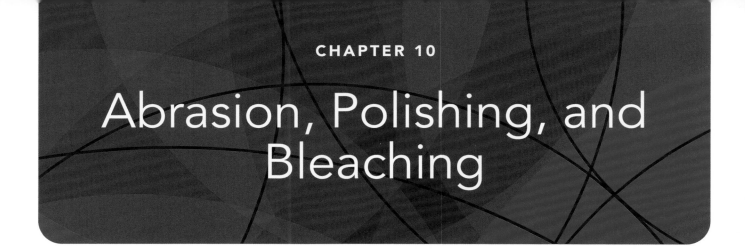

Abrasion, Polishing, and Bleaching

The surfaces of normal, healthy-looking teeth have a high gloss and an unstained white/ivory color. *Abrasion* is a process of surface roughening that can either wear away tooth structure destructively or be used to correct tooth shape or attain an optimal smooth finish on the surface of a restoration. Polishing and bleaching are two different approaches to **whitening** teeth by attacking surface stains. *Polishing* is an abrasive process of smoothing a rough surface and removing stains with very fine particles, and *bleaching* lightens or eliminates surface stains with strong peroxide solutions. This chapter deals with the basic processes of these techniques.

◼ Abrasion

Abrasion is the process of wear on the surface of one material by another material by scratching, gouging, chiseling, tumbling, or other mechanical means. The material that causes the wear is called an **abrasive**; the material being abraded is the **substrate**.

Grinding is the gross reduction of the surface of a substrate, and is usually performed with large-particle–size abrasives. After grinding, the surface texture of the substrate is usually rough to the touch and gives a diffuse reflection to incident light (Fig 10-1).

Abrasives are either bonded to a mandrel or disk for use in a rotary handpiece or are in the form of powders (or pastes) that are applied to the substrate using a cloth wheel, brush, or cup.

Factors affecting rate of abrasion

1. *Hardness.* A large difference in hardness between the abrasive and substrate (eg, tooth enamel, amalgam) allows the most efficient grinding to take place. Brinell and Knoop hardness values are functions of a material's resistance to indentation, and Mohs values indicate one material's resistance to scratching by another (Table 10-1).
2. *Particle size.* Particles are classified as *fine* (0 to 10 μm), *medium* (10 to 100 μm), and *coarse* (100 to 500 μm), according to the average particle size of the sample. Larger abrasive particles will abrade a surface more rapidly than will smaller particles; however, they tend to leave coarser scratches in the abraded surface than do fine particles. Equivalent-sized scratches can be produced by different sizes of particles by varying the applied pressure (Fig 10-2a).
3. *Particle shape.* Sharp, irregularly shaped particles will abrade a surface more rapidly and will produce deeper scratches (Fig 10-2b) than will more rounded particles with duller cutting angles. The abrasion rate of an abrasive decreases during use because of rounding of the particles and also because of contamination of the abrasive with debris from the substrate material.
4. *Speed.* The greater the speed at which the abrasive travels across the surface of the substrate, the greater the rate of abrasion. Friction at higher speeds, how-

Table 10-1 Hardness of dental abrasives and substrates

MATERIAL	HARDNESS SCALE		
	MOHS	BRINELL	KNOOP
Abrasives			
Talc	1		
Gypsum	2		
Chalk	3		
Rouge	5–6		
Pumice	6	450	560
Tripoli	6–7		
Garnet	6.5–7	550	
Tin oxide	6–7		
Sand	7	650	800
Cuttle	7	650	800
Tool steel	—	800	
Zirconium silicate	7–7.5		
Tungsten carbide	9	1,200	2,100
Aluminum oxide	9	1,700	1,900
Silicon carbide	9.–10	3,000	2,500
Boron carbide	9–10		2,800
Diamond	10	> 3,000	7,000
Substrates			
Acrylic	2–3		25
Pure gold	2.5–3	30	
Hard gold alloys	3–4		
Amalgam	4–5	90	
Dentin	3–4		
Enamel	5–6	270	
Glass	5–6		
Resin composite	5–7		200
Porcelain	6–7	400	

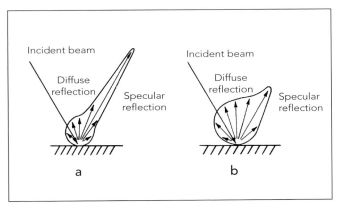

Fig 10-1 Schematic of diffuse and specular reflection: (a) high gloss; (b) low gloss. (Reprinted with permission from O'Brien et al.[1])

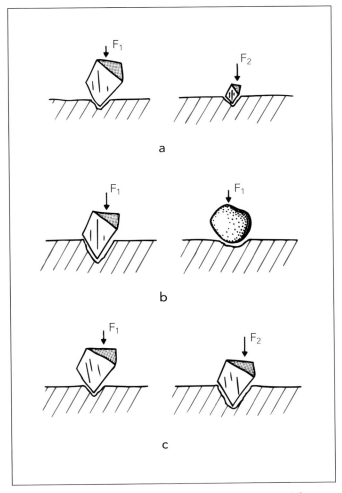

Fig 10-2 Factors affecting abrasion. (a) Large particle produces similar scratches with lesser applied force (F_1) than smaller particle with greater applied force (F_2). (b) Sharp particle produces deeper abrasion than rounder particle under equal applied force (F_1). (c) Deeper and wider scratches are produced by increasing the applied force from F_1 to F_2.

ever, tends to create higher temperatures at the surface of the substrate.

5. *Pressure*. The greater the pressure applied, the more rapid the abrasion. Greater pressure produces deeper and wider scratches (Fig 10-2c) and creates higher temperatures (and patient discomfort).

6. *Lubrication*. Lubricants, such as silicone grease, water spray, and glycerol, are used during abrasion for two purposes: to reduce heat buildup and to wash away debris to prevent clogging, or **blinding**, of the abrasive instrument. Too much lubrication can reduce the abrasion rate, however, because it may prevent some of the abrasive from coming in contact with the substrate.

Applications of abrasives

Dental prophylaxis pastes

Prophylaxis pastes are used to remove exogenous stains without damaging the underlying tooth structure or adjacent restorative materials. The abrasive selected should be harder than the surface stain and softer than the tooth surface, although it is not always practicable. If the tooth structure is excessively roughened during the procedure, it should be polished with a fine abrasive (eg, such as zirconium silicate); otherwise, plaque and food substances will easily adhere to the tooth.

The most common abrasives used in prophylaxis pastes are pumice, silica, zirconium silicate, and other silicates. They are usually supplied in various particle sizes (coarse, medium, fine), which produce different rates of abrasion and sizes of scratches. Sodium fluoride or stannous fluoride are incorporated into some prophylaxis pastes to help prevent dental caries.

Dentifrices

Dentifrices are used for removing debris and minor stains from teeth and for polishing tooth surfaces. The most commonly used abrasives are dibasic calcium phosphate dihydrate, anhydrous dibasic calcium phosphate, tricalcium phosphate, calcium pyrophospate, and hydrated alumina.

Many dentifrices contain therapeutic agents, such as sodium fluoride, stannous fluoride, or sodium monofluorophosphate; these decrease the acid solubility of tooth enamel, decrease hypersensitivity, and interrupt the mechanisms of plaque attachment and calculus formation on tooth structure. Dentifrice pastes additionally may contain a humectant to reduce evaporation of water, a surface-active detergent, binders, flavoring and sweetening agents, and a preservative. Abrasive values for dentifrice products are reported using the **abrasivity index**, which is a measure of the abrasion of dentin.

In selecting a dentifrice for a patient, the following factors should be considered: degree of staining, toothbrushing habits (force, stiffness of brush, method of brushing), the presence of relatively soft restorative materials (eg, acrylic resin veneers, silicates), and the amount of exposed cementum and dentin.

Denture cleaners

Food debris, plaque, calculus, and stains may accumulate on denture base materials as they do on natural teeth. Daily soaking in a denture cleanser solution or brushing with or without a paste or powder is usually effective.

Chemical cleansers may contain sodium perborate, which releases peroxide. As peroxide decomposes, oxygen is released, resulting in effervescence. The effervescence along with the oxidizing ability of peroxide are assumed to be responsible for the cleaning action. Dentures may also be soaked in a dilute solution of 5% sodium hypochlorite (1:3 water). Other chemical denture cleansers may contain dilute acids or enzymes. Dentures should not be soaked in hot water, which may warp the denture base material.

Brushing may be needed to remove stains and stubborn deposits. Hard-bristle brushes or brushing with much force may abrade the plastic surface of the denture and should be avoided. Dentifrices are generally too abrasive for use with dentures, although some with gentle abrasives (sodium bicarbonate or acrylic resin) can be used. Organic solvents should be avoided, as they may cause crazing and eventual cracking of the denture material. Ultrasonic vibration has not been shown to adequately remove plaque from dentures.

Handpiece instruments

Bonded abrasives attached to handpiece instruments are available for dental use in various shapes, abrasive sizes, and hardnesses:

1. **Dental stones** are composed of abrasive particles that have been sintered together or bonded with an organic resin to form a cohesive mass. These stones are available in fine, medium, and coarse grades. The color of the stone is an indication of the particular

abrasive used; green stones contain silicon carbide and white stones contain aluminum oxide. Diamond stones generally have a higher cutting efficiency than silicon carbide or aluminum oxide.

2. Dental excavating burs have a cutting action on tooth structure that is similar to grinding and polishing. Low-speed burs are composed of either carbon tool steel or tungsten carbide, and high-speed burs are almost exclusively composed of the harder tungsten carbide. Burs with eight blades produce a rather rough surface texture on the substrate, and can be used for gross reduction of tooth structure and removal of old restorations. For a surface on tooth structure and restorations, burs with 12, 20, or 40 blades should be used. The relative hardness values of the burs and the substrates should be considered (see Table 10-1). For example, hard restorative materials (eg, quartz-filled composite restorative materials and dental porcelain) will rapidly dull the sharp cutting edges of the high-speed tungsten carbide burs. Cutting efficiency and durability of the burs varies greatly among manufacturers and design types. Crosscut fissure burs have higher cutting efficiency than plain fissure burs, but they produce a rougher surface.

3. **Rubber wheels** are used for fine grinding of restorative materials (eg, removing coarse scratches from rough grinding). They are made by molding fine abrasives (eg, aluminum oxide, silicon carbide, and chromium oxide) in an elastomeric matrix.

4. **Disks** and **strips** are made by bonding abrasive particles onto a thin plastic backing. They generally wear out rapidly due to the loss of abrasive particles. They are particularly useful in finishing relatively flat surfaces. Abrasives commonly used on disks and strips are garnet, emery, aluminum oxide, and quartz (cuttle).

◼ Polishing

The process of making a rough surface smooth to the touch and glossy (mostly specular reflection of incident light) (see Fig 10-1a) is called **polishing**. Polishing is usually performed with very-small-particle–size (submicron-size) abrasives.

To produce a smooth, lustrous surface by abrasion, successively smaller particle sizes must be used. Larger particles remove large amounts of material from the substrate, and smaller particles smooth out the rough-

ness produced by the larger particles. Final polishing of a surface with a very fine abrasive produces a virtually scratch-free surface by creating a thin **microcrystalline** or **amorphous** layer on the surface of the substrate.

It is extremely important to remove all debris and abrasive particles from the surface of the substrate before using a finer abrasive during the polishing sequence. Even a single abrasive particle left on the substrate from a previous step will continue to scratch the surface during the subsequent polishing steps.

Appearance and texture of polished surfaces

A polished surface is important for esthetic and functional reasons. If the scratches produced by the abrasives are greater in width than the wavelength of visible light (ie, approximately 0.5 µm), the surface will appear to have a dull finish. If the scratches are less than about 0.5 µm in width, the surface will appear shiny. In addition, it has been found that the tongue can distinguish subtle differences in roughness; scratches more than 20 µm deep feel rough, whereas those less than 2 µm deep feel smooth.

Techniques for polishing restorative materials

Dental amalgam
A polished surface is desirable on dental amalgam to retard the collection of plaque and help retard tarnish as well. Burnishing alone does not create as smooth a surface. Although an amalgam restoration can be burnished immediately after carving, most brands should be left undisturbed for at least 24 hours before polishing to allow the amalgam to set completely. Polishing can then be performed with a rotary instrument (cup, brush, or felt) and a fine abrasive mixed with water or alcohol in a slurry or paste; flour of pumice (ground volcanic glass), extra-fine silex (various silicates, such as quartz or tripoli), or tin oxide may also be used. Care must be taken to use sufficient water or alcohol to avoid frictional heating of the restoration, which could cause pulpal damage.

Fast-setting high-copper amalgams may be successfully polished 10 to 12 minutes following placement.

Gold alloys
Coarse, medium, and fine abrasives are used in sequence for the finishing of gold alloys. First, coarse

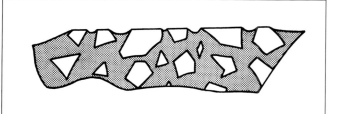

Fig 10-3 Uneven wear of composite surface produces valleys in the resin matrix between the hard filler particles.

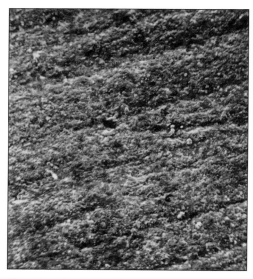

Fig 10-4 Scanning electron micrograph of a composite restorative material with conventional filler, finished with a 12-fluted bur. (Reprinted with permission from O'Brien et al.[1])

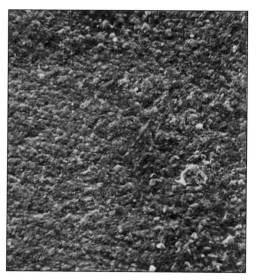

Fig 10-5 Scanning electron micrograph of a composite restorative material with smaller filler particles in the micron range, finished with the rubber-abrasive resin composite wheel. (Reprinted with permission from O'Brien et al.[1])

scratches are removed with fine pumice or coarse abrasive rubber wheels. The surface is then finished with a rubber wheel impregnated with a fine abrasive and finally polished with tripoli and rouge on rag wheels. Care must be taken to avoid overfinishing of contours and margins.

Acrylic resin denture bases and veneers

Gypsum material left on the denture base following processing and deflasking may be removed with a "shell blaster." Small blemishes and bumps on the resin surface may be scraped off or removed with an acrylic finishing bur. Denture base material is comparatively soft and can be finished easily with a rag wheel and fine pumice followed by tripoli or tin oxide. The contour of the denture should remain intact during finishing. Acrylic dentures are particularly easily abraded by pumice.

Resin composite restorations

Polishing resin composite restorations is difficult, because they are composed of a relatively soft polymeric resin and a hard filler. Relief polishing may result because of unequal wear rates of the resin and filler, leaving "valleys" between the filler particles (Fig 10-3). This problem is more apparent in the conventional, large-particle resin composites, which still look and feel rough after finishing with abrasives (Fig 10-4). The valleys and filler particles from relief polishing of microfilled resin composites are so small that the surface appears glossy (large specular component of reflection) and feels smooth (Fig 10-5). The new types of hybrid and small-particle resin composites also tend to appear shiny and smooth but cannot be polished as easily as the microfilled type.

A typical sequence for polishing resin composites would be as follows: coarse grinding with a diamond

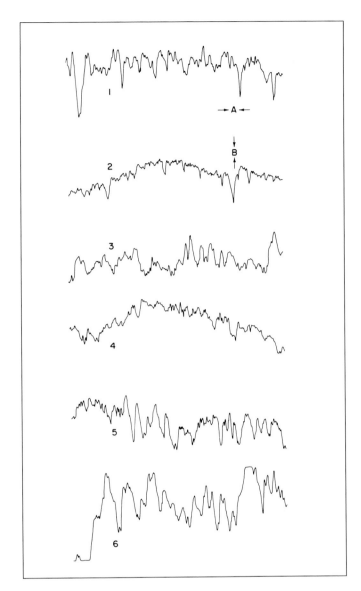

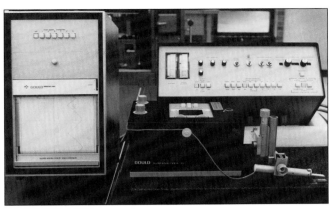

Fig 10-7 Surface analyzer using a diamond stylus to produce roughness profiles (Surfanalyzer, Gould).

Fig 10-6 Roughness profiles of conventional resin composite surfaces finished with: (1) green to white stone; (2) silicon carbide disks; (3) 12-fluted bur; (4) 40-fluted bur; (5) green to white stone to alumina paste; and (6) diamond stone. For scale: A = 50 μm; B = 2 μm. (Reprinted with permission from Tolley et al.[2])

stone or a green stone followed by a series of coarse to fine quartz or aluminum oxide abrasive disks or rubber wheels. Carbide burs with 12 or more blades have also been used. The effects of several polishing sequences on the surface roughness of resin composites are shown in Fig 10-6, which are tracings from the surface analyzer shown in Fig 10-7.

Porcelain

The best way to obtain a smooth, glossy surface on dental porcelain is by glazing in a porcelain oven. After minor adjustments of the surface, the porcelain can be polished using a series of coarse to fine abrasive rub-

ber wheels (containing silicon carbide or aluminum oxide), followed by a fine-particle–size diamond paste applied on a felt wheel.

◼ Bleaching

Since the 1800s, bleaching has been used to whiten teeth, but with the introduction of home bleaching systems in 1989, its use has widened.

Three types of bleaching treatments are currently used (Table 10-2). The first is home treatment, which involves the patient using carbamide peroxide materials

Table 10-2 Tooth bleaching options

	HOME BLEACHING	DENTIST-ASSISTED BLEACHING	POWER OR COMBINATION BLEACHING
Patient selection	Anyone with mild discolorations desiring teeth a shade or two whiter and willing to devote time to an at-home regimen	Anyone with mild to acute discolorations desiring a more dramatic whitening effect	Anyone with mild to severe discolorations desiring an immediate result
Materials used	CP (10% to 22%) or whitening gels containing no peroxide	CP (34% to 44%)	Hydrogen peroxide (30% to 50%)
Location	At home, 2 to 4 hours per day	Dental office	Dental office
Technique	A custom-fitted tray is made in a dental office; the correct strength of solution and the tray are taken home with the patient, who administers the treatment and returns periodically for follow-up	CP is applied in a customized whitening tray and placed in the patient's mouth for at least 30 minutes per treatment; additional applications are sent home with the patient	The solution is applied to the teeth by a dental professional and activated with a special light or heat source
Outcome	Takes about 3 to 4 weeks for measurable results to be seen	Some results are seen within 30 minutes of treatment	In most cases dramatic results are seen immediately
Average number of treatments	Once per day for 2 to 3 hours for 4 to 6 weeks	Can be used as a "jump-start" for daily home treatments	One visit; an at-home regimen may be suggested depending on the stains being treated

CP = Carbamide peroxide

in a custom-fitted tray overnight or for a few hours a day. The other two types are performed in the dental office. About three office appointments are usually required for dark stains. One method involves application of carbamide peroxide for about 30 minutes, while the other, *power bleaching*, uses a 30% to 50% hydrogen peroxide solution further activated by a strong light or heat. Dental office treatments may also involve microabrasion to remove superficial stains from enamel with hydrochloric acid and a fine abrasive.

The results of bleaching last about a year. Deep, dark stains are better handled with porcelain veneers. Side effects of bleaching include tooth hypersensitivity, soft tissue lesions, and sore throat and nausea from swallowing the bleach. Anesthesia should not be used during treatment, because it would mask irritation of the pulp. Considerable care is needed to protect the patient's eyes and to discontinue the treatment if painful. Although bleaching can be effective, many patients have an unrealistic view of the natural color of teeth and undergo unnecessary treatment.

■ Glossary

abrasion The mechanical process of surface wear of one material by another.

abrasive The material that causes the wear of another material.

abrasivity index A method of rating the abrasiveness of dentifrices.

amorphous Without crystalline structure; having random arrangement of atoms in space.

blinding Clogging of an abrasive wheel with debris, causing reduction of abrasive action.

dental stones Grinding instruments composed of abrasive particles bound in a hard resin matrix or sintered together into a hard mass.

disks Grinding and polishing rotary instruments composed of abrasive particles cemented to a flexible plastic backing.

microcrystalline Composed of tiny (submicron) crystals.

polishing The process of making a rough surface smooth and glossy.

rubber wheels Grinding and polishing instruments composed of abrasive particles in a flexible rubber matrix.

strips Instruments for grinding and polishing interproximal areas; composed of abrasive particles cemented to a flexible plastic backing.

substrate The material being abraded.

whitening Removal of surface discoloration by polishing or bleaching.

◼ Discussion Questions

1. Since many esthetic porcelain restorations are given a final thin layer of stain glaze for color matching, how could a dentifrice cause an undesirable change in color?

2. How could polishing teeth reduce the need for bleaching?

3. Why is trying to obtain snow-white teeth by bleaching unrealistic?

4. What are the dangers of bleaching teeth, and what are the current regulations regarding the use of these products?

◼ Study Questions

(See appendix E for answers.)

1. What is an abrasive?

2. Which factors affect the rate of abrasion?

3. Place the following in order of hardness: cuttle, rouge, silicon carbide, chalk, sand, diamond, aluminum oxide, and pumice.

4. Rouge is used to polish gold alloys. What effect do you think it would have on dental porcelain?

5. Why is it important to obtain polished surfaces on dentition?

6. During grinding and polishing, what would be the effect if coarse abrasive particles from a previous step were present during the final polishing step? How can it be avoided?

7. How sensitive is the tongue to detecting scratches?

8. What are some common abrasives found in *(a)* prophylaxis pastes; *(b)* dentifrices; and *(c)* stones, rubber wheels, and disks?

9. Which criteria would you use in selecting a dentifrice for a patient?

10. When should you polish an amalgam restoration? Which materials would you use?

11. Why are composite restorations difficult to polish? When would a rough surface on a composite restoration be desirable?

12. What evidence is provided regarding the performance of the large number of bleaching products?

◼ References

1. O'Brien WJ, Johnston WM, Fanian F, Lambert S. The surface roughness and gloss of composites. J Dent Res 1984;63(5):685–688.
2. Tolley LG, O'Brien WJ, Dennison JB. Surface finish of dental composite restorative materials. J Biomed Mater Res 1978;12:233–240.

◼ Recommended Reading

American Dental Association. Dentists' Desk Reference: Materials, Instruments and Equipment, ed 2. Chicago: American Dental Association, 1983.

Ashmore H, Van Abbé NJ, Wilson SJ. The measurement in vitro of dentine abrasion by toothpaste. Br Dent J 1972;133:60.

Council on Dental Therapeutics: Guidelines for the acceptance of peroxide-containing oral hygiene products. J Am Dent Assoc 1994;125:1140.

Gerdin PO. Studies in dentifrices. IV. Size and shape of particles in commercial dentifrices. Svensk Tandlak T 1971;64(7):447–461.

Grabenstetter RJ, Broge RW, Jackson FL, Radike AW. The measurement of the abrasion of human teeth by dentifrice abrasives: A test utilizing radioactive teeth. J Dent Res 1958;37:1060–1069.

Haywood VB, Leonard RH, Nelson CF, Brunson WD. Effectiveness, side effects and long-term status of nightguard vital bleaching. J Am Dent Assoc 1994;125:1219.

Abrasivity of current dentifrices. Council on Dental Therapeutics. J Am Dent Assoc 1970;81:1177.

Norton FH. Elements of Ceramics, ed 2. Reading, MA: Addison-Wesley, 1974:260–268.

Phillips RW. Skinner's Science of Dental Materials, ed 7. Philadelphia: WB Saunders, 1973:623–640.

Powers JM, Roberts JC, Craig RG. Wear of filled and unfilled dental restorative resins. Wear 1976;39:117–122.

Reder BS, Eames WB. The cutting rates and durability of diamond stones [abstract 499]. J Dent Res 1976;55(B):186.

Stookey GK, Muhler JC. Laboratory studies concerning the enamel and dentin abrasion properties of common dentifrice polishing agents. J Dent Res 1968;47(4):524–532.

Whitehurst JF, Stookey GK, Muhler JC. Studies concerning the cleaning, polishing, and therapeutic properties of commercial prophylactic pastes. J Oral Therm Pharm 1968;4(3):181–191.

CHAPTER 11

Structure and Properties of Metals and Alloys

A wide variety of metals is used in dentistry (Table 11-1) and each has a melting or solidification temperature that is characteristic of that element. When elements are alloyed together to change their properties, the single melting temperature is changed to a range of temperatures over which the liquid is in equilibrium with solid crystals nucleated in the liquid metal.

The upper temperature for the liquid-solid alloy range is called the *liquidus* temperature, and the lower temperature limit is called the *solidus* temperature. When a liquid alloy melt is being cooled, the liquidus temperature is the temperature at which solid crystals start to nucleate. When a mixture of an alloy liquid and crystals is being heated, the liquidus temperature is the temperature at which the crystals dissolve into liquid, and the solidus temperature is the temperature at which the last liquid solidifies on cooling or the first liquid is formed on heating.

Complete melting is needed for casting and soldering, and at least an additional 100°C superheat is needed for a fluid melt to cast. A reducing flame rich in gas should be used for casting and soldering, otherwise the liquid metal will be oxidized by the oxygen in air, which keeps the solder from wetting the surface and flowing. Note that a gas/air torch cannot be used to cast a metal with a liquidus temperature above 1,000°C because the flame does not get hot enough. To provide a margin of safety against melting the castings in a fixed partial denture, the liquidus temperature of the solder should be at least 50°C lower than the solidus temperature of the casting alloy being soldered.

Table 11-1 Metallic elements used in dentistry

ELEMENT	UNIT CELL	MELTING TEMPERATURE (°C)
Mercury	Rhombohedral	–39
Gallium	Orthorhombic	30
Indium	Tetragonal	156
Tin	Face-centered cubic	419
Aluminum	Face-centered cubic	660
Silver	Face-centered cubic	960
Gold	Face-centered cubic	1,063
Copper	Face-centered cubic	1,083
Manganese	Cubic	1,244
Beryllium	Hexagonal close pack	1,284
Nickel	Face-centered cubic	1,452
Cobalt	Body-centered cubic	1,493
Iron	Body-centered cubic	1,535
Palladium	Face-centered cubic	1,552
Titanium	Hexagonal close pack	1,668
Platinum	Face-centered cubic	1,769
Chromium	Body-centered cubic	1,875
Molybdenum	Body-centered cubic	2,610

Fig 11-1 Formation of crystal nuclei in liquid metal. ○ = atoms in liquid state; ● = atoms in solid state.

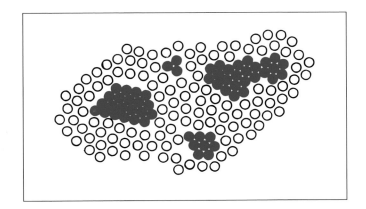

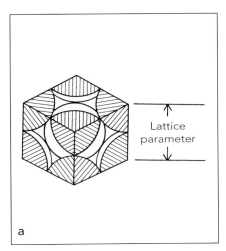

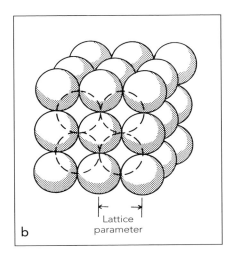

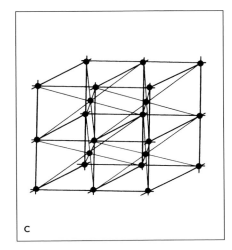

a   b   c

Fig 11-2 (a) The body-centered cubic unit cell is typical of the crystal lattice of pure iron at room temperature. The lattice parameter for iron is 2.87 Å. (b) A part of a body-centered cubic crystal lattice. It could extend in all directions. In this *hard sphere model*, the atoms are visualized as hard spheres of a definite radius in contact. (c) The body-centered cubic space lattice can be visualized as a *point skeleton* of the body-centered cubic crystal lattice.

◼ Unit Cells of Crystal Lattices

Liquid metals nucleate **crystals** on cooling (Fig 11-1). The atoms joining the crystals form a packing arrangement in space that is characteristic of that metal or alloy at equilibrium. The smallest division of the crystalline metal that defines the unique packing is called the **unit cell**. When the unit cell is repeated in space, the repeating atomic positions form the **crystal lattice** structure of a crystalline solid (Fig 11-2). The atoms at the corners of the unit cell are shared among the adjacent eight-unit cells, as shown for the body-centered unit cell. Therefore, one-eighth of the corner atom is associated with the cell; there are eight corner atoms, so they each contribute one atom to the unit cell. The body-centered atom is totally inside the

unit cell and is not shared, so it contributes the second atom to the unit cell mass. Using the **lattice parameters** to calculate the volume of the cubic cell, the density of the metal can be calculated by dividing the mass of atoms in the unit cell by its volume. The lattice parameters for metals and alloys range between 2 Å and 10 Å for the different unit cells formed.

It has been observed that the position of the neighboring atoms surrounding every atom of a crystal lattice is identical in a pure crystalline metal. When the property of identical periodic points in space was explored mathematically, it was discovered that there are 14 ways to arrange points in space, called **space lattices** (Fig 11-3). A pure metal crystal lattice is similar to one of the space lattices except that each mathematic point is the site of an atom. Complex crystal lattices like amalgam alloy and

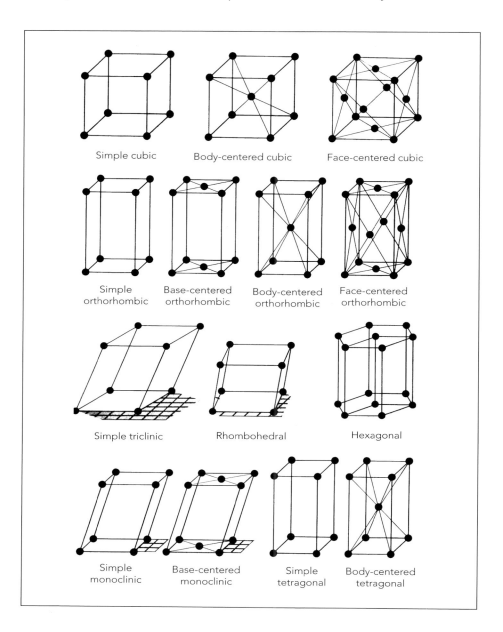

Fig 11-3 Unit cells of the 14-space lattice contain atoms arranged so that each one has identical surroundings. (Reprinted with permission from Mott.[1])

Simple cubic   Body-centered cubic   Face-centered cubic

Simple orthorhombic   Base-centered orthorhombic   Body-centered orthorhombic   Face-centered orthorhombic

Simple triclinic   Rhombohedral   Hexagonal

Simple monoclinic   Base-centered monoclinic   Simple tetragonal   Body-centered tetragonal

enamel have the points of their space lattices replaced by the different atoms of the material or by groups of atoms. The unit cell of each crystalline material, no matter how complex, corresponds with one of these 14 space lattice unit cells (see Table 11-1).

■ Nucleation and Polycrystalline Grain Structure

As the melt of metal is cooled, clusters of atoms come together from the liquid to form solid crystal **nuclei**. These nuclei will be stable and grow into **crystallites** or

grains if the energy of the system is favorable, ie, lowered by the process. The energy is lowered by an atom bonding to the solid nuclei, thereby giving up its liquid-state kinetic energy of motion. However, when an atom bonds to the nuclei, the energy can also be raised by the creation of more interfacial surface energy as a result of the increased surface area of the nuclei in contact with the liquid. The energy of the system is favorable for stable nuclei and growth when more energy is lost by bonding than is gained by increasing the interfacial surface area.

Nucleation can occur by two processes. The first, called **homogeneous** nucleation, is enhanced by rapid cooling,

Fig 11-4 Irregular polygons called *grains* or *crystallites*. An average distance measured across the faces of the crystal grains is called the *grain size*. It may be less than 1,000 Å or more than 1 cm, depending on the number of nuclei present during solidification. (Reprinted with permission from Guy.[2])

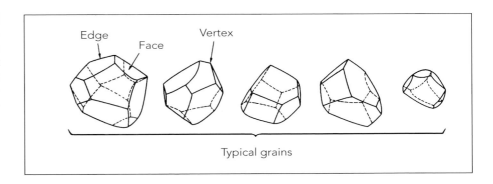

Fig 11-5 The grain structure of a metal is revealed by polishing the surface to a mirror finish and etching lightly in acid. To study the grain structure of metals used for dental appliances, a light or scanning electron microscope is needed for magnification because of the small grain sizes. (Reprinted with permission from Guy.[2])

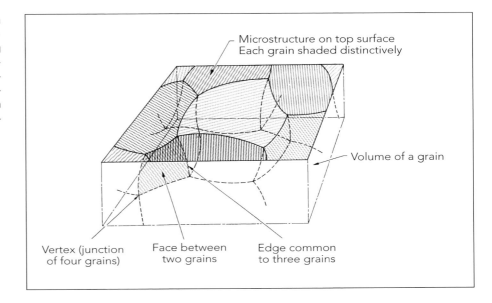

or supercooling, of the nuclei. The result is that more energy is lost when an atom of the liquid bonds to the solid. With rapid cooling (quenching in water), more nuclei are formed per unit volume. These nuclei grow together to form the irregular **polycrystalline** grains or crystallites that fit together like a three-dimensional puzzle to form the bulk of the metal shape (Figs 11-4 and 11-5). The more nuclei that are formed by rapid cooling, the smaller the grain size or crystallite dimensions. Another means of decreasing the grain size (*grain refining*) is by adding to the melt a foreign solid particle or surface to which the atoms are attracted, such as a very fine high-melting metal or oxide powder. This process of seeding the nuclei is called *heterogeneous nucleation*.

Grain size and properties

Decreasing the grain size can have a number of beneficial effects on the cast alloy structure of a crown or removable partial denture. The finer grain size can raise the yield stress, increase the ductility (percent elongation), and raise the **ultimate strength**. The change in these properties according to changes in grain size is related to the processes of plastic **deformation** and fracture and how the boundaries between grains relate to these processes. The size of metal grains in different metals may range from less than 1,000 Å to more than 1 cm. Grains contain large numbers of unit cells—even grains that are only 1,000 Å across. The lattices of the grains are formed in random directions when they grow from the melt. A boundary is formed where the grains grow into contact, because the atoms in one grain's crystal lattice are not in position to mesh with the repeating atoms in the crystal lattices of adjacent grains. These **grain boundaries** are several atom layers thick that are distorted from normal atomic positions to bridge the mismatch in the lattice orientations of adjacent grains.

Only metals with simple body-centered or face-centered cubic unit cells have enough densely packed planes of atoms in their lattices to allow plastic deformation at **yield stress**. These lattice types permit shearing of the densely packed planes of atoms like cards of a microscopic deck sliding over each other. However, the lattice of adjacent grain can be viewed as a second microscopic card deck at a different angle. To get the metal to deform, it is necessary to force the cards of one deck into other decks at an angle. But the more grains per unit volume, the more difficult it is to get the planes (cards) to slide because the dislocated slipping planes run against the grain boundaries sooner. Thus, a greater resistance to slippage is created by more grain boundaries, and higher yield stress results.

On the other hand, a material will fracture because a crack opens up on a grain boundary. This situation is more likely to occur in large-grain metals, when the planes cannot be slipped into the adjacent grains. Many smaller grains in various orientations can divide the plastic strain among the grains more easily, with more of them oriented for slipping. Large grains must each accommodate a larger strain and will have fewer planes properly oriented to slip. The result is lower ductility and lower ultimate strength for large-grain metals, which open cracks more readily at grain boundaries because the plastic deformation cannot be accommodated. For these reasons, grain-refined or *micrograin* alloys produced by heterogeneous nucleation are advantageous for developing fixed partial denture alloys with higher yield stress, better ductility, and improved ultimate strength.

◨ Alloy Systems

Most pure metals are miscible when melted together. When two metals form a solution in the liquid state so their atoms mix randomly on the atomic scale, they are said to form an **alloy**. As the alloy liquid freezes, the atoms may remain randomly distributed on the unit-cell lattice sites in each crystal grain. This random distribution in the solid alloy is called a **solid solution**. But, if like atoms prefer to bond among themselves, the atoms of different elements may segregate in different grains.

Different grains may be practically pure if their elements are insoluble in each other's lattices in the solid state. Or they can have a limited solubility in the other's crystal lattice if the elements exhibit partial solubility in one another. Metal atoms of two different metal elements are more likely to be soluble in each other's lattices if they (1) have the same atomic lattice type, (2) have similar atomic radii (ie, a difference of less than 10%), (3) have the same valence number, and (4) form bonds to other atoms with strengths similar to those they form among themselves. On the other hand, if these rules are not followed and the unlike atoms have a strong affinity to each other, grains of an **intermetallic compound** may be formed at definite ratios of the alloying elements (eg, dental amalgam alloy Ag_3Sn).

The energetically stable crystal lattice structures and their compositions for an alloy that is preferred by "nature" varies with temperature and ratio of the alloying elements. It is not possible to calculate the equilibrium composition and structures and the temperatures at which they change. They must be determined experimentally by measuring the temperatures at which the latent heat is liberated when the alloy solidifies or solid lattices transform to different crystal lattices. The type of crystal lattice is determined by x-ray diffraction from the crystal atomic planes. The angle and intensity of the x-ray beam reflections (ie, diffraction) are characteristic of the atomic composition, type of crystal lattice, and position of atoms in their unit cell. Thus, experimental detection of the temperature when heat is liberated indicates when an alloy is changing its structure, and x-ray scattering identifies what lattices are present. This information is portrayed in a **binary phase diagram** of the alloy system (Figs 11-6 and 11-7). The alloy system represents all possible ratios of the elements.

When two elements are alloyed, the system is called a **binary alloy**; when three elements are alloyed, the system is a **ternary alloy**, and so on. An alloy is named by listing its elements in descending order of percent composition. For example, Ag_3Sn is called *silver-tin alloy*. If more than two elements are involved, the number of phase changes and their representation becomes complex, but their description follows the same principle.

An *equilibrium phase* is defined as a homogeneous body of matter that is physically distinct and mechanically distinguishable. For a pure material like water, the vapor, liquid, and solid **phases** are physically distinct and mechanically distinguishable in properties like hardness, compressibility, and elastic modulus. However, when the phase definition is applied to an alloy system, it is important to recognize that if two different types of unit cells nucleate from the melt—as, for example, at the **eutectic** (lowest melting) point in Fig 11-7—a two-phase re-

Fig 11-6 Copper-gold phase diagram. The disordered solid solution (softer) and ordered solid solutions (harder) are produced by heat treatment. FCC = face-centered cubic.

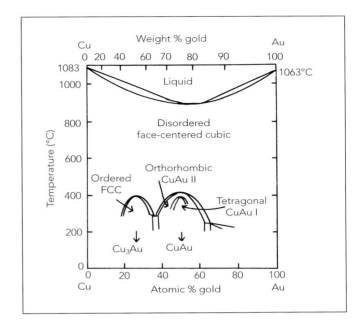

Fig 11-7 Silver-copper phase diagram showing a eutectic (lowest melting) point at 28.1% copper.

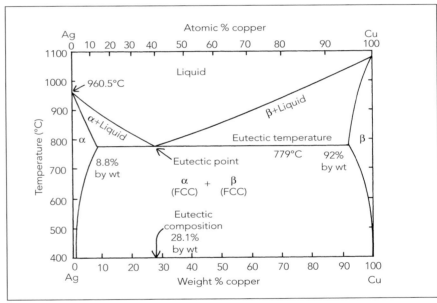

gion is formed. These two phases nucleate as separate grains. They are physically distinct, as indicated by grain boundaries that define their limits, and their mechanical properties differ, as can be measured by a microhardness tester impinging on individual grains. Note that two-phase alloys are not as corrosion resistant as like single-phase alloys, because microscopic galvanic corrosion cells are set up between the grains of the different phases. Also, porcelain bonding to multiphase alloys is considered potentially weaker because of composition differences of the grains.

◼ Deformation in Metals

There are three types of deformations that can occur in metals, which arise from different mechanisms. The simplest deformation, *elastic strain*, is the elastic stretching of lattice in which all of the atoms are shifted from their equilibrium positions by a fraction of their atomic spacing. The strain is directly proportional to the applied stress (ie, force area or force intensity) up to the proportional limit stress. When the stress is removed, the atoms

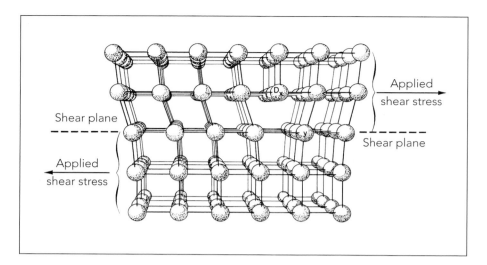

Fig 11-8a Distortion (strain) around a dislocation in a simple cubic crystal lattice. The size of the atoms has been reduced so the perspective can be seen. The row of atoms of the dislocation is D_x. (Reprinted from Zinman.[3])

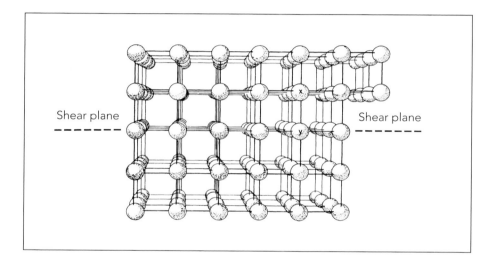

Fig 11-8b The crystal lattice as it would appear after the yield stress has been exceeded and the dislocation has moved through the lattice. The solid has been deformed to this new shape. (Reprinted from Zinman.[3])

return to equilibrium spacing. Compared with most polymeric materials, metals generally have strong metallic bonds and resist elastic stretching. This stiffness or resistance to elastic strain is indicated by the high elastic moduli of metals. Stiffness is desirable for removable partial dentures, so forces can be transmitted by the framework across an arch to better distribute the load. It is desirable for the alloy of resin-bonded fixed partial dentures to resist flexing of the bond.

Another type of deformation is *plastic deformation*, a permanent deformation that begins when the elastic limit stress or its approximation, yield stress, is reached. This mode of deformation requires that atoms be shifted to new atomic sites on the lattice. These lattice sites must be identical to the old sites and not far away, so the en-

ergy to shift atoms is not too great. Thus, ductility is associated with face-centered and body-centered cubic metal lattices, which have more identical sites and more closely packed planes, so atoms do not have to slide far to reach the new lattice sites. Intermetallic compounds are usually brittle because the atomic sites are specific to the different atoms of the compound and are not interchangeable.

The mechanism of plastic deformation is called **dislocation motion**, which is the slipping of the closely packed planes over each other. A **dislocation** (Fig 11-8a, D_x) is the line of atoms that denotes the edge of an additional half-plane of atoms that appears to be wedged into the lattice. The lattice is distorted (strained) by the presence of the dislocation line of atoms. Dislocation motion shifts atoms from one lattice site to the next, rather than moving all of the atoms of the plane at one time, which would take much more energy (Fig 11-8b).

Any process that impedes dislocation movement tends to harden a metal, raise its yield stress, and often lower its ductility. Some processes are reversible, allowing the hardness to be low when making an appliance, for example, after which the metal can be hardened to provide better service if necessary.

One process for **hardening** metal is called **cold working**, or *work hardening*—any plastic deformation of metal by hammering, drawing, cold forging, cold rolling, or bending. These processes produce many dislocations in the metal that cannot slip through each other as easily as the lattice becomes more distorted. The yield stress can be raised more than 100% when a drawn orthodontic wire is compared with the as-cast metal. In dentistry, cold working occurs when gold foil is compacted, a denture clasp is bent, an inlay margin is burnished, or a deformed metal layer forms on a crown during finishing and polishing.

A second process for hardening a metal is *precipitation hardening*, in which a second phase of finely dispersed clusters of atoms are precipitated from a metastable supersaturated solid solution by reheating an alloy that was quench-cooled to form the metastable supersaturated solid.

Heat treatment can also be used to harden gold-copper alloys by a slightly different process. Because the gold-copper system forms a complete solid solution at all compositions, the atoms can be interchanged on the lattice sites. However, as the atoms are cooled, the copper and gold atoms tend to separate on alternating planes of the lattice in ordered arrangement. This ordering makes dislocation motion more difficult, raising the yield stress. These alloys are soft if quenched but hard if cooled slowly on the bench top or held in the furnace at the ordering temperature range (350°C for 30 minutes).

Other heat treatments are used to homogenize the grains of an alloy that have developed composition gradients by rapid cooling and **crystallization** of the melt. When cooled rapidly, the grains of the alloy cannot maintain an equilibrium or uniform composition in the grain. The first part of the grain to cool will be richer than the average composition of the higher-melting-temperature element, and the last part of the grain to solidify is richer in the low-melting alloy component. This inhomogeneity tends to reduce corrosion resistance of the metal be-

cause of the galvanic cell created between the center of the grain and the grain boundary. Heating the solid at a temperature and for a duration that allows the atoms to reach equilibrium will improve corrosion resistance.

Diffusion in Metals

Atoms of a crystalline solid vibrate about their fixed lattice positions. As they absorb heat with increasing temperature, they vibrate at greater amplitude. Also, a small fraction of the atom sites are vacant in a metal. As the temperature increases, an atom may momentarily experience an increase in vibrational energy, which will be sufficient to permit it to jump from one lattice site to another. As the temperature and time increase, more atoms will be able to jump or diffuse to new lattice sites. This random jumping during heat treatment allows the rearrangement of the crystal lattice. Atomic diffusion also permits rearrangement of cold-worked metals and permanent deformation of metals at stress levels far below the yield stress if the stress lasts long enough. In general, these rearrangements by diffusion begin to occur at a significant rate as the temperature of metal exceeds one half of its absolute melting temperature. The rate of rearrangement accelerates rapidly as the metal or alloy approaches its solidus temperature.

There are several heat treatment processes for metals that utilize the process of diffusion. Among them is an **annealing** heat treatment to release **residual stress**, allowing the dislocations and atomic vacancies to move and realign to lower the internal residual stress fields in a cold-worked metal at a relatively low temperature and short heating time.

If the temperature and heating times are extended for a cold-worked metal, the metal can experience **recrystallization**, in which stress-free grains are crystallized out of the deformed grains. A *recrystallization temperature* is the temperature at which it would take 1 hour for the cold-worked metal to recrystallize. This temperature is between one-third and one-half of the absolute melting temperature for most metals (Fig 11-9). As the temperature and time are further extended, **grain growth** occurs, during which the stress-free grains grow larger at the expense of the disappearing small grains.

The residual stress heat treatment relaxes the internal stress, which may cause warpage over time. The chance of corrosion related to residual stress differences

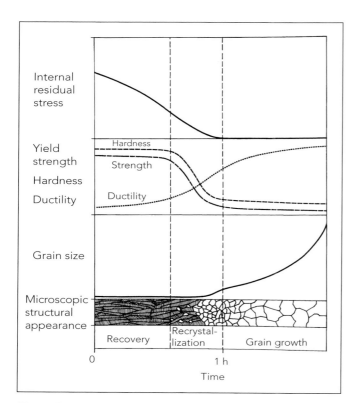

Fig 11-9 A microscopic view of the stages that a cold-worked metal, such as an orthodontic wire, goes through when subjected to prolonged heating. The higher the temperature and the greater the cold working, the more quickly the transitions occur. This figure shows recrystallization being completed in 1 hour, which means the temperature of heating was the recrystallization temperature as per the definition. The changes in properties can be compared with the structural changes. (Reprinted with permission from Jastrzebski.[4])

on the metal surface are reduced. Recrystallization heat treatment lowers the yield stress and increases the ductility. Grain growth further reduces yield stress and increases ductility yield stress. When soldering a cold-worked wire in which a high-yield stress is desired (eg, a partial denture wire clasp or an orthodontic appliance), a low-melting solder and a short soldering time are desirable to minimize recrystallization and grain growth.

▣ Glossary

alloy An atomic mixture of metallic elements.

annealing A relatively low-temperature heat treatment for removing residual stress.

binary alloy An alloy composed of two elements.

binary phase diagram A map with temperature and composition as coordinates, which displays the regions where each stable phase exists.

cold working Deforming a metal at temperatures that are low compared with its melting temperature. Also called *work hardening*.

crystal A solid with periodic arrangement of atoms in space, usually with atomic planes forming facets on the surface.

crystal lattice The periodic arrangement of atoms in three-dimensional space.

crystallite A crystal with irregularly shaped surfaces instead of facets.

crystallization The process of crystal and crystallite formation.

deformation The process of changing the shape of a metal by applied stresses.

dislocation A row of atoms displaced from their normal positions in the lattice.

dislocation motion The movement of a dislocation through a crystal under an applied stress.

eutectic alloy An alloy that is easily melted with respect to its component elements and that can transform at one temperature from liquid to two phases separated as distinct grains in solid metal.

eutectic composition The alloy composition at which the eutectic transformation occurs.

eutectic temperature The temperature at which the eutectic transformation occurs.

grain Another name for crystallite.

grain boundary The interface or junction of adjacent grains.

grain growth Enlargement of grains by heating.

hardening A process in which the yield stress and resistance to indentation are increased.

homogeneous Having uniform composition throughout.

intermetallic compound An alloy phase with a composition usually near a definite fixed atomic ratio of the elements.

lattice parameters The distances between corners of the unit cell.

nuclei The embryos of the crystallites formed from the liquid.

phase A homogeneous body of matter that is physically distinct and mechanically distinguishable.

polycrystalline Composed of many crystallites.

recrystallization The process of forming new crystallites from existing crystallites by heating.

residual stress Internal stress remaining between parts of a solid after the applied stress is removed.

solid solution An alloy phase in which one alloying element enters the lattice of the other.

space lattice A pattern of points in space that satisfies the condition that each point is surrounded by the same arrangement of points.

ternary alloy An alloy composed of three elements.

ultimate strength The maximum stress a solid can support based on its original cross-sectional area.

unit cell The minimum grouping of atoms of a homogeneous crystalline solid that gives the geometric relationships, composition, and distance between the atoms in space.

yield stress The stress at which dislocation motion, permanent deformation, and plastic flow begin.

◼ Discussion Questions

1. Gold and copper are completely soluble in each other in the liquid state. What is the connection between this mutual solubility and their lattice structure?

2. Which mechanical properties of a metal are affected if dislocation motion in the lattice is impeded?

3. How can both the strength and ductility of gold castings be raised by alloying and process control?

4. Why does overheating orthodontic wires lead to brittleness?

◼ Study Questions

(See appendix E for answers.)

1. How does the melting of a pure metal differ from the melting of an alloy?

2. What effect does incomplete melting have on dental castings and solder joints?

3. What is the relationship between the density of a molten alloy and its crystalline solid? Is it the same, less, or greater? Why?

4. How can the density change from liquid to solid damage a dental casting?

5. How many atoms are contained in a face-centered cubic unit cell?

6. Outline how the density of a face-centered cubic metal can be calculated from knowledge of the composition of the unit cell, the atomic weight of the atoms present, the type of unit cell, and the lattice parameters for the unit cell.

7. Which of the following metals are capable of experiencing a large amount of ductility? (Their unit cell types are provided.)

   Ag_3Sn—orthorhombic
   beryllium—hexagonal
   copper—face-centered cubic
   gold—face-centered cubic
   iron—body-centered cubic

8. List several ways in which the yield stress of a metal or alloy may be increased.

9. How can dislocation motion be impeded so as to raise the yield stress?

10. Is it better to have large or small crystallites in order to have a high yield stress and ultimate strength?

11. The grain boundaries of the crystallites at the surface of a metal can be made visible by polishing to a mirror finish with fine abrasives and etching the surface lightly with an acid. *(a)* If 0.5 µm is the resolution of a light microscope, how small a crystal grain might one see? *(b)* Why does acid etch the grain boundaries more than the interior of the grain? Why are different grains etched at different rates?

12. What are the eutectic temperature and composition for the silver-copper system?

13. At what temperatures does solidification begin and end for an alloy containing 40% by weight copper and 60% by weight silver?

14. The composition of an alloy can be specified by the weight percentages or the atomic percentages of its elements. Given the alloy Ag_3Sn, calculate the atomic percentage of silver and the weight percentage of silver if the gram atomic weight of silver is 107.9 and the gram atomic weight of tin is 118.7.

15. How do a crystal lattice and a space lattice differ?

16. Discuss how the yield strength and percentage elongation change with time during the heating of a drawn wire.

17. If the recrystallization temperature of an iron wire is 450°C, how long would it take a drawn iron wire to recrystallize at that temperature? What fraction of the absolute melting temperature (ie, degrees kelvin) of iron is 450°C?

References

1. Mott N. The solid state. Sci Am 1967;217:80–89.
2. Guy AG. Introduction to Materials Science. New York: McGraw-Hill, 1971.
3. Ziman J. The thermal properties of materials. Sci Am 1967;217: 180–1884.
4. Jastrzebski ZD. Nature and Properties of Engineering Principles. New York: John Wiley & Sons, 1959.

● Recommended Reading

Brandt DA, Warner JC. Metallurgy-Fundamentals. Tinley Park, IL: Goodheart-Willcox, 2005.

Flinn RA, Trojan PK (eds). Engineering Materials and Their Application. Boston: Houghton-Mifflin, 1990.

Greener EH, Harcourt JK, Lautenschlager EP. Materials Science in Dentistry. Baltimore: Williams & Wilkins, 1972.

Guy AG. Elements of Physical Metallurgy. Reading, MA: Addison-Wesley, 1959.

Jere H, Rose RM, Wulff J. The Structure and Properties of Materials, vol 2. New York: John Wiley & Sons, 1965.

Moffatt WG, Pearsall GW, Wulff J, et al. The Structure and Properties of Materials, vol 1. New York: John Wiley & Sons, 1965.

Moniz BJ Metallurgy, ed 2. Homewand, IL: American Tech, 1994.

Mott N. The solid state. Sci Am Sept 1967:80–90.

Reed-Hill RE. Physical Metallurgy Principles, ed 2. New York: Van Nostrand Reinhold, 1973.

Rose RM, Shepard LA, Wulff J. The Structure and Properties of Materials, vol 4. New York: John Wiley & Sons, 1965.

Van Vlack LH. Materials Science for Engineers. Reading, MA: Addison-Wesley, 1970.

CHAPTER 12

Dental Amalgams

Amalgam has been an accepted part of dental therapeutics for more than 150 years and is still used for more than 75% of direct posterior restorations. The reasons for its popularity lie in its ease of manipulation, relatively low cost, and long life. Some concern has arisen with reference to mercury from both a biologic and an environmental viewpoint; however, it is believed that dental amalgam presents an acceptable risk-to-benefit ratio when properly used. An exception to this position has been taken in northern Europe, where concerns have been raised regarding amalgam use in vulnerable populations, such as pregnant women and pedodontic patients.

Amalgam's primary application in dentistry is in the restoration of posterior teeth and, to some degree, for cores in fixed partial denture buildups. Small Class V restorations are now virtually always carried out using composite and hybrid glass-ionomer restorative materials. Posterior lesions are restored primarily by amalgam, although composites have been used successfully in small cavities as a result of recent improvement in their clinical handling.

Chemical Composition and Microstructure

The general classification of **dental amalgam** alloys is presented in Fig 12-1 and Table 12-1. Contemporary amalgams are mainly classified as **high-copper amalgams** and have existed since the 1960s. In an attempt to circumvent the problems with mercury, a radically new composition was introduced, replacing mercury with a gallium-indium-tin liquid. To understand the significance of these

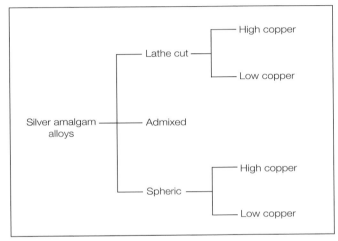

Fig 12-1 A general classification of amalgam alloys.

Table 12-1 Classification of amalgam alloys

COMPOSITION	MORPHOLOGY	EXAMPLE
Traditional	Lathe cut	Aristaloy (Goldsmith & Revere)
Traditional	Spheric	Spheraloy (Kerr/Sybron)
High copper	Lathe cut (single composition)	Epoque 80
High copper	Spheric (single composition)	Tytin (Kerr/Sybron)
High copper	Admixed (traditional + Ag-Cu eutectic)	Dispersalloy (Dentsply Caulk)

materials and how the solid-state reactions in amalgams has made them superior clinical materials, it is first necessary to look at the so-called traditional amalgams.

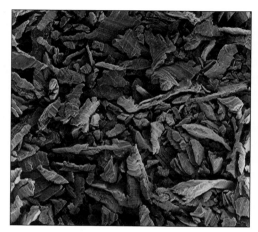

Fig 12-2 Traditional lathe-cut amalgam alloy (original magnification ×100).

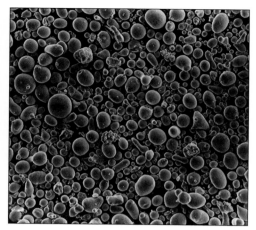

Fig 12-3 Traditional spheric alloy (original magnification ×500).

Traditional amalgam alloys

Lathe cut

Until the 1960s, the chemical composition and microstructure of available amalgam alloys were essentially the same as those of the most successful systems investigated by G.V. Black.[1] **Traditional alloys** were delivered to the dentist as filings, which were lathe cut from a cast **ingot**. Milling and sifting produced the ultimate particle-size distribution, as well as the final form of the amalgam alloy particles. Figure 12-2 illustrates a typical traditional **lathe-cut** alloy.

The commercial alloy evolved into a blend of different particle sizes to optimize packaging efficiency. The particles in a commercial lathe-cut alloy might range in length from 60 to 120 µm, in width from 10 to 70 µm, and in thickness from 10 to 35 µm. The particle size has become still smaller (less than 30 µm) due to the introduction of spheric alloys. By weight, the traditional alloys contain 66% to 73% of silver and 25% to 29% of tin, with about 6% of copper, up to 2% of zinc, and up to 3% of mercury.

The structures of these traditional alloys are phase mixtures of the **gamma (γ) phase** of the silver-tin system (Ag_3Sn) and the **epsilon (ε) phase** of the copper-tin system (Cu_3Sn). It has been shown that Ag_3Sn produces the best physical properties when alloys of the silver-tin system react with mercury.[2] Some of these traditional alloys are still available, but they represent a minor component of the overall amalgam market.

Spheric

Spheric alloys were introduced on the market during the 1960s. These alloys lowered the necessary **mercury-alloy ratios** and dramatically reduced **condensation** pressures. Their particle shape is created by means of an atomizing process whereby a spray of tiny drops is allowed to solidify in an inert gaseous (ie, argon) or liquid (ie, water) environment. Although all alloys produced in this way are classified as spheric, their particle shape might be irregular (Fig 12-3). The maximum particle size in a spheric alloy powder is generally 40 to 50 µm or less, although there usually is a particle size distribution.

High-copper blended and single-composition amalgam alloys

During the late 1960s, alloys with a significantly different chemical composition were introduced on the market. All of these alloys could be characterized by their higher copper content. A list of current high-copper alloy products is presented in Table 12-1.

The first alloy of this type (Dispersalloy)[3] was a mechanical mixture of a traditional lathe-cut alloy with a spheric alloy in a ratio of 2:1 (Fig 12-4). The chemical composition of the spheric particle was 72% silver and 28% copper by weight, which corresponds to the **eutectic composition** of the silver-copper system. The overall composition of this alloy contained approximately 13% copper by weight, more than twice the maximum amount permitted in the American Dental Association's (ADA's)

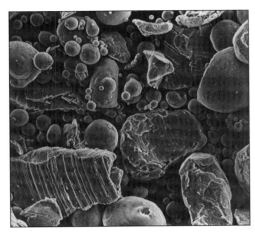

Fig 12-4 Blended high-copper amalgam alloy with spheres of silver-copper and lathe-cut particles of a traditional alloy (original magnification ×1,000).

Table 12-2 Typical compositions of amalgam alloys (% by weight)

TYPE	AG	SN	CU	AN	OTHER
TL	70.9	25.8	2.4	1.0	—
TS	72.0	26.0	1.5	0.5	—
HCS	41.0–61.0	24.0–30.5	13.0–28.3	0–0.5	In 3.4
HCAd	62.0–69.7	15.1–18.6	12.0–22.7	0–0.9	In 10
HCL	43.0	29.0	25.0	0.3	Hg 2.7
GA	50.0	26.0	15.0	—	Pd 9

TL = traditional lathe cut; TS = traditional spheric; HCS = high-copper spheric; HCAd = high-copper admixed; HCL = high-copper lathe cut; GA = alloy for gallium amalgam.

specifications for amalgam alloy at that time. Amalgams made from this alloy, however, were clinically superior to traditional amalgams with respect to marginal integrity,[4] and consequently, other manufacturers developed similar compositions, some with a copper content greater than that found in traditional amalgam. At present, the copper content varies up to approximately 30% by weight in some commercial amalgam alloys (Table 12-2).

The structures of several high-copper alloys are similar to that of Dispersalloy. They can be classified as **blended alloys** in which the traditional and high-copper phases are mechanically blended. Other alloys are produced by melting together all components of a high-copper system and creating a single-composition spheric or lathe-cut alloy, rather than a mechanical mixture of two distinct powders. Depending on the number of components involved, these systems are also referred to as **ternary, quaternary,** or **single-composition alloys.**

In an effort to improve clinical handling properties, some amalgam alloy manufacturers supply **admixed alloys.** The chemical compositions and physical forms of the basic powders (lathe cut or spheric) in these alloys are varied. This system further differs from those using Dispersalloy in that both blended components represent copper-enriched alloys. It is important to stress that all of these copper-enriched alloys contain more than 10% copper by weight in the form of either the silver-copper eutectic or the copper-tin system. Several typical classifications and compositions of high-copper systems are presented in Table 12-2. The dynamics of the current

marketplace preclude a comprehensive listing, as a great number of alloys appear and disappear worldwide in response to local demand.

Although amalgam alloys containing many other metals have been proposed or investigated on an experimental basis, at present only palladium, selenium, and indium have been used as commercial additives. Because of economic reasons, the alloys intended for mercury amalgamation and containing palladium feature a relatively low (less than 1%) concentration. Selenium has been added in an attempt to improve **biocompatibility,**[5] and indium has been admixed in large concentrations (10% by weight) in metallic form to high-copper amalgam to reduce the mercury vapor released during mastication.[6,7]

Gallium alloys

The melting temperature of gallium can be suppressed below room temperature with the addition of appropriate amounts of indium and tin, resulting in **gallium alloys.** This liquid can then be triturated with a silver-tin-copper alloy powder (spheric) in the same fashion as dental amalgam. Significant amounts of palladium are added to the alloy powder in current commercial compositions to improve corrosion properties. A current composition marketed in Japan, known as *Gallium alloy GF* (Tokuriki Honten), comes in powder form and contains the following elements (by weight): silver, 50%; tin, 25.7%; copper, 15%; palladium, 9%; and traces, 0.3%. It is also available as a liquid containing gallium, 65%; indium, 18.95%; tin, 16%; and traces, 0.5%.

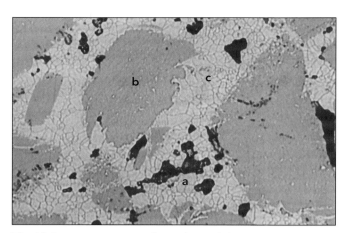

Fig 12-5 Microstructure of a traditional dental amalgam containing (a) γ2 and (b) unreacted γ in (c) a γ1 matrix.

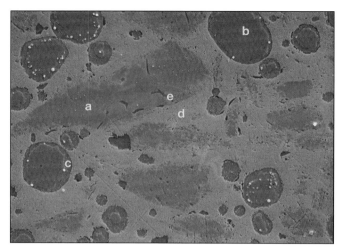

Fig 12-6 Scanning electron micrograph of Dispersalloy amalgam. (a) Ag₃Sn; (b) silver-copper eutectic; (c) η′ phase (Cu₆Sn₅); (d) γ1 phase (Ag₂Hg₃); (e) ε phase (Cu₃Sn). (Original magnification ×1,000. Courtesy of T. Okabe.)

■ Setting Reactions and Microstructure

Traditional amalgams

The **amalgamation** reaction of the traditional alloy with mercury (known as **trituration**) as well as its microstructure after setting are described on the basis of a reaction of Ag_3Sn (γ) with mercury. Copper and/or zinc are not usually taken into account, but their presence has important effects. During hardening, new reaction products with mercury are formed at the cost of the original alloy particles. The main reaction products formed are the **gamma 1 (γ1)** (silver-mercury) and **gamma 2 (γ2)** (tin-mercury) phases. Formation of a network is completed before all the original reactant is consumed. This amalgamation reaction can be symbolized as follows:

$$Ag_3Sn + Hg \rightarrow Ag_2Hg_3 + Sn_7Hg + Ag_3Sn$$
$$\gamma + Hg \rightarrow \gamma1 + \gamma2 + \gamma \text{ (remnant)}$$

After the amalgamation reaction is complete, the remnants of the high-melting-point silver-tin particles are embedded in a matrix of reaction products with mercury (Fig 12-5). In most traditional amalgams, the γ1 and γ2 phases form a continuous network. The formation of such an interconnecting structure is extremely important, because the γ2 phase is prone to corrosion and should

be considered the weak link in many traditional dental amalgams. The copper contained in the original alloy will react with tin during trituration to form the **eta prime (η′) phase** Cu_6Sn_5. The presence of copper has long been associated with improving the physical properties of amalgam, particularly its flow or deformation under static load. This effect is magnified in high-copper amalgams. The presence of zinc appears to extend the working time and, hence, the plasticity of the traditional amalgam.

High-copper amalgams

All high-copper amalgams are characterized by the γ2 phase being either absent or substantially reduced, because tin preferentially reacts with copper rather than with mercury, preventing the formation of the tin-mercury reaction product. During amalgamation of blended alloys, Cu_6Sn_5 is created from copper and tin. The same process occurs in traditional amalgams, but to a lesser extent, because the copper concentration is less. Because most of the reactive copper is present in the silver-copper spheres, the Cu_6Sn_5 phase is formed at the surface of these particles, creating a reaction zone that is easily identified in the microstructure (Fig 12-6). The mechanism to form Cu_6Sn_5 can be described by:

$$6Cu + 5Sn \rightarrow Cu_6Sn_5$$

In single-composition systems, Cu_6Sn_5 also will be formed during amalgamation reactions. In this case, however, the reaction is thought to be:

$$2Cu_3Sn + 3Sn \rightarrow Cu_6Sn_5$$

because the source of copper is the ϵ phase in single-composition alloys. It is obvious that in dental amalgam alloys where equivalent amounts of copper and Cu_3Sn are present, both reactions may be equally important in the formation of Cu_6Sn_5. It should be stressed that some high-copper amalgams may initially contain the $\gamma2$ phase if the mercury content is higher than a certain critical percentage. In these amalgams, the elimination of $\gamma2$ may occur over a substantial period because the reactions are diffusion controlled. In general, in lathe-cut and blended alloys, the mercury-alloy ratios are greater than or equal to 1.0, whereas in spheric alloy systems, the mercury-alloy ratios are less than 1.0 and may be as low as 0.7. As mentioned earlier, the $\gamma2$ phase is considered the weak link in a traditional low-copper amalgam. However, because the $\gamma2$ phase is absent in high-copper amalgams, attention should be focused on the least resistant phase in the multiphase structure associated with these amalgams. Preferential corrosion of the Cu_6Sn_5 phase reportedly has been shown to be significant both in vivo[8] and in vitro.[9]

Evidence has been presented for the presence of an additional tin-mercury phase, **delta 2 ($\delta2$)**,[10] at the grain boundaries of the resulting $\gamma1$ network. This phase results from the lower tin concentration in the last of the mercury to solidify. Its location at grain boundaries makes this phase important for determining the structure-sensitive properties of amalgam. Since copper and tin will preferentially combine in dental amalgam, the higher copper concentrations will also reduce the formation of $\delta2$.

As mentioned earlier, admixing of indium has lowered the amount of mercury vapor released from amalgam. This phenomenon has also been verified recently for amalgams prepared from a mercury-indium liquid in which the indium concentration was as high as 30%.[11] It is possible that through solid solution, indium may increase the stability of the $\gamma1$ phase (Sarkar NK, personal communication, 1994).

Gallium amalgams

The structure of gallium amalgams has been interpreted in terms of a reaction zone of $CuGa_2$ and $PdGa_5$ sur-

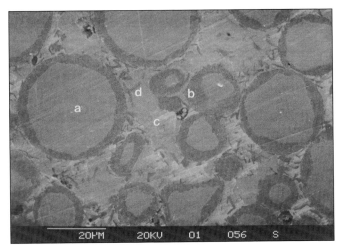

Fig 12-7 Scanning electron micrograph of gallium amalgam (GF Alloy). (a) Unreacted alloy particle; (b) reaction zone (copper-gallium and palladium-gallium compounds); (c) matrix (silver-indium); (d) β tin. (Original magnification ×1,000. Courtesy of S-Y Lee.)

rounding the unreacted alloy particles, which are held together by a matrix of Ag_9In_4 containing islands of Ag_9Ga_3 and **beta (β) tin.** The structure of set gallium amalgam (GF alloy) is shown in Fig 12-7.

Physical Properties

The physical properties of dental amalgam are usually compared with those specified in the American National Standards Institute/American Dental Association (ANSI/ADA) specifications for dental amalgam. These properties are (1) 1-hour compressive strength, (2) **creep**, or resistance to static load, and (3) dimensional change. The ANSI/ADA limits are (1) 1-hour compressive strength of at least 80 MPa (11,000 psi), (2) dental creep of no more than 3%, and (3) dimensional change of ± 20 µm/cm. The corresponding properties of several commercial alloys are presented in Table 12-3. The rationale for these properties is that high early strength is important to withstand dental finishing procedures and occlusal stresses. Low creep is desirable for maintaining marginal integrity, and dimensional change must be controlled to prevent excessive marginal leakage.

Continual reaction occurs as a function of time. The 24-hour compressive strengths shown in Table 12-3 are adequate for most occlusal loadings. If the bite force is assumed to be 750 N (170 lb) and the contact area 2 mm², the compressive stress offered to the amalgam

Table 12-3 Physical properties of amalgam

TYPE	COMPRESSIVE STRENGTH (MPa) (30 MIN/1 H/1 D)	TENSILE STRENGTH (MPa)	KNOOP HARDNESS	CREEP (%)	DIMENSIONAL CHANGE (MM/CM)
TL	53 / 89 / 430	52	146	2.05	8
TS	170 / 265 / 444	55	174	0.21	0
HCS	122 / 220 / 486	63	173	0.07	−7
HCL	59 / 97 / 477	45	174	0.17	5
HCB	79 / 123 / 434	50	155	0.24	−7
GA	— / 343 / 383	57	—	0.17	16

TL = traditional lathe cut; TS = traditional spheric; HCS = high-copper spheric; HCL = high-copper lathe cut; HCB = high-copper blend; GA = alloy for gallium amalgam.

would be on the order of 380 MPa (55,000 psi). As can be seen in Table 12-3, this value is similar to the compressive strengths of most set amalgams. Little additional hardening occurs beyond 24 hours, although additional phase changes are possible.

The amount of residual mercury is very important in the determination of mechanical properties. In general, the compressive strength will decrease 1% with each 1% increase in mercury above 60%. Low mercury-alloy ratios after condensation are therefore desired. In addition to the effects of residual mercury, compressive strength will also decrease 1% with each 1% of porosity. Adequate condensation of amalgam is, therefore, mandatory in achieving maximum strength.

It should also be emphasized that amalgam, in both traditional and high-copper compositions, is a brittle material. Generally, the tensile strength of a brittle material is much less than its corresponding value in compression. For amalgam, the tensile strength values are about one-seventh of the compressive strength values (see Table 12-3). This means tensile failure is much more likely to occur than compressive failure. Tensile failure is particularly apt to occur in the margins where the amalgam may be unsupported or the mercury concentration is higher due to the condensation process. Obviously, the last bit to condense will have the higher mercury concentration because mercury expression occurs as the amalgam is packed. Because of the higher mercury concentration at the margin, this area may contain greater amounts of the δ2 phase, contributing to weakness in this region. Tensile failure may also occur at the isthmus of mesio-occlusodistal restorations with too little bulk at the step.

Creep and **flow** are both deformations produced by constant load. The creep of amalgam is important because amalgam at oral temperatures is at 0.9 Tm, where Tm is the melting temperature. At these temperatures, atomic diffusion occurs easily, and deformation under static load is possible. As seen in Table 12-3, the creep of high-copper amalgam is at least an order of magnitude lower than the upper limit of 3% for traditional amalgams. This lower creep has been associated with the presence of Cu_6Sn_5 in the γ1 network and the decreased amount of available tin.[12] The lower creep of high-copper amalgams may also be related to the absence of the δ2 phase. Furthermore, the lower creep of high-copper amalgam has been suggested as a possible reason for its demonstrably better marginal integrity.

The wear of amalgams is approximately the same magnitude as that of tooth enamel. The wear resistance of amalgams exceeds that of most posterior composite restorative materials; therefore, amalgams are much more likely than most composite restorative materials to maintain occlusal contacts.

The physical properties of gallium amalgam are intermediate compared with traditional and high-copper amalgams (see Table 12-3).

■ Corrosion

Traditional amalgams are susceptible to **corrosion,** with chlorides attacking the γ2 phase. This phase has been shown to corrode according to:

$$8Sn_7Hg + 21O_2 + 42H_2O + 28Cl^- \rightarrow$$
$$14Sn_4(OH)_6Cl_2 + 8Hg$$

This process then leads to two deteriorating effects: *(1)* the corrosion of interconnected γ2 further weakens the amalgam, particularly the tensile strength; and *(2)* the mercury liberated by the corrosion process can react with the remaining unreacted γ in the amalgam to produce additional reaction products (γ1 + γ2). The formation of these new reaction products could produce an additional dimensional change (**mercuroscopic expansion**), leading to unsupported amalgam at the margin, which can easily fracture in tension. The entire mechanism has been associated with the phenomenon of amalgam ditching (Fig 12-8), which was prevalent in the clinical use of traditional amalgam. The liberation of mercury as a corrosion by-product of amalgam has created additional concerns from a bicompatibility point of view.

In high-copper amalgams, corrosion associated with γ2 is eliminated or reduced because of the absence or reduction of the γ2 phase; the η′ phase (Cu_6Sn_5) occurrs instead. However, the η′ phase has also proven to be susceptible to corrosion in the oral cavity, with the following reaction:

$$4Cu_6Sn_5 + 19O_2 + 18H_2O + 12Cl^- \rightarrow$$
$$6[CuCl_2 \cdot 3Cu(OH)_2] + 20SnO$$

This reaction will not substantially affect the strength of the high-copper amalgam in the margin because the Cu_6Sn_5 is not an interconnected phase. However, the corrosion of Cu_6Sn_5 has raised questions as to the biocompatibility of the copper-containing corrosion products of high-copper amalgams.

Amalgams that appear to have superior corrosion behavior have been produced by adding less than 1% (by weight) of palladium to a commercial high-copper single-composition amalgam alloy and 5% to an experimental dispersed-phase high-copper amalgam alloy.[13] Palladium may be soluble in γ1, with a resultant improvement in the corrosion behavior of that phase.

Recent studies have also shown that mercury is released during free corrosion of amalgam in vitro in various artificial salivas. Over the short term, this mercury burden was found to be in the range of 4 to 20 μγ/day, or about the same value as the dietary intake; over longer periods, the mercury released from amalgams was considerably lower than dietary intake.[14] The concentration of the dissolved mercury found in such in vitro tests may be unre-

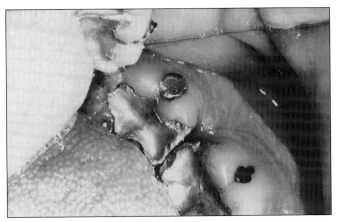

Fig 12-8 Marginal breakdown of traditional amalgam (original magnification ×2.5).

alistically high compared with that found in vivo, because the natural buffering capacity of saliva, along with the attendant organic proteins, may appreciably lower corrosion kinetics. Porosity will have a significant effect on corrosion of both traditional and high-copper amalgams in effecting increases in surface area and surface energies.

Corrosion of gallium amalgams

In vitro corrosion studies have shown that gallium amalgams corrode at rates similar to those of traditional amalgams, with the attendant release of cations of gallium, copper, tin, indium, and silver. This finding is understandable in terms of the high concentrations of β tin present in the matrix. In addition, substantial amounts of gallium were leached out into neutral and acidic saline solutions.[15]

◼ Clinical Performance

The clinical success of amalgam can only be achieved when careful technique is applied to all parts of the restorative process, such as cavity preparation, mixing of the alloy and mercury (trituration), packing of the plastic amalgam mix into the preparation (condensation), and finishing. The most significant factor in amalgam behavior under oral conditions is the choice of amalgam alloy. Estimated median clinical lifetimes vary from 6 years for some of the traditional products to more than 20 years for the best contemporary high-copper systems.

Unfortunately, the long-term clinical function has been documented for only a few of the available commercial

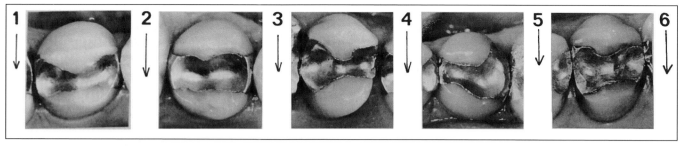

Fig 12-9 Categoric ranking scale for clinical evaluation of marginal breakdown. (Courtesy of H. Letzel and M. M. A. Vrijhoef.)

systems for two reasons: (1) the tradition of clinical research is relatively young, and (2) many of the high-copper systems have only recently been put on the market. However, a comprehensive analysis of laboratory and clinical research studies by Marshall and Marshall[16] supports the long-term performance superiority of high-copper amalgam alloys.

The choice of the alloy is the most prominent factor in marginal deterioration. Marginal deterioration is measured in vivo by comparison of intraoral photographs with a graded scale of marginal failure (Fig 12-9). When treated with appropriate statistics, a quantitative measurement of marginal deterioration may be obtained. These techniques have also allowed for measurement of the kinetics of marginal breakdown (Fig 12-10).

High-copper amalgams tend to give less marginal fracture, although the best traditional systems available might be as good as, or even better than, the least effective high-copper amalgams. The admixing of up to 10% indium by weight did not adversely affect the marginal integrity or luster of a high-copper amalgam.[17] Other factors, such as cavity preparation, application of a cavity varnish, mode of packing, and type of finishing, reportedly may have an influence on marginal fracture in a statistical sense. However, their influence is moderate when compared with the differences due to alloy type.

Several investigators have shown that the risk of marginal fracture increases with increasing cavity size.[18] An investigation of the influence of the cavosurface angle (CSA) on marginal fracture indicated that a CSA of 90 degrees produced slightly less marginal fracture than a CSA of less than 90 degrees,[19] which is consistent with published theoretic considerations.[20] Finishing the margins with tungsten carbide burs or chisels did not have any detectable influence; however, amalgam restorations with an applied layer of cavity varnish have been shown to have slightly more marginal fracture than those without it.[21] It has also been shown that from the standpoint of marginal fracture, careful application of cotton rolls in combination with vacuum ejection was equivalent to restorations made using rubber dam.[22] Similarly, different modes of packing or condensing (hand versus four distinct commercial mechanically and air-driven vibrators) did not reveal any marginal deterioration differences.[23]

Commercial amalgamators are available for the mechanical trituration of the alloy and mercury (Fig 12-11). In the case of modern high-copper amalgams, different types of postcarving **burnishing** produce some differences in marginal fracture compared with the traditional polishing methods (carried out after 1 day). These differences are smaller than those between the distinct amalgam systems that are available commercially.[24]

Thus, the differences in marginal fracture due to operative variables are small compared with differences between amalgam systems and patients. The clinician may, therefore, seem to have only a small influence on the results of clinical reports found in the literature. However, caution must also be taken in extrapolating clinical literature results to the general practice situation, because neither the clinicians nor the patients in these published studies may be representative. In this regard, cross-sectional clinical performance data from general practices show a dramatic reduction in lifetimes as compared with controlled clinical trials in academic centers.[25] It is thus necessary to realize that the manufacturer makes the amalgam alloy, but the clinician makes the amalgam restoration. It is of ultimate importance to control the clinician factor, as well as the patient factor, in a general practice situation.

Clinical behavior of gallium amalgams

Changes in marginal integrity, surface texture, luster, and color were measured clinically over periods of up to 2 years by several Japanese clinical studies (eg, Sakai et al[26]).

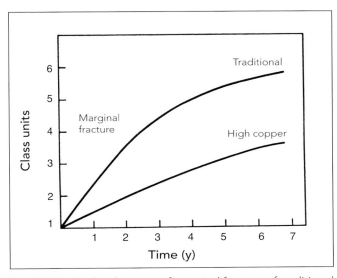

Fig 12-10 Idealized version of marginal fracture of traditional and high-copper amalgams as a function of time.

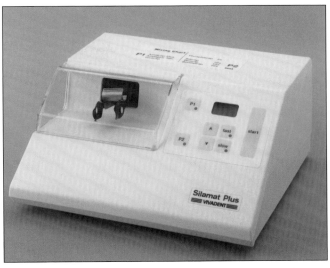

Fig 12-11 A programmable amalgamator available for the mechanical trituration of the alloy and mercury. (Courtesy of Ivoclar Vivadent.)

It was found that significant changes in luster and surface roughness occur within periods as early as 4 months after placement, with more severe occlusal changes than buccal changes. In light of the significant corrosion behavior associated with the presence of free tin and the selective attack of gallium in the current commercial formulation, this finding is probably not too surprising.

Correlations Between Laboratory Properties and Clinical Data

Creep

In 1970, the correlation between creep and the susceptibility of both traditional and high-copper amalgam restorations to marginal fracture was reported, with a higher creep corresponding to more marginal breakdown.[4] This correlation was subsequently verified in a large number of published studies. It still attracts attention among researchers and in product advertisements. Frequently, statements can be found in contemporary literature expressing, either explicitly or implicitly, that a low-creep amalgam would solve the marginal fracture problem. This statement is not necessarily true, however. Several investigators have shown that there is no correlation between creep and marginal deterioration for the $\gamma 2$-free amalgams. However, there are indications of a posi-

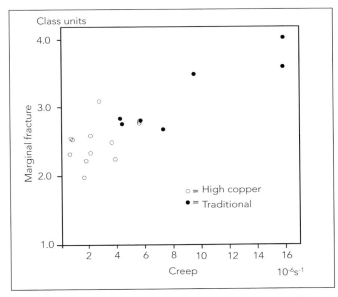

Fig 12-12 Correlation of marginal fracture and creep for traditional and high-copper amalgams. (Adapted with permission from Vrijhoef and Letzel.[27])

tive correlation between creep and marginal fracture for the group of traditional amalgams containing $\gamma 2$ (Fig 12-12). Enough clinical and laboratory studies support this correlation to stress that caution is required not to overestimate creep as a selection criterion for the prediction of marginal fracture. General practitioners should not buy their alloy on the basis of creep data alone but rather as

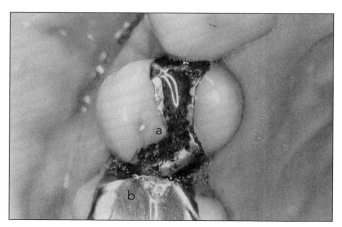

Fig 12-13 Corroding amalgam (a) in interproximal contact with gold casting alloy (b).

part of a complete picture in which clinical evidence from a controlled clinical study plays a substantial role.

Creep will also be affected by porosity. An increase in creep of 30% for a 1% increase in porosity was noted for traditional amalgams.

Corrosion

A well-known and frequently recognized phenomenon in the early life of an amalgam restoration is the "galvanic pain" caused by the **galvanic action** of amalgam restorations in combination with other metallic restorations in interproximal or occlusal contact (Fig 12-13). Clinical studies have found that this type of pain occurred only in a small percentage of cases and was generally not serious; it usually occurred in the first hours and in no instance did it last longer than a few weeks after the placement of the material. It is also possible that the galvanic currents produced could have a harmful effect on the soft tissues or on the organism as a whole; however, the frequency of the occurrence of these effects is supposed to be low or absent.

Galvanic corrosion can adversely affect both the amalgam and the dissimilar metal in contact with it. For example, if the amalgam is in interproximal contact with a gold restoration, the amalgam will corrode as the anode. The surface wear will cause it to lose luster and become rough. Mercury, when produced as a corrosion product, will amalgamate with the gold alloy, producing a color change as well as an embrittling effect.

Galvanic effects with dissimilar metals in occlusion are often greater, because occlusal forces at points of contact are usually great enough to rupture protective films of corrosion products that would form in the absence of contact. Thus, mixed metals in contact, either permanent or intermittent, should be avoided in clinical practice.

The loss of luster and the discoloration of the restoration's surface, the first indications of surface deterioration of the amalgam restoration and the bulk of material underneath, have been the subject of many clinical studies. A rough restoration surface is prone to the formation of plaque and can cause irritation to adjacent soft tissues. The aggressive attack of the oral environment on amalgam is primarily due to the chloride ions in saliva. In addition, the silver in amalgam can tarnish because of the action of sulfide ions. This damage is confined to the surface layers and can easily be removed by polishing. Further, the sulfide ion concentration is controlled by such factors as the patient's diet and health.

The corrosion products at the cavosurface margin are phosphates, whereas the corrosion products seen within the bulk of the restoration are oxides and hydroxychlorides. Corrosion products may have a positive effect. If these products precipitate in the space between the cavity wall and the restoration (Fig 12-14), less saliva can penetrate it, and percolation may be minimized. Sealing of the cavosurface margin takes place within the first several days. Both traditional and high-copper amalgams display this effect.

Sensitivity and amalgam bonding

Clinical experiences indicate that many of the modern high-copper spheric amalgams produce more postoperative sensitivity than other systems. It is speculated that these materials, which universally contract on setting, produce large gaps at the cavosurface margins that cannot be sealed by the resulting formation of corrosion products. In addition, the dynamic dimensional changes produced by thermal and mechanical stresses to the margin may potentiate this phenomenon. Obviously, an open margin is a preferred pathway for bacterial invasion. For these reasons, the sealing of amalgam cavity walls with a dentin adhesive or glass ionomer has become popular. Traditional dentin adhesives, newer amalgam/dentin adhesives, and hybrid glass ionomers have all shown the ability to reduce leakage and, in some cases, reduce caries when used under amalgams.[28,29] The bond strength of these products ranges from a few MPa for traditional dentin adhesives and ionomers to 10 MPa for newer products. Choice should not be based solely on

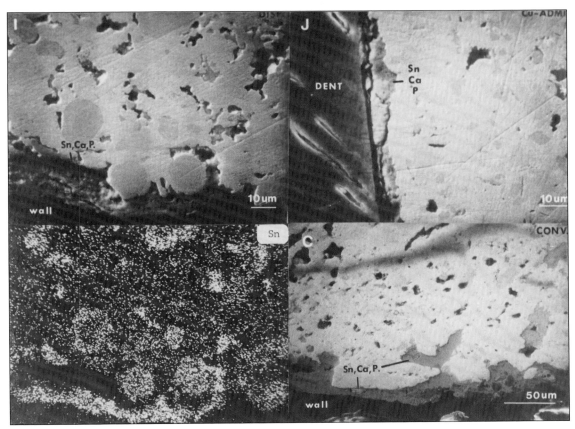

Fig 12-14 Scanning electron micrographs of Dispersalloy, high-copper admixed, and conventional amalgams, that have been retrieved from failed clinical restorations. Note buildup of tin, calcium, and phosphorous corrosion products at the cavodentinal wall. (Reprinted with permission from Marshal et al.[8])

strength values, however, because some of the products that are lower in strength have been more effective in sealing the margin.[30]

Biocompatibility

The contribution of mercury to the environmental burden of dental amalgam is of great concern. A report submitted to the US Public Health Service (USPHS) summarizes the risk-to-benefit ratio involved in amalgam usage.[31] From a risk standpoint, there is no doubt that the presence of amalgams will increase mercury levels in blood, urine, and tissue. The level of increase, however, is currently thought to be below that associated with clinical symptoms. Table 12-4, adapted from the USPHS report, summarizes what is currently known about mercury uptake from a wide variety of sources and includes, as benchmarks, the World Health Organization (WHO) total

mercury uptake and the Occupational Safety and Health Administration (OSHA) workplace limit. Values for mercury intake from amalgam are around one-half to one-tenth of these levels. Mercury uptake from amalgam is similar to that absorbed from food associated with normal saliva.

Biologic testing procedures have revealed some interaction within cell cultures that has been associated either with unreacted mercury or with copper leached out during corrosion of high-copper amalgam systems. Implantation studies have demonstrated that traditional and high-copper amalgams are well tolerated by connective tissue and bone.

Inflammatory reactions and formation of secondary dentin have been noted, but proper use of lining materials in deep cavities should minimize possible pulpal and dentinal reactions.

Amalgam may also produce gingival reaction due to corrosion or to "tattoos" caused by the accidental sub-

Table 12-4 Estimated absorption of mercury[31]

SOURCE	TYPE	ABSORPTION (NG/D)
WHO	Total	43,000
OSHA (air workplace)	Elemental	429,000
Amalgam	Elemental	1,240–29,000
Water	Inorganic	5
Food	Organic + organic	2,220–5,572
Saliva	Inorganic	180–1,400
Air (home)	Elemental	4,160
Air (ambient)	Elemental	32–96

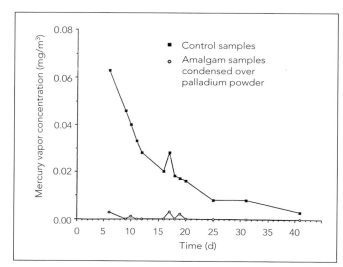

Fig 12-15 Reduction of mercury vapor released from amalgam samples (Tytin) into bottle by condensation over palladium powder, compared with control. (Reprinted with permission from O'Brien.[33])

gingival condensation of amalgam. The use of amalgams with superior corrosion resistance is indicated to minimize these effects.

Under normal service conditions, amalgam restorations are covered by a film of saliva that reduces the vapor pressure and reroutes the mercury from the respiratory tract to the esophageal tract, which has a greater tolerance to mercury.

Elevated serum mercury levels have been identified in populations of dental practitioners after 20 years of clinical practice. However, these levels were far below those producing clinical toxicity, and the practitioners were symptom free.

Recent research has found that the greatest amount of mercury vapor released from amalgam is during setting, which probably accounts for increased mercury levels in urine after the placement of restorations.[32] The presence of palladium during setting greatly reduces the amount of mercury vapor released (Fig 12-15). Palladium has the strongest bond with mercury of any of the transition metals of the periodic table and reduces the mercury vapor pressure of the amalgam.

The US Food and Drug Administration held a public meeting of its Panel on Dental Products in September 2006[34] to review a literature search on the health safety of dental amalgam. Several findings supported the relative safety of using dental amalgam, but there was a lack of data regarding children, pregnant women, and other vulnerable groups. The data presented indicated that dental amalgam restorations do release mercury vapor, but the daily amount released in a patient with seven amalgam fillings is about 1 γ compared with 5 to 6 γ from food and water sources. Data further indicated that the use of amalgam fillings has dropped from 66% to about 30% in the past 15 years, with composite materials serving as replacement.

None of the data presented supported a link between amalgam restorations and the incidence of systemic medical conditions as claimed by anti-amalgam consumer groups who participated in the public phases of the meeting. The panel voted that more studies in more diverse populations were needed to come to any conclusions about the health safety of dental amalgams.

■ Clinical Decision Scenarios for Dental Amalgams

This section presents one approach for choosing dental cements for specific situations. Each of the following scenarios uses the same format as that presented in chapter 7. Advantages and disadvantages of each material are prioritized using the following codes: • of minor importance, •• important, and ••• very important.

Materials Glass ionomer vs amalgam for cores

Situation A patient comes to the office complaining of a broken tooth. On examination the clinician finds that the lingual cusps of the mandibular right first molar have fractured right at the gum line. The tooth already has a large mesio-occlusodistal amalgam in it, and the facial cusps are not sturdy. The treatment plan is to prepare a pin-retained core buildup and then a full gold crown. The clinician has both amalgam and a glass-ionomer core material available.

Critical Factor Strength

AMALGAM	GLASS IONOMER
ADVANTAGES	ADVANTAGES
••• High strength • Long clinical history • Bonds to tooth	• Immediate set Fluoride release
DISADVANTAGES	DISADVANTAGES
• 24-hour set • No fluoride release • No bond to tooth	••• Low strength

Analysis/Decision Despite the advantages for the glass ionomer, its low strength makes it unsuitable for a full buildup, so the amalgam was selected. Glass ionomers have been advertised for this use, but time has shown that they do not hold up well if they are the entire support for the crown. Glass ionomers are useful for filling in small depressions in the preparation but not for the complete core.

◼ Glossary

admixed alloy An amalgam alloy containing particles of different composition, that is, silver-tin particles and silver-copper particles.

alloy for dental amalgam A silver-tin alloy containing other metals, usually copper and zinc, that will be mixed with mercury to form dental amalgam.

amalgamation Reaction that occurs between mercury and an amalgam alloy.

beta (β) tin An allotropic form of tin.

biocompatibility The ability of a material to provide successful service in a host while causing minimal response.

blended alloy An alloy containing both spheric and lathe-cut particles.

burnishing Smoothing the surface of a dental amalgam after initial carving by rubbing it with a metal instrument having a broad surface.

condensation Packing dental amalgam into a prepared cavity.

corrosion Degradation due to the electrochemical process.

creep Permanent (plastic) deformation under constant load after the material has set.

delta 2 (δ2) phase A tin-mercury compound that is a reaction product in dental amalgam.

dental amalgam An alloy that results when mercury is combined with a silver alloy; initially a plastic mass that hardens after placement in a prepared cavity.

epsilon (ε) phase A copper-tin compound (Cu_3Sn) that occurs in particles in traditional alloys.

Materials Amalgam vs glass ionomer for crown margin repair in patient with low caries risk

Situation A patient with several all-ceramic crowns comes to the office for a checkup. He has had the crowns for about 15 years, and gingival recession has resulted in supragingival margins around these crowns. His oral hygiene is good, but a small caries lesion can be seen on the buccal margin of the crown on his mandibular right first molar. A new crown could be made, but the patient does not want to pay for it. The clinician decides to place a small repair restoration on the margin after removal of the caries lesion. She compares amalgam and glass-ionomer restorative material.

Critical Factors Low cost, durability of restoration, ease of placement

AMALGAM	GLASS IONOMER
ADVANTAGES	ADVANTAGES
••• Easy to place ••• Excellent durability ••• Low cost Long history of success	••• Resonably easy to place Tooth colored ••• Low cost • Fluoride release •• Bonds to tooth
DISADVANTAGES	DISADVANTAGES
Not tooth colored • No fluoride release • Difficult interproximal placement •• No bond to tooth	••• Less durable • More plaque retentive ••• Isolation is critical

Analysis/Decision The durability and ease of placement of amalgam, combined with its low cost, made it the best choice for this restoration. The access was easy, and the patient was not too concerned with the appearance of the repair. The patient's low risk for caries was also significant in making the decision.

eta prime (η') phase A copper-tin compound (Cu_6Sn_5) that is a reaction product in dental amalgam.

eutectic composition An alloy or solution whose components are proportioned so the melting point is the lowest possible for those components. On cooling, the single liquid phase is transformed into two or more solid phases, the number of solid phases being equal to the number of components.

flow Permanent (plastic) deformation that occurs while the material is setting and in the process of developing its final strength.

gallium alloy A product formed by the reaction of an alloy powder (silver-tin-copper) with a gallium-based liquid alloy (gallium-indium-tin).

galvanic action Electric potentials in the mouth caused by the contact of dissimilar metals in interproximal or occlusal contact.

gamma (γ) phase A silver-tin compound (Ag_3Sn) that forms a substantial part of the amalgam alloy and is also present in the resulting amalgam structure after reaction with mercury has occurred.

gamma 1 (γ_1) phase A silver-mercury compound (Ag_2Hg_3) that is a reaction product in dental amalgam.

gamma 2 (γ_2) phase A tin-mercury compound (Sn_7Hg) that is a reaction product in dental amalgam.

high-copper amalgam Dental amalgam alloy with a relatively high copper content (10% by weight). This alloy is characterized by the corrosion-prone $\gamma 2$ phase being either absent or substantially reduced.

Materials Amalgam vs glass ionomer for repair of a proximal margin on a metal crown in patient with high caries risk

Situation The same patient as in the previous scenario returns to the same clinician 6 years later for a dental hygiene appointment. He is now 72 years old and is starting to show the signs of advancing age. He is more frail, forgetful, and is taking medication for high cholesterol, which has a side effect of slight xerostomia (reduced saliva output). The result of these new circumstances is a lowered hygiene level. There is quite a bit of plaque buildup interproximally, and several all-ceramic crowns show small areas of decay around the margins. Cost remains a problem.

Critical Factors Caries resistance, low cost

AMALGAM	GLASS IONOMER
ADVANTAGES	ADVANTAGES
•• Easy to place •• Excellent durability ••• Low cost •• Long history of success	•• Resonably easy to place •• Tooth colored ••• Low cost ••• Fluoride release Bonds to tooth
DISADVANTAGES	DISADVANTAGES
•• Not tooth colored ••• No fluoride release •• Difficult interproximal placement No bond to tooth	•• Less durable •• More plaque retentive Isolation is critical

Analysis/Decision This time the clinician chose the glass-ionomer material because it is capable of preventing recurrent decay due to its reliable and high fluoride release. New crowns are not feasible because of the patient's poor financial situation and insurance, which would pay a small fraction of the total cost. The clinician explained to the patient the need for supplementation with artificial saliva and the possible need to replace the restorations every 3 years because of erosion.

ingot Cast rod of alloy.

lathe-cut alloy Amalgam alloy made by machining small, irregularly shaped chips from a large cast bar of alloy.

mercuroscopic expansion The expansion that occurs when mercury, released by the corrosion of the $\gamma 2$ phase, reacts with the remaining amalgam alloy particles, producing an unsupported wedge at the margin of the restoration.

mercury-alloy ratio The ratio of the amount of mercury to be mixed with an amount of amalgam alloy.

quaternary alloy An alloy containing four elements.

single-composition alloy Each alloy particle contains the same components in the same ratios.

spheric alloy An alloy whose particles are created by means of an atomization process whereby a spray of tiny drops is allowed to solidify in an inert gaseous or liquid environment.

ternary alloy An alloy containing three elements.

traditional (or conventional) alloys An alloy with the following composition: 66% to 73% silver by weight, 25% to 29% tin by weight, 2% to 6% copper by weight, 0% to 2% zinc by weight, and 0% to 3% mercury by weight.

trituration Mixing dental amalgam alloy with mercury.

■ Discussion Questions

1. Are dental amalgams a health hazard?

2. Why is dental amalgam so popular, even though it is not esthetic?

3. What are the advantages and disadvantages of using a bonding agent with amalgam restorations?

4. How does copper affect the set microstructure of amalgam?

■ Study Questions

(See appendix E for answers.)

1. How can the working time of amalgam be controlled?

2. Should a zinc-free amalgam be used?

3. Can some amalgams be finished the same day they are placed?

4. Why are spheric amalgams difficult to condense?

5. Does creep predict marginal fracture?

6. Why are seal/bond amalgam restorations of particular interest?

7. How safe are amalgams?

■ References

1. Black GV. An investigation of the physical characters of the human teeth in relation to their diseases, and to practical dental operations, together with the physical characters of filling materials. III. Filling materials. Dent Cosmos 1895;37:553–571.

2. Gruber R, Skinner EW, Greener EH. Some physical properties of silver-tin amalgams. J Dent Res 1967;46:497.

3. Innes DBK, Youdelis WV. Dispersion strengthened amalgams. J Can Dent Assoc 1963;29:587–593.

4. Mahler DB, Terkla LG, Van Eysden J, Reisbick MH. Marginal fracture versus mechanical properties of amalgam. J Dent Res 1970;49:1452–1457.

5. Sato A, Kumei Y. New selenium-containing silver amalgam. Bull Tokyo Med Dent Univ 1982;29:19.

6. Powell LV, Johnson GH, Bales DJ. Effect of admixed indium on mercury vapor release from dental amalgam. J Dent Res 1989;68:1231–1233.

7. Youdelis W. Amalgam as restorative material: Is there anything new? J Esthet Dent 1992;4:61–63.

8. Marshall GW, Jackson BL, Marshall SJ. Copper rich and conventional amalgam restorations after clinical use. J Am Dent Assoc 1980;100:43–47.

9. Averette DF, Hochman RF, Marek M. The effects of corrosion in vitro on the structure and properties of dental amalgam. J Dent Res 1978;57(spec issue A):165.

10. Sarkar NK. Intergranular structure in dental amalgams. J Mat Sci (Mater Med) 1994;5:171–175.

11. Okabe T, Yamashita T, Nakajima H, Berglund A, Zhao L, Ferracane JL. Mercury release from amalgams prepared with binary Hg-In liquid alloys [abstract 27]. J Dent Res 1994;73(special issue):105.

12. Okabe T, Mitchell R, Wright AH, Fairhurst CW. Amalgamation reaction on high copper single composition alloys. J Dent Res 1977;56(spec issue A):79.

13. Greener EH, Szurgot K. Properties of Ag-Cu-Pd dispersed phase amalgam. J Dent Res 1982;61:1192–1194.

14. Brune D. Metal release from dental biomaterials. Biomater 1986;7:163–175.

15. Herø H, Jørgensen RB. Corrosion of gallium alloys [abstract B-23]. Trans Acad Dent Mater. 1993;6:327.

16. Marshall SJ, Marshall GW Jr. Dental amalgam: The materials. Adv Dent Res 1992;6:94–99.

17. Johnson GH, Bales DJ, Powell LV. Effect of admixed indium on the clinical success of amalgam restorations. Oper Dent 1992;17:196–202.

18. Mahler DB, Marantz RL. Marginal fracture of amalgam: Effect of type of tooth and restorations. J Dent Res 1980;59:1497–1500.

19. Akerboom HBM. Amalgamrestauraties nader bekeken. De caviteitspreparatie [thesis]. Amsterdam: Free Univ, 1985.

20. Jørgensen KD. The mechanism of marginal fracture of amalgam fillings. Acta Odontol Scand 1965;23:347–389.

21. Borgmeijer PJ. Amalgamrestauraties nader bekeken. De caviteits behandeling [thesis]. Amsterdam: Free Univ, 1985.

22. Letzel H, Fick JM, Aardening CJMW, Van Leusen J, Vrijhoef MMA. Influence of rubber dam use on clinical behavior of amalgam restorations. J Dent Res 1979;58:180.

23. Letzel H, Vrijhoef MMA. Condensation methods vs. the clinical behavior of amalgam restorations. J Dent Res 1982;61:567.

24. Letzel H, Vrijhoef MMA. The influence of polishing on the marginal integrity of amalgam restorations. J Oral Rehabil 1984;11:89–94.

25. Letzel H, Van Hof MA, Vrijhoef MMA, Marshall GW, Marshall SJ. Failure, survival and reasons for replacement of amalgam restorations. In: Anusavice KJ (ed). Quality Evaluation of Dental Restorations. Chicago: Quintessence, 1989:83–92.

26. Sakai T, Kaga M, Oguchi H. Two-year clinical observation of gallium alloy in pediatric patients [abstract P-053]. Trans Acad Dent Mat 1993;6:327.

27. Vrijhoef MMA, Letzel H. Creep versus marginal fracture of amalgam restorations. J Oral Rehabil 1986;13:299–303.

28. Pashley EL, Comer RW, Parry EE, Pashley DH. Amalgam buildups: Shear strength and dentin sealing properties. Oper Dent 1991:16:82–89.

29. Manders CA, Garcia-Godoy F, Barnwell GM. Effect of copal varnish, ZOE or glass ionomer cement bases on the microleakage of amalgam restorations. Am J Dent 1990;3:63–66.

30. Clinical Research Associates. Clin Res Associates Newsletter 1994;18(2):3.

31. United States Public Health Service. Dental Amalgams: A Scientific Review and Recommended Public Health Strategy for Research, Education and Regulation. Final Report of the Subcommittee on Risk Management of the Committee to Coordinate Environmental Health and Related Programs. January 1993.

32. Frykholm KO. On mercury from dental amalgam. Acta Odont Scand 1957;15:(suppl 22):7–108.

33. O'Brien WJ, inventor. Method and composition for removing mercury vapor from dental restorations. US patent 5242305. 1993

34. US Food and Drug Administration Dental Products Panel. Transcript and Meeting Minutes, September 6 and 7, 2006. Available at http://www.fda.gov/ohrms/dockets/ac/cdrh06.html. Accessed 16 April 2008.

■ Recommended Reading

Langan DC, Fan PL, Hoos AA. The use of mercury in dentistry: A critical review of the recent literature. J Am Dent Assoc 1987;115:867–880.

Neme AM, Wagner WC, O'Brien WJ. Effects of palladium addition on emission of mercury vapor from dental amalgam. Dent Mater 1999;15:382–389.

Parker-Pope T. Mercury in fillings—Are they a problem? Wall Street Journal September 17, 2006.

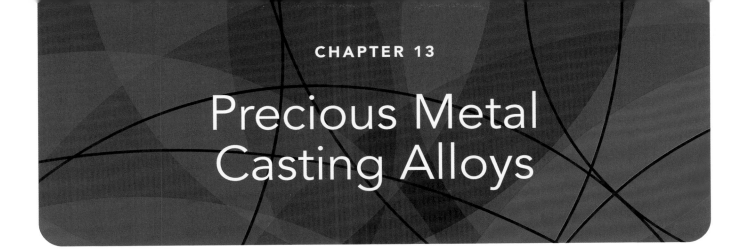

Precious Metal Casting Alloys

Since the introduction of investment casting to dentistry by Taggart in 1907, precious metal alloys have traditionally been used for several types of restorations. High-gold alloys are still used for inlays because soft alloys that can be burnished are desirable. Full-cast crowns and three-quarter crowns are still cast from gold alloys as well. However, most crowns and fixed partial dentures for the anterior part of the mouth are of the porcelain-fused-to-metal (PFM) type. Alloys for PFM fixed partial dentures have revolutionized this field and include palladium and nickel alloys, as well as high-gold alloys. Another change has been the introduction of lower-gold alloys to replace the traditional 18-carat American Dental Association (ADA)–certified alloys developed during the 1930s. The tarnish resistance of these lower-gold-content alloys is sufficient for some oral environments but not for others.

■ Composition and Properties

Precious metal casting alloys contain mainly gold, palladium, platinum, and silver, which are classified as **noble metals**. They also contain limited amounts of non-precious alloying elements such as copper, indium, iron, tin, and zinc (Table 13-1). The **carat** scale expresses the relative amount of gold in an alloy, with 24 carat being pure gold. Twelve- and 18-carat alloys contain 50% and 75% gold, respectively. The **fineness** of a gold alloy is the percentage of gold content multiplied by a factor of 10 (eg, 75% is 750 fine). Fineness is used with dental gold solders, but the carat scale is seldom used in dentistry. Copper, silver, palladium, and platinum generally serve

as hardening elements in alloys with high gold content. Iron and tin, at much lower concentrations, are hardening additions in PFM alloys. Indium, iron, and tin also serve to promote bonding of porcelain to PFM alloys by formation of stable, adherent oxides.

High-gold alloys

Traditional dental casting alloys contain 70% by weight or more of gold, palladium, and platinum, and they are categorized in accordance with their Vickers hardness number (VHN). The *Vickers hardness test*, or the *136-degree diamond pyramid hardness test*, is a microindentation method in which the indenter produces a square indentation, the diagonals of which are measured. The diamond pyramid hardness is calculated by dividing the applied load by the surface area of the indentation.

The American National Standards Institute/American Dental Association (ANSI/ADA) specification[2] divides these alloys into four types based on mechanical properties:

Type I—Soft (VHN 60 to 90)
Type II—Medium (VHN 90 to 120)
Type III—Hard (VHN 120 to 150)
Type IV—Extra hard (quenched VHN minimum 150; hardened VHN minimum 220)

Table 13-2 identifies currently available alloys and their mechanical properties.

Type I alloys are weak, soft, highly ductile, and do not harden by heat treatment. They are useful only in areas not subject to occlusal stress and thus are not widely used. Type IV alloys are relatively strong, hard, and non-

Table 13-1 Role of alloying elements in dental gold alloys[1]

PROPERTY	GOLD	PLATINUM	PALLADIUM	COPPER	SILVER	ZINC	IRIDIUM
Specific gravity	19.32	21.45	12.0	8.96	10.49	7.31	22.4
Melting point in °C (°F)	1,063 (1,945)	1,769 (3,224)	1,552 (2,829)	1,083 (1,981)	961 (1,761)	420 (787)	2,443 (4,429)
Atomic diameter (Å)	2.88	2.77	2.74	2.55	2.88	2.66	3.32
Space lattice	Face-centered cubic	Face-centered cubic	Face-centered cubic	Face-centered cubic	Face-centered cubic	Close-packed hexagonal	Face-centered cubic
Chemical activity	Inert	Inert	Mild	Very active	Active	Very active	Active
Color	Yellow	White	White	Red	White	White	White
Approximate content	50%–95%	0%–20%	0%–12%	0%–17%	0%–20%	0%–2%	0.005%–0.1%
Density (specific gravity)	Increases markedly	Increases markedly	Lowers slightly	Lowers	Lowers	Lowers	Increases slightly
Effect of color on alloy	Lends yellow color	Whitens slowly; 12% required; not pure white	Whitens rapidly; as little as 5%	Lends red color; dark plate high in Cu	Whitens very slowly, counteracts redness of Cu; creates green gold	Percentages too low to have effect	White
Melting	Raises melting point mildly	Raises melting point fairly rapidly	Raises melting point rapidly	Lowers melting point even below its own	Slight effect; may raise or sometimes lower mildly	Lowers melting point rapidly; in most solders	No effect
Tarnish resistance	Essential to good tarnish resistance	Contributes importantly to tarnish resistance	Increases tarnish resistance but less than Au and Pt	Contributes to tarnish in flame or with sulfurous food	Tarnishes in presence of sulfur	Will tarnish, but in low percentage has little effect	Increased
Heat hardening	Contributes importantly with Cu	Increases with Cu	Some increase with Cu	Essential if alloy heat hardens	Increases with Cu	Slight with Cu	No effect
Gas absorption	—	—	Rather high for hydrogen	—	Rather high for oxygen	A good deoxidizer	No effect
Castability	—	—	(Effects not critical)	(Effects not critical)	—	Decreases surface tension and increases fluidity	No effect

Table 13-2 Composition and properties of precious metal alloys

TYPE	APPROXIMATE COMPOSITION (%)				VHN		YIELD STRENGTH PSI (MPa)		DUCTILITY (% ELONGATION)
	Au	Pt	Pd	Ag	AS CAST	HARDENED	QUENCHED	HARDENED	
I. Soft: one- and two-surface inlays	82	—	2	12	85	—	20,000 (140)	—	45
II. Medium: inlays, MOD, crowns	77	—	2	12	120	145	33,000 (225)	42,000 (290)	43
III. Hard: inlays, crowns, fixed partial dentures	73	2	2	12	130	200	37,000 (255)	50,000 (345)	40
	60	—	4	25	140	240	56,000 (385)	100,000 (690)	20
IV. Extra-hard: thin crowns, fixed partial dentures, removable partial dentures	63	0	4	17	220	280	105,000 (725)	115,000 (790)	12
	71	6	—	12	245	270	70,000 (480)	110,000 (760)	9
	63	1	4	20	240	300	100,000 (690)	120,000 (825)	10

ductile. They are intended for high-stress applications such as partial dentures. These alloys also are not widely used.

The intermediate type II and type III alloys are used for most restorations. Type II alloys are used for inlays in which **burnishability** of margins is more important than high strength. Type III alloys are used in higher-stress applications for inlays, onlays, and three-quarter crowns, and for fixed partial denture (FPD) retainers and pontics where the restoration design makes burnishability less important than strength.

Typical composition ranges for high-gold alloys are shown in Table 13-2. Iridium in small amounts, around 0.1%, is added as a grain refiner by several manufacturers. Type III and type IV alloys may contain a high percentage of both palladium and platinum as hardening elements, as shown in the table, while retaining a light gold color. Type III and type IV alloys are susceptible to heat treatment and may be hardened or softened by appropriate heating cycles. Alloys containing more than 6% palladium are normally white (silver colored).

Typical composition ranges of these alloys are presented in Table 13-2. They are hard, strong, and heat treatable and have mechanical properties characteristic of type III and type IV alloys.

Low-gold alloys

The main incentive for the use of these alloys is financial; when the price of gold increases, the use of low-gold alloys increases relative to that of high-gold alloys. Low-gold alloys are composed mainly of gold, silver, and copper, with a small percentage of palladium. Gold content ranges from 45% to 60%.

Few alloys are marketed with gold contents between 55% and 70% because the cost savings are not high enough, and few alloys contain less than 45% gold because of **tarnish** and **corrosion** problems with use. Alloys in this group may contain additional palladium to partially make up for the low gold content (Table 13-2).

The mechanical properties of the low-gold alloys generally correspond to the properties of ANSI/ADA type III alloys. Thus, the alloys are strong and hard and have only moderate ductility.

Low-gold alloys are rarely used for inlays but can be suitable for full-cast crowns.

Palladium-silver alloys

Alloys with palladium as their main ingredient have several applications. Palladium-silver alloys provide mechanical properties similar to those of type III gold alloys. A greater silver content increases the ductility and lowers the hardness, but it increases corrosion problems. These alloys are more commonly used for crowns than for inlays. Unless other alloying elements are added, these materials are not heat treatable, because they form a continuous solid solution at all compositions (Fig 13-1).

High-palladium alloys contain a small percentage of other precious metals. They have been used as PFM alloys, but the formation of silver oxide and volatilization of

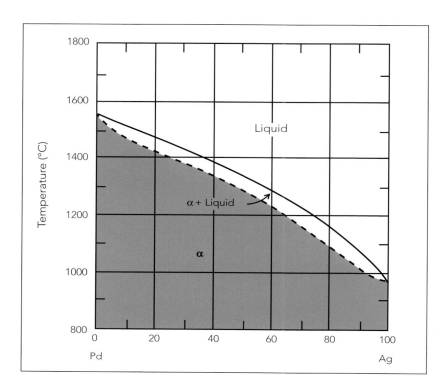

Fig 13-1 Palladium-silver phase diagram. Below about 900°C, a solid solution (α) is formed at all compositions in the solid state.

the silver with these alloys has caused discoloration of the porcelain.

PFM alloys

Alloys that are used as bases for porcelain need to develop and maintain strength at the required temperature, to provide a firm bond to the applied porcelain, to be able to cast thin sections, and to have high yield strength. Three groups of precious alloys are used for PFM application:

Type I—Alloys containing over 90% gold, platinum, and palladium, with small amounts of iron, indium, and tin as hardening and bonding agents

Type II—Alloys containing approximately 80% gold, platinum, and palladium, with trace additions of iron, indium, tin, and silver making up the balance

Type III—Palladium-silver alloys

PFM alloys are the most widely used alloys in commercial laboratories, constituting approximately 70% of all cast units currently in use. Precious PFM alloys are now in direct competition with nonprecious PFM alloys.

The ability to produce good casting precision in cross sections, high yield strength, controlled thermal expansion, and suitable surface characteristics for bonding to

dental porcelain are properties that make PFM alloys desirable. Burnishability is a secondary consideration.

Normally, bonding involves the use of a precious metal alloy containing small quantities of iron, indium, and tin. Controlled oxidation of the castings during a "degassing heat treatment" produces an oxide coating on the alloy surface to which the porcelain adheres.

The properties of PFM alloys are improved by heat treatment. A precipitation reaction during the porcelain firing procedure strengthens and hardens the alloys. Iron-platinum and gold-tin phases are common precipitates.

The high-precious-metal alloys are still widely used. Nickel-chromium and other base metal alloys also used for PFM applications are, in general, less desirable because of problems with casting accuracy, fit, finishing, and porcelain bonding.

■ Heat Treatment

Except for type I and type II high-gold alloys, precious metal casting alloys respond to heat treatment by changes in properties and microstructure.

Homogenizing (softening) **heat treatment** consists of heating the alloy to a temperature approximately 75°C below the solidus temperature, holding at that tempera-

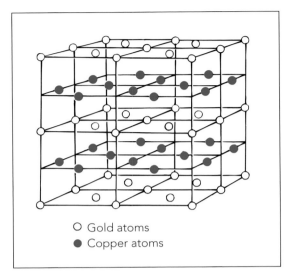

Fig 13-2 Lattice arrangement in an ordered gold-copper alloy with a regular alternation of unlike atoms in layers.

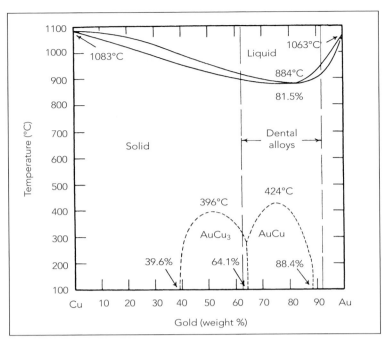

Fig 13-3 Gold-copper phase diagram. The ordered phases $AuCu_3$ and $AuCu$ may be formed by heat treatment. The formation of these phases results in hardening. Quenching from 700°C avoids their formation and hardening.

ture for 10 to 30 minutes, and then quenching to room temperature. Hardening can be produced by one of two methods: slow cooling or a constant-temperature heat treatment. In either case, the important factor is the time spent in a critical temperature range between the softening range and room temperature. This critical temperature varies among alloys; it generally lies about halfway between room temperature and the alloy's softening temperature. Typical cycles for a type III high-gold alloy are as follows: The softening treatment consists of holding the alloy at 700°C to 750°C for 10 minutes, followed by quenching to room temperature. The hardening treatment consists of 10 minutes at 350°C to 400°C, followed by quenching or low cooling to room temperature.

High-fusing alloys may require more time as well as higher temperatures for both softening and hardening heat treatments.

Basic Crystal Structure

All precious metal casting alloys are based on metallic elements having face-centered cubic crystal structures.

With the appropriate homogenizing heat treatment, most of them can be converted to a single phase. Hardening heat treatment results in **precipitation** of phases with other crystal structures, and hardening alloys may contain several different phases. A rearrangement of atoms within the unit cells of the crystal structure, called **ordering**, can occur in many alloys, resulting in a characteristic microstructure. This mechanism is important in the hardening of binary gold-copper alloys but is of secondary importance in dental alloys (Figs 13-2 and 13-3).

Cast Microstructure

The cooling and nucleation rates are high for most dental castings. Thus, the typical cast structure consists of fine uniform **grains**. Large-grain structures are found more often with PFM white alloys unless a **grain refiner** (eg, iridium) is used (Figs 13-4 and 13-5). Single-phase structures are usually found in alloys that have received a thorough softening (homogenizing) heat treatment. Hardening produces the appearance of a discontinuous grain boundary precipitate. However, at a submicro-

199

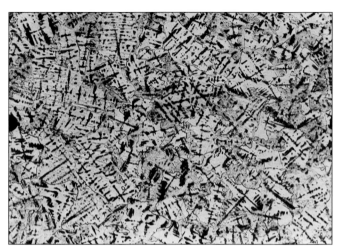

Fig 13-4 Dendritic (skeleton- or needle-shaped) grain structure of precious metal alloy as cast (original magnification ×100).

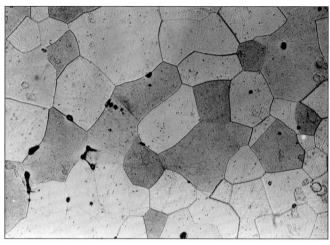

Fig 13-5 Normal grain structure of cast gold alloy after softening heat treatment (original magnification ×100).

scopic level, hardening causes a continuous precipitate throughout the grains due to the separation of silver-rich and copper-rich gold alloy phases. Alloys that undergo ordering during hardening exhibit changes in microstructure.

◖ Glossary

burnishability Ability of a metal to undergo surface deformation (stretching) with a special tool (burnishing instrument).

carat A measure of the gold content of an alloy, with 24 carat indicating 100% gold.

corrosion Attack on a metal surface involving loss of material (eg, rusting of iron).

fineness The percentage of gold content in an alloy multiplied by a factor of 10 (eg, 75% gold is 750 fine).

grain A single crystal of metal as seen in the microstructure.

grain refiner An ingredient of an alloy (eg, gold alloys) that helps form smaller grains when the alloy is cast.

homogenizing heat treatment A process of heating an alloy to produce a more uniform distribution of elements by diffusion, usually resulting in softening of the alloy.

noble metal A metal that is resistant to oxidation; includes gold, platinum, palladium, and the other platinum group metals.

ordering The regular arrangement of atoms of an element in a lattice structure rather than a random distribution.

precious metal A metal that is relatively high in cost; includes gold, platinum, palladium, and silver.

precipitation The separation of a phase from a solution on cooling, due to reduced solubility.

tarnish The formation of objectionable reaction products on the surface of an alloy (eg, black oxides or sulfides on silver).

white gold alloy An alloy containing gold and white metals (eg, silver, palladium) that impart a white appearance to the entire mass.

◖ Discussion Questions

1. What is the relationship between carat and platinum metal content and the tarnish of gold restorations?

2. How have the high price of gold and patients' desire for esthetic restorations affected the use of precious metal restorations?

3. What major effect does iridium have on the microstructure of gold alloys?

4. How would the temperature of quenching a gold casting mold affect its mechanical properties?

Study Questions

(See appendix E for answers.)

1. List the elements classified as *noble*.

2. Which elements contribute to the hardening of dental gold alloys?

3. Give the main applications of the ANSI/ADA type I, II, III, and IV alloys.

4. Which three elements are added in fractional amounts to harden high-gold alloys to be used with porcelain?

5. What effect does palladium content have on the color of gold alloys?

6. Describe a softening heat treatment for the ANSI/ADA type III and IV alloys.

7. Describe a hardening heat treatment for the ANSI/ADA type III and IV alloys.

8. Which element is used as a grain refiner in gold casting alloys? Why is it added?

9. Describe the purpose of the heat treatment given to alloys prior to porcelain application.

10. Which five elements are usually present in the white gold alloys used with porcelain (PFM)?

11. What is *ordering* in the gold-copper system?

12. What process is currently believed to be responsible for the hardening of gold-copper-silver alloys by heat treatment?

13. What is the main risk involved in using low-gold (less than 45%) fixed partial denture alloys?

14. Which mechanical property is usually considered a measure of the burnishability of a soft inlay alloy?

15. What has been the main problem with high-silver alloys for use with porcelain?

References

1. Brumfield RC. Role of Allowing Elements in Dental Gold Alloys. New York: Jelenko, 1955.

2. American National Standards Institute/American Dental Association. ANSI/ADA Specification No. 5-1997. Dental Casting Alloys. Chicago: American Dental Association, 1997.

Recommended Reading

Burse AB, Swartz ML, Phillips RW, Dykema RW. Comparison of the in vitro and in vivo tarnish of three gold alloys. J Biomed Mater Res 1972;6:267–277.

Civjan S, Huget EF, Dvivedi N, Cosner HJ Jr. Further studies on gold alloys used in fabrication of porcelain fused to metal restorations. J Am Dent Assoc 1975;90:659–665.

Civjan S, Hugel EF, Marsden JE. Characteristics of two gold alloys used in fabrication of porcelain fused to metal restorations. J Am Dent Assoc 1972;85:1309–1315.

Coleman RL. Physical properties of dental materials (gold alloys and accessory materials). Nat Bur Stand J Res 1928;1(6):867–938.

Fuys RA, Fairhurst CW, O'Brien WJ. Precipitation hardening in gold-platinum alloys containing small quantities of iron. J Biomed Mater Res 1973;7:471–480.

German RM, Guzowski MM, Wright DC. The colour of gold-silver-copper alloys. Gold Bull 1980;113–116.

Kurnakow N, Zemezuzny S, Zasadetelev M. The transformation in alloys of gold with copper. Inst Metals J 1916;15:305.

Kurnakow NS, Ageew NW. Physicochemical study of the gold-copper solid solutions. Inst Metals J 1931;46:481–501.

Leinfelder KF. An evaluation of casting alloys used for restorative procedures. J Am Dent Assoc 1997;128:37–45.

Leinfelder KF, O'Brien WJ, Ryge G, Fairhurst CW. Hardening of high-fusing gold alloys. J Dent Res 1966;45:393.

Leinfelder KF, O'Brien WJ, Taylor DF. Hardening of dental gold-copper alloys. J Dent Res 1972;51:900–905.

Naylor WP. Introduction to Metal Ceramic Technology. Chicago: Quintessence, 1992.

O'Brien WJ, Kring JE, Ryge G. Heat treatment of alloys to be used for the fused porcelain technique. J Prosthet Dent 1964;14:955–960.

Rapson WS. The metallurgy of the coloured carat gold alloys. Gold Bull 1990;23:125–133.

Schoonover IC, Sauder W. Corrosion of dental alloys. J Am Dent Assoc 1941;28:1278.

Shell JS. Some factors influencing specific gravity determinations of gold cast alloys. J Dent Res 1966;45:337.

Sims JR, Blumenthal RN, O'Brien WJ. An electrical resistance study of the precipitation reaction in an Au-Pt-Fe alloy. J Biomed Mater Res 1973;7:497–507.

Smith DL, Burnett AP, Brooks MS, Anthony DH. Iron-platinum hardening in casting golds for use with porcelain. J Dent Res 1970;49:283.

Swartz ML, Phillips RW, El Tannir MD. Tarnish of certain dental alloys. J Dent Res 1958;37:837.

Taggart WH. A new and accurate method of making gold inlays. Dent Cosmos 1907;49:1117.

Valega TM (ed). Alternatives to Gold Alloys in Dentistry. Washington, DC: United States Department of Health, 1977:77–1227.

Wise EM. Cast gold dental alloys. In: ASM Metals Handbook. Cleveland: American Society for Metals, 1948:1120.

Wise EM, Crowell WS, Eash JT. The role of the platinum metals in dental alloys. I & II. Trans Metallurgical Soc AIME 1932;99:363.

Wise EM, Eash JT. The role of the platinum metals in dental alloys. III. The influence of platinum and palladium and heat treatment upon the microstructure and constitution of basic alloys. Trans Metallurgical Soc AIME 1933;104:276.

Yasuda K. Age-hardening and related phase transformations in dental gold alloys. Gold Bull 1987;20:90–103.

CHAPTER 14

Alloys for Porcelain-Fused-to-Metal Restorations

In response to the fluctuating prices of gold and other precious metals, many alternative **alloys** have been introduced into the dental profession. Although the development of these alternative systems was largely motivated by economics, the resultant properties of these alloys often make them superior choices even when compared with more costly alternatives. Selection of the optimal alloy to use for crowns and fixed partial dentures should be based on a rational appraisal of the properties relevant to the intended use of the alloy. A classification of current alloy systems is shown in Fig 14-1.

The proliferation of alloy systems has complicated the practitioner's choice of products for specific restorative situations. As a result, many practitioners rely solely on the advice of dental laboratories for their selections, and many laboratories base their choices on cost factors rather than on a material's properties. In addition, many less significant criteria for alloy selection are used by clinicians, such as alloy color, gold cement, "precious only," "high cost," or "looks, feels, or is cast like gold."

Rational selection of a casting alloy for porcelain-fused-to-metal (PFM) restorations should be based on the following criteria:

1. Physical properties
2. Chemical properties
3. Biocompatibility
4. Laboratory workability
5. Porcelain compatibility

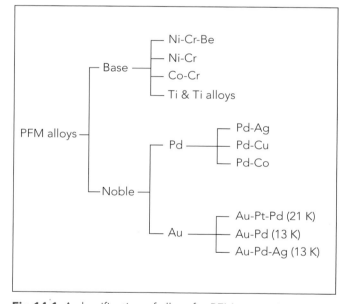

Fig 14-1 A classification of alloys for PFM restorations.

Last, in a balanced decision, cost should be considered relative to these criteria. Factors such as single-unit or multiple-unit, presence or absence of metal occlusal surfaces, span length, and porcelain brand often indicate different alloy choices. A practitioner using only one alloy is unlikely to make an optimal choice in every clinical situation.

Table 14-1 Composition (%) of alloys for PFM restorations*

ALLOYS	Au	Pt	Pd	Ag	Sn	In	Ga	OTHER METALS
High gold	74–88	0–20	0–16	0–15	0–3	0–4	—	Zn < 2; Fe < 0.5; Ta <1
Gold-palladium (no silver)	45–68	0–1	22–45	—	0–5	2–10	0–3	Zn < 4
Gold-palladium-silver	42–62	—	25–40	5–16	0–4	0–6	0–2	Zn 0–3
Palladium-copper	0–2	0–1	66–81	—	0–8	0–8	3–9	Cu 4–20; Zn 0–4
Palladium-silver	0–6	0–1	50–75	1–40	0–9	0–8	0–6	Zn 0–4; Mn 0–4
Nickel-chromium								Ni 59–74; Cr 10–22
Nickel-chromium-beryllium								Ni 70–80; Cr 12–15; Be 0.6–2
Cobalt-chromium								Co 54–65; Cr 24–32
Titanium								CP Grades 2 and 4
Titanium alloys								Ti-6Al-4V; Ti-Nb-Al

*Courtesy of A. Prasad.

Classifications

Before discussing alloy characteristics, it is worth reviewing the terms *noble*, *precious*, *semiprecious*, and *nonprecious*. **Noble metals** are defined on the basis of their chemical properties; that is, they resist oxidation and are not attacked by acids. Eight metals meet this definition but only four are widely used in dental alloys: gold, palladium, silver, and platinum. (See appendix C for all noble metals, including gold, platinum, palladium iridium, rhodium, ruthenium, osmium, and silver.) These metals give noble metal alloys their inert properties in the mouth.

The term **precious** refers only to cost, which is controlled by supply and demand. Many elements in the periodic table, including the eight noble metals, are precious by today's standards.

The term **semiprecious** was originally coined for noble metal alloys that contained significant amounts of silver, and it subsequently has been applied to a variety of alloys, some of which are mixtures of precious and nonprecious ingredients. It is advisable to drop the term *semiprecious* from the dental vocabulary, as it is not well defined and leads to much confusion.

Nonprecious alloys are composed of nonprecious ingredients, except for the common inclusion of 1% to 3% beryllium, a precious but ignoble metal. Most nonprecious alloys are based on a combination of nickel and chromium, although cobalt-chromium and iron-based alloys also exist. See Table 14-1 for the compositions of alloys commonly used in PFM restorations.

When an alloy is chosen for a particular clinical situation, a number of characteristics have clinical significance and should be considered. Among the most important of these characteristics are physical and chemical properties, casting accuracy, and porcelain-metal compatibility.

Physical and Chemical Properties

Color is one of the most obvious physical properties of an alloy. Although the color has no biologic significance, it is equated with quality in the minds of many clinicians. Sometimes this factor seems to matter more to the clinician than to the patient.

When the gold content of an alloy is decreased and metals such as silver and palladium are substituted, yellow color is lost. These less yellow dental alloys are not yet widely accepted. The profession's desire for gold color is so strong that gold-colored semiprecious and nonprecious alloys are commercially available, even though their other physical and chemical properties fall far short of those of even the cheapest white alloys. In some countries, yellow alloys of copper and nickel are currently popular.

If an alloy is gold colored, it must contain copper, gold, or both. However, an alloy can contain substantial amounts of gold or copper without appearing yellow. Examples of this apparent contradiction are jewelers' white gold and some popular gold alloys for PFM restorations (eg, Degudent U, Evonik Degussa; SMG-3, Ney Dental). The latter products contain more than 80% gold, yet no yellow color is seen because of the strong whitening effects of palladium and platinum. Color can be a misleading indicator of composition; dentists should consider other physical and chemical properties as more important than color when a casting alloy is selected.

Some important physical and chemical properties to consider when choosing a cast alloy are:

1. *Noble metal content:* the weight (or better, the atomic) percentage of the eight noble metals contained in an alloy
2. *Hardness:* the Vickers hardness number (VHN), a measure of resistance to indentation
3. *Yield strength:* a measure of the stress required to cause permanent deformation under tension
4. *Elongation:* the amount of permanent deformation a metal undergoes when loaded to its fracture point
5. *Fusion temperature:* the approximate temperature at which an alloy separates under its own weight from partial melting

All of these characteristics have clinical significance. The noble metal content determines, to a large extent, the corrosion resistance and inert properties of the alloy. Hardness is important in relation to occlusal wear resistance and finishing and affects polishing properties. Yield strength is necessary in determining load-bearing ability, especially in fixed partial dentures. Elongation relates to margin-finishing properties, especially important in partial veneer crowns and abutments. However, the elongation value for an alloy may be clinically irrelevant if the yield strength is high. To use the potential elongation, stresses exceeding the yield strength must be applied to move the metal. Within each group of alloys, yield strength generally increases with increasing hardness. Fusion temperature is important in relation to solder melting ranges and correlates with **sag resistance**.

Porcelain-Metal Compatibility

Thermal expansion, bond strength, and composition are also properties to consider when choosing among alloys for PFM restorations, as these characteristics determine porcelain-metal compatibility. Thermal expansion is important because a state of zero residual stress is desirable for porcelain in the final restoration. Such a state is achieved when the total expansions and contractions of the porcelain and metal are matched between the porcelain firing temperature and room temperature.

Porcelain-to-metal bond strength ensures retention of porcelain both in the oral environment and during thermal processing, when the induced thermal stresses can be high.

Composition is a key factor in porcelain-metal compatibility because some components of an alloy can affect the color of the porcelain, perhaps compromising the esthetics of a restoration. Among the alternative alloys, those containing silver are often associated with porcelain color changes and can cause "greening" of some brands of porcelain. The mechanism behind this discoloration is an exchange between silver from the alloy and sodium from the porcelain. The exchange process requires an oxidizing atmosphere, but a subsequent reducing atmosphere is required to produce the colloidal precipitate responsible for color changes in the porcelain.

Other Properties

Because the cross-sectional area of metal used in PFM restorations is usually smaller than that used in all-metal restorations, physical properties such as yield strength of the alloy are crucial in design. Stress in turn controls the minimum allowable dimensions of critical areas like connectors. The elastic modulus is equally important because it determines the flexibility of the metal framework. Flexibility is inversely proportional to elastic modulus; an alloy with a high elastic modulus will flex less under load than an alloy of low elastic modulus.

Chemical properties are important because they affect tarnish resistance, corrosion resistance, and thermal stability. Thermal properties are critical in alloys for PFM restorations because the alloy must have a sufficiently elevated melting temperature range to provide dimen-

Table 14-2 Typical properties of alloys for PFM restorations

GROUP	VHN	ELASTIC MODULUS PSI × 10⁶ (GPa)		YIELD STRENGTH PSI (MPa)		SPECIFIC GRAVITY
High gold	182	13	(90)	65,000	(448)	18.3
Gold-palladium (no silver)	220	18	(124)	83,000	(572)	13.5
Gold-palladium-silver	218	16	(110)	63,600	(439)	13.8
Palladium-copper	425	14	(96)	166,000	(1,145)	10.6
Palladium-silver	242	20	(138)	77,000	(531)	11.1
Nickel-chromium	257	29	(207)	58,000	(400)	8.7
Nickel-chromium-beryllium	357	31	(213)	116,000	(800)	7.8

sional stability during the porcelain firing cycle. Thermal creep results in distortions such as sag in fixed partial denture frameworks and margin opening during the porcelain firing cycles.

Casting accuracy must, of course, be sufficient to provide clinically acceptable castings. In addition to dimensional accuracy (a strong function of technique), the mold-filling ability also contributes to casting accuracy.

Biocompatibility involves a number of factors, among them cytotoxicity and tissue irritation. Potential biologic hazards from the **base metal** alloys, particularly nickel and beryllium, are controversial. These potential hazards may affect not only the patient but also the clinician or technician who makes the restoration. The lack of data and long-term clinical experience suggests caution in using base metal alloys, particularly for people with known sensitivity to base metals. To date, however, neither experimental data nor clinical experience unequivocally contraindicate the use of alloys containing these potentially toxic elements, even in patients known to be sensitive to them.

The following discussion of each alloy group is intended to be general and not necessarily specific to the proprietary products. The product examples were chosen based on their status as the historic forerunners of each alloy group. Table 14-2 lists properties of alloys used in dentistry for crowns and copings.

High-Gold Alloys

PFM technology was introduced to the dental profession with Ceramco no. 1 alloy in 1958. The alloy was a forerunner of the improved high-gold alloys that remain on the market today, such as Jelenko O (Jelenko).

The high-gold alloys are composed principally of gold and platinum group metals. The gold content in these alloys varies from 78% to 87% by weight, and total noble metal content is about 97%. Small amounts of tin, indium, and iron are added for strength and to promote a good porcelain bond to metal oxide. Because of their high nobility, these alloys tend to be costly, both in terms of their cost per ounce and their high density, resulting in heavy castings.

High-gold alloys are usually light yellow in color, although some are white. Some are very yellow, apparently in response to the gold mystique previously discussed. The properties of the very yellow alloys are usually inferior to other products in the group, and their low tensile strength, in particular, makes them a questionable choice for fixed partial dentures.

The hardness of alloys in this group is considered ideal for working characteristics and ease of finishing, and the tensile strength for all but the very yellow products is good. Corrosion resistance is excellent because of the high nobility. Porcelain discoloration is not a problem because the alloys contain little or no silver.

Besides cost, the principal disadvantages of the high-gold alloys are low elastic modulus and poor sag resistance during the porcelain firing cycle. These factors are also troublesome for fixed partial dentures and suggest the use of alternative alloys for these situations.

■ Gold-Palladium-Silver Alloys

Gold-palladium-silver alloys were the first alternative systems, introduced in 1970 as Will-Ceram W (Ivoclar Vivadent), and they remain on today's market. The addition of substantial amounts of silver (10% to 15%) and a relatively high palladium content (20% to 30%) reduces the cost compared with those of higher gold content. The elastic modulus is higher, and the alloys are less susceptible than the high-gold group to dimensional changes during the porcelain baking cycle. Corrosion resistance and clinical working characteristics are generally good.

The principal disadvantage of these alloys is their tendency to induce color changes in porcelain because of their silver content. Silver transport into the porcelain results in a yellow-green color change, depending on the brand of porcelain.

The gold-palladium-silver group has been largely superseded by silver-free gold-palladium alloys, which eliminate problems with porcelain color change. Although gold-palladium-silver alloys are successfully used by many practitioners and have had excellent commercial success, they are used less since the introduction of the cost-competitive silver-free alloys.

■ Palladium-Silver Alloys

The first palladium-silver alloy was introduced to the dental profession in the 1970s, but the one that has remained on the market the longest is Will-Ceram W-1, introduced in 1975 and at one time the largest-selling alloy in the United States.

Palladium-silver alloys usually include 50% to 60% palladium, with most of the balance being silver. The physical and chemical properties are favorable for PFM restorations and are comparable with those of other noble metal alloys. The 50% to 60% nobility assures a satisfactory degree of tarnish and corrosion resistance and good clinical working characteristics.

The elastic modulus for this group is the most favorable of all the precious metal alloys and results in the least flexible castings. Only nonprecious alloys have superior elastic moduli. Palladium-silver alloys solder well and have the lowest sag tendency of the precious metal alloys. Porcelain bond strength is also excellent.

The principal disadvantage of this group is a porcelain color change to green—which occurs to a greater degree in this group than in alloys with lower silver content, such as the gold-palladium-silver alloys. Color problems vary considerably, depending on the brand of porcelain; with some brands this disadvantage is eliminated. Will-Ceram and Ivoclar (Ivoclar Vivadent) porcelains are more resistant to discoloration than others.

Some manufacturers recommend the use of metal surface coupling agents to reduce porcelain color problems. Some of these coupling agents are modified porcelains and others are 24-carat gold. The colloidal gold agents are reasonably effective in reducing surface activity of silver in the alloy, thus preventing diffusion into the porcelain. However, if these gold coupling agents are used in excessive amounts, the gold interferes with surface oxidation necessary for a porcelain-metal bond. Selecting a brand of porcelain that does not change color is a more reliable solution to the problem than using coupling agents.

The palladium-silver group can be a good alternative to the gold-containing group. If the porcelain is one that shows minimal (or no) color change in the presence of silver, it is difficult to find fault with these alloys. Mechanical properties are often superior to even the most costly noble metal alloys.

■ Gold-Palladium Alloys

The gold-palladium silver-free alloys were developed in the mid-1970s to alleviate the color problems caused by silver. The first silver-free alloy was introduced in 1975 as Olympia (Jelenko). These alloys generally contain about 50% gold and 40% palladium. They have had considerable commercial success. Yield strength and hardness are favorable, and elastic modulus is increased significantly compared with high-gold alloys. Cost is comparable with that of the gold-palladium-silver group.

The only recognized disadvantage of the gold-palladium group is thermal expansion incompatibility with some of the higher-expansion porcelains. The silver-free alloys tend to have lower expansion values than the silver-containing group. Some incompatible combinations are well known and are readily acknowledged by the respective manufacturers.

In the absence of thermal expansion incompatibility, there are no disadvantages and several recognizable advantages to using alloys from this group. Rigidity is improved for partial dentures, and the porcelain-metal bonds are adequate. Corrosion resistance is excellent because of the high nobility. Sag tendencies are about the same as for gold-palladium-silver alloys and, again, much better than for high-gold alloys. Gold-palladium alloys can be an excellent choice when their relatively high cost is not a major consideration.

Relatively recently, small amounts of silver have been added to otherwise silver-free compositions. The resulting alloys are probably superior to the silver-free compositions. Because the silver content is low (usually less than 5%, compared with 10% to 15% in the gold-palladium-silver group), there is no porcelain discoloration. However, marketing appeal may be lacking because of the impression created by advertising "silver-free, trouble-free" alloys. The best way to test the efficacy of these products is through clinical experience. These alloys seem promising because thermal expansion is increased and castability is better than with the silver-free alloys. The increase in expansion tends to eliminate the incompatible porcelain-metal combinations previously mentioned.

Palladium-Copper Alloys

The palladium-copper alloys are a relatively recent development, first introduced to the dental profession in 1982 as Option (Ney Dental).

Palladium-copper alloys are usually composed of 70% to 80% palladium and contain little or no gold, up to 15% by weight of copper, and around 9% of gallium. Copper was an unusual addition to porcelain-bonding alloys; such large amounts of copper would cause problems with bonding and porcelain color in gold-based alloys, but apparently do not cause these problems in alloys rich in palladium. Some palladium-copper alloys have a rather heavy oxide that is difficult to cover with opaque porcelain. High hardness values in some of the alloys are offset by a relatively low elastic modulus, resulting in better working characteristics than would be expected with a high hardness value. Strength is good, and some alloys exhibit extremely high yield strengths.

Palladium-copper alloys generally do not melt or cast as easily as palladium-silver alloys, but they are acceptable in this regard. Presoldering has been associated with problems for some, but not all, of these alloys. In addition, the sag resistance of most of them is not as high as in the palladium-silver alloys, again tending to contraindicate their use in large-span fixed partial dentures.

Palladium-Cobalt Alloys

Palladium-cobalt alloys, with around 88% palladium and 4% to 5% cobalt by weight, have been in limited use. The main advantages of these alloys is a higher **coefficient of thermal expansion**, which is useful with certain porcelains. However, the main disadvantage is the formation of a dark oxide that may be difficult to mask at thin margins. Also, these alloys may be more susceptible to hot tearing and embrittlement from carbon if no silver is present. Commercial palladium-cobalt alloys on the market are Jelenko PTM (Jelenko) and Jeneric/Pentron APF (Jeneric/Pentron).

Base Metal Alloys

Developed in the early 1970s, most of the base metal alloys are based on nickel and chromium, but a few cobalt-chromium and iron-based alloys are also available. Because they are not noble metals, their corrosion resistance depends on other chemical properties. A thin, invisible chromium oxide layer provides a complete and impervious film that passivates the surface of the alloy. The passive layer is so thin, it does not dull the surface finish. A similar passive oxide layer limits surface corrosion in ordinary stainless steel.

In addition to noticeable differences in chemical properties, the nonprecious alloys have different physical properties than the noble metal alloys. The most significant of these are high hardness, high yield strength, and high elastic modulus. Elongation is about the same as for gold alloys but is negated by the high yield strength, which makes it difficult or impossible to work the metal.

When used for metal occlusal restorations, the non-precious alloys have only a few recognizable advantages: they are low in cost and some have high hardness values, which can be important when wear resistance is needed. Some nickel-chromium alloys in this group, especially those containing beryllium, have mold-filling abilities that are superior to all other groups. This mold-filling ability permits easier casting of thin sections and produces sharp margins on castings.

However, base metal alloys have many disadvantages when used for metal occlusal restorations. Their hardness makes occlusal adjustments, polishing, crown removal, and endodontic opening difficult. Laboratory labor costs are often higher for crowns made from non-precious alloys because their hardness increases working time. Increased labor costs offset the slight savings in the cost of material. Although casting accuracy can be excellent, the high casting shrinkage (approximately 2.3%) must be accommodated, usually through modification of the casting techniques used for gold alloys, which have a lower casting shrinkage (1.4%). Soldering is unreliable in areas where stresses are involved, although soldering of contacts and minor repairs presents no problem. For the latter, white palladium–based solders work well.

Properties that are considered disadvantageous for metal occlusal applications can be used to advantage in porcelain occlusal restorations. Examples include high tensile strength (up to 120,000 psi, or 830 MPa) and high elastic modulus (about 30 million psi, or 200,000 MPa). The high tensile strength permits the use of thinner metal sections than would be possible if noble metal alloys were used (with the possible exception of some high-palladium alloys). Nickel-chromium alloys have the highest elastic moduli of all dental alloys, which decreases flexibility to a significant degree. The flexibility of a fixed partial denture framework constructed of nickel-chromium is less than half that of a framework of the same dimensions made from a high-gold alloy. Unlike the relatively thick metal crowns, PFM crowns can be easily removed by penetrating the porcelain with rotary diamond instruments, followed by separating the thin metal with proprietary carbide burs made for this purpose.

The addition of beryllium to some nickel-chromium alloys results in more favorable properties. Beryllium increases fluidity and improves casting performance.

Beryllium also controls surface oxidation and results in more reliable, less technique-sensitive porcelain-metal bonds. Generally, these bonds are satisfactory when the alloy contains beryllium but are often questionable when beryllium is lacking. Beryllium-containing alloys require strict control of grinding dust in dental laboratories according to the Occupational Safety and Health Administration.

Nickel-chromium alloys show sag resistance that is uniformly superior to all noble metal alloys. This characteristic, along with increased stiffness and high tensile strength, make them useful in fixed partial dentures. The problems with presoldering, often necessary for fixed partial dentures, can be easily overcome by using the cast-joining techniques described by Weiss and Munyon.[1]

Some nickel-chromium alloys have been chemically modified to overcome certain objectionable properties of this group as compared with noble metal alloys. Examples include products that are advertised to "feel like gold," "cast like gold," or "process like gold." In general, such modified alloys fall short in mechanical or physical properties, or in casting behavior, when compared with the better nickel-chromium-beryllium alloys in this group. The latter alloys are simply different from gold or other noble metal alloys, but their differences can be used to advantage.

The allergenic properties of nickel and nickel-containing alloys are well documented.[2–5] Clinicians must take a careful history with patients and/or consult with an allergy specialist on how to test for nickel sensitivity before recommending the use of nickel alloys for PFM restorations. In addition, consulting with dental laboratories about their use of nickel alloys is important, since many brands of nickel alloy are just labeled as "nonprecious" alloys (see chapter 16).

In summary, base metal alloys are a useful alternative in PFM restorations. Disadvantages associated with metal occlusal restorations are largely overcome when these alloys are used for thin copings under porcelain. Until more long-term data are available, the practitioner should keep in mind the potential biologic hazards associated with base metals and should always follow recommended safety precautions when using these materials. Such precautions include strict control of grinding dust (eg, with suction, masks) and screening patients for allergy to nickel (eg, pierced earring posts and other jewelry).

Titanium Alloys

Although titanium is not a noble or precious metal, it is often not classified with the base metals in dentistry because of its high biocompatibility. The main problem with the use of titanium for PFM restorations is difficult processing. Casting of titanium alloys requires a high casting temperature (2,000°C), rapid oxidation, and reactions with investments. Titanium melting is best done in specially designed furnaces with an argon atmosphere. Investments for use with titanium are described in chapter 19. A titanium alloy, Ti-6Al-4V, has been used for PFM restorations with special low expansion porcelains (coefficient of expansion of $9 \times 10^{-6}/°C$). Pure titanium is used and formed by machining and spark erosion with a process developed by NobelBiocare for their Procera porcelain. Jeneric/Pentron markets a Ti-Al-V alloy (R/2) with an ultimate tensile strength of 1,000 MPa (145,000 psi) and elongation of 9%.

Criteria for Selecting Alloys

Rational selection of a specific alloy should be based on a balanced consideration of cost and the properties relevant to the intended use of the alloy. For single crowns, properties such as strength and sag resistance are less important than they are for fixed partial dentures. Castability, biocompatibility, tarnish and corrosion resistance, porcelain color, and hardness are usually equally important for both alloy uses. For fixed partial dentures, solder and joining behavior, sag resistance, strength, and elastic modulus become increasingly important as the span increases. Porcelain thermal expansion compatibility also increases in importance as the span width increases because of the complexity of geometry and consequent stress fields due to porcelain and alloy mismatch.

When cost is not a major factor, the clinician has a wide spectrum of alloys from which to choose for PFM restorations. Selection of the best alloy for a particular case necessitates consideration of many factors, including the brand of porcelain selected. Whereas it is difficult to rationalize the use of high-gold alloys because of their disadvantages, gold-palladium alloys are considered ideal noble metal alloys by many clinicians. If the clinician were forced to use only one alloy for all PFM restorations, the gold-palladium alloys would prob-

ably be the most logical selection. Mechanical and physical properties are good, and there are no biologic objections. Porcelain compatibility and castability are good with minor (less than 5%) silver additions to the gold-palladium alloys.

Gold-palladium-silver alloys are comparable in cost with gold-palladium alloys, but unfortunately they cause discoloration of porcelain due to the substantial silver content (10% to 15%). The silver-free alloys and the very low-silver palladium-gold alloys seem to be better choices, in most cases.

When cost is a major factor, the nonprecious nickel-chromium-beryllium alloys are alternative candidates. Considering all factors, including labor, cost may not be significantly different among the alloy groups. The nickel-chromium-beryllium alloys are often the alloys of choice where large-span fixed partial dentures are involved, high castability is needed, or esthetic considerations are important. The question of biocompatibility with base metal alloys has yet to be resolved.

Palladium-silver alloys have excellent clinical working characteristics and—provided the porcelain is not one susceptible to discoloration in the presence of silver—have no real disadvantages. Long-term clinical success is well known with palladium-silver.

The newer palladium-copper alloys appear to have many of the advantages of palladium-silver alloys without the porcelain color problems. Limited experience indicates slightly more difficult melting and casting than with palladium-silver but generally good working characteristics and excellent strength. These palladium-copper alloys may replace the palladium-silver alloys as more clinical evidence is accumulated and soldering techniques are developed.

Some clinicians have found that the very yellow high-gold alloys lead to better porcelain color because their oxides are more readily opaqued with porcelain, allowing thinner opaque porcelain layers and, consequently, better esthetics. In such situations, the lack of strength and poor sag resistance are probably of minor importance and the high-gold yellow alloys should be considered a rational choice for single crowns.

When metal occlusal restorations are present, or when partial veneer abutments are cast in the same alloy, metal hardness and ductility can become important. In these situations, rational alloy choices may be more restricted.

Clinical indications for PFM alloys

LONG-SPAN FPDs	SHORT-SPAN FPDs AND SINGLE CROWNS
RATIONAL SELECTIONS	RATIONAL SELECTIONS
1. Nickel-chromium-beryllium 2. Palladium-silver 3. Gold-palladium, perhaps with minor silver additions	1. Palladium-copper 2. Palladium-silver 3. Nickel-chromium-beryllium 4. Gold-palladium, perhaps with minor silver additions
IRRATIONAL SELECTIONS	IRRATIONAL SELECTIONS
1. High gold, especially the very yellow ones, due to their high cost, poor sag resistance, and, for the very yellow examples, poor strength 2. Palladium-copper, due to soldering or joining problems 3. Gold-palladium-silver for the combination of cost and porcelain color problems 4. Nickel-chromium without beryllium, because the addition of beryllium greatly enhances its properties without increasing biocompatibility concerns	1. Gold-palladium-silver, due to the combination of cost and porcelain color problems 2. High gold, due to cost and lack of desirable properties 3. Nickel-chromium without beryllium, because the addition of beryllium greatly enhances its properties

FPD = Fixed partial denture

■ Glossary

alloy A mixture of two or more metals.

base metal A metal that oxidizes readily.

coefficient of thermal expansion A measure of the dimensional change on heating or cooling, expressed as length change per degree of temperature change.

noble metal A metal that is resistant to oxidation; includes gold, platinum, palladium, and other platinum group metals.

nonprecious metal Relatively inexpensive base metal, such as nickel, chromium, and cobalt.

precious metal An expensive metal; includes gold, platinum group metals, and silver.

sag resistance The amount a bar of the material will distort at high temperatures.

semiprecious Alloys containing silver as well as precious metals.

■ Discussion Questions

1. Why are the melting temperatures of these alloys so high?

2. What is the role of minor alloying elements in the bonding of these alloys with porcelain?

3. Why does the silver content of these alloys cause a problem with the color of applied porcelains? What has been done about this problem?

4. What is the main biologic concern with the use of nickel alloys in the mouth?

Study Questions

(See appendix E for answers.)

1. What are precious and semiprecious alloys?

2. What are nonprecious alloys?

3. What are the rational considerations for the selection of an alloy?

4. What is the advantage of palladium-silver alloys?

5. What are the advantages and disadvantages of palladium-copper alloys?

6. Which base metal alloys may be used with porcelain?

7. How do nonprecious alloys compare with precious metal alloys?

8. What are gold-palladium alloys, and what are their advantages and disadvantages?

9. What are the necessary precautions for using base metal alloys in place of precious metal alloys?

References

1. Weiss PA, Munyon RE. Repairs, corrections and additions to non-precious ceramo-metal frameworks (II). Quintessence Dent Technol 1980;7:45–58.
2. Bergman M, Bergman B, Söremark R. Tissue accumulation of nickel released due to electrochemical corrosion of non-precious dental casting alloys. J Oral Rehabil 1980;7:325–330.
3. Moffa JP. Biological effects of nickel-containing dental alloys. Council on Dental Materials, Instruments, and Equipment. J Am Dent Assoc 1982;104:501–505.
4. Moffa JP. Biocompatibility of nickel based dental alloys. CDA J 1984;12:45–51.
5. Peltonen L. Nickel sensitivity in the general population. Contact Dermatitis 1979;5:27–32.

Recommended Reading

Anusavice KJ. Noble metal alloys for metal-ceramic restorations. Dent Clin North Am 1985;29:789–803.

Anusavice KJ, et al. Interactive effect of stress and temperature on creep of PFM alloys. J Dent Res 1985;64:1094–1099.

Baran GR. Selection criteria for base metal alloys for use with porcelain. Dent Clin North Am 1985;29:779–787.

Bertolotti RL. Calculation of interfacial stress in porcelain-fused-to-metal systems. J Dent Res 1980;59:1972–1977.

Bertolotti RL, Fukui H. Measurement of softening temperatures in dental bake-on porcelains. J Dent Res 1982;61:180–183.

Cai Z, Bunce N, Nunn ME, Okabe T. Porcelain adherance to dental cast CP titanium. Biomaterials 2001;22:979–983.

Cascone PJ. Effect of thermal properties on porcelain in metal compatibility. J Dent Res 1979;58:263.

Darque-Ceretti E, Helary D, Aucouturier M. An investigation of gold/ceramic and gold/glass interfaces. Gold Bull 2002;35:118–129.

German RM. Gold alloys for porcelain-fused-to-metal dental restorations. Gold Bull 1980;13:57–62.

Reese JA, Valega TM (eds). Restorative Dental Materials. London: Quintessence, 1985:108–133.

Tuccillo JJ, Cascone PJ. The evolution of porcelain-fused-to-metal (PFM) alloy systems. In: McLean JW (ed). Dental Ceramics. Proceedings of the First International Symposium on Ceramics. Chicago: Quintessence, 1983:347–370.

Valega TM Sr (ed). Alternative to Gold Alloys in Dentistry [publication no. (NIH) 77-1227]. Washington, DC: US Department of Health and Human Services, 1977:40–67.

Whitlock RP, Hinman RW, Eden GT, Tesk JA, Dickson G, Parry EE. A practical test to evaluate the castability of dental alloys. J Dent Res 1981;60:404.

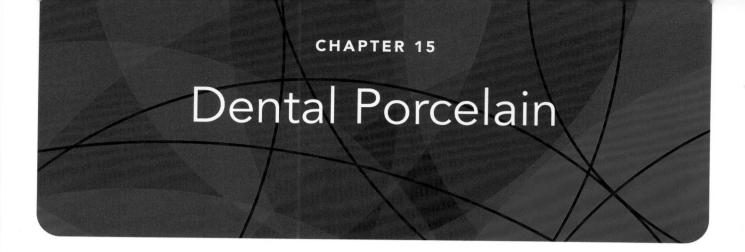

CHAPTER 15

Dental Porcelain

Porcelain has been used for denture teeth since 1790. The main advantages of porcelain are its excellent esthetic properties, durability, and biocompatibility. Today it is used mainly for individual jacket crowns and for veneering metal crowns and fixed partial dentures. There is also increasing use of porcelain **veneers** bonded to teeth to cover unsightly areas. Porcelain has also been used to fabricate inlays, but this practice has fallen into disuse.

Porcelain is defined as a white, translucent ceramic that is fired to a glazed state. Dental porcelains are classified according to fusion temperature as follows:

High fusing	1,288°C to 1,371°C (2,350°F to 2,500°F)
Medium fusing	1,093°C to 1,260°C (2,000°F to 2,300°F)
Low fusing	660°C to 1,066°C (1,220°F to 1,950°F)

Denture Teeth

The raw materials for porcelain denture teeth are mainly **feldspar**, about 15% quartz, and, to improve moldability, Kaolin (4%). A plastic mass made from this mixture and additional pigments is formed into metal molds and fired under vacuum to reduce porosity. During firing, the teeth are glazed by the glass produced from the feldspar. Metal pins or holes are then placed in the teeth for mechanical attachment to the denture base. Improvements in acrylic denture teeth have increased their use as an alternative to porcelain.

Advantages

1. Excellent biocompatibility
2. Natural appearance
3. High resistance to wear and distortion

Disadvantages

1. Brittle
2. No bond to acrylic denture bases; requires mechanical attachments
3. Produces clicking sound on contact
4. Cannot be polished easily after grinding
5. Higher density increases weight of teeth
6. Mismatch in coefficient of thermal expansion (TE) produces stresses in acrylic denture base

Porcelain Enamels Used With Metals

Composition

Dental porcelains are used to bond with metals for a natural-appearing outer layer, as shown in Fig 15-1. These porcelains were developed during the 1950s by raising the coefficient of TE of feldspar to match the values of gold alloys, which are 13 to 14 $\times$ 10^{-6}°C. This modification was accomplished by heating orthoclase feldspar with alkali metal carbonates (eg, K_2CO_3, Li_2Co_3) to approximately 1,093°C (2,000°F) to form a glass and

Table 15-1 Chemical analysis (%) of dental porcelains[2]

COMPOUND	BIODENT OPAQUE	CERAMCO OPAQUE	VMK OPAQUE	BIODENT DENTIN	CERAMCO DENTIN	VMK DENTIN
SiO_2	52.0	55.0	52.4	56.9	62.2	56.8
Al_2O_3	13.55	11.65	15.15	11.80	13.40	16.30
CaO	—	—	—	0.61	0.98	2.01
K_2O	11.05	9.6	9.9	10.0	11.3	10.25
Na_2O	5.28	4.75	6.58	5.42	5.37	8.63
TiO_2	3.01	—	2.59	0.61	—	0.27
ZrO_2	3.22	0.16	5.16	1.46	0.34	1.22
SnO_2	6.4	15.0	4.9	—	0.5	—
Rb_2O	0.09	0.04	0.08	0.10	0.06	0.10
BaO	1.09	—	—	3.52	—	—
ZnO	—	0.26	—	—	—	—
UO_3	—	—	—	—	—	0.67
B_2O_3, CO_2, H_2O	4.31	3.54	3.24	9.58	5.85	3.75

a high-expansion ceramic phase identified as leucite ($K_2O \cdot Al_2O_3 \cdot 4SiO_2$).[1] An analysis of several of these high-expansion porcelain enamels is presented in Table 15-1.

During manufacture, the fused glass containing the leucite is quenched or "fritted" in water, freezing it in an amorphous state. The **frit** is then ground up by ball milling and pigmented with colored ceramic compound such as iron oxide to shade the porcelain. Each kit of porcelain supplied to dental technicians contains about a dozen shades in at least three translucency levels for forming layers to build up the crown. Layers of opaque porcelain screen out the underlying metal oxide surface color. Opaque porcelain contains approximately 15% tin oxide, zirconium oxide, or titanium dioxide. A highly translucent porcelain, called *incisal* or *enamel porcelain*, gives the crowns a natural translucent appearance at the incisal edge. The main layer, above the opaque layer, is the *body* or *dentin* layer.

Condensation and sintering

Porcelain crowns are built up by applying a paste of porcelain powder to a metal casting or a platinum foil matrix with a small brush. Generally, distilled water or special liquids are used to form the paste with the porcelain powder on a glass slab. As each layer of paste

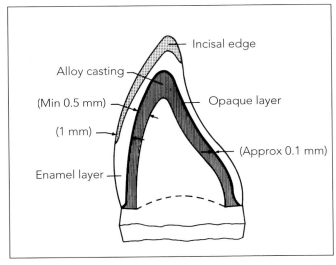

Fig 15-1 Cross section of a metal-ceramic crown with full coverage.

is added, most of the water is removed by a vibrator and absorbent tissue paper. This step gives the wet crown more strength and increases the density of the compact.

As each layer of the crown is built up, it is fired in a porcelain furnace. The wet crown is first dried in front of the furnace to remove the residual water and then fired under vacuum. As the porcelain is heated, adja-

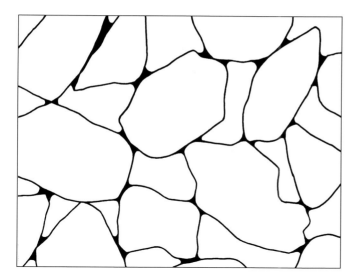

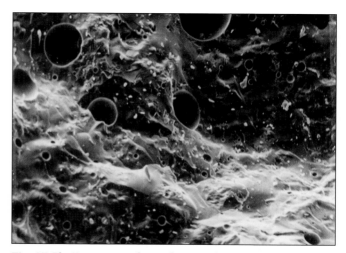

Fig 15-2 Biscuit stage of vitreous sintering, involving flow of glass to form bridges between particles. (Reprinted with permission from Van Vlack.[3])

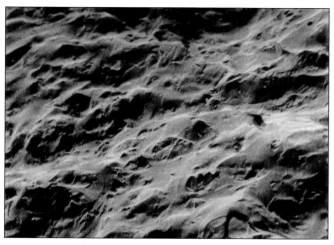

Fig 15-3a Fracture surface of gingival porcelain fired under vacuum (scanning electron micrograph; original magnification ×300). (Reprinted with permission from Meyer et al.[4])

Fig 15-3b Fracture surface of gingival porcelain fired under normal atmospheric pressure (scanning electron micrograph; original magnification ×300). (Reprinted with permission from Meyer et al.[4])

cent particles bond together in a process called **sintering**. Although there is no meeting of the porcelain powder particles, they join together by flow on contact as a result of surface energy (Fig 15-2).

Firing in a vacuum furnace greatly reduces the porosity of the final product, as shown in Figs 15-3a and 15-3b. The first firing of porcelain is called the **bisque** or *biscuit bake*. After the incisal layer is added, the porcelain is brought to the final stage, called the **glaze bake**. When the glazing temperature of the porcelain is reached, a layer of glass is formed on the surface. After glazing, the crown is removed from the furnace and cooled under an inverted glass or beaker. An alterna-

tive approach is to add a thin layer of a low-fusing glass or glaze to the surface and fire to the flow temperature of the glaze.

Properties

Porcelain enamels have a **vitreous** structure consisting of an irregular network of silica produced by the presence of large alkali metal ions, such as sodium, potassium, and lithium (Fig 15-4a). This amorphous structure produces physical properties typical of a glass, including brittleness and lack of a definite melting temperature. Glasses are brittle due to their irregular structure and the absence of slip planes, which are present in a

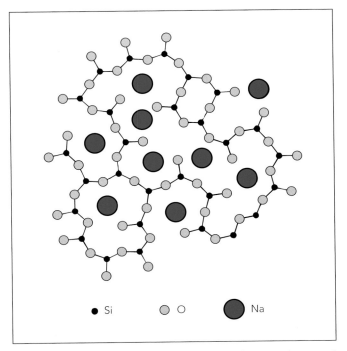

Fig 15-4a Irregularity of glass structure (silicon and oxygen) due to the presence of large alkali cations (sodium). (Modified with permission from Warren.[5])

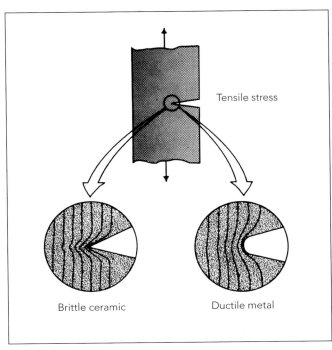

Fig 15-4b Effects of tensile forces on crack propagation in ceramics and metals, resulting in brittleness and ductility, respectively.

true crystalline material. The strength of glasses and brittle materials is governed by the presence of small flaws or cracks. When stressed in tension, according to the **crack propagation theory**, small flaws tend to open up and propagate, resulting in a low tensile strength. This is less of a factor with ductile metals because the stress concentration around the tip of the flaws is reduced by elongation of the metal, as illustrated in Fig 15-4b. However, glasses are much stronger in compression, because **residual compressive stresses** tend to close up flaws. Therefore, the tensile strengths of vitreous dental porcelains are around 35 MPa (5,000 psi) as compared with compressive strengths of 517 MPa (75,000 psi).

The strength of dental porcelains is traditionally tested in flexure as a beam and reported as **modulus of rupture**. The modulus of rupture of a vitreous body or enamel porcelain is about 90 MPa (13,000 psi). The strengths of vacuum-fired porcelains are higher due to fewer flaws.

Vitreous dental porcelains do not have a definite melting temperature but undergo a gradual decrease in viscosity when heated. A sharp decrease in viscosity occurs around the **glass-transition temperature** (T_g), as shown in Fig 15-5. Below T_g, the glass has the properties of a solid. Above T_g, glass flows more readily, and vitreous sintering takes place.

A typical TE curve of a porcelain bar is shown in Fig 15-6. The TE is linear up to around T_g, but above T_g there is a rapid increase in the rate of expansion when the glass has a more liquid structure. If heating is continued, the bar will reach the softening temperature and collapse. The TE of dental porcelains for bonding to metals is especially important in relation to the TE of the metal involved. Generally, the metal and porcelain should be matched in coefficients of TE values. If the TE curves of the metal and porcelain are too far apart, undesirable thermal stresses will result in fracture of the porcelain, which is the weaker material. The porcelain and metal are therefore said to be incompatible.

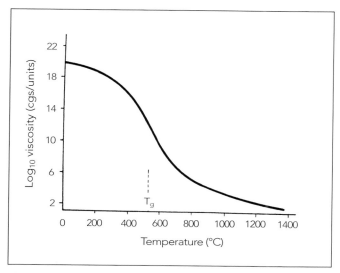

Fig 15-5 Viscosity (rigidity) increasing rapidly below glass-transition temperature. (Reprinted with permission from Jones.[6])

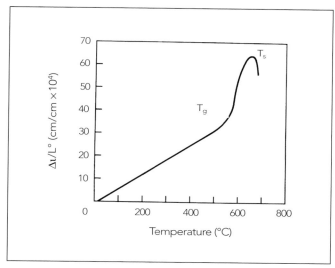

Fig 15-6 TE curve for glass with a T_g and softening temperature (T_s).

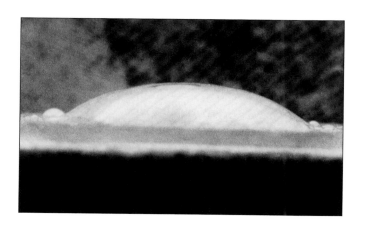

Fig 15-7 Good wetting of molten porcelain on alloy.

Adhesion to metals

Several factors have been identified as promoting good adhesion or bonding of a porcelain enamel to a metal, including wetting, adherent oxide, and mechanical retention.

Wetting
Good wetting of the porcelain on the metal is indicated by a low contact angle of a drop of the porcelain when fired on the solid, as shown in Fig 15-7. It promotes penetration of the glass into surface irregularities and, therefore, a greater area of contact. Good wetting also indicates chemical compatibility between the porcelain and the metal.

Adherent oxide
The presence of an adherent oxide on the metal surface that is wet by the porcelain provides a beneficial transition layer. The diffusion of atoms from the metal and porcelain into this oxide is cited as evidence of a chemical bond. A nonadherent oxide, however, can lead to a weak boundary and failure.

Mechanical retention
The presence of surface roughness on the metal oxide surface can result in mechanical retention on a microscopic level, especially if undercuts are present.

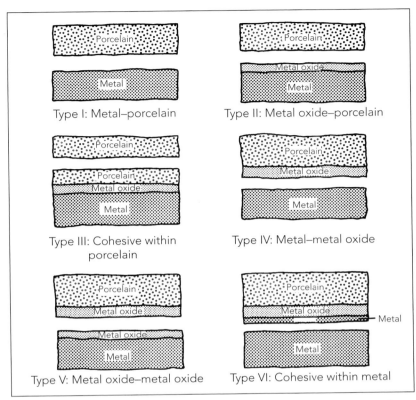

Type I: Metal–porcelain

Type II: Metal oxide–porcelain

Type III: Cohesive within porcelain

Type IV: Metal–metal oxide

Type V: Metal oxide–metal oxide

Type VI: Cohesive within metal

Fig 15-8 Classification of porcelain enamel failures according to interfaces formed. Type III represents cohesive failure indicative of a proper bond. (Reprinted with permission from O'Brien.[7])

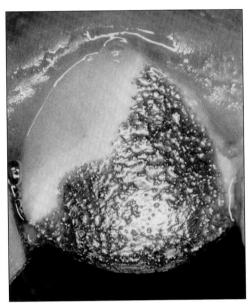

Fig 15-9 Type I failure in gold casting coated with pure gold.

Fig 15-10 Example of type V failure with fracture through oxide layer of nickel-chromium alloy.

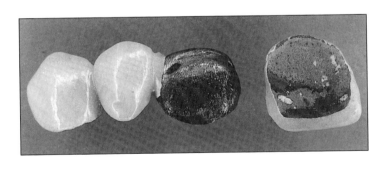

Bond failure classification

Figure 15-8 illustrates several types of failure that may occur. The type I failure shown in Fig 15-9 was the result of using a thick, pure gold coating agent on the alloy surface. Such a coating blocks formation of the trace metal oxide layer necessary for strong bonding.

Figure 15-10 shows a type V failure in a nickel-chromium alloy. If the oxide layer on nickel alloys becomes too thick, a weak boundary layer is formed. Figure 15-11 shows a nickel alloy surface with microscopic cohesive attachment sites where the bond was stronger than the porcelain. The relationship between the density of these sites to bond strength is depicted in Fig 15-12.

When density is low, mixed types of bond failures are observed. However, when the **cohesive plateau** is reached, the bond strength is equal to the strength of the porcelain (S_p) and cohesive failure is observed. Because the bond strength in tension has been found to be about 35 MPa (5,000 psi) with properly oxidized gold alloys, and the tensile strength of the porcelain has been measured to be about the same, higher bond strengths lack practical significance. Shear bond strength tests indicate values of 111 MPa (16,000 psi) to 147 MPa

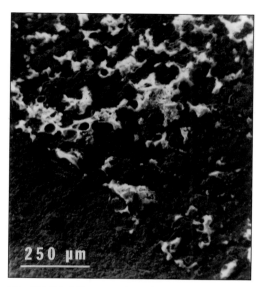

Fig 15-11 Microscopic cohesive attachment sites on fracture interface between nickel alloy and porcelain; a mixed failure.

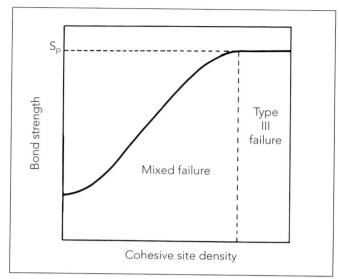

Fig 15-12 Relationship between density of cohesive attachment sites and observed bond strengths.

(21,000 psi), which represent the shear strengths of the porcelains.

Advantages

1. High strength
2. Potential for fixed partial dentures
3. Excellent fit

Disadvantages

1. Appearance of metal margins
2. Discoloration by metal
3. Difficulty producing an appearance of translucency
4. Bond failure with metals
5. Possible disadvantages of alloy used

■ All-Ceramic Crowns

A classification of porcelain crowns according to composition is shown in Fig 15-13. **Jacket crown** is the traditional, accepted term for all-ceramic crowns used for restoring the entire clinical crown portion of a tooth.

The most significant developments for dental ceramics in the 1980s were the emergence of new materials and processes for fabricating ceramic jacket crowns. Porcelain jacket crowns were used widely in dentistry since Land developed the platinum foil technique in 1903. They were fabricated with high-fusing feldspathic porcelains and were known for natural esthetics resulting mainly from high translucency and the use of specialized laboratory techniques. However, they have not been used extensively for decades. Failures of these porcelain crowns include fracture and breakage. Although it has been suggested that failures are caused by the low strength of the porcelain or possibly poor adaptation to the tooth resulting in high-stress areas, such evidence has not been documented.

In 1965, alumina-reinforced porcelain crowns were introduced with a coping or core of a ceramic material containing 40% to 50% alumina with an outer layer of translucent porcelain (Fig 15-14). The alumina ceramic core material has a flexural strength of approximately 131 MPa (19,000 psi), which is twice that of feldspathic porcelain. The clinical failure rate for anterior crowns made with alumina ceramic cores has been established to be below 2%, which is considered an acceptable risk. However, the 15.2% failure rate for molar crowns is unacceptable. Therefore, core materials for anterior crowns should not have flexure strengths significantly below 131 MPa (19,000 psi); the strength required for posterior crowns is still to be determined.

Magnesia core crowns, developed in the 1980s, had a high-expansion core based on magnesia instead of alumina and allowed the use of body and incisal porce-

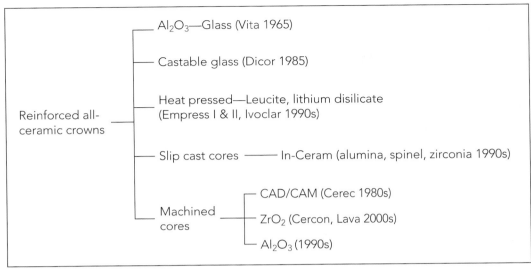

Fig 15-13 A classification of porcelain crowns according to composition.

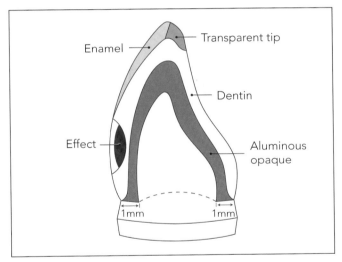

Fig 15-14 Aluminous porcelain crown with strong ceramic core. (Modified with permission from McLean.[8])

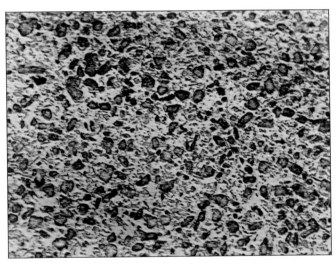

Fig 15-15 Microstructure of high-expansion magnesia core material. (Reprinted with permission from O'Brien.[9])

lains used for porcelain-fused-to-metal (PFM) (Fig 15-15). The coefficient of TE for this core material is $14.5 \times$ ppm/°C, and the modulus of rupture is 269 MPa (39,000 psi) when glazed. Although clinical testing of these crowns was successful, they have had limited use because of their fabrication using the platinum foil technique, which has declined in practice.

Castable ceramics

Castable ceramic systems are used to cast crowns via the lost wax process. They are indicated for use in single anterior and posterior crowns. Tooth preparation is either a 90-degree shoulder with a rounded internal line angle or a 120-degree chamfer with adequate tooth

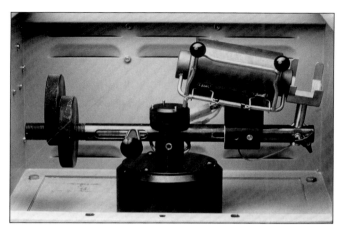

Fig 15-16 Centrifugal casting machine for castable ceramic crown.

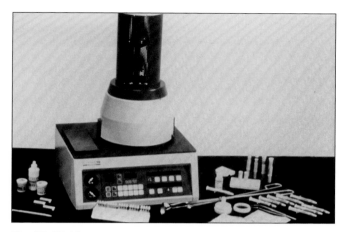

Fig 15-17 Heat pressing system.

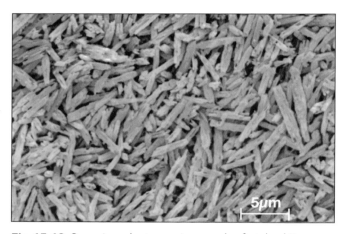

Fig 15-18 Scanning electron micrograph of etched Empress II core showing lithium disilicate crystals.

reduction—from 1 mm minimum on the gingivo-axial surfaces to 1.5 to 2 mm incisally and occlusally.

Impressions, models, and dies are made in the usual manner. The restoration is waxed on the die, and the wax pattern of the crown is invested in a phosphate-bonded investment following the same procedure used for some metal crowns. An ingot of the ceramic material is placed in a special crucible and melted and cast with a motor-driven centrifugal casting machine at 1,380°C (2,500°F) (Fig 15-16). The cast crown is a clear glass that must be heat treated to form a crystalline ceramic, which is essentially a fluorine mica silicate. The crystallization procedure takes several hours in a heat-

treating or "ceramming" furnace, with a final temperature of 1,075°C (1,967°F).

The fired ceramic crown has a "universal" white shade with a translucency of around 50%. It has a flexure strength of 152 MPa (22,000 psi) and a coefficient of TE of $7.2 \times 10^{-6}/°C$. Final shading is achieved using a series of light coats of colored surface porcelains. Shaded zinc phosphate cements are suggested by the manufacturer. Because the entire crown is translucent, these colored cements may also be used to achieve the final shade. Before seating the crown, tight contacts may be adjusted with an abrasive stone or wheel and then polished with rubber wheels. Although there are many cast ceramic crowns in service, the major system (Dicor, Dentsply International) is being phased out commercially.

Heat-pressed ceramics

In this process, high-leucite porcelain ingot cylinders are heated to 115°C to a plastic state. Then, the ingots are pressure-injected into investment molds formed by the lost wax process for crowns, inlays, onlays, and veneers (Fig 15-17). Two compositions are available for heat pressing. The original composition (Empress I, Ivoclar Vivadent) introduced in the early 1990s is a high-leucite porcelain. Due to the high leucite content and pressure forming process, the flexural strength of porcelain formed by this process is around 125 MPa. The more recent composition is a lithium disilicate glass-ceramic (Empress II) with a flexural strength of around 350 to 400 MPa produced by heat treatment. The heat treatment produces a fine structure of lithium disilicate crystals

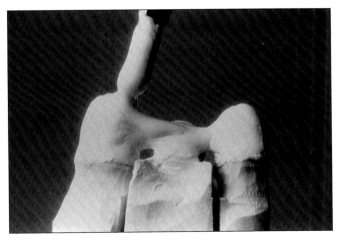

Fig 15-19 Application of alumina-liquids slip to plaster cast that absorbs water by capillary action. (Courtesy of Ivoclar Vivadent.)

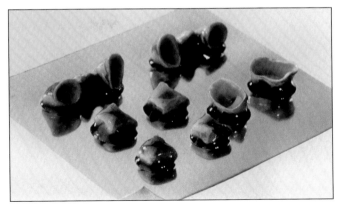

Fig 15-20 Glass infiltration of alumina copings fired on platinum foil.

(Fig 15-18). The advantages of the process are good fit and higher strength for the resulting restorations. A disadvantage is the initial high cost for the equipment.

Slip casting

This process for forming ceramic cores gives very high strength values depending on the material used. For example, the value for alumina is 400 MPa; for spinel, 375 MPa; and for zirconia, 600 MPa. To form the alumina cores, a slurry of fine ceramic particles is painted on plaster dies, which absorb the water to form a green state core. Next, the green core is sintered at 1,120°C to form a dense mass. Glass is then applied and fused at 1,100°C for 4 hours to allow glass infiltration (Figs 15-19 and 15-20). The rest of the crown is formed by firing a translucent body porcelain over the cores by traditional firing.

Although the strength of the glass-infiltrated alumina cores is high, alumina cannot be etched and silane treated for resin bonding; the same general process is used for the other materials. In the 1990s, alumina was the first composition sold. Spinel is a compound of alumina and magnesia with a greater translucency, and zirconia has the highest strength.

Advantages
1. High strength
2. Good fit

Disadvantages
1. High initial cost
2. Long processing time
3. Lack of bonding to the tooth structure

Milled ceramic restorations
Chairside CAD/CAM

A number of systems for machining ceramics to produce inlays, onlays, veneers, and crowns have been introduced. The first of these uses computer-aided design and computer-assisted manufacture (CAD/CAM) technology. In making a restoration with the Cerec CAD/CAM chairside system (Sirona) (Fig 15-21), the following sequence is carried out. First, a powder is applied to the patient's prepared tooth to provide contrast for the optical scanner. Next, the prepared tooth is scanned with an optical probe, and the image is stored in a computer. The restoration is then designed on a monitor screen with computer assistance, after which a block of a machinable ceramic is selected by shade. With information from the computer, the restoration is milled in a few minutes in a compartment of the chairside unit. The restoration is then acid etched, and a silane agent is applied in preparation for bonding to the tooth preparation. After cementing with a resin cement, the main surfaces are contoured with a diamond contour instrument and polished.

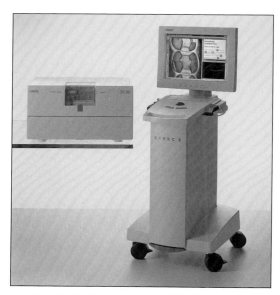

Fig 15-21 CAD/CAM system for chairside inlay fabrication. (Courtesy of Sirona Dental.)

Table 15-2 Flexural strengths of high-strength dental ceramics

MATERIAL	FLEXURAL STRENGTH (MPa)	TYPICAL PRODUCT
Cast glass-ceramic	125	Dicor
Alumina core	140	Vitadur, Vident
Magnesia core, glazed	269	Magcor
Heat pressed (leucite)	151	Empress, Ivoclar Vivadent
Heat pressed (lithium disilicate)	350	Empress II
Slip cast (alumina)	400	In-Ceram, Vita
Slip cast (spinel)	350	In-Ceram
Slip cast (zirconia)	650	In-Ceram
Machined alumina	650	Procera, Nobel Biocare
Machined leucite	135	Pro-Cad, Sirona Dental
Machined zirconia	900	Cercon, DeguDent

Although more recent CAD/CAM models (eg, Cerec 3) can fabricate crowns as well as inlays, onlays, and veneers, the expensive equipment, extensive training, and longer chairside time make the chairside CAD/CAM units useful for special practices only.

Advantages
1. Work can be done chairside
2. Requires only one visit

Disadvantages
1. High initial equipment costs
2. Reported lack of marginal accuracy
3. Labor intensive for the dental practitioner, including extensive training

Laboratory-based CAD/CAM
Several laboratory-based systems have been introduced where the expensive and complicated equipment is located in the dental laboratory, and fabrication is based on a traditional addition silicone impression taken by the clinician. These systems use machine milling to make ceramic core copings that have higher strength and greater marginal accuracy. One of the early systems (Procera) uses a dry-pressed alumina that is milled and sintered at a high temperature to form a ceramic coping, which is then covered with a translucent layered body/incisal feldspathic porcelain to produce an all-ceramic crown. More recent systems use super-strong stabilized zirconia core copings milled to have strengths approaching 900 MPa (eg, Cercon, DeguDent; Lava, 3M ESPE). These opaque porcelains are also covered with sintered translucent feldspathic body and incisal porcelains that are esthetically favorable but relatively weak.

The high strength of the stabilized zirconia ceramics comes from the addition of around 3 mol% of yttrium oxide, which stabilizes the high-temperature tetragonal crystal form of zirconia even when cooled down to room temperature. However, if a stress crack begins to spread under tensile stress, a transformation to the monoclinic room temperature crystal structure occurs, with a 3% volume expansion and a residual compressive stress, thereby stopping the crack propagation. The net result of this "transformation toughening" is strengthening of the zirconia. Table 15-2 presents the flexure strengths of several dental porcelains for comparison.

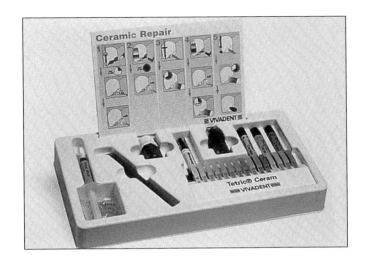

Fig 15-22 Porcelain repair kit with etchant, bonding resins, and repair composite. (Courtesy of Ivoclar Vivadent.)

◼ Porcelain Repair

Since dental porcelains are brittle, fractures occasionally occur. Fortunately, they can be repaired without replacement of the entire restoration. A number of repair systems have been developed for chairside use (Fig 15-22), and the general method for repair is as follows:

1. Establish a dry field.
2. Remove the surface of adjacent remaining porcelain with an abrasive bur.
3. Treat the area to be repaired with etching gel, and then clean it off.
4. Silanize the ceramic surface with a silane component.
5. Apply a metal bonding component over exposed metal surfaces.
6. Apply bonding resin to the entire area.
7. Repair the restoration with a composite component and cure.

The shear bond strengths of repair systems usually range from 10 to 15 MPa after storage in water for 1 day and thermocycling.

◼ Surface Treatments for Strengthening Porcelain

Polishing

Surface treatments to increase strength are appealing because they do not require major investments in new technology. The simplest method is polishing, which reduces the size of surface flaws and thus dramatically increases strength. In experimental strength testing, dental materials manufacturers and researchers have found that highly polished ceramic specimens can have strength values 50% to 100% greater than unpolished specimens.[10]

It is foolish to place an expensive high-strength ceramic material in a patient's mouth in a roughened state. A study of crown fractures showed that failure was often initiated by scratches on the internal surface of the crown.[11] Deep scratches may be clinically induced during routine procedures, such as when coarse burs are used to roughen ceramic crowns to improve occlusion and fit. Porcelain can be polished and flaws removed with Sof-Lex (3M ESPE) or finishing disks by Shofu Dental. Reglazing is another option but is not as convenient. Metals in PFM restorations are much less sensitive to these flaws.

Ion-exchange treatment

The process of ion-exchange treatment (Tuf-Coat, GC International) is carried out in the dental laboratory and consists of heating the porcelain restoration, which has been coated with a potassium salt, in a low-temperature oven. As a result, sodium ions from the porcelain surface are exchanged for potassium ions. Since potassium ions are about 35% larger in diameter than sodium ions, the surface layer develops a residual compressive stress (Fig 15-23). Consequently, the flexural strength of the porcelain is increased as long as the surface is not damaged by grinding.

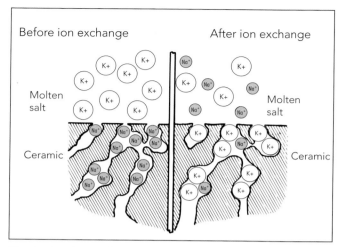

Fig 15-23 Strengthening of porcelain by replacing sodium ions with larger potassium ions. (Reprinted with permission from Dunn.[12])

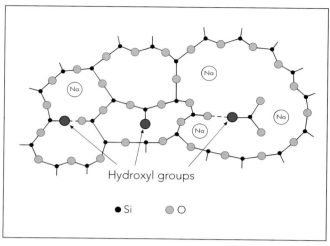

Fig 15-24 Structure of hydrated glass. (Modified with permission from O'Brien.[13])

This procedure is a simplification of the original process of immersing the porcelain restoration in a bath of molten potassium salt. It is especially useful for the internal surface of an all-ceramic porcelain crown but is not recommended for use with the new high-strength porcelains (ie, **aluminous porcelain**, Procera, In-Ceram). An anterior porcelain jacket crown made from a feldspathic porcelain without a core may be the only major application.

Hydrothermal porcelains

Hydrothermal porcelains (eg, Ducera LFC) have a special nonfeldspathic composition that forms a plasticized surface layer when hydrated. This characteristic is unusual in that the surface hardness of the porcelain is significantly reduced and flexural strength is significantly increased. The increase in strength is due to the plastic nature of the hydrated surface, which allows for deformation of surface flaws and prevents them from propagating through the bulk. Raman spectroscopy and scanning electron microscopy verify hydration of the glass structure (Fig 15-24). The reaction occurs as an ion exchange between the alkali ion and a proton:

$$Si–O–Na^+ + HOH \rightarrow Si–OH + Na^+OH^-$$

Molecular water has also been detected in the glass structure.

■ Selection Criteria

The gold standard for selecting a new all-ceramic crown system is the 5-year clinical failure rate of a system for its intended application, not the reported strength of the ceramic. The clinical failure rate is about 2% for all-ceramic anterior crowns; it is higher for posterior crowns.[14] The clinical failure rate for posterior PFM restorations is also about 2%.[15] Therefore, any of the new ceramic systems (eg, Empress, Procera, In-Ceram) are acceptable for anterior crowns but are riskier for posterior restorations. Clinical longevity data for the higher-strength ceramic core crowns are still not available.

In addition to porcelain strength, other factors that are important for clinical survival of posterior crowns include adhesive bonding of porcelain to teeth and bonding of the porcelain layers to each other. Bonding to dentin is significant because it reduces stress concentrations within the ceramic crown; this factor is much more important for ceramics than for metals. Also, bonding of the weaker outer body and incisal porcelains to a high-strength core is important to distribute stress and prevent fracture of the outer layers. Therefore, a well-documented clinical failure rate of no more than about 2% is the standard for replacing posterior PFM restorations with all-ceramic restorations.

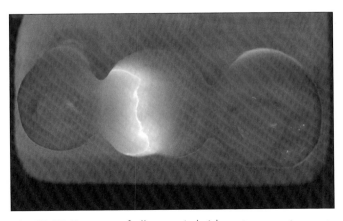

Fig 15-25 Fracture of all-ceramic bridge at connector area. (Courtesy of Dr Won Oh.)

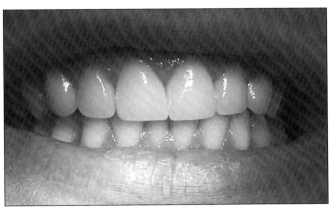

Fig 15-26 Ceramic veneers on anterior maxillary teeth. (Courtesy of Dr Wayne Yee.)

The use of newer and stronger ceramics for all-ceramic fixed partial dentures depends on the mechanical stresses in a specific patient's mouth. Posterior bridges are the riskiest, and studies have shown that they usually fail at connector areas when flexural strengths are exceeded (Fig 15-25).[16] The length and radius of curvature at the gingival embrasure of the connector is critical.

Selection of ceramic systems for veneers must allow for thin translucent restorations that can be bonded to the facial and incisal surfaces of anterior teeth to cover discolorations and fill in unsightly gaps between teeth. Traditional body and incisal feldspathic porcelains used for PFM restorations as well as newer fluorapatite translucent porcelains (eg, IPS e.max Ceram, Ivoclar Vivadent) are usually used with a refractory die technique (Fig 15-26).

Clinical Decision Scenarios for Dental Porcelain

This section presents an approach for choosing materials and a system for specific situations. It uses the same format as that presented in chapter 7. Advantages and disadvantages of each material/system are prioritized using the following codes: • of minor importance; •• important; and ••• very important.

Materials IPS Empress vs Vita In-Ceram

Situation* Clinicians in a large practice have decided to buy an all-ceramic crown system for their in-house dental laboratory. They are choosing between the IPS Empress and Vita In-Ceram systems.

Critical Factors Etchability, cost, and flexural strength

IPS EMPRESS	VITA IN-CERAM
ADVANTAGES	ADVANTAGES
••• Ability to be etched and bonded to dentin •• Marginal fidelity of < 50 μm ••• High flexural tensile strength •• Versatility (anterior crowns, veneers, inlays, and onlays) •• Relatively simple process using a modified lost wax technique •• Biocompatiblility	••• High flexural tensile strength •• Marginal fidelity of 20 to 25 μm ••• Versatility (single crown; anterior fixed partial dentures; and inlays, onlays, and veneers with spinel In-Ceram) •• No thermal sensitivity •• Biocompatibility •• Flexibility of provisional cementation
DISADVANTAGES	DISADVANTAGES
•• Learning period required for technicians	••• Long learning period required for technicians because of the complexity of slip-cast fabrication ••• Cannot be etched or bonded to dentin ••• Time and labor intensive

Analysis/Decision The clinicians chose the IPS Empress equipment. Although both systems have merit, the IPS Empress system requires less time and labor and has a shorter learning period for technicians. In addition, IPS Empress allows bonding to dentin, which is permanent and lowers stress concentrations.

*Scenario courtesty of Dr Waletha Wasson, DDS, MS.

■ Glossary

aluminous porcelain A porcelain-containing alumina (Al_2O_3) as an opacifier and strengthener.

bisque The first firing of a porcelain; also called *biscuit bake*.

cohesive plateau The apparent bond strength between porcelain and alloy equal to the strength of the porcelain, attained when the bond is stronger than the porcelain.

crack propagation theory The theory that glasses and other brittle materials fail by the propagation of minute flaws or cracks when under stress.

feldspar A crystalline mineral of the general formula $X_2O \cdot Al_2O_3 \cdot 6SiO_2$, where X may be sodium or potassium.

frit A powdered glass.

glass-transition temperature The temperature below which a glass behaves like a solid.

glaze The shiny layer of surface glass produced on a porcelain by firing. The glass may either come from within the porcelain or be added to the surface before the final firing; also called *glaze bake*.

Materials CAD/CAM inlays vs Empress inlays

Situation* A patient had a number of routine restorations placed over the years. They consist basically of Class 1 and 2 amalgam restorations and some anterior composites. The patient has been very satisfied with these restorations but is now seeking more esthetic, but still long-lasting, alternatives to replace the amalgams. She also indicates that she is leaving on vacation in 2 weeks and would like to have all of the dental work done beforehand.

Critical Factors Good esthetics, speed of completion

CAD/CAM INLAYS	EMPRESS INLAYS
ADVANTAGES	ADVANTAGES
••• Good esthetics ••• Can be completed in one appointment • No impressions required • No temporization required •• Not dependent on laboratory availability	••• Excellent esthetics •• Good marginal adaptation
DISADVANTAGES	DISADVANTAGES
• More expensive equipment •• Variability in marginal adaptation	••• At least two appointments required for completion • Impressions required • Temporization required •• Dependent on laboratory availability

Analysis/Decision The clinician chose the CAD/CAM porcelain inlays because they can be made chairside, which is much faster than Empress inlays, which must be sent to an outside dental laboratory.

*Scenario courtesty of Dr Gisele de Faira Neiva.

jacket crown An all-porcelain crown.

modulus of rupture The flexural strength of a material determined by loading a beam-shaped specimen.

porcelain A white, ceramic-containing glass with a glazed surface.

residual compressive stress Stress frozen in a material that is independent of an applied force.

sintering The densification of a powdered material, usually by heating.

veneer A restoration consisting of a thin layer of translucent porcelain or composite that covers the facial and incisal portions of teeth to improve esthetics.

vitreous Glass-like in properties.

■ Discussion Questions

1. What is the biocompatibility of porcelain to soft and hard tissues that it contacts?

2. Compare the advantages of PFM with all-ceramic crowns.

3. What is the nature of the bond between porcelain and metal?

■ Study Questions

(See appendix E for answers.)

1. What is the difference between vitreous and crystalline ceramics?

2. Which ions form glasses by their incorporation into silicate systems?

3. What is the nature of the coloring agents used in dental porcelains?

4. How is a frit made?

5. How does sintering differ from complete fusion?

6. What is the role of surface tension in sintering?

7. Why are porcelains fired under vacuum?

8. Why is glazing not produced during the biscuit bake?

9. How much shrinkage occurs during the firing of porcelain?

10. Define *glass-transition temperature*.

11. Why are glasses considerably weaker under tensile stresses than under compressive stresses?

12. Why can residual stresses in ceramics be either beneficial or harmful?

13. How does the bond strength of porcelains to alloys compare with the strength of the feldspar glass alone?

14. What effect does the addition of oxide-forming elements to gold have on the wetting and bonding of porcelain enamels?

15. Using the hierarchy of evidence discussed in the book's introduction, identify the common belief that all-ceramic crowns will last longer if the core materials of the crown have a very high flexural strength.

■ References

1. O'Brien WJ, Ryge G. Relation between molecular-force calculations and observed strengths of enamel-metal interfaces. J Am Ceramic Soc 1964;47:5–8.
2. Nally JN, Meyer JM. Experimental study on the nature of the ceramic-metallic bonding [in French]. Schweiz Monatsschr Zahnheilkd 1970;80:250.
3. Van Vlack LH. Elements of Materials Science. Reading, MA: Addison-Wesley, 1959.
4. Meyer JM, O'Brien WJ, Yu R. The sintering of dental porcelain. J Dent Res 1976;52:580.
5. Warren BE. X-ray diffraction of silicate glasses. J Am Ceram Soc 1941;24:256.
6. Jones GO. Glass. London: Metheun, 1956.
7. O'Brien WJ. Dental porcelains. In: Craig RG (ed). Dental Materials Review. Ann Arbor: University of Michigan Press, 1977:123–135.
8. McLean J. The Science and Art of Dental Ceramics. Vol I. The Nature of Dental Ceramics and Their Clinical Use. Chicago: Quintessence, 1979.
9. O'Brien WJ (ed). Magnesia ceramic jacket crowns. Dent Clin North Am 1985;29:719–723.
10. Griffith AA. The phenomenon of rupture and flow in solids. Phil Trans Roy Soc 1921;A221:163–198.
11. Hullerström AK, Bergman M. Polishing systems for dental ceramics. Acta Odontol Scand 1993;51:229–234.
12. Dunn B. Applications of ceramic science to dental porcelain. In: Yamada HN (ed). Dental Porcelain: The State of the Art—1977. Los Angeles: Univ of Southern California, 1977:41–45.
13. O'Brien WJ. Strengthening mechanisms of current dental porcelains. Compend Contin Educ Dent 2000;21:625–632.
14. Glantz P-OJ. The clinical longevity of crown and bridge prostheses. In: Anusavice KJ (ed). Quality Evaluation of Dental Restorations. Chicago: Quintesscence, 1989:343–354.
15. Coornaert J, Adriaens P, DeBoever J. Long-term clinical study porcelain-fused-to-gold restorations. J Prosthet Dent 1984;51:338–342.
16. Oh W, Anusavice KJ. Effect of connector design on the fracture of all-ceramic fixed partial dentures. J Prosthet Dent 2002;87:536–542.

■ Recommended Reading

Anusavice KI, Shen C, Vermost B, Chow B. Strengthening of porcelain by ion exchange subsequent to thermal tempering. Dent Mater 1992;8:149–152.

Denry IL. Recent advances in ceramics for dentistry. Crit Rev Oral Biol Med 1996;7:134–143.

Duke S (ed). Cerec Symposium 2001. Compend Contin Educ Dent 2001;22(suppl):S3–S54.

Evans DB, O'Brien WJ. Fracture strength of glass-infiltrated–magnesia core porcelain. Int J Prosthodont 1999;12:38–44.

Felcher FR. Dental porcelains. J Am Dent Assoc 1932;19:1021.

Hodson JT. Some physical properties of three dental porcelains. J Prosthet Dent 1956;9:235.

Kelly JR. Dental ceramics: Current thinking and trends. Dent Clin North Am2004:513-530.

Kelly M, Asgar K, O'Brien WJ. Tensile strength determination of the interface between porcelain fused to gold. J Biomed Mater Res 1969;3:403–408.

Kingry WD. Introduction to Ceramics, ed 2. New York: John Wiley, 1996:791.

Lewis AF, Natarajan RT. Adhesion Science and Technology. New York: Plenum Press, 1975.

Mackert JR Jr, Ringle RD, Parry EE, et al. The relationship between oxide adherence and porcelain-metal bonding. J Dent Res 1988;67:474.

McLean JW. A higher strength of porcelain for crown and bridge work. Br Dent J 1965;119:268.

Mumford G. The porcelain fused to metal restorations. Dent Clin North Am 1965;9:241.

O'Brien WJ, Boenke KM. Properties of a hot-pressed lithium disilicate glass-ceramic [abstract]. J Dent Res 2000;79:179.

O'Brien WJ, Ryge G. Contact angles of drops of enamels on metals. J Prosthet Dent 1965;15:1094.

O'Brien WJ, Ryge G (eds).Ceramic Engineering and Science Proceedings. Columbus, OH: American Ceramic Society, Jan-Feb 1985.

Piche PW, O'Brien WJ, Groh CL, Boenke KM. Leucite content of selected dental porcelains. J Biomat Res 1994;28:603–609.

Preston JD (ed). Perspectives in Dental Ceramics. Proceedings of the Fourth International Symposium on Ceramics. Chicago: Quintessence, 1988:53.

Rekow ED. A review of the developments in dental CAD-CAM systems. Curr Opin Dent 1992;2:25.

Ryge G. Current American research on porcelain-fused-to-metal restorations. Int Dent J 1965;15:385.

Shell JS, Nielsen JP. A study of the bond between gold alloys and porcelain. J Dent Res 1962;41:1424–1437.

Sherrill CA, O'Brien WJ. The transverse strength of aluminous and feldspathic porcelains. J Dent Res 1974;53:683.

Shoher I, Whiteman A. Captek—a new capillary casting technology for ceramometal restorations. Quintessence Dent Technol 1995; 18:9.

Siervo S, Pampalone A, Siervo P, Siervo R. Where is the gap? Machinable ceramic systems and conventional laboratory restorations at a glance. Quintessence Int 1994;25:773–776.

van Dijken, Jan WV. All-ceramic restorations: Classification and clinical evaluations. Compend Cont Educ Dent 1999;20:1115–1136.

Vergano PJ, Hill DC, Uhlmann DR. Thermal expansion of feldspar glasses. J Am Ceram Soc 1967;50:59.

Vines RF, Semmelman JO. Densification of dental porcelains. J Dent Res 1957;36:950.

Weinstein M, Katz S, Weinstein AB, inventors. Fused porcelain-to-metal teeth. US Patent 3,052,982. 1962.

Weinstein M, Weinstein AB, inventors. Porcelain-covered metal-reinforced teeth. US Patent 3,052,983. 1962.

CHAPTER 16

Base Metal Casting Alloys

Chromium-containing **base metal casting alloys** have been used in dentistry for almost 80 years. The attractiveness of these materials stems from their corrosion resistance, high strength and modulus of elasticity, low density, and low cost.

Chromium-type alloys are the principal materials used in the fabrication of removable partial denture (RPD) frameworks, and they enjoy wide use in fixed prosthodontic procedures as well. Alloys of similar composition to those used in removable and fixed dental restorations are available for use in dental, maxillofacial, and orthopedic implants. Figure 16-1 indicates which chromium-containing alloys are recommended for these procedures.

Alloys for Removable Partial Dentures

Alloys based on cobalt or nickel and containing a substantial amount of chromium are suitable for construction of RPD frameworks, full denture bases, and temporary tooth-borne surgical and periodontal splints. Table 16-1 shows the base metal RPD alloys that are currently available.

Alloy compositions

Cobalt-chromium

The major constituents of most available materials are about 60% cobalt and 25% to 30% chromium, which im-

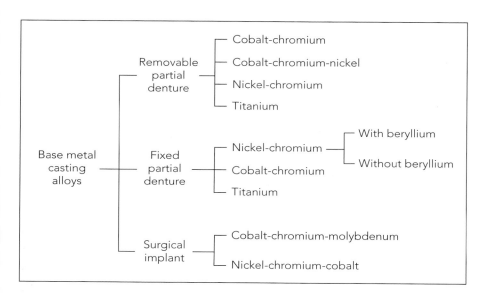

Fig 16-1 A classification of base metal casting alloys.

part corrosion resistance. They may also contain minor quantities of molybdenum, aluminum, tungsten, iron, gallium, copper, silicon, carbon, and platinum. Manganese and silicon enhance fluidity of the molten alloys; molybdenum, tungsten, and carbon are the principal hardening and strengthening elements.

Cobalt-chromium-nickel

The base of this variant of the cobalt-chromium system consists of about 50% cobalt, 25% chromium, 19% nickel, and minor components that are found in other cobalt-based products. In addition, the molybdenum level of about 3.7% and carbon level of about 0.2% in cobalt-chromium-nickel alloys are significantly lower than those of the more conventional cobalt-chromium alloys.

Nickel-chromium

A representative proprietary nickel-chromium alloy contains about 70% nickel and 16% chromium. Important minor components are about 2% aluminum and 0.5% beryllium. Aluminum and nickel form an **intermetallic compound** (Ni_3Al) that contributes to strength and hardness; and beryllium lowers the melting range, enhances fluidity, and improves grain structure. Other minor elements include molybdenum, tungsten, manganese, cobalt, silicon, and carbon.

Physical properties

Melting temperatures of the base metal RPD alloys are significantly higher than those of dental golds; a fusion temperature range of 1,399°C to 1,454°C (2,550°F to 2,650°F) is common. Chromium-type casting alloys are lighter than their gold alloy counterparts. Polished cobalt-chromium and nickel-chromium prostheses are lustrous and silvery white. Densities of the cobalt-chromium and nickel-chromium materials lie between 8 and 9 g/cm³. Lightweight materials are especially useful for the construction of large and bulky maxillary removable appliances. Linear casting shrinkage is relatively high, 2.05% to 2.33%.

Mechanical properties

Chromium-containing RPD alloys are about 30% harder than type IV golds. Usually, indentation hardness is measured on the **Rockwell hardness scale** (R-30N), and a Vickers hardness number (VHN) of 370 is typical. Appliances cast from alloys exhibiting such hardness values

Table 16-1 Chromium-type RPD alloys

ALLOY	MANUFACTURER
Vitallium	Austenal Dental
Vitallium 2	Austenal Dental
Dentorium	Dentorium Products
Regalloy	Dentsply International
JD Alloy: LG Alloy	Jelenko
Neoloy "N" Partial Alloy-Regular	Neoloy
Nobilium Alloy	Nobilium/American Gold
Ticonium Premium 100*	Ticonium
Premium Hard	Ticonium
Master Tech	Ivoclar Vivadent

*Nickel-chromium–based alloy.

must be finished and polished with special laboratory equipment.

Ultimate tensile strength values range from 90,000 to 120,000 psi (621 to 828 MPa). Values for yield strength fall between 60,000 and 90,000 psi (414 and 621 MPa) and are comparable with the yield strengths of type IV golds. When comparing yield strengths of base metals with those of golds, the amount of offset (0.1% or 0.2%) used in analysis of stress-strain diagrams must be the same for both types of materials. Use of a 0.2% offset in the evaluation of base metals is common; resulting values may be as much as 10% higher than those obtained with a 0.1% offset.

The modulus of elasticity (stiffness) of cast base metal alloys is approximately twice that of cast dental gold alloys. Thus, under a given load within the elastic limit, a structure cast from a chromium-type alloy will be deflected only half as much as a structure of comparable thickness cast from a gold alloy. Modulus of elasticity values of the cobalt-chromium and nickel-chromium RPD alloys approach 30 million psi (207 GPa).

Chromium-type alloys are brittle. Elongation values depend on casting temperature and mold conditions. Available cobalt-chromium alloys exhibit elongation values of 1% to 2%, whereas cobalt-chromium-nickel alloy, which contains lesser amounts of molybdenum and carbon than the other cobalt-based materials, shows an elongation of 10%.

The mechanical properties of cobalt-chromium–based RPD alloys can be neither improved nor controlled by heat treatment. On the other hand, the strength and ductility of some nickel-chromium alloys can be altered markedly by high-temperature heat treatment. A softening treatment (15 minutes at 982°C [1,800°F] followed by water quenching) may be used to improve workability, and subsequent rehardening (15 minutes at 704°C [1,300°F] followed by water quenching) increases the toughness of dental castings.

Chemical properties

Clinical experience indicates that RPD alloys containing a total of no less than 85% by weight of chromium, cobalt, and nickel exhibit a reasonable degree of intraoral corrosion resistance. The surfaces of these alloys are made passive in air by the spontaneous development of a thin, transparent, and contiguous chromium oxide film. This protective film reduces the corrosion rate to a relatively low level.

Recently, it was shown that thin coatings of electrolytic zirconium oxide (ZrO_2) deposited on cobalt-chromium alloys reduce chromium-release levels in artificial saliva, as compared with uncoated cobalt-chromium alloys. The coated alloys also exhibit better corrosion resistance than their uncoated counterparts.

Modification or repair of a cobalt-chromium-molybdenum RPD framework should not be accomplished with a different alloy (cobalt-chromium-nickel, for instance). If a gold braze were used to join these dissimilar alloys, the least noble component (cobalt-chromium-nickel) would undergo corrosion in a galvanic couple with the gold brazing alloy.

All chromium-type alloys are attacked vigorously by chlorine; household bleaches should not be used for cleaning appliances made from chromium alloys.

Manipulation

Alloys melting above 1,300°C (2,372°F) should not be cast in gypsum investments. High-fusing alloys require the use of **ethyl silicate–** or **phosphate-bonded investment** materials. These investments preclude the possibility of harmful sulfonation of the cast alloy, which could occur on breakdown of a conventional gypsum (calcium sulfate dihydrate) investment. The thermal expansion of ethyl silicate– and phosphate-bonded investments compen-

sates, in part, for the relatively high linear casting shrinkage of cobalt-chromium alloys. The manufacturer of one high-fusing nickel-chromium RPD alloy suggests that this product be cast into molds made from a special oxalate-protected gypsum-bonded investment.

Entrapped gases can produce voids in large castings. Care must be exercised to ensure adequate spruing and mold venting, complete wax elimination, and proper melting and casting practices to facilitate the escape of mold gases.

High-temperature equipment (oxygen/acetylene, oxygen/natural gas, or electric induction) is required. An induction melting unit equipped with an **optical pyrometer** provides the most reliable means for attaining proper melting and casting temperatures. Oxidation of the metal and the formation of brittle nitrides must be avoided.

Casting temperatures affect the microstructure and mechanical properties of chromium-type alloys. Excessive temperatures and overheating can lead to production of casting porosity and interaction between the alloy and constituents of the investment.

Simple "broken-arm" machines are not recommended for the centrifugal casting of lightweight, base metal RPD frameworks. The most satisfactory results are obtained with more complex equipment that allows for adjustment and control of acceleration, centrifugal force, and speed.

Cast molds should be set aside and bench cooled to room temperature before further handling. Investment molds can be cleaved with a small pneumatic mallet for retrieval of the castings. Oxide coatings and remnants of investment should be removed by liquid honing or abrasive blasting, rather than by "pickling" in mineral acids.

High hardness and strength make the use of high-speed laboratory equipment necessary for sprue removal, gross grinding, and finishing operations. Special stones and abrasive wheels are available.

Disadvantages

Allergic responses to the constituents of base metal alloys, especially nickel, are observed occasionally. Most adverse tissue reactions attributed to the wearing of a base metal removable prosthesis, however, are manifestations of improper design or poor fit.

Although certain physical and mechanical features of the chromium-type alloys are superior to those of RPD golds, clinical application of the chromium-containing materials may be burdened by the following occurrences:

1. Clasps cast from relatively nonductile base metal alloys can experience fatigue and break in use; some fail within a short period of time. When tested in the dry state, cobalt-chromium-molybdenum specimen bars can sustain 78,000 loading cycles. Similar tests performed in artificial saliva or water showed resistance to fatigue up to 59,000 and 36,000 loading cycles, respectively. These reductions in resistance to fatigue are attributable to corrosion of the alloy (Co-Cr-Mo) in aqueous mediums.

2. Minor but necessary adjustments required on delivery of a base metal RPD can be made difficult by the alloy's high hardness, strength, and accompanying low elongation. Such adjustments consume inordinate amounts of the clinician's valuable chair time.

3. High hardness of the alloy can cause excessive wear of restorations or natural teeth that contact the cast framework.

◼ Alloys for Fixed Partial Dentures

Castings of chromium-containing alloys are used as substructures for porcelain-veneered fixed restorations and, to a lesser extent, as all-metal restorations. Numerous varieties of chromium-type alloys are available for fixed partial denture (FPD) applications (Table 16-2).

Minor compositional differences can produce significant variations in the microstructures and properties of chromium-containing FPD alloys. Thus, previous experience with one commercial product cannot be used to predict the handling characteristics and clinical behavior of another.

Alloy compositions

Nickel-chromium
Available nickel-chromium products contain 62% to 82% nickel and 11% to 22% chromium. Common minor constituents are molybdenum, aluminum, manganese, silicon, cobalt, gallium, iron, niobium, titanium, and zirconium. Beryllium, in amounts ranging from 0.5% to 2% by weight, is a constituent of several commercial alloys.

The ease with which certain nickel-chromium alloys can be etched electrochemically has led to the wide clinical use of resin-bonded fixed prostheses, commonly known as *Maryland bridges* (Fig 16-2).

Electrochemical etching (Fig 16-3) creates a large bonding area for a resin cement and thereby precludes the concentration of occlusal stresses in narrow tags of luting medium that protrude from perforated frameworks. Also, etching minimizes exposure of the resin luting medium to untoward events that may lead to abrasion or microleakage between the resin and the metal framework.

Cobalt-chromium
Typically, these products contain about 53% to 65% cobalt and about 27% to 32% chromium. Some members of the cobalt-chromium alloy family contain 2% to 6% molybdenum. Other minor components include tungsten, iron, copper, silicon, tin, manganese, and ruthenium, a platinum group metal.

Properties

Melting ranges of the nickel-chromium and cobalt-chromium alloys are between 1,232°C and 1,454°C (2,250°F and 2,650°F). When polished, the surfaces of nickel-chromium and cobalt-chromium castings are lustrous and silvery white. These alloys are light, with densities slightly greater than 8 g/cm^3.

Available chromium-type alloys for casting single- and multiple-unit fixed restorations offer broad ranges of hardness and strength. Most, however, are harder and stronger than their noble metal FPD counterparts. Typical Rockwell values and VHNs are in the vicinity of 50 and 3,000, respectively. Ultimate tensile strength ranges from 80,000 to 150,000 psi (552 to 1,034 MPa), and yield strength is between 32,000 and 110,000 psi (221 and 779 MPa).

Modulus of elasticity values are close to 30 million psi (207 GPa). High stiffness coupled with relatively high yield strength suggests the usefulness of chromium-type alloys for the fabrication of conventional long-span fixed prostheses and thin resin-bonded cast restorations. The elongation of most chromium-containing FPD alloys is low (2% to 3%).

Bond strengths of many base metal–porcelain combinations are comparable with those of noble alloy–porcelain couples. Nevertheless, nickel-chromium-beryllium alloys produce significantly better bonding to porcelain than beryllium-free nickel-chromium alloys. Bonding of porcelain to chromium-type alloys without beryllium is in-

Table 16-2 Chromium-type FPD alloys

ALLOY	MANUFACTURER	MAJOR ELEMENTS	CONTAINS BERYLLIUM
Vera Bond	AalbaDent	Ni-Cr	Yes
Vera Soft	AalbaDent	Ni-Cr	Yes
Beta	Sterngold	Ni-Cr-Mo	Yes
Microbond NP2*	Dentsply Austenal	Ni-Cr-Ga	No
Vi-Comp	Dentsply Austenal	Co-Cr-Mo	No
Biobond II	Dentsply International	Ni-Cr-V	Yes
Neptune	Jeneric Industries	Ni-Cr-Mo	No
Novarex	Jeneric Industries	Co-Cr-W	No
Rex V	Jeneric Industries	Ni-Cr-Mo	Yes
Rexalloy	Jeneric Industries	Ni-Cr-Mo	No
Rexillium III	Jeneric Industries	Ni-Cr-Mo	Yes
Crown Cast*	Jeneric Industries	Co-Cr-Si	No
Albond	Jensen Industries	Ni-Cr-Mo	No
Unitbond	Jensen Industries	Ni-Cr-Mo	Yes
Neobond II	Neoloy	Co-Cr-W	No
Neobond II Special	Neoloy	Co-Cr-W	No
NPX III*	Nobilium/American Gold	Ni-Cr	Yes
NuPent	Pentron	Co-Cr-W	No
Pent V	Pentron	Ni-Cr-Mo	Yes
Pentillium	Pentron	Ni-Cr-Mo	Yes
PNP	Pentron	Ni-Cr-Mo	No
Safety Bond	Pentron	Ni-Cr-Mo	No
Wonder White*	Pentron	Co-Cr-Si	No
Ultra NP	3M ESPE	Ni-Cr	No
Ultra 100	3M ESPE	Co-Cr	No
Will-Ceram Litecast B	Ivoclar Vivadent	Ni-Cr-Mo	Yes
Will-Ceram Litecast	Ivoclar Vivadent	Ni-Cr-Mo	No

*Not used with fused porcelain.

hibited by thick oxides that accrue on the underlying cast framework. Usually bond failure occurs within the oxide layer.

Nickel-chromium and cobalt-chromium alloys have higher in vitro corrosion rates than dental golds. The clinical significance of this finding, however, is not known. Overall, nickel-chromium and cobalt-chromium FPD alloys are sensitive to routine dental laboratory procedures. Castings of these alloys are not as accurate as those cast from type III and type IV golds and low-gold alloys. However, when castings are oversized, discrepancies involving margins are relatively small. Thus, it is difficult to produce a cast chromium-type crown with acceptable retention and proper margins.

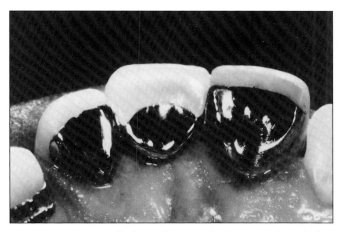

Fig 16-2 Resin-bonded prosthesis with abutments bonded to enamel. (Courtesy of Dr Van P. Thompson.)

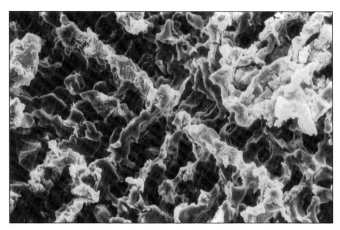

Fig 16-3 Microstructure of an etched Ni-Cr-Mo-Al-Be alloy showing dendritic structure. (Courtesy of Dr Van P. Thompson.)

Manipulation

The alloys' high melting and casting temperatures mandate the use of phosphate-bonded investments. Burnout temperatures of 732°C to 927°C (1,350°F to 1,700°F) are required, and 815°C (1,500°F) is most commonly used.

The thermal expansion of some available "high-heat" investments does not compensate adequately for the casting shrinkage of chromium-type FPD alloys. Often, copings and crowns tend to be undersized. Many of the problems encountered in the adjustment and seating of undersized, tight-fitting copings and crowns, however, can be obviated by the judicious use of a so-called die spacer. Researchers and clinicians agree that the castability of nickel-chromium-beryllium alloys is better than that of beryllium-free chromium-type alloys.

High-temperature equipment (acetylene/oxygen, natural gas/oxygen, or electric induction) is required for melting. Oxides that form during heating of the alloy prevent coalescing of the molten ingots. After casting, the lightweight oxides formed on melting the alloy will remain in the crucible as slag.

High hardness and strength necessitate the use of high-speed laboratory engines and special abrasive disks and stones for sprue removal and finishing. The use of inappropriate equipment and metal-removing instruments is time-consuming and ineffective.

The refractory oxides that form on chromium-type alloys, especially those containing beryllium, make soldering a difficult task. Solder joints exposed to high masticatory forces are unreliable. Whenever possible, multiple-component fixed frameworks should be cast in one piece.

Surface preparation of substrate castings is critical. The porcelain-bearing surface of the cast framework must be ground and finished with successively finer ceramic-bonded aluminum oxide stones. The use of resin-bonded disks and other resin-bonded metal removal devices may deposit a resin-rich layer of debris on the metal's bonding surface, which may preclude the future development of the proper surface oxide.

The ground surfaces of the framework should be pressure blasted with clean, unrecycled fine-grit aluminum oxide until all scratches made by grinding are obliterated. Then the framework must be cleaned ultrasonically in an industrial detergent. The use of household detergents for the cleaning of cast frameworks should be avoided because they tend to bleach tenacious surface debris rather than facilitate its removal.

After cleaning, the frameworks should be transferred with a hemostat to a beaker containing deionized water and rinsed ultrasonically. All subsequent handling of the cleaned and rinsed framework must be accomplished with a clean metallic instrument to prevent contamination of the bonding surface by organic materials.

Manufacturers' instructions regarding thermal conditioning (*desorbing* or *degassing*), choice of porcelain, and fusion procedure should be followed explicitly.

Biologic effects

Alloys containing nickel are risky due to the high inci-dence of nickel allergenic sensitivity, especially among women.[1,2] Many patients become aware of allergic re-sponses to alloys through wearing jewelry. In recognition of this problem, hypoallergenic pierced earrings do not contain nickel. Therefore, it is essential for clinicians to take a careful health history of patients before consider-ing the use of alloys containing nickel for either crowns or fixed or removable partial dentures. Clinicians should also discuss the use of nickel alloys with the dental tech-nicians working with them. It is not unusual for dental lab-oratories to categorize alloys containing nickel in a gen-eral category of nonprecious dental alloys without taking sufficient caution with regard to their use.

Nonetheless, with respect to biologic safety, it must be understood that corrosion is the most relevant be-havior of base metal dental alloys. Elements released in the mouth during corrosion can cause local toxicity, al-lergy, and carcinogenesis. Worries concerning systemic effects of casting alloys are based on meager evidence. On the other hand, local toxic effects are not well docu-mented but involve high risk, because local tissues are exposed to high concentrations of released metal ions. Beryllium, a component of several chromium-type base metal casting alloys, is a mutagen and, in different forms, is a known carcinogen.

Auger electron microscopy and electrochemical tests concerning four nickel-chromium FPD alloys demonstrated that beryllium-free alloys are more resistant to acceler-ated corrosion than beryllium-containing alloys. After cold sterilization, all four alloys showed lower corrosion rates in cell culture solutions.

Corrosion products of nickel-based alloys released to cell culture media do not alter cellular morphology or viability of human gingival fibroblasts, but they reduce cellular proliferation. However, metal ions released from nickel-based dental casting alloys interfere with cellular energy metabolism. Ion release stops glucose-6-phosphate dehydrogenase activity and reduces cellular **adenosine triphosphate (ATP)**.

Dusts from grinding nickel- and beryllium-containing alloys should be avoided. Work areas must be equipped with adequate air-exchange systems and kept free from dust. In addition, laboratory personnel should be equipped with individual respirators.

Advantages and disadvantages

The nickel-chromium alternatives to noble FPD alloys offer high strength, stiffness, and hardness at a seemingly low cost. Nonetheless, some significant disadvantages accompany their selection and clinical application. High hardness complicates occlusal adjustment, polishing, restoration removal, and endodontic opening. Usually, laboratory labor is more costly for base metal fixed restorations than for noble alloy restorations because the former's properties and technique sensitivities increase working time. Often, material cost savings are negated by increased labor costs and risks for allergic reactions.

◉ Surgical Alloys

Presently, most permanent dental implants are machined from highly biocompatible, commercially pure titanium. Nonetheless, chromium-type casting alloys exhibiting a sufficient degree of electropassivity are available for use in bone surgery as plates, screws, **intermedullary** bars and trays, and posts for anchorage of fixed and remov-able dental prostheses.

Alloy compositions

Two chromium-type alloy systems are available. One is based on about 60% cobalt and 32% chromium (Vital-lium, Dentsply Austenal) and the other contains about 54% nickel, 25% chromium, and 15% cobalt (surgical ticonium, Ticonium). These alloy systems use about 4% molybdenum, 0.5% silicon, and 0.6% iron, and both con-tain manganese and carbon. In the cobalt-chromium–based alloy, however, the contents of manganese (about 0.7%) and carbon (about 0.4%) are 24 and 30 times greater, respectively, than in the nickel-chromium-cobalt alloy.

Properties

Liquidus temperatures of chromium-type surgical alloys are in the vicinity of 1,554°C (2,650°F). When highly pol-ished, the surfaces of cast surgical devices are lustrous and silvery white. Most implant devices, however, are left with a dull matte finish. The surgical alloys are light; their densities (about 8 g/cm^3) are comparable with those of chromium-type RPD alloys.

Chromium-type surgical alloys offer a wide choice of mechanical properties (Table 16-3). Chemically, these alloys are not inert, although in vivo and in vitro testing has shown that these materials are more resistant to corrosion than many stainless steels used in implants. Placement of cast screws and pins requires the use of instruments made from the same alloy to prevent corrosion by the interaction of dissimilar metals.

Manipulation

The same factors that are important to the proper handling of chromium-containing RPD alloys must be considered with respect to the selection of investment materials, melting and casting techniques, and finishing procedures for chromium-type surgical alloys.

Biologic effects

Implanted metallic bodies can stimulate both generic and specific local responses. A **generic tissue response** is evidenced by fibrous encapsulation of the implant. This reaction may be a manifestation of rejection or merely a reparative response to surgical trauma. **Specific tissue responses** are induced by identifiable chemical, physical, and mechanical factors.

Chemical responses are traceable to corrosion of the implant. Regardless of alleged corrosion resistance, any metal or alloy placed in contact with tissue will exhibit some degree of ionization or solubility. The severity of a chemical response is related directly to the concentration of metal ions released into the tissue. Ions in local tissues can be transported to various distant organs, particularly the lungs, liver, and spleen, regardless of the implant site.

Mass, size, and configuration of the implant can influence biologic tolerance. The availability of casting alloys suitable for implantation has encouraged the use of massive forms with greater surface areas. Large surface areas create potential spaces at implant-tissue interfaces, which can be transformed into **adventitious bursae**. Large metallic implants are more likely to elicit signs of clinical failure than are smaller ones. Sharp edges and protuberances can injure intervening soft tissue, and movement of the implant resulting from improper stabilization may produce painful bursae and **decubitus ulcers**.

The formation of an adventitious bursa is an early sign of implant rejection. Continued irritation by corrosion or movement can cause pain, swelling, and necrosis, thereby necessitating removal of the implant. Complete rejection is manifested by the formation of fistulae or by frank extrusion.

Solutions containing nickel ions are known to elicit expression of inflammatory mediators. Also, it is known that exposing keratinocytes, monocytes, or endothelial cells to solutions containing nickel ions causes expression of inflammatory mediators, such as **interleukin 1β**, **tumor necrosis factor α**, and **intercellular adhesion molecules**.

Advantages and disadvantages

The availability of surgical casting alloys makes possible the on-site preoperative construction of customized replacements for various parts of the mandible and the facial bones. Cobalt-chromium-molybdenum, the most commonly used chromium-type surgical alloy, is especially suited for the management of situations with high strength requirements. On the other hand, the nickel-chromium-cobalt–based material offers good ductility and lower hardness and yield strength. These features may allow adjustment or shaping often required during the placement of cast implant devices.

Over the years, problems associated with surgical alloy–tissue interaction have catalyzed the search for alloplasts that exhibit a greater degree of inertness. Today, the need for this feature in dental endosteal implants is being met by the remarkable metal titanium.

Table 16-3 Mechanical properties of surgical alloys[3]

PROPERTY	COBALT-CHROMIUM	NICKEL-CHROMIUM-COBALT
Tensile strength (psi)	130,000	68,000
Yield strength* (psi)	100,000	48,000
Proportional limit (psi)	69,000	38,000
Modulus of elasticity ($\times 10^6$ psi)	36	29
Elongation (%)	2	20
Hardness (R-30N)	54	19

*0.2% offset

● Commercially Pure Titanium and Its Alloys

Commercially pure titanium

The following features make commercially pure titanium (CPTi) an attractive alternative to chromium-type surgical, RPD, and FPD alloys: low cost, low density, nonstrategic geopolitical status, mechanical properties that resemble those of hard and extra-hard casting golds, high corrosion resistance, and remarkable biocompatibility.

"Commercially pure" disclaims 100% purity and acknowledges that small amounts of oxygen (0.18% to 0.40% by weight) and iron (0.20% to 0.50% by weight) are combined with titanium. On the basis of varying oxygen and iron contents, CPTi is obtainable in four different grades.

Titanium crowns, multiple-unit fixed restorations, and RPD frameworks are being cast in research laboratories and in a growing number of commercial dental laboratories. Fortunately, the nucleus of trained titanium technicians continues to grow, as continued improvements in melting and casting technologies and mold fabrication procedures are needed in this area. The titanium learning curve is steep and comparable with the curve involving the substitution of chromium-type alloys for conventional golds. Clearly, continuous progress is being made in developing solutions to problems encountered in casting a low-density (4.5 g/cm^3) metal that melts at temperatures in the vicinity of 1,700°C (3,092°F); possesses a strong affinity for oxygen, hydrogen, and nitrogen; and reacts with the components of most investment materials. Thus, attempts to minimize the effects of these untoward factors are starting to improve casting efficiency by favorably affecting the filling of molds with molten metal. Complete "mold fills" ensure the production of complete castings.

Attainment of a small marginal gap width between the restoration and tooth structure requires a complete mold fill. In a clinical study of margin quality, the marginal discrepancies for titanium and gold restorations were 72 ± 18 μm and 64 ± 18 μm for titanium and gold, respectively. Although gap widths in titanium restorations did not match the gold standard, the data justify the use of titanium as an alternative to gold for inlay and onlay restorations.

However, it appears that little or no progress is being made toward improvement of the soundness of castings. Micro- and macroporosity remain consistent features of dental restorations cast from titanium. One study reports that the use of a double-sprue technique for titanium copings produces smoother cast surfaces and less internal porosity than a single-sprue design. Also remaining to be resolved definitively is the inordinate amount of difficulty experienced in making relatively thin castings.

To make a suitable titanium coping for a porcelain-fused-to-metal restoration, the pattern is usually waxed to a thickness of about 0.6 mm. The resultant casting must be machined to the desired thickness. When heated in air at temperatures in the vicinity of 750°C (1,382°F), titanium becomes embrittled through the absorption of oxygen, hydrogen, and nitrogen. Such embrittlement may cause thin margins of restorations to fracture during burnishing. When heated at temperatures below 800°C (1,472°F) for short periods, titanium of high purity (or CPTi) forms a compact, adherent oxide scale. Moreover, at higher temperatures and extended periods of heat treatment, titanium forms a porous and poorly adherent scale.

During a few successive firings of a low-fusing (750°C), low-expansion (7.1 × 10^{-6}/°C on cooling) porcelain to titanium, the smooth adherent oxide produced on degassing at 750°C thickens and becomes flaky. An oxide of this type precludes attainment of a reliable porcelain-to-metal bond.

A study comparing titanium and titanium alloy (Ti-6Al-4V) with cobalt-chromium RPD clasps placed in 0.75-mm undercut specimens produced the following results[4]:

1. Over 3 years of simulated clinical use, there was less loss of retention for clasps made from CPTi and Ti-6Al-4V than for cobalt-chromium clasps.
2. Porosity in pure titanium and Ti-6Al-4V clasps was greater than for cobalt-chromium clasps.
3. The observed porosity in the titanium clasps did not provide proof of fracture or permanent deformation.

In another study, fatigue resistance of cast clasps made from an experimental titanium alloy (Ti-50.8Ni) was compared with clasps cast from CPTi, cobalt-chromium alloy, and a gold-silver-palladium-copper alloy.[2,5] The clasp tips were engaged in 0.25- and 0.50-mm undercut areas of abutments. No significant changes in retentive force were observed for Ti-nickel clasps in 1,010 repeated cycles. During testing, the other three clasp types showed a significant decrease in the force required for removal from the retentive undercuts.

Properties

At room temperature, the lattice configuration of virgin CPTi is hexagonal close packed. This atomic arrangement, known as the α *phase*, persists until the metal is exposed to high temperatures. On reaching its transus temperature of 833°C (1,531°F), titanium's entire habit becomes body-centered cubic. This crystal lattice is known as the β *phase*. Fabricated titanium structures consisting mainly of β phase are stronger but less ductile than comparable structures with a dominant α phase. Thus, to obtain consistently reproducible mechanical properties, the solidified metal's cooling rate and the time and temperature of subsequent heat treatments must be controlled.

The tensile strength and elongation of pure titanium are about 36,250 psi (250 MPa) and 50%, respectively. However, seemingly slight variations in oxygen and iron content exert substantial and lasting effects on titanium's properties. Generally, as oxygen or iron content increases, strength increases and ductility decreases. Furthermore, the consequences of titanium-oxygen interactions seem to vary according to melting and casting practices. When melted and cast with the use of an argon arc–centrifugal casting machine, yield strength (0.2% offset), ultimate tensile strength, and elongation for grade 1 CPTi are about 84,000 psi (579 MPa), 101,600 psi (701 MPa), and 18%, respectively. Comparatively, castings made in an argon-tungsten arc vacuum pressure machine exhibit greater ductility (elongation = 31%), but yield strength and tensile strength drop to 11,300 psi (285 MPa) and 53,000 psi (365 MPa), respectively.

Titanium's elastic modulus of about 17 million psi (117 GPa) is higher than those of type III and type IV casting golds (~100 GPa), but lower than those of most chromium-type alloys (171 to 218 GPa). The VHN of cast CPTi is 210.

Titanium alloys

Only a few titanium alloys are being used in the United States for the commercial production of fixed or removable dental prostheses. Nevertheless, there is a high level of interest within the dental research community. Titanium alloys of interest include Ti-30Pd, Ti-20Cu, Ti-15V, and Ti-6Al-4V.

Alloying other metals with titanium requires lower melting and casting temperatures. Also, it provides a means to stabilize, or expand, either the α phase field or the β phase field. In Ti-13Nb-13Zr, niobium and zirconium expand the β phase field by decreasing the α + β transus temperature. Conversely, in Ti-6Al-4V, aluminum is an α stabilizer because it increases the α + β to β transformation temperature and thereby expands the α phase field. Accordingly, Ti-13Nb-13Zr is a near-β alloy with a substantially lower β transus (735°C) than Ti-6Al-4V (1,000°C), which has an α + β structure.

The effects of interactions with atmospheric gases during melting, casting, and other high-temperature laboratory procedures are as destructive to titanium alloys as they are to unalloyed titanium. Thus, the problems encountered in producing cast dental restorations from titanium alloys are not unlike those experienced with titanium of high or commercial purity.

Properties

The ultimate tensile strength, 0.2% offset yield strength, and modulus of elasticity of various titanium alloys range from 101,500 to 142,800 psi (700 to 985 MPa); 81,200 to 124,700 psi (560 to 860 MPa); and 16 million to 17 million psi (110 to 117 GPa), respectively. Except for modulus of elasticity, the tensile properties of titanium alloys are similar to those of chromium-type alloys.

Biologic effects

The corrosion resistance and biocompatibility of titanium at room, oral, and body temperatures are attributed to the formation of a stable oxide film with a thickness of less than 1 nm (10^{-9} m). If the film is scratched or abraded, the involved area repassivates instantaneously. At high temperatures, the oxide film is not protective because it thickens and becomes nonadherent.

Numerous reports document the superior biocompatibility of titanium.[6] The reaction of tissue that contacts titanium or its alloys, Ti-6Al-4V and Ti-13Nb-13Zr, is extremely mild, and direct bone ingrowth or osseointegration does occur. See chapter 23 for further information on osseointegration with titanium.

The need for simple, reliable, and reasonably priced technology that would make the routine production of titanium dental restorations in any dental laboratory possible may be fulfilled through computer-aided design and computer-aided manufacturing (CAD/CAM). These technologies are being used routinely to produce customized titanium valvular and titanium hip prostheses.

◉ Glossary

adenosine triphosphate (ATP) A nucleotide compound occurring in all cells but chiefly in striated muscle tissue; it represents the energy reserve of the cell.

adventitious bursa Fluid-filled cyst formed between two parts as a result of friction.

base metal alloy An alloy composed of metals that are neither precious nor noble.

decubitus ulcer Superficial loss of tissue on the surface of skin or mucosa, usually with inflammation, caused by pressure.

ethyl silicate–bonded investment A silica refractory bonded by hydrolysis of ethyl silicate in the presence of hydrochloric acid.

generic tissue response A reaction that cannot be attributed to a specific characteristic of a foreign body or substance.

intercellular adhesion molecules Chemokines that regulate lymphocyte and leukocyte migration, roles of integrins involving interactions of lymphocytes with intestinal mucosa, lymphocyte movement through the central nervous system, and tumor immunotherapy.

interleukin 1β A cytokine produced especially by monocytes and macrophages that regulates immune responses by activating lymphocytes and mediates other biologic processes such as inflammation and infection.

intermedullary Between bone marrow spaces.

intermetallic compound A definite combination by weight between metals. These compounds have specific, reproducible physical characteristics.

optical pyrometer A device to measure temperature by matching the color of an electrically heated wire to the color of the surface being tested. The current required is calibrated against temperature.

phosphate-bonded investment Used in casting high-melting alloys. Contains a mixture of silica with a metallic oxide and a phosphate that combine to bind the silica together. On heating, forms complex silicophosphates that increase the strength of the mold.

Rockwell hardness scale (R-30N) An indication of resistance to penetration of balls or metal cones of differing diameters under different loads.

specific tissue response A reaction caused by a definite characteristic of a foreign body or substance.

tumor necrosis factor α A cytokine (one of a class of immunoregulatory substances secreted by cells of the immune system) produced mainly by monocytes and macrophages. It is found in synovial cells and macrophages in the tissues.

◉ Discussion Questions

1. What are the biocompatibility problems associated with high nickel and cobalt alloys?

2. What are the advantages and disadvantages of Ni-Cr alloys for porcelain-fused-to-metal restorations?

3. Compare the relative clinical advantages and disadvantages of gold and Co-Cr alloys for RPDs.

4. What are the advantages and disadvantages of titanium as an alloy for porcelain-fused-to-metal FPDs?

◉ Study Questions

(See appendix E for answers.)

1. What are the three major types of chromium-containing dental casting alloys?

2. How do the mechanical properties of chromium-type FPD alloys differ from those of dental gold alloys?

3. Which properties of the chromium-type alloys make these materials suitable for the fabrication of long-span FPDs?

4. What effect do excessive surface oxides have on the bonding of porcelain to chromium-type alloys?

5. How do the tensile properties of cast titanium alloys compare with those of chromium-type alloys?

RPD alloys: true/false statements

1. Certain minor components strengthen cobalt-chromium–based alloys.

2. The performance potential of cobalt-chromium castings is enhanced by nitride inclusions and excessive metallic carbides.

3. Low density is a useful characteristic of chromium-type RPD alloys.

4. The hardness and strength of chromium-type RPD alloys are essentially the same as those of type IV gold alloys.

5. In function, a chromium-type RPD framework is more likely to flex than one cast from a type IV gold alloy.

6. Chromium-containing removable prostheses should be cleaned regularly in household bleaches.

7. Gypsum investments are not recommended for the casting of cobalt-chromium alloys.

8. Casting temperatures for cobalt-chromium alloys must be controlled carefully.

9. Conventional laboratory equipment and techniques can be used to finish cobalt-chromium and nickel-chromium castings.

10. Sensitivity to one or more alloy components accounts for a significant incidence of adverse tissue response among wearers of nonprecious-type RPDs.

FPD alloys: true/false statements

1. Chromium-containing FPD alloys are based entirely on the nickel-chromium system.

2. The mechanical properties of the chromium-type FPD alloys are slightly inferior to the properties of dental gold alloys.

3. Certain properties of chromium-type alloys make them suitable for fabrication of long-span fixed restorations.

4. Except for modulus of elasticity, the tensile properties of some titanium alloys are comparable with those of chromium-type alloys.

5. The ability of chromium-type alloys to form surface oxides when exposed to temperatures used in the porcelain firing cycle ensures the development of a strong and reliable porcelain-to-metal bond.

6. The biocompatibility of CPTi, certain titanium alloys, and chromium-type FPD alloys is well documented.

Surgical casting alloys: true/false statements

1. The tensile properties and hardness of nickel-chromium-cobalt and cobalt-chromium surgical alloys are comparable.

2. Chemical factors alone influence tissue response to alloy implants.

3. Metallic ions liberated from an alloy implant can be transported to distant organs.

4. The surface area of a metallic implant plays a prominent role in biologic acceptance.

5. Certain clinical signs signal complete rejection of an implant device.

References

1. Peltonen L. Nickel sensitivity in the general population. Contact Dermatitis 1979;5:27–29.
2. Wataha JC. Biocompatibility of dental casting alloys: A review. J Prosthet Dent 2000;83:223–234.
3. Civjan S, Huget EF, Godfrey GD, Lichtenberger H, Frank WA. Effects of heat treatment on mechanical properties of two nickel-chromium-based casting alloys. J Dent Res 1972;51:1537–1545.
4. Bridgeman JT, Marker VA, Hummel SK, Benson BW, Pace LL. Comparison of titanium and cobalt-chromium removable partial denture clasps. J Prosthet Dent 1997;78:187–193.
5. Kotake M, Wakabayashi N, Ai M, Yoneyama T, Hamanaka H. Fatigue resistance of titanium-nickel alloy cast clasps. Int J Prosthodont 1997;10:547–552.
6. Wataha JC, Lockwood PE, Marek M, Ghazi M. Ability of Ni-containing biomedical alloys to activate monocytes and endothelial cells in vitro. J Biomed Mater Res 1999;45:251–257.

Recommended Reading

Chromium-type RPD alloys

Asgar K, Techow BO, Jacobson JM. A new alloy for partial dentures. J Prosthet Dent 1970;23:36–43.

Bates JF. Studies related to the fracture of partial dentures: Flexural fatigue of a cobalt-chromium alloy. Br Dent J 1965;118:532–537.

Bumgardner JD, Lucas LC. Cellular response to metallic ions released from nickel-chromium dental alloys. J Dent Res 1995;74:1521–1527.

Carter JJ, Kidd JN. The precision casting of cobalt-chromium alloys. Part I. The influence of casting variables on dimensions and finish. Br Dent J 1965;118:383.

Earnshaw R. Further measurements of the casting shrinkage of dental cobalt-chromium alloys. Br Dent J 1960;109:238.

Hsu HC, Yen SK. Evaluation of metal ion release and corrosion resistance of ZrO2 thin coatings on the dental Co-Cr alloys. Dent Mater 1998;14:339–346.

Kotake M, Wakabayashi N, Ai M, Yoneyama T, Hamanaka H. Fatigue resistance of titanium-nickel alloy cast clasps. Int J Prosthodont 1997;10:547–552.

Lassila LV, Vallittu PK. Effect of water and artificial saliva on the low cycle fatigue resistance of cobalt-chromium dental alloy. J Prosthet Dent 1998;80:708–713.

Luthy H, Marinello CP, Reclaru L, Scharer P. Corrosion considerations in the brazing repair of cobalt-based partial dentures. J Prosthet Dent 1996;75:515–524.

Osborne J. Improvement in cobalt-chromium alloys. Rev Belge Med Dent 1966;21:303–310.

Paffenbarger GC, Caul HJ, Dickson G. Base metal alloys for oral restorations. J Am Dent Assoc 1943;30:825.

Taylor DF, Leibfritz WA, Alder AG. Physical properties of cobalt-chromium alloys. J Am Dent Assoc 1958;56:343.

Taylor TD, Morton TH Jr. Ulcerative lesions of the palate associated with removable partial denture castings. J Prosthet Dent 1991;66:213–221.

Chromium-type FPD alloys

American Dental Association, Council on Dental Materials, Instruments, and Equipment. Report on base metal alloys for crown and bridge applications: Benefits and risks. J Am Dent Assoc 1985;111:479–483.

Anusavice KJ, Shafagh I. Inert gas presoldering of nickel-chromium alloys. J Prosthet Dent 1986;55:317–323.

Bertolotti RL. Alternative casting alloys for today's crown-and-bridge restorations. Part I. All metal restorations. J Calif Dent Assoc 1983; 11:37.

Bezzon OL, de Mattos M, Ribeiro RF, Rollo JM. Effect of beryllium on the castability and resistance of ceramometal bonds in nickel-chromium alloys. J Prosthet Dent 1998;80:570–574.

Bumgardner JD, Doeller J, Lucas LC. Effect of nickel-based dental casting alloys on fibroblast metabolism and ultrastructural organization. J Biomed Mater Res 1995;29:611–617.

Bumgardner JD, Lucas LC. Corrosion and cell culture evaluations of nickel-chromium dental casting alloys. J Appl Biomater 1994;5: 203–213.

Hansson O. Casting accuracy of a nickel and beryllium-free cobalt-chromium alloy for crown and bridge prostheses and resin-bonded bridges. Swed Dent J 1985;9:105–115.

Huget EF, Dvivedi N, Cosner HE Jr. Properties of two nickel-chromium crown-and-bridge alloys for porcelain veneering. J Am Dent Assoc 1977;94:87–90.

Huget EF, Vilca JM, Wall RM. Characterization of two ceramic-base metal alloys. J Prosthet Dent 1978;40:637–641.

Livaditis GJ, Thompson VP. Etched castings: An improved retentive mechanism for resin-bonded retainers. J Prosthet Dent 1982;47: 52–58.

Messer RL, Lucas LC. Cytotoxicity of nickel-chromium alloys: Bulk alloys compared to multiple ion salt solutions. Dent Mater 2000; 16:207–212.

Moffa JP. Physical and mechanical properties of gold and base metal alloys. Alternatives to Gold Alloys in Dentistry. Bethesda, Md: National Institutes of Health, 1977;81–87.

Moffa JP, Guckes AD, Okawa MT, Lilly GE. An evaluation of non-precious alloys for use with porcelain veneers. Part II. Industrial safety and biocompatibility. J Prosthet Dent 1973;30:432.

Moffa JP, Jenkins WA. Status report on base-metal crown and bridge alloys. J Am Dent Assoc 1974;89:652–655.

Morris HF. Veterans Administration Cooperative Studies Project No. 147/242. Part VII: The mechanical properties of metal ceramic alloys as cast and after simulated porcelain firing. J Prosthet Dent 1989;61:160–169.

Morris HF, Manz M, Stoffer W, Weir D. Casting alloys: The materials and the clinical effects. Adv Dent Res 1992;6:28–31.

O'Connor RP, Mackert JR Jr, Myers ML, Parry EE. Castability, opaque masking, and porcelain bonding of 17 porcelain-fused-to-metal alloys. J Prosthet Dent 1996;75:367–374.

Sandrik JL, Kaminski EJ, Greener EH. Biocompatibility of nickel-base dental alloys. Biomater Med Devices Artif Organs 1974;2:31.

Sarkar NK, Greener EH. In vitro corrosion resistance of new dental alloys. Biomater Med Devices Artif Organs 1973;1:121–129.

Sced IR, McLean JW. The strength of metal-ceramic bonds with base metals containing chromium. A preliminary report. Br Dent J 1972;132:232–234.

Vermilyea SG, Tamura JJ, Mills DE. Observations on nickel-free, beryllium-free alloys for fixed prostheses. J Am Dent Assoc 1983; 106:36–38.

Wataha JC. Biocompatibility of dental casting alloys: A review. J Prosthet Dent 2000;83:223–234.

Winkler S, Morris HF, Monterio JM. Changes in mechanical properties and microstructure following heat treatment of a nickel-chromium base alloy. J Prosthet Dent 1984;52:821–827.

Chromium-type surgical alloys

Civjan S, Huget EF, Erhard WL, Vaccaro GJ. Properties of surgical casting alloys. J Prosthet Dent 1972;28:77–81.

Cohen J. Corrosion testing of orthopaedic implants. J Bone Joint Surg 1962;44:307–316.

Ferguson AB, Akahoshi Y, Laing PG, Hodge ES. Characteristics of trace ions released from embedded metal implants in the rabbit. J Bone Joint Surg Am 1962;44:323–336.

Ferguson AB, Akahoshi Y, Laing PG, Hodge ES. Trace metal ion concentration in the liver, kidney, spleen, and lung of normal rabbits. J Bone Joint Surg Am 1962;44:317–322.

Hicks JH, Cater WH. Minor reactions due to modern metal. J Bone Joint Surg Br 1962;44-B:122–128.

Shettlemore MG, Bundy KJ. Toxicity of aqueous metal solutions representative of ionic degradation products using a bioluminescent bacterial assay. J Biomed Mater Res 1999;45:395.

Titanium and titanium alloys

Adachi M, Mackert JR Jr, Parry EE, Fairhurst CW. Oxide adherence and porcelain bonding to titanium and Ti-6Al-4V alloy. J Dent Res 1990;69:1230.

Albrektsson T, Brånemark PI, Hansson HA, Lindstrom J. Osseointegrated titanium implants. Requirements for ensuring long-lasting, direct bone-to-implant anchorage in man. Acta Orthop Scand 1981;52:155–170.

Al-Mesmar HS, Morgano SM, Mark LE. Investigation of the effect of three sprue designs on the porosity and the completeness of titanium cast removable partial denture frameworks. J Prosthet Dent 1999;82:15–21.

Besimo C, Jeger C, Guggenheim R. Marginal adaptation of titanium frameworks produced by CAD/CAM techniques. Int J Prosthodont 1997;10:541–546.

Blackman R, Baez R, Barghi N. Marginal accuracy and geometry of cast titanium copings. J Prosthet Dent 1992;67:435–440.

Cai Z, Bunce N, Nunn ME, Okabe T. Porcelain adherance to dental cast CP titanium. Biomaterials 2001;22:979–984.

Chan D, Guillory V, Blackman R, Chung KH. The effects of sprue design on the roughness and porosity of titanium castings. J Prosthet Dent 1997;78:400–404.

Davidson JA, Mishra AK, Kovacs PT. A new low modulus, high strength, biocompatible Ti-13Nb-13Zr alloy for orthopaedic implants. Trans Soc Biomater 1993;16:145.

Donachie MJ (ed). Titanium. A Technical Guide. Metals Park, OH: ASM International, 1988;11, 105.

Goodman SB, Davidson JA, Fornasier VL, Mishra AK. The local and systemic response to cylinders of a low modulus titanium alloy (Ti-13Nb-13Zr) and a wear resistant zirconium alloy (Zr-25Nb) implanted in the rabbit tibia. Trans Soc Biomater 1993;16:76.

Hamanaka H, Doi H, Yoneyama T, Okuno O. Dental casting of titanium and Ni-Ti alloys by a new casting machine. J Dent Res 1989; 68:1529–1533.

Hero H, Syverud M, Waarli M. Mold filling and porosity in castings of titanium. Dent Mater 1993;9:15–18.

Lintner F, Zweymuller K, Brand G. Tissue reactions to titanium endoprostheses. Autopsy studies in four cases. J Arthroplasty 1986;1: 183–195.

Lyman WS. Titanium, properties of pure metals. In: Baker H, Benjamin D (eds). Metals Handbook, ed 9, vol 2. Metals Park, OH: ASM International, 1979:815.

Menis DL, Moser JB, Greener EH. Experimental porcelain compositions for application to cast titanium [abstract 1565]. J Dent Res 1986;65:343.

Sunnerkrantz P, Syverud M, Hero H. Effects of casting atmosphere on the quality of Ti-crowns. Scand J Dent Res 1990;98:268–272.

Vallittu PK, Kokkonen M. Deflection fatigue of cobalt-chromium, titanium, and gold alloy denture clasps. J Prosthet Dent 1995;74: 412–415.

Wolf BH, Walter MH, Boening KW, Schmidt AE. Margin quality of titanium and high-gold inlays and onlays: A clinical study. Dent Mater 1998;14:370–374.

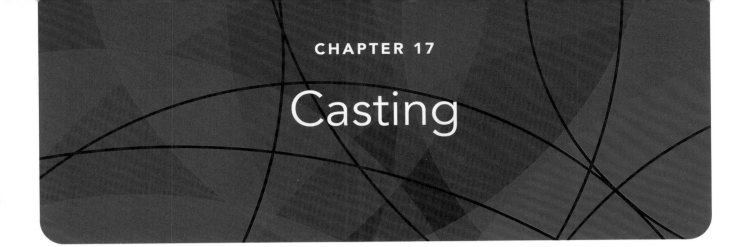

CHAPTER 17

Casting

The **lost wax casting process**, though one of the oldest existing technologies, is still the preferred and most common method for casting dental restorations. This mode of **casting** is favored because asymmetric castings incorporating extremely fine detail can be fabricated conveniently and inexpensively compared with other modes of casting.

In brief, a metal casting is made using a **refractory** mold made from a wax replica or pattern. The procedure includes the following steps:

1. Prepare the tooth or teeth to receive a cast restoration.
2. Make an impression of the prepared tooth.
3. Pour **gypsum** slurry into the impression to make a positive cast, which is an exact replica of the dental arch from which the individual **die**(s) representing the prepared tooth or teeth is sectioned.
4. Make a wax pattern that will be representative of the lost tooth structure.
5. **Sprue** the wax pattern (fix it in space) (Fig 17-1).
6. Invest the wax pattern.
7. Eliminate the wax pattern by burning the wax out of the investment in a furnace, thus making the mold.
8. Force molten metal into the mold.
9. Clean the cast.
10. Remove the sprue from the casting.
11. Finish and polish the casting on the die.
12. Cement the finished cast restoration on the prepared tooth.

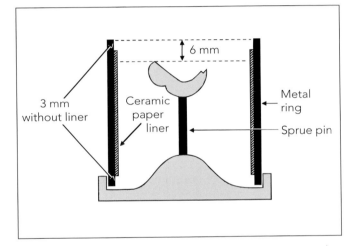

Fig 17-1 Arrangement of a pattern in a ring prior to pouring the investment material. (Modified from Craig and Peyton.[1])

When the direct technique—in which the pattern is made on the tooth rather than on the die—is used, steps 2 and 3 are omitted. The desired accuracy of the casting is about 0.1%; therefore, the lost wax procedure requires specially developed materials that compensate for the dimensional changes indicated by the following equation:

$$\text{Shrinkage (wax + alloy)} = \text{Investment expansion}$$

Table 17-1 Expansion requirements of casting

RESTORATION	EXPANSION (%)
Thin three-quarter crown	1.80
Classes 1 and 2, small MOD	1.85
Large MOD, three-quarter crown	1.90
Overlay, pin pontic	1.95
Bulky three-quarter crown	2.00
Small Class 5, full crown	2.10
Large Class 5	2.40

MOD = mesio-occlusodistal

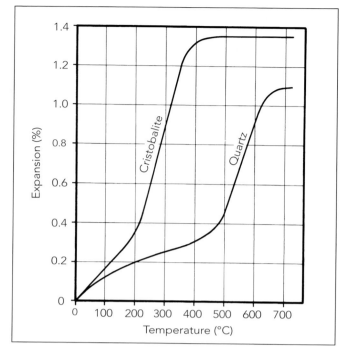

Fig 17-2 Typical TE curves for cristobalite and quartz.

■ Thermal Shrinkage

Wax

A wax pattern prepared directly in a patient's mouth will shrink about 0.4% when cooled from oral temperature. In the indirect method of preparing the wax pattern on a die, the wax shrinkage is about 0.2%.

Gold alloy

The casting shrinkage takes place as the solidified metal cools to room temperature. The values for this shrinkage depend on the geometry of the casting. For example, the gold shrinkage ranges from 1.25% for a thin three-quarter crown to 1.75% for full crowns and 2% for Class 5 restorations. Table 17-1 summarizes the average amount of mold expansion required for typical types of restorations to compensate for wax and metal shrinkages.

■ Thermal Expansion

Gypsum-bonded investment

High-heat technique

This method uses cristobalite (a high-expansion form of silica) **investment** materials (Fig 17-2). After the investment has been mixed according to the manufacturer's instructions and allowed to set for at least 45 minutes and no longer than 60 minutes, the mold is placed in a 200°C oven for 20 to 30 minutes to burn out the wax pattern. The temperature of the mold is further elevated by transferring the mold to a second oven and holding at 700°C for no longer than 20 to 30 minutes to obtain the maximum thermal expansion (TE) of 1.25% (Table 17-2). Because this type of investment is weak by nature, a metal ring must be used. To increase the setting expansion (SE) of 0.35%, the inside of the ring should be lined with a dampened liner strip that also acts as a cushion against which expansion can take place. This greater expansion caused by the uptake of water from the liner, referred to as *hygroscopic expansion* (HE), is double the normal SE (see Table 17-2). The HE cited in Table 17-2 includes the SE. Adding the 0.70% HE to the 1.25% TE gives the maximum expansion one can expect—about 1.95%. Most of the compensation is the TE that takes place after the wax pattern is eliminated from the mold. (See chapter 4.)

Water-immersion hygroscopic technique

Investments made for water immersion are much stronger than the high-heat types; therefore, a metal ring is not necessary. Instead, a rubber ring is used to contain the

Table 17-2 Mold expansion

TECHNIQUE	SETTING EXPANSION (%)	HYGROSCOPIC EXPANSION (%)	THERMAL EXPANSION (%)
High heat (cristobalite)	0.35	0.70*	1.25 (700°C)
Hygroscopic immersion (Beauty-Cast, Whip Mix)	0.30	1.50	0.55 (480°C)
Hygroscopic water added (Hygrotrol, Jelenko)	0.75	2.00	0.55 (480°C)
Phosphate–high heat (Ceramigold , Whip Mix)	0.23–0.50	0.35–1.20	1.33–1.58 (700°C)

*Wet liner.

mixed investment. Maximum HE is obtained by immersing the invested pattern and rubber ring, allowing the investment to set under water. Most of the compensatory expansion is HE (1.50%), which again includes the normal SE of 0.3% (see Table 17-2). This expansion takes place with the pattern present in the mold, which may cause distortion in certain pattern configurations (eg, mesio-occlusodistal). After the investment has set, the rubber ring is removed from the mold, and the mold is placed directly into a 480°C oven for 30 to 45 minutes to eliminate the wax and acquire the additional necessary TE of 0.55%. With a water-immersion investment, one can expect an overall expansion of 2.10%. (See chapter 4.)

Phosphate-bonded investment

This type of investment is supplied as a powder containing silica, primary ammonium phosphate ($NH_4H_2PO_4$), and magnesium oxide (MgO). The setting reaction in aqueous solution is:

$$NH_4H_2PO_4 + MgO \rightarrow NH_4MgPO_4 + H_2O$$

A phosphate investment such as Ceramigold (Whip Mix) may be mixed with a liquid containing a silica sol in water, which increases setting and HE. The expansion of a phosphate investment is adjusted by varying the amount of silica sol liquid used in mixing and by using HE and high-heat expansion methods. These investments are used for high-fusing gold alloys used with porcelain. (See chapter 19.)

Other investment systems

With the advent of alloy systems that do not incorporate any of the noble metals, a very different investment material is required because of the higher fusion or melting temperatures of the alloys. To overcome the decomposition of the gypsum- and phosphate-type investment systems, silicate investments, zircate investments and various magnesia investments may be used.

◼ Spruing

The purpose of spruing the wax pattern is fourfold:

1. To form a mount for the wax pattern and fix the pattern in space so a mold can be made
2. To create a channel for elimination of wax during burnout
3. To form a channel for the ingress of molten alloy during casting
4. To compensate for alloy shrinkage during solidification

Sprue size and design

The sprue must be large enough so that it remains open until the casting solidifies and short enough to allow rapid filling of the mold cavity. Large and small inlays require sprues that are 14 gauge (4 to 5 mm long) and 16 gauge (3 to 4 mm long), respectively. Large and small crowns require 10- and 12-gauge sprues, respectively, with an average sprue length of 4 to 5 mm.

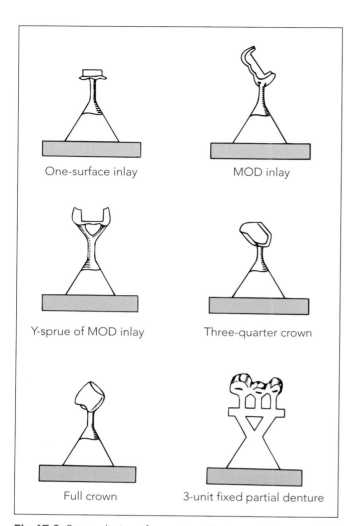

One-surface inlay

MOD inlay

Y-sprue of MOD inlay

Three-quarter crown

Full crown

3-unit fixed partial denture

Fig 17-3 Sprue designs for castings (not to scale).

Point of attachment

Sprue attachment must always be made at the bulkiest portion of the pattern (Fig 17-3). If two bulky portions of the castings are separated by a thin cross section (eg, for a mesio-occlusodistal inlay) a Y-shaped sprue (see Fig 17-3) must be used. Turbulence of the molten gold as it enters the mold causes porosity, which is due to entrapped gases and an inappropriate angle of sprue attachment. All attachments, both the sprue pattern and sprue/crucible former, must therefore be "trumpeted" or "filleted" to eliminate all sharp corners, angles, and instrument marks.

Sprue selection

The wax sprue is most common. Plastic sprues are not recommended because their higher flow temperatures and TE characteristics make it difficult to eliminate the sprue. Because the wax melts at a much lower temperature than the plastic sprue and the TE of the wax is five times that of plastic, excessive wax pressure may build up in the mold during burnout before the plastic sprue softens. A hollow metal sprue pin is preferable to a solid metal pin because of its stronger attachment. Sticky wax must be used to fill the hollow sprue core before use.

Orientation in mold

The wax pattern is mounted on the sprue pin, which in turn is mounted on a clean sprue/crucible former, as indicated in Fig 17-1. It is essential that, when the investment ring is placed over the assembly of the pattern and sprue/crucible former, the pattern be 6 mm from the end of the ring. If the pattern is less than 6 mm from the end, there is not enough thickness of investment to keep the molten gold from breaking through. If there is more than 6 mm of space, the gold will solidify before the entrapped air can escape, resulting in rounded margins, incomplete casting, or mold fracture.

Liner

A liner is placed inside the ring to allow lateral expansion of the investment, and 3 mm of clearance is allowed at each end of the ring so the mold is sealed and anchored in place. After the liner is placed in the ring, it is dipped in water until saturated, and the excess water is shaken off.

■ Melting

New metal

Since gold alloys and other alloys change composition during casting, at least one-third of new gold by weight must be used for each melt.

Contamination

Clean melting crucibles are essential to prevent alloy contamination. Copper-containing gold alloys and noncopper alloys for use with porcelain should not be melted in the same crucible. Previously cast metal must be thoroughly cleaned using appropriate fluxes to remove all gases, oxides, and investment before remelting.

Table 17-3 Methods of alloy melting

TORCH	ELECTRIC
Gas-air	Resistance
Gas-oxygen	Induction
Air-acetylene	Electric arc
Oxygen-acetylene	

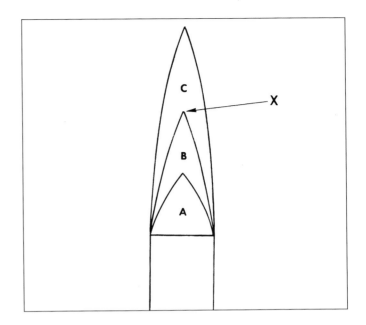

Fig 17-4 Zones of torch flame. The innermost cone (A) consists of unburnt gases and is not hot enough to melt gold. The second cone (B) is blue with burning gases and forms a reducing atmosphere. Point X is best for melting or soldering, because it is the hottest zone of the flame. The outer cone (C), which contains burnt gases, forms an oxidizing atmosphere and should be avoided.

Methods of melting

The various modes available for melting alloys may be grouped into two categories: (1) those using a torch and (2) those using some form of electric assistance, as shown in Table 17-3. Each mode has unique advantages and disadvantages, and, in general, the modes requiring some form of electric energy are more costly than those requiring a torch.

Torch melting

The natural gas/air method is the most common for melting gold alloys intended for inlays and fixed partial dentures. Such alloys require the maximum heat production that a gas/air torch is capable of generating (Fig 17-4). For gold alloys with higher fusion temperatures, such as those intended for porcelain-fused-to-metal applications, palladium alloys and some base metal alloys can be melted by the higher temperatures provided by the natural gas/oxygen torch.

Air-acetylene and oxygen-acetylene flames generate much higher temperatures, with the latter providing the hottest flame. Although air-acetylene and oxygen-acetylene modes have the advantage of melting the alloys faster than gas-air or gas-oxygen modes, the disadvantages outweigh their advantages for the following reasons:

1. Excessive heat may distill lower melting components, thus changing the composition of the alloys.
2. Overheating some alloys allows environmental gases to be dissolved in the melt, resulting in porous castings.
3. Some alloys, particularly base metal, may be excessively hardened and made too brittle due to the uptake of carbon from the acetylene flame.
4. Since the environment cannot be controlled, the extremely high temperature may cause excessive oxidation of the alloy. The newer titanium alloys cannot be melted by torch. The air-acetylene and oxygen-acetylene modes should be used only by a highly skilled technician.

Electric melting

Electric resistance melting, induction melting, and electric arc melting are types of electric melting. The former is suitable for all gold alloys, and the latter two types are capable of melting cobalt-chromium and titanium alloys. Gold and palladium alloys require a reducing atmosphere as supplied by the middle blue cone of the torch (see Fig 17-4), with flux being added to the melt. The electric resistance furnace uses a carbon (rather than ceramic) crucible, thus providing a reducing environment throughout the melting regime.

The electric resistance furnace also provides the best means of temperature control. The torch adjustment is always variable, with no means of monitoring the temperature, and the induction and electric arc modes are less controllable than the resistance mode because melting is achieved so rapidly. Attempts to control the melt temperature when using induction or electric arc require a pyrometer to be focused on the melt. However, since each alloy has its a unique emissivity, the pyrometer is only reliable when calibrated to a given alloy; when a different alloy is used, the pyrometer must be recalibrated.

◖ Casting Machines

Casting machines provide the means for transferring the molten alloy from the melting crucible to the mold. They vary greatly, from the most elementary to the complex, with corresponding variations in cost. The casting machines can be divided into two broad categories: (1) those that use pneumatic forces and (2) those that provide primarily centrifugal forces to transfer the molten alloy to the heated mold.

Pneumatic forces

A very old method still practiced to a limited extent throughout the world uses steam pressure to drive the melt into the mold. The alloy is melted in the sprue/crucible former part of the mold. A simple handheld device fitted with a wet asbestos plug is quickly placed over the melt, making a seal with the mold ring. When the device is pressed down firmly, the wet asbestos makes contact with the molten alloy, generating sufficient steam pressure to complete the casting.

The pressure/vacuum casting machine produces pressure over the molten alloy. At the same time, a vacuum is applied to the bottom of the mold; thus, the molten alloy is "pushed and sucked" into the mold. In variance, the vacuum/pressure types of casting machines first evacuate the melting chamber to reduce oxidation and then apply air pressure uniformly about the casting ring, forcing the alloy into the mold. An innovative variation of the pneumatic mode is the jet casting machine, which depends on combustion gas to provide the casting force.

Casting results from these machines are comparable. One factor must be taken into consideration when using the pneumatic-type casting machines: They all provide good castings when a porous gypsum investment is used, but when a denser investment—such as a phosphate investment or an investment that tends to sinter

on heating—is used, castings may be incomplete. Since the melting procedure is usually done directly in the sprue/crucible former part of the investment mold, which may be subject to thermal decomposition, thin sprues must be used to prevent premature entrance of the alloy into the sprue opening of the mold during melting.

Centrifugal forces

Two considerations are fundamental to any casting procedure: (1) the casting force, be it pneumatic pressure or centrifugal (speed of the rotating arm), and (2) the rate of time required to fill the mold. In most cases the two are inversely related—the greater the casting force used, the less time required to fill the mold.

The **castability** of an alloy is determined by a number of variables: its melting range, the mold temperature, and the initial acceleration of the casting machine or applied force, among them. The rotation speed of the spring-driven casting machines can be increased by increasing the number of windings of the casting arm. The vertical rotating casting machines reach their maximum revolutions per minute before the horizontal rotating casting machines. The pneumatic modes require less time to fill the mold, however. Even more time is required to fill the mold with the motor-driven casting machine because of the longer time needed to achieve maximum rotation.

A large posterior full crown with a thick occlusal surface cross section, large adjoining cusps, and feathered margins can hinder the maximizing of the casting force. As the molten metal under a given centrifugal force enters the thickest cavernous area of the mold, a pressure drop is realized before the molten alloy is forced into the feathered margin area. The greatest difficulty in the casting process is the initial acceleration of the casting machine's arm. To improve the castability of an alloy, the initial acceleration of the rotation must be increased so that the mold is filled quickly; the ultimate rotation speed of the casting machine becomes relatively unimportant compared with the initial acceleration.

With the advantage of increased acceleration, casting of finer detail and thinner cross sections can be made. This function has clinical significance, because the ability to cast thin sections is critical for maximum marginal integrity and is especially important with alloys intended for porcelain bonding. When casting alloys with a high modulus of elasticity are used, a coping thickness of only

0.1 mm will provide sufficient strength to support the porcelain and allow increased thickness of body porcelain to cover the opaque porcelain, thus greatly improving the esthetics.

Cleaning and Finishing the Casting

After the casting has been made, the mold is removed from the cradle of the casting machine as soon as the arm stops rotating. It is then immersed in cold water when the button (the excess gold left in the crucible above the sprue) turns a dark red. This step softens the gold casting, which can then be hardened in a controlled manner by heat treatment. As the mold is plunged into the water, the water in contact with the mold boils, breaking most of the investment away from the casting. The rest can be removed easily with careful use of any suitable hand instrument or brush.

The cleaned casting may have a dark or tarnished appearance due to oxide or sulfide deposits on the surface. These deposits can be removed by immersing the casting in a pickling solution, usually comprising an acid or a combination of acids with a hydrogen chloride base. It is highly recommended that the pickling solution be acquired from the alloy supplier, because their formulations are usually nonfuming and emanate no corrosive vapors.

The casting is placed in a small porcelain casserole, and just enough solution is added to cover the casting. The solution may be heated carefully until the characteristic gold luster develops. The pickling solution is then flushed from the casserole with copious quantities of tap water. Plastic or quartz tongs are not required for this method, eliminating the risk of dropping the casting. Also, since only a small quantity of solution is needed (10 mL), new pickling solution can be used each time.

Pickling solution should never be used if the color has changed even slightly, nor should metal tongs be used. The gold casting should never be heated directly or indirectly in a flame before immersing it in pickling solution because the casting may be dropped or become distorted, or the margins may become rounded from overheating. Furthermore, grain growth is possible, making the casting weak and difficult or impossible to polish. Ultrasonic cleaners and abrasive spray devices (ie, sandblasting) can also play a useful role in the overall cleaning procedure.

Polishing is the final step after precision of fit and marginal integrity have been established on the die. Rubber, rag, or felt wheels impregnated with abrasives are used in the initial stages of finishing. Final polishing is accomplished with various oxides of tin and aluminum used in conjunction with a small rag or chamois buffing wheel, followed with an iron oxide rouge. Since these oxides are often supplied in stick form for convenience of handling and confining the abrasive to the wheel, residual traces of the rosin or wax-like matrix must be removed with a suitable solvent or a polishing compound remover followed by a hot, soapy water rinse.

Other Casting Alloys

The metals used for partial denture frameworks are usually alloys of cobalt, with chromium being the primary additive. Lesser quantities of nickel, molybdenum, and carbon are added in varying amounts. Gold alloys have been used for this purpose; however, since they possess a relatively low modulus of elasticity and proportional limit, are relatively soft, and have a density about twice that of cobalt alloys, gold alloys are not preferred for partial denture fabrication. Both types of alloys, however, possess excellent corrosion-resistance properties.

The casting technique for cobalt alloys is very similar in most respects to that described for gold alloys. Although the demands for accuracy may not be as stringent, the principles set forth for gold casting are still valid. Only the primary differences between the gold and cobalt alloy techniques will be presented here. Because the general practitioner is not likely to have the appropriate casting facilities, the technical manuals supplied by the manufacturers should be consulted for further details.

The investment used must be of the phosphate- or silica-bonded type. Cobalt alloys melt in the temperature range of 1,250°C to 1,450°C (2,280°F to 2,640°F), well above the decomposition temperature of calcium sulfate. Gypsum investment therefore cannot be used.

Induction is the preferred method for melting cobalt alloys. An oxygen-acetylene torch may be used, but the control of the flame is critical. If the flame is acetylene-rich, carbon is picked up by the alloy, embrittling it; if the flame is oxygen-rich, the metal is oxidized. The melting range of these alloys is well above the upper limits of an air-gas or an oxygen-gas flame, and therefore these mix-

Gold Casting Troubleshooting

GENERAL PROBLEMS

1. Problems with accuracy

Water/powder ratio Higher values reduce setting, thermal, and HE, giving smaller casting.

Spatulation Increased spatulation increases setting expansion, giving larger castings.

Burnout temperatures Lower temperatures result in less TE and smaller castings.

Immersion time Delays results in decreased HE and smaller castings.

Water-added technique Decreased amounts of water added to investment result in decreased HE and smaller castings.

Water bath Temperatures below 37°C (100°F) reduce HE and result in smaller castings.

2. Problems with distortion

Wax too hot Excessive shrinkage results on cooling.

Wax too cool The pattern undergoes stress release with a change in shape.

Insufficient pressure during waxing The pattern distorts because of thermal shrinkage.

Delayed investment The sooner the investment is complete, the less distortion there will be.

Heating pattern during spruing Distortion could result.

Overheating casting during soldering procedure Warping or melting of the margins results.

3. Problems with bubbles

Inadequate vacuum or ineffective painting procedure The vacuum must have at least 26 in of mercury for vacuum investing.

Water/powder ratio If the investment is too thick, it will not cover the pattern completely.

Excessive vibration of the ring Small nodules are consequently produced.

4. Problems with surface roughness

Water/powder ratio A high ratio increases the roughness of the mold.

Excess wetting agent or salivary contamination A resulting film may form on the pattern surface and be reproduced on the casting surface. Generally the roughness is localized on the exterior and is mass-like in appearance.

Prolonged heating or overheating of the mold Prolonged heating may cause investment disintegration, whereas overheating may cause a reaction between the alloy and casting investment. Roughness appears general and feels sharp.

Premature heating of casting investment Wait a minimum of 45 minutes for burnout.

5. Problems with fins on the surface or margins

Prolonged heating Cracks in the investment that radiate out from the surface of the pattern may result.

Heating rate is too rapid Cracks may appear in the investment, caused by nonuniform heating of the investment.

Water/powder ratio A high ratio produces a weak investment that may crack.

Excessive casting pressure Metal impact may cause investment fracture.

Cooling of the investment prior to casting Cracks in the investment could result.

6. Problems with short, rounded margins

Investment or alloy is too cold In this case, solidification is completed prior to completion of the mold.

Casting pressure The casting pressure is inadequate to fill the mold because of trapped air. The situation depends on the pattern position and the porosity of the investment.

Incomplete burnout Residual carbon at peripheral portions of the pattern may result.

7. Problems with miscasting

Casting is nearly or entirely missing The pattern detaches from the sprue pin due to excessive vibration.

Pattern fractured during investing

Gold alloy was too cold during casting

Incomplete burnout

Sprue pin was too small If the sprue freezes before the alloy fills the mold completely, incomplete casting results.

8. Problems with pits

Inclusions of investment, asbestos, or other debris are carried to the margin by molten alloy Pits generally exhibit angular edges. They may be rounded if they are the result of flux inclusion.

PROBLEMS WITH INTERNAL POROSITY

9. Problems with localized shrinkage porosity

Sprue pin diameter is too small The sprue channel solidifies simultaneously with or before the casting. Additional molten alloy is prevented from entering the mold to compensate for solidification shrinkage.

Alloy or mold temperature is too low Rapid solidification of the alloy results here.

10. Problems with subsurface porosity

Short, thick sprue pin Rapid entry of the alloy causes skin formation; the bulk of alloy pulls away, forming subsurface porosity.

Alloy or mold temperature is too high The first portion of gold to contact the investment will solidify and form a thin skin. The alloy behind it shrinks during solidification and pulls away, forming small porosities.

11. Problems with microporosity

Alloy or mold temperatures are too low If solidification occurs more rapidly than normal, shrinkage may develop throughout the casting.

PROBLEMS WITH EXTERNAL POROSITY

12. Problems with back pressure porosity

Insufficient alloy mass Air is entrapped in the solidifying alloy.

Insufficient turns on the casting machine The denser the investment, the greater the force needed to eliminate the gas within the mold chamber.

Pattern is too far away from the end of the ring The situation is aggravated by dense investments and lower burnout temperatures.

tures cannot be used. Because of the relatively great hardness of the cobalt alloys, sandblasting and electrolytic polishing techniques are used. Rouges can often be used for final polishing.

Nickel alloys used for fixed partial dentures are melted with gas-oxygen or acetylene-oxygen torches or by electric induction. Phosphate-bonded investments are required, since these alloys are cast at about 1,260°C (2,300°F). They are handled similarly to the cobalt-chromium alloys. Titanium-based alloys must be melted in a highly controlled inert environment (ie, argon or nitrogen) using either the induction or electric arc mode. Because titanium alloys have such extremely high fusion temperatures, only zircate or magnesia investments can be used.

◗ Glossary

castability The ability of an alloy to completely fill a mold.

casting A process for forming objects by pouring molten metals in molds that are cooled to cause solidification.

die A replica of a tooth or prepared tooth onto which a wax pattern is formed. The die is usually made of a gypsum material.

gypsum The hydrated product formed when plaster is mixed with water: $CaSO_4 \cdot 2H_2O$.

investment A molding material that surrounds the pattern and subsequently hardens and forms the mold after the wax pattern is eliminated.

lost wax casting process A method of casting metals that uses a wax model of the object to form the mold and, after wax elimination, the mold cavity.

refractory Any material that has an extremely high melting point. In gold casting, some form of silica (usually cristobalite) would be the refractory.

sprue Part of a casting that acts as a channel for the molten metal to flow into the mold cavity.

◗ Discussion Questions

1. For an inlay casting, how close is the tolerance at the margins?

2. If an inlay or crown casting is too small, what factors in the process may be responsible?

3. How can porosity, which is a problem in polishing, be reduced?

4. Compare the advantages and disadvantages of the high-heat and hygroscopic mold expansion techniques.

5. Why are the properties of the wax pattern so important in the accuracy of the lost wax process?

◗ Study Questions

(See appendix E for answers.)

1. Describe the lost wax technique of casting.

2. What equation must be satisfied to make a casting that will fit?

3. What are the two primary techniques used in fabricating a wax pattern?

4. What primary factor determines the amount of gold shrinkage?

5. What is cristobalite?

6. Why is it necessary to use an asbestos liner when making a cristobalite investment?

7. Name four common investing techniques.

8. Which investment is designed for the higher-fusing casting golds, as used in porcelain-fused-to-gold techniques?

9. How can the expansion of phosphate investment best be controlled?

10. What are the four primary functions of the sprue?

11. Why must gold alloys be cleaned by melting on a charcoal block before being used for the second time?

12. Name three types of casting machines commonly used in gold casting.

13. What is the nature of pickling solutions used for cleaning gold alloys?

14. What are the primary components of the base metals used for partial denture frameworks?

15. Why is gold not the metal of choice for fabricating a partial denture framework?

16. Name two types of investment used for casting cobalt-chromium alloys.

■ Reference

1. Craig RG, Peyton FA. Restorative Dental Materials, ed 5. St Louis: Mosby, 1975.

■ Recommended Reading

Asgar K, Arfaei AH. Castability of crown and bridge alloys. J Prosthet Dent 1985;54:60.

Asgar K, Lawrence WN, Peyton FA. Further investigations into the nature of hygroscopic expansion of dental casting investments. J Prosthet Dent 1958;8:673.

Craig RG, Eick JD, Peyton FA. Strength properties of waxes at various temperatures and their practical applications. J Dent Res 1967; 46:300.

Delgado VP, Peyton FA. The hygroscopic setting expansion of a dental casting investment. J Prosthet Dent 1953;3:423.

Docking AR. The hygroscopic setting expansion of dental casting investments. Parts I–IV. Aust Dent J Jan 1948:6.

Docking AR. The hygroscopic setting expansion of dental casting investments. Part II. Aust Dent J May 1948:160.

Docking AR. The hygroscopic setting expansion of dental casting investments. Part III. Aust Dent J Sept 1948:320.

Docking AR. The hygroscopic setting expansion of dental casting investments. Part IV. Aust Dent J Sept 1949:261.

Donovan TE, White LE. Evaluation of an improved centrifugal casting machine. J Prosthet Dent 1985;53:609.

Dootz ER, Graig RG, Peyton FA. Influence of investments and duplicating procedures on the accuracy of partial denture castings. J Prosthet Dent 1965;15:679.

Eames WB, MacNamara JF. Evaluation of casting machines for ability to cast sharp margins. Oper Dent 1978;3:137.

Earnshaw R. Investments for casting cobalt-chromium alloys. Br Dent J 1960;108:1.

Ida K, Daita K, Kawai S, Yamaga R. Casting force in several casting methods. Part I. Casting pressure produced by gaseous pressure casting apparatus and speed of revolution of centrifugal casting machine. J Osaka Univ Dent Sch 1970;10:35.

Ida K, Kuroda T, Yamaga R. Casting force in several casting methods. Part II. Comparison of casting time in several casting methods. J Osaka Univ Dent Sch 1970;10:47.

Ida K, Tsutsumi S, Togaya T. Titanium or titanium alloys for dental casting. Microfilmed Paper no. 397. Presented at the Annual Meeting of the International Association for Dental Research, Dental Materials Group, Osaka, Japan, 5–7 June, 1980.

Jones DW, Wilson HJ. Variables affecting the thermal expansion of refractory investments. Br Dent J 1968;125:249.

Jørgensen KD. Study of the setting expansion of gypsum. Acta Odontol Scand 1963;21:227.

Mahler DB, Ady AB. An explanation for the hygroscopic setting expansion of dental gypsum products. J Dent Res 1960;39:576.

Mahler DB, Ady AB. The influence of various factors on the effective setting expansion of casting investments. J Prosthet Dent 1963; 13:365.

Mahler DB, Ady AB. The effect of the water bath in hygroscopic casting techniques. J Prosthet Dent 1965;15:1115.

Mahler DB, Asgarzadeh K. The volumetric contraction of dental gypsum materials on setting. J Dent Res 1953;32:354.

Nielsen JP. Pressure distribution in centrifugal dental casting. J Dent Res 1978;57:261–269.

Peyton FA, et al. Controlled water-addition technic for hygroscopic expansion of dental casting investment. J Am Dent Assoc 1956; 52:155.

Ryge G, Fairhurst CW. Hygroscopic expansion. J Dent Res 1956;35: 499.

CHAPTER 18

Soldering, Welding, and Electroplating

◼ Soldering

Soldering is often used in the construction of dental appliances. To improve the dimensional accuracy, larger fixed partial dentures (FPDs) are frequently cast in parts that are soldered together after careful fitting to the master cast. Wrought-wire clasp arms can be soldered in place for partial dentures using investment soldering techniques. Orthodontic wires and bands are often soldered together. Soldering can be used to build up certain regions of crowns and inlays where the dimensions should be increased, such as for missing contact points. In addition, some casting defects can be corrected with soldering.

Clean oxide-free metal surfaces brought into intimate contact will bond together as a consequence of metallic bonding forces. However, bonding does not occur in most practical situations because of surface contamination and/or oxidation. Also, metallic bonding forces are of a very short range compared with the surface roughness of polished flat surfaces. Only small areas will be sufficiently close for bonding to occur, even when clean and oxide free.

The first step in soldering is to make sure that metal surfaces are free of contamination by cleaning and using **fluxes**, which also prevent oxidation during the soldering process. Second, a metal or alloy with a lower melting point than the parts to be joined must be chosen. Finally, the parts and **solder** should be brought to the solder's melting temperature. If the molten metal wets the solid metal, it will spread between the flux and the metal part, providing intimate contact. The solder penetrates joints by capillary action. On solidification, the solder will still be in contact and metallic bonding will be established.

Solder compositions

The proportion of pure gold in gold solders is specified by its *fineness*. Usually, the fineness of a solder is less than that of the alloy being soldered. Some manufacturers give a carat designation indicative of the gold alloy for which the solder is to be used (eg, an 18-carat solder is intended for soldering an 18-carat alloy); the proportion of gold in the solder may be less than 18 carat. The compositions of several solder alloys are presented in Table 18-1.

Copper is added to a solder to lower the fusion temperature, improve its strength, and make it amenable to age hardening. Silver, added in a larger proportion than copper, improves the wetting (spreading and penetration) of gold solders and also whitens the alloy. Tin and zinc are present in relatively fixed amounts (2% to 4%) to lower the fusion temperature, and nickel may be added instead of copper if a white alloy is desired.

Preceramic solders for soldering porcelain-fused-to-metal (PFM) appliances must withstand the high sintering temperatures of porcelain and so contain more noble metals and less tin and zinc. Copper is not used because it colors the porcelain green, as does silver.

Silver solders contain 10% to 80% silver, 15% to 50% copper, 4% to 35% zinc, and small amounts of cadmium, tin, and phosphorus to lower the fusion temperature.

Flux and antiflux compositions

Borax flux for soldering gold can be made from dehydrated borax ($Na_2B_4O_7$), boric acid (H_3BO_3), and silica (SiO_2). The fused borax flux produces oxide-free surfaces over which the solder will flow easily. The flux can be applied as a powder, a liquid (flux mixed with alcohol), or a paste. A paste gives the most control in application and

Table 18-1 Composition of gold solders[1]

SOLDER NO.	COMPOSITION (WEIGHT %)				
	GOLD	SILVER	COPPER	ZINC	TIN
A	65.0	16.3	13.4	3.9	1.7
B	65.4	15.4	12.4	3.9	3.1
C	66.1	12.4	16.4	3.4	2.0
D	72.9	12.1	10.0	3.0	2.0
E	80.9	8.1	6.8	2.1	2.0

is formed by mixing the powdered flux with petrolatum or a similar inert base.

Fluoride fluxes are used for soldering alloys containing chromium, because fluorides dissolve the chromium oxide. A flux consisting of potassium fluoride, boric acid, borax glass, and sodium carbonate or silica is typical. The ingredients are fused and ground to fine powder, which is used either directly or as a liquid in alcohol or a paste in petrolatum.

An **antiflux** prevents the flow of solder and is used to confine the solder to the work area. Graphite from a lead pencil is a convenient antiflux; however, it is removed by oxidation at higher temperatures. An effective antiflux for prolonged heating or higher temperatures can be made from a suspension of rouge (ferric oxide) or chalk (calcium carbonate) in alcohol.

Investment materials

Soldering investments should not expand as much as casting investments because soldering requires lower temperatures. Consequently, quartz-based rather than cristobalite-based gypsum investments are used for soldering with typical low-fusing gold solders. Phosphate-bonded soldering investments are used for preceramic soldering.

Manipulation of solder

Selection is made on the basis of the solder's corrosion resistance, strength, fusion temperature, and color (to give an inconspicuous joint). The fusion range of the solder must be at least 100°C (212°F) below that of the parts to be soldered. In addition, the selection of solder is based on how permanent the appliance will be and if the appliance can be removed for cleaning. A solder of 580 fine has been suggested as the lowest fineness to be used in permanent restorations; higher-fineness solders are generally recommended. Removable appliances can be removed for cleaning and polishing, so a lower-fineness solder may be used.

In soldering appliances such as orthodontic wires and bands, recrystallization or softening of the wires must be avoided. Lower-melting-point solders (eg, silver solders or low-fineness gold solders) that also improve the mechanical properties of the joint are preferable. Silver solders are used for stainless steel and other base metal wires.

Gold solders used with nickel-chromium and cobalt-chromium-nickel wires are generally about 450 fine and seldom above 650 fine. Solders with higher fineness have inferior mechanical properties.

Cleaning

Surface films of inorganic gases, organic material, and metallic oxides separate the two surfaces and prevent the solder from wetting the metal's surfaces. Parts must be thoroughly clean to obtain a good joint, and the use of fluxes will prevent oxidation during the soldering process.

Casting oxides are removed by pickling in acids. If the parts are polished before soldering, they must be thoroughly washed with soap and water and then pickled to remove residual polishing materials. Rubber-bonded finishing wheels and points are useful for removing oxides and contamination from the region to be soldered.

Investment soldering

Investment soldering is recommended for precise arrangement of parts for fixed partial dentures or partial dentures with wrought-wire clasp arms. The general procedure is as follows:

1. To prevent warping or porosity, the parts are placed on the master cast so that the **gap distance** between them is at least 0.1 mm. Excessive gap distance can lead to distortion and pitting. A typical business card, which ranges in thickness from 0.20 to 0.34 mm, can be used as a gauge for maximum gap distance. Sheets of paper should not be used as a gauge because they are often too thin, ranging from 0.05 to 0.1 mm in thickness.

2. The parts are securely fastened together with **sticky wax** before removal from the master cast and subsequent placement in the soldering investment.

3. Investment should cover metal parts not to be soldered, but no investment should be at the joint.

4. Antiflux may be applied to confine the flow of solder.

5. To obtain dimensional accuracy, the investment is preheated to eliminate moisture and to provide enough thermal expansion to compensate for the thermal expansion of the crowns. Overheating may cause sulfur contamination.

6. Flux can be applied to the joint area before or after preheating.

7. Soldering is accomplished with a reducing flame when the parts are at 750°C to 870°C (1,382°F to 1,598°F), giving them a yellowish red color. The solder should immediately flow smoothly into the joint area if the surfaces are clean.

8. The investment and appliance are allowed to cool for about 5 minutes before quenching to allow some age hardening and prevent warping that could result if the investment were quenched immediately. Total bench cooling, however, would make the solder too brittle through age hardening.

9. The flux cools to a glass that can be removed through pickling. Generally, finishing instruments should not be used to remove the flux because the glass is harder than the metal, and the surrounding metal would be removed along with the flux. Small amounts of flux can, however, be chipped or crushed off with a hard instrument (eg, no. 7 spatula or knife).

Free-hand soldering

Soldering of orthodontic appliances is usually accomplished without the use of an investment. Orthodontic torches can be placed on the bench so that both hands are free to hold the parts in position. Solder is generally melted onto one of the parts, and then they are held together and the joint is heated.

Thin wire parts must be held in contact to avoid narrowing of the joint caused by the surface tension of the solder. This decrease in diameter concentrates stress and is much more significant than for larger appliances.

Orthodontic torches, which develop small needle-like flames, are used to limit the heating to a small area around the joint. The wires can easily be overheated, however, which results in deterioration of mechanical properties. Overheating of stainless steel wires can lead

to carbide precipitation, which may soften the wire. Orthodontic silver solders with low soldering temperatures (620°C to 665°C) are recommended.

Defective soldering

Overheating of wrought wires during soldering can lead to diffusion between solder and wire and to recrystallization and grain growth. Microstructural changes due to heating or overheating, surface pitting, and internal porosity all serve to weaken the joint.

When the solder does not flow properly, resulting in an incomplete joint, it is usually due to one or more of the following:

1. The parts were too cool when the solder was applied.

2. If the parts were not at similar temperatures, the solder would flow over the hotter part, leaving an incomplete joint.

3. Flux was insufficient to cover the joint.

4. Contamination was present due to improper cleaning, poor placement of flux, sulfur released from overheated investment, oxidation from an improperly adjusted torch, or oxidation caused by removing the reducing portion of the flame from the joint before the solder flowed.

5. The gap distance was too small (< 0.1 mm) for the solder to penetrate between the parts. The joint may appear complete, but there will be a void at the center of the soldered joint that could result in premature failure.

6. If the gap distance was too large, the solder may not bridge the gap or, if it does, the diameter of the joint will be too small for adequate strength. Parts should be shaped to fit together with a proper gap distance separating them.

Properties of solder

Fusion temperature

The melting ranges of several gold solders are presented in Table 18-2. The difference in melting range between high- and low-fineness solders is not great. Silver solders begin to melt between 600°C and 700°C (1,112°F and 1,292°F), with a range of about 10°C to 40°C.

Mechanical properties

Gold solders have different properties for their soft and hard conditions (Table 18-3). The proportional limit can be doubled for these solders at the expense of elonga-

Table 18-2 Melting range of gold solders

SOLDER NO.	°C	°F
A	765–800	1,410–1,470
B	745–785	1,375–1,445
C	750–805	1,385–1,480
D	755–835	1,390–1,534
E	745–870	1,375–1,597

Table 18-3 Tensile properties of gold solders[1]

SOLDER NO.*	HEAT TREATMENT	PROPORTIONAL LIMIT		TENSILE STRENGTH		ELONGATION
		KG/CM²	PSI	MPa	PSI	(%)
A	Soft	2,100	30,000	302	44,000	9
	Hard	5,400	77,000	632	92,000	< 1
B	Soft	1,890	27,000	283	42,500	14
	Hard	3,850	55,000	431	63,000	1
C	Soft	2,060	29,500	306	44,500	12
	Hard	5,420	77,500	573	83,500	< 1
D	Soft	1,680	24,000	247	36,000	7
	Hard	4,300	61,500	480	70,000	< 1
E[†]	Soft	1,440	20,500	257	37,500	18

*Composition given in Table 18-1.
[†]No appreciable age hardening.

tion and, therefore, toughness. Age-hardened solder joints are very brittle.

Silver solders have mechanical properties comparable with gold solders in the soft condition.

Corrosion resistance

Since there is a composition difference between the solder and the parts, the joint is susceptible to galvanic corrosion.

Interfacial properties

The relationship of the interfacial energies among the metal parts, solder, and flux determines how well the solder will flow. The fluxes used in dentistry will remove surface oxides and protect the parts from further oxidation. Solders penetrate the flux and wet the metal surfaces beneath.

Soldering of metal-ceramic fixed partial dentures

Metal-ceramic FPDs can be soldered together before placement and firing of the ceramic (preceramic soldering) or after firing of the ceramic (postceramic soldering). The two methods require different procedures and materials.

In preceramic soldering, a high-fusing precious metal solder must be used to avoid melting or distortion during firing of the porcelain. Usually a single-orifice gas/oxygen torch is used for soldering. Except for the use of a phosphate-bonded soldering investment, the procedure is similar to the previously described investment soldering.

A lower-fusing gold solder is used for postceramic soldering so as to avoid thermal damage to the porcelain or its shape. To avoid overheating the porcelain, the parts are oven soldered. Except for the oven heating, the procedure is the same as for investment soldering. Following oven drying and fluxing, the correct amount of solder is placed on the joint, and the dried invested pieces are placed in a furnace heated to the upper fusion range of the solder.

Preceramic and postceramic soldering have been successfully used with base metal–ceramic fixed partial dentures. The main difference between soldering of gold and base metal alloys is that special fluoride fluxes must be used for the latter to dissolve the chromium oxides. However, not all fluoride fluxes work equally well. It is important to use the manufacturer's recommended fluxes for these alloys.

Commercial soldering materials

A number of companies supply gold ranging from 450 to 800 fine. In addition, most companies carry white gold solders for soldering white gold. Some companies also have special gold solders made to match the colors of their popular gold alloys. A liquid flux, "T" Flux (Evonik Degussa), is recommended for both postceramic and conventional soldering of precious metal alloys.

Some soldering investments (Whip Mix) can be used for both high-temperature alloys and conventional low-temperature gold alloys. Chromium-containing orthodontic wires are soldered with special silver wires and with fluxes containing potassium fluoride, which dissolves chromium oxide. These products are available from orthodontic wire suppliers.

◉ Welding

Bonding will occur between two metallic surfaces placed in contact if they are free of surface films (including oxides and films of adsorbed gases) and surface roughness. The three methods of **welding** used in dentistry achieve metal-to-metal contact differently.

Spot welding

In **spot welding**, the two clean metal surfaces to be welded are placed together under pressure (Fig 18-1). Metal-to-metal contact is obtained by passing a current through the joint to cause interfacial melting. If a pulse of sufficient voltage and duration is applied by means of copper electrodes, melting will begin at the interface between the parts and will spread outward to form a weld.

The equation

$$Heat = I^2R$$

gives the amount of heat in watts generated per second by a current of I amperes passing through a structure with a resistance of R ohms. The resistance of the joint is much higher than that of the rest of the parts because of the small contact area at the joint and the surface films present. Because the current is constant, more heat will be generated at the contact areas than in the interior parts. Therefore, the metal will melt first at the contact points.

Liquid contact is established because of the applied pressure and the expansion on melting. Molten areas spread because the resistance of the metal in its liquid state is greater than in its solid state. Similar conditions exist at the electrode interface, but a higher-energy pulse would be required to cause melting because of the low resistance and high thermal conductivity of copper.

Small welds are generally considered better, because bonding is achieved with a minimum of change in the original grain structure.

Spot (resistance) welding is used to join flat structures, such as orthodontic bands and brackets, and to join orthodontic wires. The work is pressed together between two copper electrodes, and an electric pulse is applied. The magnitude of the pulse depends on the metals and their size and shape at the welding point, and on the size of the electrodes. Typical values for the pulse are 2 to 6 V for 0.04 to 0.02 seconds at 250 to 750 Å.

Pressure welding

If two metal parts are placed together and a sufficiently large force is applied perpendicular to the surface, **pressure welding** occurs. Pure gold is extremely malleable and, in the form of thin foils, can be pressure welded by hand. Pure gold has no surface oxides, but adsorbed gases prevent metal-to-metal contact. The applied force must be sufficiently large to produce permanent distortions parallel to the surface so as to expose film-free metal. The force must be applied rapidly so the exposed surfaces can be compressed together before surface gases adsorb. In pressure welding, the problems of surface roughness are overcome by compressive forces.

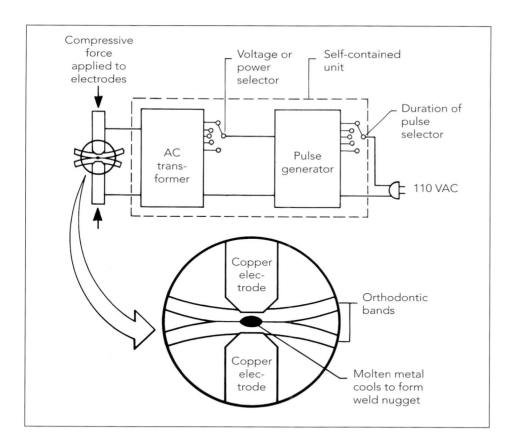

Fig 18-1 Schematic of a dental spot welder. Adjustable parameters are the magnitude and duration of the pulse, electrode size and shape, and pressure applied at the electrodes. Typical pulse parameters are 2 to 6 V for 0.04 to 0.02 sec, which generally results in an applied current of 250 to 750 Å, depending on the metal, size and shape of the work, electrodes, and pressure.

Gold foil, which is extremely thin and clean, may be welded under the pressure of dental instruments known as gold foil condensers to form gold foil restorations. Although rarely used today, gold foil restorations were popular during the 19th century. The absence of an oxide or contamination on the surface of pure gold allows room temperature welding.

Laser welding

A laser generates a coherent, high-intensity pulse of light that can be focused. By selecting the duration and intensity of the pulse, metals can be melted in a small region without extensive microstructural damage to surrounding areas. In **laser welding**, the beam is focused at the joint to melt the opposing surfaces. Due to expansion from the locally high temperature and the change of state, the two liquid surfaces contact and form a weld on solidification.

The intensity and duration of the laser pulse are such that a weld can be achieved before much heat is conducted away. Thus, there is very little heating of the total appliance except at the point of application, so the procedures can be performed on the master cast.

Properties of welds

Strength

In engineering applications, spot and pressure welds have strengths comparable with other forms of joining metals, such as soldering or arc welding. Laser welds are comparable with soldered joints between cast structures. Spot welding of work-hardened structures, such as bands and wires, destroys the grain structure and softens the metal at and around the weld.

Corrosion resistance

In general, welds are more susceptible to corrosion than are the metals surrounding them. Spot welding in dentistry has been confined to provisional appliances, where the results have been satisfactory. Pressure-welded gold foil restorations are not subject to corrosion in the oral environment.

Electroplating

Dies formed by **electroplating** are used in the construction of ceramic and PFM restorations, particularly for full-mouth reconstruction. The chances for abrasion of the die surface are higher for construction of appliances involving ceramics than for all-metal ones. Consequently, a more durable die is desired when ceramic restorations are involved. Metal-plated dies are more abrasion resistant than stone dies and are therefore often used for making PFM restorations as well as for platinum-bonded alumina crowns.

Galvanic corrosion, in which the anode is corroded by oxidation and ionic dissolution, plays a role in the process of electroplating. Under proper conditions—dependent on electrolyte, composition, potential difference between electrodes, and the metals involved—the dissolved ions from the anode can plate onto the cathode.

Plating solutions vary in their ability to plate concave surfaces, such as tooth surfaces of impressions. This plating ability is referred to as **throwing power**. Considering the size, depth, and shape of impressions of teeth, solutions with considerable throwing power are required for dental applications.

Plating manipulation

Impressions from compound or elastomeric materials can be electroplated. The basic procedure for construction of electroformed dies is to plate an impression with an appropriate metal, which is then poured in stone or acrylic resin. The impression is then removed, leaving the metal firmly attached to the die material. Generally, compound impressions are plated with copper, whereas silver is used for elastomeric impressions. Nickel may also be used.

To establish electric contact with a direct current power supply and the inner surface of the impression, a copper wire is threaded through nonvital regions of the impression. The impression is made electrically conductive by a process called **metallizing**, whereby a camel-hair brush is used to burnish a fine powder of metal onto the impression. Wax is then applied over areas that need not be plated.

The plating solution must contain the same metal ion as the plating electrode. The impression is made cathodic to the plating anode by connection to a direct current power supply. At the proper voltage—dependent on the size of the impression and the materials in-volved—the process requires about 10 to 15 hours. Approximately 1 mm of metal is deposited on the impression, and the impression is rinsed thoroughly in running water and other appropriate solutions to neutralize the plating electrolytes. The impression is then poured in stone or acrylic resin and removed as usual, leaving the metal attached to the stone or acrylic resin.

There are potential inaccuracies associated with electroformed dies that do not occur with properly made stone dies, especially if self-curing acrylic resin is used instead of stone. The duration of the plating process may cause distortion of the impression, and the plated metal layer can slightly distort the impression's surface. In addition, curing shrinkage of the acrylic resin may distort the metal.

Platinum-bonded alumina crowns

Jacket crowns are generally made by firing porcelain to a thin platinum coping that has been adapted to a die. This coping is not bonded to the porcelain and must be removed before cementation, which results in a thick cement layer between the crown and the tooth. Electroplating the platinum coping with tin and oxidizing the electroplated coping in a furnace has been found to produce a tin oxide layer to which the alumina core will adhere. This process allows the platinum coping to be left in place during cementation and likely improves the strength of the crown.

Electroformed gold copings

Nearly pure gold copings for PFM restorations can be made by an electroplating process similar to that used to make electroplated dies. In this case, an accurate die is metallized and plated with gold to a thickness of 0.2 to 0.3 mm. The die material is then removed from the gold by grinding and dissolving the remainder in an acid solution, and the gold is trimmed and fitted to the master die to give an accurate coping. Gold particles and organic binders are then applied to the outer surface of the coping before it is electroplated with tin so as to obtain a good bond with dental porcelains that have fusion temperatures below 927°C. Thin, accurate-fitting gold copings result. These copings are too weak to support porcelain FPDs, however.

Commercial products

Silver plating solutions are difficult to obtain. They contain silver cyanide and, therefore, should only be used under a hood. Silver plating has been largely discontinued, but copper plating is still used. Apparatus and materials for making electroformed gold copings are available (Captek).

● Glossary

antiflux Material placed on the work area before the flux to confine the flow of solder.

electroplating The formation of a metallic surface coating on another by an electrochemical solution.

fluoride flux Fluoride-containing flux for chromium alloys.

flux A substance that promotes the flow of solder over the metal parts by cleaning the surfaces and removing oxides.

gap distance Space between parts to be soldered that will be filled with solder.

laser welding A form of welding in which the heat for melting the metal is supplied by a focused beam of light generated by a laser.

metallizing Coating an impression material with a powdered metal to make it electrically conductive.

pressure welding A form of welding in which the weld is made by pressure.

solder Metal or alloy melted to unite adjacent, less fusible metal parts.

soldering investments Similar in composition to quartz casting investments; may be used for soldering.

spot welding A form of welding in which the heat for melting the metal is generated by the flow of electricity through the parts to be welded.

sticky wax Brittle wax-containing resin used to hold metal parts during investment soldering. It fractures rather than deforms under stress.

throwing power A measure of the uniformity in plating thickness of irregular surfaces.

welding The joining of metal surfaces directly by the application of heat or high compressive forces.

● Discussion Questions

1. Why do fixed partial dentures often fail clinically at solder junctions?

2. How do the processes of soldering and welding differ on a basic level?

3. What precautions need to be taken when soldering or welding wrought metals?

4. What problems might be expected in the clinical use of pure electroplated gold PFM dentures? What evidence might be needed?

5. What are the consequences of using too much solder or making too large a spot weld when joining orthodontic wire?

● Study Questions

(See appendix E for answers.)

1. What are the two main components of gold solder, besides gold, and why are they added?

2. What would be expected to happen if a porcelain-gold appliance were presoldered with an ordinary gold solder?

3. Why is a special fluoride flux required to solder alloys containing chromium?

4. What is an antiflux?

5. Give two examples of an antiflux.

6. To avoid melting gold parts, what fineness does the solder usually have relative to the parts?

7. What is the recommended minimum fineness for soldering permanent restorations?

8. Why is silver solder recommended for soldering stainless steel wires?

9. Why is cleaning the parts important to successful soldering?

10. When is investment soldering recommended?

11. What would happen with investment soldering if the sticky wax fractured but the soldering operations were continued?

12. What is the purpose of preheating the investment, and what will happen if it is overheated?

13. How does one determine if all parts are at the proper temperature for soldering?

14. Why is it important to have uniform heating at the joint?

15. What are some of the major differences between investment soldering of relatively large parts and freehand soldering of wires?

16. What microstructural changes are expected if wrought wires are overheated?

17. What difficulties might occur if soldering were performed in a dark room?

18. A soldered joint of an appliance that failed in service had the following defects: surface porosity, flux incorporated into the solder, and a large pore at the center of the joint. What were the likely causes?

19. If a joint becomes oxidized during soldering, what will happen?

20. What are causes of oxidation?

21. What errors in soldering procedure could lead to a poorly fitting appliance?

22. Why is flux important to successful soldering?

23. Referring to Table 18-3, what property of solders is seriously reduced by age hardening, and how is this avoided in the investment soldering procedure?

24. Why would it be impractical to spot weld flat copper structures together using orthodontic spot welders?

25. Why is it unlikely that thin foils of copper could be pressure welded by gold foil condensers?

26. Why can laser welding be accomplished on the master cast?

27. Can pressure welding be applied to nongold alloys?

28. Why might an organic film prevent welding during spot welding of orthodontic appliances?

29. What is the main application of electroplating in dentistry?

30. What are the advantages and disadvantages of electroplated dies?

31. Why is the throwing power of a plating solution important?

Reference

1. Coleman RL. Physical Properties of Dental Materials. National Bureau of Standards Research Paper No. 32. Washington, DC: US Government Printing Office, 1928.

Recommended Reading

Bailey JH, Donovan TE, Preston JD. The dimensional accuracy of improved dental stone, silverplated, and epoxy resin die materials. J Prosthet Dent 1988;59:307–310.

Coleman RI. Some effects of soldering and other heat treatment on orthodontic alloys. Int J Orthod 1933;19:1238.

Crowell WS. Dental gold solders. In: Lyman T (ed). Metals Handbook, ed 5. Cleveland: ASM, 1948:1104.

Erpenstein H, Borchard R, Kerschbaum T. Long-term clinical results of galvano-ceramic and glass-ceramic individual crowns. J Prosthet Dent 2000;83:530–534.

Gordon TE, Smith DL. Laser welding of prostheses—An initial report. Quintessence Int 1972;3:63–64.

McLean JW. The Science and Art of Dental Ceramics. Vol 2: Bridge Design and Laboratory Procedures in Dental Ceramics. Chicago: Quintessence, 1980.

Meyer FS. The elimination of distortion during soldering. J Prosthet Dent 1959;9:441.

Milner DR, Apps RI. Introduction in Welding and Brazing. New York: Pergamon Press, 1968.

O'Brien WJ, Hirthe WM, Ryge G. Wetting characteristics of dental gold solders. J Dent Res 1963;42:675.

Peyton FA, Craig RG. Restorative Dental Materials, ed 4. St Louis: Mosby, 1971.

Phillips RW. Skinner's Science of Dental Materials, ed 8. Philadelphia: Saunders, 1982.

Rogers OW. The gold solder, gold alloy interface. Aust Dent J 1977;22:168–171.

Rogers OW. The dental application of electroformed pure gold. I. Porcelain jacket crown technique. Aust Dent J 1979;24:163–170.

Ryge G. Dental soldering procedures. Dent Clin North Am 1958:747–757.

Sloan RM, Reisbick MH, Preston JD. Post-ceramic soldering of various alloys. J Prosthet Dent 1982;48:686–689.

Smith DL, Burnett AP, Gordon TE Jr. Laser welding of gold alloys. J Dent Res 1972;51:161–167.

Stade EH, Reisbick MH, Preston JD. Preceramic and postceramic solder joints. J Prosthet Dent 1975;34:527–532.

Traini T. Electroforming technology for ceramometal Restorations. Quintessence Dent Technol 1995;18:21–25.

Vence BS. Electroforming technology for galvano-ceramic restorations. J Prosthet Dent 1997;77:444–449.

Vrijhoef MM, Spanauf HJ, Renggli HH, Wismann H, Somers GA. Electroforming as an alternative to casting: A preliminary report. Restorative Dent 1985;1:143, 145–146.

Willis LM, Nicholls JI. Distortion in dental soldering as affected by gap distance. J Prosthet Dent 1980;43:272–278.

Zietsman ST, Fidos H. Electrical resistance welding or orthodontic wires. J Dent Assoc S Afr 1982;37:880–884.

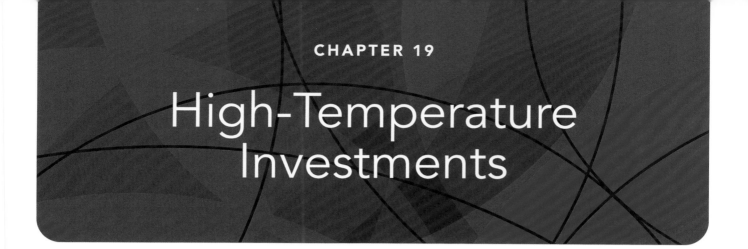

CHAPTER 19

High-Temperature Investments

High-temperature **investments** are used for numerous processes in the fabrication of dental alloy prostheses that require stability of the investment at temperatures in excess of about 1000°C to 1,200°C (1832°F to 2,192°F), approximately 65°C to 150°C (150°F to 300°F) above the top of the melting range for most dental alloys. The International Organization for Standardization (ISO)[1] classifies investments according to their intended use:

Type 1: For fabrication of inlays, crowns, and other fixed restorations.
Type 2: For fabrication of partial dentures or other removable appliances.
Type 3: For fabrication of casts used for joining or repairing prosthetics by soldering, brazing, or welding procedures.
Type 4: For fabrication of refractory dies.

There are two classes of casting investments and **refractory** die materials, classified according to their recommended burnout process:

Class 1: Recommended for burnout and thermal expansion by a slow or step heating method.
Class 2: Recommended for burnout and thermal expansion by a quick (rapid) heating method.

Among the processes for which high-temperature investments are used are the casting of dental alloys that need to be heated to temperatures of 1,200°C (2,192°F) or higher, including type 1 and 2 investments—many high-gold and palladium-based alloys used for the fabrication of porcelain-veneered fixed partial dentures and dental alloys based on nickel, cobalt, or titanium. Some

of the latter alloys are also used for crowns, inlays, onlays, and removable partial dentures in addition to fixed partial dentures (FPDs). High-temperature investments are also used as soldering investments (type 3) and for fabrication procedures (type 4) such as the construction of dies on which metal frameworks are placed for the application of porcelain, the firing of porcelain-fused-to-metal (PFM) prostheses, and for direct construction of all-ceramic restorations.

Two significant changes have occurred in the processing of dental alloy prostheses in the last 6 years:

1. Rapid-heating investments (Class 2 investments) are now used for the casting of dental alloys. Invested **molds** are inserted directly into a hot furnace to achieve burnout of the pattern and sprue system (an all-wax sprue is required because distortion and cracking of the investment occurs with the use of plastic sprues) and to rapidly raise the temperature at which the mold is held (soaked) to achieve uniform thermal expansion of the mold. After soaking, thermal expansion compensates for the shrinkage of the cast alloy prosthesis on cooling. The rapid-heat processing saves considerable time in the total process of pattern formation, investing, and heating of investment to the casting temperature. It is estimated that about 50% of the castings made now use rapid-heating investments.

2. Titanium alloys have not achieved the widespread use that had been hoped for by some in the dental industry and profession. Their lower densities, high corrosion resistance, and exceptionally high biocompatibility made them an intriguing candidate for use in dental oral prostheses. However, these alloys require special investments and processing methods because they are

cast at higher temperatures than other alloys. Titanium alloys are highly reactive; they can easily degrade the more conventional molds at elevated temperatures and, as a result, produce poor surface finishes. Further, they can be contaminated by degradation of the investment components, such as silica and carbon, and by oxygen and nitrogen present in the atmosphere. These contaminants harden and embrittle the surface of titanium castings. Routine casting of high-quality, cost-effective, cast prosthetic components became an obstacle in many dental laboratories. Because of the difficulties in processing cast titanium and the lower esthetics of titanium crowns compared with all-ceramic crowns, little attention is now given to using titanium alloys for the applications mentioned. However, for use as a denture base, titanium and its alloys remain attractive outside the United States, and research on these alloys continues, especially in Japan.

Because of the innovative approaches used in the development of investments for casting of titanium alloys, the subject is presented here for historic purposes.

High-temperature investments are not gypsum based as are those used for the casting of alloys that have casting temperatures less than approximately 1,200°C (2,192°F). The predominate compositions used for casting high-temperature alloys, creating veneering dies, and for **fixtures** for soldering, brazing, or welding operations are based on the use of a phosphate binder. Silicate-bound systems are also used,[2] but because of the greater difficulty involved, these systems tend to be restricted to the casting of cobalt-chromium alloys at temperatures above 1,425°C (2,600°F). Entirely new systems or modifications of the aforementioned ones needed to be created for the casting of titanium-based alloys.

◼ Phosphate-Bonded Investments

Applications

Casting of alloys

Phosphate-bonded investments (PBIs) have been used in dentistry for many years to make molds for casting high-melting-temperature dental alloys. Type 1 casting investments traditionally have been used for the casting of inlays, crowns, and other restorations, especially for alloys based on gold, platinum, palladium, cobalt-chromium, and nickel-chromium, to which porcelain is fused in the construction of esthetic fixed restorations. Type 2 investments are used for the casting of removable partial dentures. These applications are still in use, but the number of alloy applications has grown. Some variations are used for cast titanium alloys, discussed later in this chapter.

For the burnout process of the conventional Class 1, type 1 investments (inlays, crowns, and fixed partial dentures), it is generally recommended that the mold at room temperature be set in a furnace, 1 hour after spatulation, heated to 800°C (1,471°F) or higher over a period of 1 to 2 hours (depending on the size of the mold) and held at the upper temperature for about 30 minutes before casting. The newer Class 2 investments allow insertion of a mold, after about 30 minutes of setting time, directly into a furnace at the burnout temperature (near 800°C or higher), with additional raising of the temperature, if needed, to the casting temperature. A soak time of about 30 minutes is needed at the highest temperature before casting. When casting titanium alloys, however, the investment temperature is often lowered to somewhere between ambient room temperature and 400°C to 500°C in an attempt to reduce reaction of the alloy with the investment.

Soldering (joining) and porcelain veneering

Another traditional use of PBIs (type 3) is to make "soldering" fixtures that hold prosthetic components in alignment while they are being joined with solders, brazing alloys, or welding alloys. Since the 1980s some newer modifications have been used to make refractory dies for the fabrication of custom veneer facings from dental porcelains (type 4).

Composition

These investments are available as two-component systems that react to form a solid when mixed together.[3] One component consists of a powder, and the other is an aqueous solution of stabilized **colloidal** silica.

The powders have a variety of ingredients. Powdered ammonium dihydrogen phosphate, $NH_4H_2PO_4$ (provided in excess), reacts with water in the presence of **calcined** magnesium oxide (MgO) powder, to provide for the binding of the particles at ambient temperatures. Particles of refractory materials such as quartz, cristobalite, or a mixture of the two, in a mass fraction of about 80% con-

Table 19-1 Properties of phosphate-bonded investments used for high-temperature operations with dental materials (except titanium alloys)[6]

Casting investments	
Compressive strength	2.5 MPa minimum, type I (for inlays, crowns, etc)* 3 MPa minimum, type II (for removable appliances)*
Setting expansion (linear)	Within 15% of manufacturer's stated value* With use of full-strength liquid, about 0.4% can be attained with some investments; when a **hygroscopic** technique is used, about another 0.6% to 0.8% can be realized[†]
Thermal expansion	Within 15% of manufacturer's stated value* About 0.8% can be attained with a 50:50 mixture of liquid and water; about 1% to 1.2% can be attained with the use of undiluted liquid[†]
Modulus of rupture	0.1 to 0.5 MPa (14.4 to 72.5 psi), green; about 0.8 MPa (116 psi), as fired[†]
Refractory die stones	
Compressive strength	13 MPa minimum
Setting expansion (linear)	Within 30% of manufacturer's stated value*
Thermal expansion	Within 15% of manufacturer's stated value* Manufacturers state that their materials are designed to be compatible with their porcelain at temperatures in the vicinity of the glass-transition temperature. Values of about 12 to 13 × 10^6/°C would be expected.

*The ISO standard[1] provides more general guidelines: compressive strength of 2 MPa minimum and thermal expansion within 20% of the manufacturer's stated value.
[†]Approximate values attainable with some of the commercial brands.

trol **thermal expansion** and thermal stresses related to the phase transformations of cristobalite that occur during heating of the investment. These particles, along with glasses and fine particles of other metal oxides, provide bulk and help achieve a smooth surface finish. Rapid-heating (Class 2) investments are modified versions of the more conventional slow-heating (Class 1) investments. They must be more permeable to allow the escape of vaporizing water and other volatile components of the investment so that the mold does not crack, spill, or explode during the heating process. One way to ensure this property is to alter the particle sizes and their distribution.[4] The powders of rapid-heating investments may also contain some insoluble raw starch to provide setting expansion by water absorption and swelling of the starch. The starch burns out along with the patterns during the burnout process, and the empty spaces left behind increase the permeability of the investment. Rapid-heat investments may also contain some soluble starch[5] or fiber to control viscosity of the mixed investment while pouring around a pattern and to maintain a uniform dispersion of the fine particles during the mixing and investing procedures.

The liquid component provides the water needed for the room-temperature setting reaction as well as silica, which increases the setting and thermal expansion. If less expansion is needed, the liquid may be diluted with water before being mixed with the powder. The setting reaction of the $NH_4H_2PO_4$ with calcined magnesium oxide in the presence of water is:

$$NH_4H_2PO_4 + MgO + 5H_2O \rightarrow NH_4 MgPO_4 \cdot 6H_2O$$

After a mixed **slurry** sets to form a mold, it is fired to burnout consumable patterns (mostly waxes, but some polymers, such as preformed sprues and/or thermoplastic sheets for forming of single-unit patterns, may also be used).

Properties

The ISO standard[1] requires that the compressive strength be no less that 2 MPa for any application. The American National Standards Institute and American Dental Association (ANSI/ADA)[6] gave the properties of PBIs as shown in Table 19-1. High-temperature mold strength is achieved by the formation of complex silicophosphates from the reaction of some of the silica with the excess dihydrogen

Fig 19-1 Example of setting expansion and thermal expansion of phosphate-bonded investments. (Courtesy of Shofu Dental.)

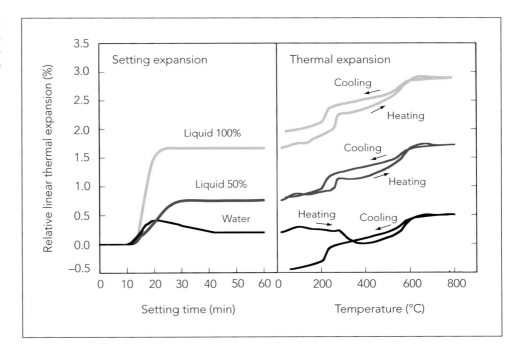

phosphate. Liquid that is supplied with the investment may be used either full strength or, as previously stated, diluted with water to provide some degree of control over the setting and thermal expansions (Fig 19-1).

Although the basic binding reaction is the same for all of the PBIs, there are some important differences in properties due to composition. Those used for the casting of high-temperature alloys and for making dies used in the fabrication of porcelain veneers contain quartz and cristobalite to achieve expansion, which compensates for the shrinkage of the cast alloy during cooling from elevated temperatures. Graphite is found in some of these investments to render them more permeable after burnout and/or to provide a reducing atmosphere, but these investments are not recommended for the casting of base metal alloys. Investments used for joining operations do not require especially fine powders and are designed without high-expansion fillers so that parts that are to be joined do not shift their relative positions while they and the surrounding investment are heated to the joining temperature.

Advantages and disadvantages

There are several advantages associated with PBIs. They have both high **green strength** and **fired strength**, which makes them easy to handle without breaking before they are placed in a furnace for the wax burnout

process and strong enough afterward to withstand the impact and pressure of centrifugally cast molten alloy. They can also provide setting and thermal expansions high enough to compensate for the thermal contraction of cast-metal prostheses or porcelain veneers during cooling. Finally, they have the ability to withstand the burnout process with temperatures that reach 900°C (1,650°F) or higher, and they can withstand temperatures up to 1,000°C (1,831°F) for short periods of time (useful for fabricating porcelain veneers or performing metal-joining operations).

These investments are at a disadvantage when used for alloys with casting temperatures higher than about 1,375°C (2,500°F). These temperatures, coupled with high mold temperatures, result in mold breakdown and rougher surfaces on castings. The high strength of these investments, although an advantage during casting, can make devesture a difficult and tedious task without the use of a simple tool, such as a press, to force the investment out of the metal casting **ring** if one is used. Further, when higher expansion is required, more of the silica liquid is used, resulting in a denser and less porous mold. Consequently, there may be incomplete castings if a release for trapped gases is not provided.

When the powder is supplied in bulk form rather than in sealed, premeasured packages, it can react over time with moisture in the air and result in either a lower expansion during setting or a loss of the ability to set to a strong mass. The temperature at which the triturated mixture is held markedly affects setting expansion.

● Ethyl Silicate–Bonded Investments

Applications

Ethyl silicate–bonded investments (ESBIs) have been used since the early 1930s to make molds for the casting of removable partial dentures of cobalt-chromium alloys. This continues to be their primary use, although they are occasionally used for the casting of nickel-based alloys.

Composition

ESBIs rely on binding by the formation of a gel from silicic acid, which is derived from the **hydrolysis** of tetraethyl orthosilicate, $Si(OC_2H_5)_4$. As with the PBIs, ESBIs are supplied as a powder that requires mixing with a liquid to bind the mixed mass via a setting reaction at room temperature. The powder consists of refractory particles of silicas and glasses in various forms along with calcined magnesium oxide and some other refractory oxides in minor amounts.

The liquid used for the setting reaction may be supplied as a stabilized alcohol solution of silica gel, or it may be supplied as two liquids (ethyl silicate and usually an acidified solution of denatured ethyl alcohol) that need to be mixed. Three-component systems are also available and may consist of stabilized colloidal silica, ethyl silicate, and denatured ethyl alcohol. Regardless of the number of liquids provided, the active species is the hydrated silica that is formed by the reaction of ethyl silicate with water in the presence of the acid (or a base) according to the reaction:

$$Si(OC_2H_5)_4 + 4H_2O \text{ acid/base} \rightarrow SiOH_4 + 4C_2H_5OH$$

Binding is by the reaction of the hydrated silica in the presence of MgO to form a gel according to the reaction:

$$nSi(OH)_4 + MgO \rightarrow MgO[Si(OH)_4]_n$$

A wetting agent is added to at least one of the liquid components to reduce the formation of gaseous bubbles on the surface of a pattern.

Properties

The ANSI/ADA specification[7] gave the properties of ESBI investments as shown in Table 19-2. The most important features of the ESBIs are their ability to withstand higher temperatures than the PBIs and to achieve sufficient expansion to compensate for the cooling shrinkage that results from the higher solidification temperatures of the higher-casting-temperature alloys with which they are used (ie, cobalt-chromium alloys). During the vibration of the investment slurry into a casting ring around a pattern, a separation occurs between the finer and coarser particles. The finer particles of the investment rise to the top of the mold (header) where the slurry acquires more liquid. The portion of the header near the bottom of the pattern, opposite the sprue end, is prone to cracking due to greater shrinkage from the evaporation of ethyl alcohol, which results from the formation of the silica gel. These cracks must be removed before the firing process by grinding the header down to a region without cracks so that when the mold achieves thermally induced expansion, the cracks will not grow. There should be a sufficient header to allow for this process. The remaining investment undergoes virtually no solidification shrinkage and is free of critical cracks. The expansion of the investment is all due to thermal expansion. Thus, distortion of patterns (such as those that can occur with **setting expansion**) is minimized, and these investments are well suited for producing large, precise castings.

Because of the low dimensional changes during setting (see Table 19-2), casts made from these investments may be **articulated** directly against gypsum casts of opposing dentition. However, the green strength of these investments is low, and refractory casts are best handled by reinforcing them with a resin dip. A fine-grained **surface coat** is sometimes applied to the reinforced cast and to the pattern on the cast to achieve a superior surface finish on the cast appliance.

Advantages and disadvantages

ESBIs offer the ability to cast high-temperature cobalt-chromium and nickel-chromium alloys and attain good surface finishes, low distortion, and high thermal expansion (good fit). They are less dense (more permeable) than the PBIs, and thin sections with fine detail can be reproduced. Also, their low fired strength makes devesting easier than with PBIs.

Table 19-2 Properties of ESBIs used for high-temperature operations with dental materials[7]

Casting investments	
Compressive strength	1.5 MPa, minimum*
Setting expansion (linear)	There is no requirement for setting expansion Setting contractions of 0% to 0.4% have been reported This value will depend on the method of measurement One manufacturer reports virtually no (0% to 0.05%) contraction[†]
Thermal expansion (linear)	Within 15% of manufacturer's stated value* About 1.5% to 1.8% can be attained between room temperature and 1,000°C to 1,177°C (1,800°F to 2,150°F)[†]

*The ISO standard[1] provides more general guidelines: compressive strength of 2 MPa minimum and thermal expansion within 20% of the manufacturer's stated value.
[†]Approximate values attainable with some of the commercial brands.

The disadvantages of ESBIs lie primarily in the added processing attention (resin-model reinforced dies, pattern coats) and the extra precaution needed in handling the low-strength fired molds. The low strength and high thermal expansion require a more precise burnout process and firing schedule to avoid cracking and, hence, destruction of the mold.

◼ Other Systems

Applications

Between 1980 and 2000, some manufacturers sought to introduce titanium-based alloys for use in the dental industries in Japan, Europe, and the United States. During continuing industrial research and development, it became apparent that the conventional, unmodified PBIs and ESBIs were not suitable materials for investments for titanium casting. Molten titanium is highly reactive with oxygen and is capable of reducing some of the oxides commonly found in these investments. Titanium can also dissolve residual oxygen, nitrogen, and carbon from these investments, and these elements can in turn harden and embrittle the cast titanium restorations. As a result, either modifications of existing refractory formulations and their binders or new refractory formulations and binder systems were required. However, it appears that the problem of developing a hard, brittle surface layer of around 80 μm to 200 μm thick has not yet been overcome. Because of this and other special processing con-

ditions, the commercial use of cast titanium-based alloys never became an important factor in the dental laboratory, and their investments are not widely used either. However, much was learned during the attempts to produce viable processes, and this knowledge may prove to be useful for developers of new dental casting processes in the future.

Composition

A variety of investment formulations for the casting of titanium were developed for casting of titanium alloys (Table 19-3).[8,9] These investments might be classified as PBIs, ESBIs, or "cemented" investments according to the source of the binder. Many kinds of refractories such as silica (SiO_2), alumina (Al_2O_3), magnesia (MgO), and zirconia (ZrO_2) have been used.

Properties

The ISO standard[1] specifies that the properties for investments must meet the properties claimed by the manufacturer. This standard applies to any dental investment regardless of the binders used, including investments used for all applications of titanium and titanium alloys in dentistry. It is reasonable to expect that the mechanical properties of those investments would be like those of the conventional PBIs and ESBIs, because experience revealed the latter investments to be strong enough for the casting process yet not too strong as to impede the devesting process.

New refractory compositions and binders were necessarily investigated for the casting of titanium prosthe-

Table 19-3 Titanium investments available in Japan and Germany

MOLD-CASTING TEMPERATURE (°C)	BINDER	REFRACTORY	BURNOUT TEMPERATURE (°C)	COUNTRY
RT	MgO, phosphate	Al_2O_3, ZrO_2	900	Japan
RT		Al_2O_3, ZrO_2	1,100	Japan
800		Al_2O_3, ZrO_2	1,150–1,200	Japan
RT		Al_2O_3, ZrO_2	900–1,000	Japan
200		Al_2O_3, SiO_2	1,100	Both
500		Al_2O_3, SiO_2	950	Both
100		$ZrSiO_4$, SiO_2	1,100	Japan
RT		Al_2O_3, $LiAlSi_2O_6$	1,050	Japan
600–700	Ethyl silicate	MgO, Al_2O_3	900	Japan
600–700		MgO, SiO_2, Al_2O_3	900	Japan
100		MgO, Zr*	850	Japan
100	Aluminous cement	MgO, Zr*	850	Japan
600–700		MgO, Al_2O_3	900	Japan

RT = room temperature.
*Addition for attaining expansion by volume change through oxidation.

ses. The objectives were to reduce breakdown of the investment and to avoid the contamination of titanium by the investment. One approach to reducing the reaction with the investment was to use molds that had been expanded by the burnout process and then cooled back to near-ambient temperatures before the casting process. This approach reduced the time that the alloy was in contact with the mold at elevated temperatures, and thus, the overall reactivity was reduced. However, lowering of the mold temperature required that either nonreversible expanders such as metals that expand by oxidation at the elevated temperatures be used, or that the temperature of the mold be kept just above the temperature at which a reversal of expansion due to crystalline phase changes takes place.

To avoid contamination of titanium by oxygen through the reduction of refractory oxides of the investment, refractory materials that are less easily reduced by titanium were necessary. The **Gibbs free energy of formation (FEF)** per mole of oxygen[10] for titanium oxide (TiO) at 1,727°C is –716 kJ/mol of oxygen, and that for titanium

dioxide (TiO_2) at 1,727°C (3,138°F) is –580 kJ/mol of oxygen. The corresponding FEFs of SiO_2 in the forms of cristobalite and quartz are –550 and –549 kJ, respectively. Therefore, it is clear that titanium would be expected to be oxidized by SiO_2, which would then be reduced.

Some modifications of PBIs were explored for the purpose of rendering them more compatible with molten titanium metals. One investment consisting of a phosphate binder, magnesia, and quartz was developed under the hypothesis that quartz would not be as reactive as silica.[11] On the basis of FEFs, there is little advantage in the use of one form of SiO_2 over another; any advantages would have to lie elsewhere (perhaps their decomposition kinetics are sufficiently different?). This investment was recommended for use as a room-temperature mold, ostensibly to reduce reaction with titanium. However, contamination of castings by reaction with the investment was still encountered.

To make use of the setting expansion of a phosphate binder, alumina (FEF = –687 kJ/mol of oxygen at 1,727°C) and magnesia (FEF = –640 kJ/mol of oxygen

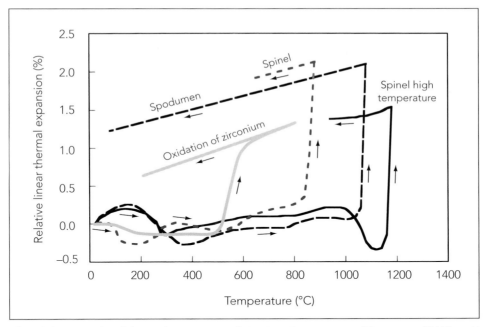

Fig 19-2 Example of thermal expansion of titanium investments. (Courtesy of Y. Tamaki and T. Miyazaki.)

at 1,727°C), both of which have good heat resistance, could be used as refractories; however, the thermal expansions of these oxides are low. If either of their powders was mixed with colloidal silica to raise the expansion, some contamination from the silica would be a possibility.

To achieve expansion without the use of reactive powders, a PBI that contained both magnesia and alumina as refractories was developed. This investment can attain large expansion by the spinel reaction of alumina and magnesia (MgO + Al$_2$O$_3$ → MgO–Al$_2$O$_3$) when it is burned out at 1,150°C to 1,200°C. The spinel is, of course, also highly refractory. The spinel-forming temperature can also be reduced by mixing with magnesia acetate. An alternative approach to obtaining the needed expansion is through the use of spodumen (Li$_2$O – Al$_2$O$_3$ – SiO$_2$).[12] Spodumen expands irreversibly on heating from 900°C to 1100°C. Figure 19-2 shows the thermal expansion curves of these titanium instruments.

The reaction of ESBIs with liquid titanium has been reported to be somewhat less than that of PBIs, most likely due to the use of highly refractory oxides in the powder (see Table 19-3). Regardless, these investments require a more complex procedure.

An early development of an investment using new binder systems was that of magnesia refractory bonded by an aluminous cement (CaO–Al$_2$O$_3$), which contains a mass fraction of 5% zirconium powder.[13] The aluminous cement serves as a binder for the magnesia refractory, and it sets by mixing with water. Oxidation of the zirconium powder to zirconia during the burnout process provides irreversible expansion to compensate for shrinkage of the casting during cooling from the solidification temperature. The zirconia formed is highly stable; it has an FEF of –728 kJ/mol of oxygen, and it should not contaminate the titanium. Titanium castings from this investment were reported to have smooth surfaces free of contamination from mold reaction.[13]

◧ Glossary

articulate To join the maxillary and mandibular dentition or a replica of it.

calcined Rendered a powdery, friable, dry substance by the application of heat.

colloidal The state of finely divided particles that are in suspension in a liquid. The particles acquire special properties (electric, gelatinous, etc) as a result of their fine size and interaction with each other and the liquid. Colloidal silica consists of fine particles of hydrated silicas that can form a gel and bind larger particles of noncolloidal nature.

fired strength The strength of an investment following a burnout process. This strength is often measured by resistance to breakage under three-point loading or bending. Compare with *green strength*.

fixture A device that is firmly fastened in place in a mechanical sense, often used to secure other devices.

Gibbs free energy of formation (FEF) Gibbs free energy is the thermodynamic function $\Delta G_f = \Delta H - T\Delta S$, where H is enthalpy, T is absolute temperature, and S is entropy. Also called *free energy*. FEF is the free energy change for formation of a particular compound at a temperature T.

green strength The prefired strength of an investment, acquired through some chemical reaction at or near room temperature. Compare with *fired strength*.

hydrolysis Decomposition of a compound by water, or the interaction of positive and negative ions of a salt with hydroxyl and hydrogen ions to form an acid and a base.

hygroscopic Pertaining to the absorption of water.

investment A heat-resistant material used to form a mold around a wax pattern.

mold A cavity into which molten metal is cast.

refractory A heat-resistant material.

ring A thin-walled structure used to contain an investment slurry before it sets; also provides support for set or fired investments that have poor strength.

setting expansion The volumetric or linear increase in physical dimensions of an investment, caused by the chemical reactions that occur during hardening to a rigid structure.

slurry A thin mixture of liquid and powder.

surface coat The first coating that is applied to a wax pattern or the surface of the mold that comes into direct contact with a cast metal.

thermal expansion The increase in dimension of a set investment due to temperature increase during burnout.

◧ Discussion Questions

1. Which developments in clinical dentistry have led to a switch from the use of gypsum to more refractory materials?

2. What are the matrix compositions of the two major high-heat investments?

3. How can additional expansion be obtained with magnesia and ESBIs?

4. Which of the two high-heat investments gives more accurate models for casting applications?

5. What are two composition changes to phosphate investments that have led to improved gas permeability and allowed rapid-heat processing for burnout?

6. What are the obstacles that have impeded the use of titanium castings for use as dental prostheses?

◧ Study Questions

(See appendix E for answers)

1. Given a multicomponent system that includes ethyl silicate as a reacting component, how can the reaction time for hydrolysis be altered?

2. Cooling hydrated ethyl silicate to 4.4°C (40°F) extends its shelf life. *(a)* Would the shelf life be extended by refrigeration to lower temperatures? *(b)* To what extent may the liquid be cooled without encountering adverse effects?

3. Why is denatured ethyl alcohol used rather than 95% ethyl alcohol as a component of an ethyl silicate system?

4. List advantages and disadvantages of phosphate-bonded investments.

5. List advantages and disadvantages of ethyl silicate–bonded investments.

6. For the casting of nonprecious fixed partial denture alloys, which technique would be recommended with a phosphate-bonded investment?

7. What are the investments of choice for casting *(a)* ceramic gold alloy; *(b)* cobalt-chromium partial denture alloy; *(c)* nickel-based fixed partial denture alloy?

8. List the six approaches to altering the fit of a casting.

9. What might be an advantage of a mixed colloidal silica–ethyl silicate system over a straight ethyl silicate system?

10. A carbon-filled and a noncarbon-filled phosphate investment are available to you for casing ceramic-veneering alloys. (a) Can both be used for casting a gold alloy? (b) Which one is recommended for casting of a nonprecious alloy and why?

11. What recent (after the year 2000) significant shift in processing has occurred and led to improved productivity with phosphate bonded investments?

● References

1. International Organization for Standardization. ISO 15912:2006. Dentistry—Casting Investments and Refractory Die Materials. Geneva: International Organization for Standardization, 2006.

2. Kondic V. Metallurgical Principles of Foundry. Amsterdam: Elsevier, 1960:193.

3. Takahashi J, Kimura H, Lautenschlager EP, Lin JHC, Moser JB, Greener EH. Casting pure titanium into commercial phosphate-bonded SiO2 investment molds. J Dent Res 1990;69(12):1800–1805.

4. Pineda RP and Chadwick TC, inventors. Phosphate investment compositions. United States patent 6551396, 2003.

5. Kamohara H, Hayashi S, Ohi N, inventors. Investments for dental casting. United States patent 4814011 1989.

6. American National Standards Institute/American Dental Association Specification No. 42. Dental Phosphate-Bonded Casting Investments. Chicago: American Dental Association, 2002.

7. American National Standards Institute/American Dental Association. ANSI/ADA Specification No. 91-1999. Ethyl Silicate Investments. Chicago: American Dental Association, 1999.

8. Togaya T. Selection of investments for improving fits of titanium castings [in Japanese]. Shika Gikou 1993;21(9):909–917.

9. Miyazaki T, Tamaki Y. Current situation of investment materials for casting of titanium [in Japanese]. Quintessence Dent Technol 1993;16:25–30.

10. Chase MW, Davies CA, Downey JRJ, Frurip DJ, McDonald RA, Syverud AN. JANAF Thermochemical Tables, vol 14, ed 3. New York: American Institute of Physics for the National Bureau of Standards, 1985.

11. Takahashi J. Can we use phosphate-bonded silica investment for casting pure titanium [in Japanese]? Quintessence Dent Technol 1993;16:24.

12. Okuda R, Satou H, Satou M, Matsui A. Assessment of an experimental investment specified for titanium casting by the observation of the castings. Dent Jpn 1991;28:71–83.

13. Togaya T, Suzuki M, Ida I, Nakamura M, Uemura T. Studies on magnesia investment for casting of titanium—Improvement of fitness on castings by utilizing an expansion due to oxidation of additive Zr powder in the investment. J Dent Mater 1985;4(4):344–349.

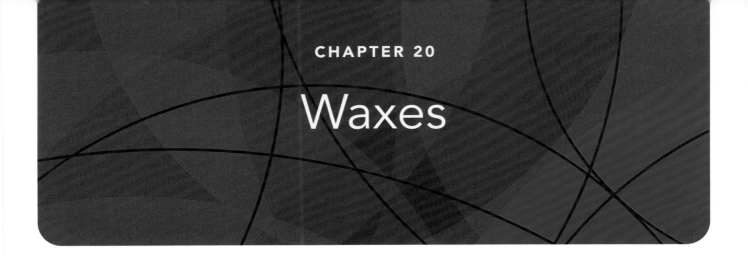

CHAPTER 20

Waxes

Many applications in restorative dentistry use waxes, such as patterns for inlays, crowns, pontics, and partial and complete dentures. Waxes are also very useful for bite registration and can be used to obtain impressions of edentulous areas.

Composition

Waxes are organic polymers consisting of hydrocarbons and their derivatives (eg, esters and alcohols). The average molecular weight of a wax blend is about 400 to 4,000, which is low compared with structural acrylic polymers. Dental waxes are blends of ingredients, including **natural waxes**, **synthetic waxes**, **natural resins**, oils, **fats**, **gums**, and coloring agents.

Natural waxes are of mineral (petroleum oil), plant, insect, or animal origin. Paraffin wax, obtained from refined crude oil, is relatively soft with a low melting range (50°C to 70°C) and is used in inlay and modeling waxes. Beeswax is brittle, with an intermediate melting range (60°C to 70°C [122°F to 158°F]). This insect wax is obtained from honeycombs and is added to many types of waxes because of its desirable **flow** properties at oral temperature. Carnauba wax is a plant wax obtained from carnauba palm trees and is hard and tough, with a high melting range (65°C to 90°C [149°F to 194°F]). It is added to toughen paraffin wax and raise its melting range. Microcrystalline waxes are obtained from petroleum. Because they have a high melting range (65°C to 90°C), they are added to modify the softening and melting ranges of wax blends and also serve to reduce stresses that occur on cooling.

Synthetic waxes, such as low-molecular-weight polyethylene, have specific melting points and are usually blended with natural waxes. Natural waxes vary more depending on their sources and need to be monitored more for properties than synthetic waxes, which are more uniform in composition.

Classification

Dental waxes are classified according to their applications into pattern, processing, and impression waxes (Fig 20-1).

Pattern waxes

Inlay, resin, casting, and base plate waxes are all pattern waxes. Inlay waxes (Kerr Dental) are used to make inlay, crown, and pontic replicas used in the lost wax casting technique. Type I inlay waxes are soft and used for the indirect inlay technique and sometimes for the attachment of miscellaneous parts. Type II inlay waxes are hard waxes used for preparing direct patterns in the mouth. The flow of these waxes and other properties are covered by the International Organization for Standardization[1] (ISO). Inlay waxes are supplied in geometric and anatomic forms as well as in bulk.

Pattern resins are characterized by higher strength and resistance to flow than waxes, good dimensional stability, and burnout without residue. Full-crown patterns fabricated from pattern resins and inlay waxes have similar marginal discrepancies.

A **pattern** is fabricated by applying the resin in 3- to 5-mm layers and curing in a light chamber or with a hand-held light-curing unit. Resin is completely eliminated from the mold before casting by heating at 690°C (1,273°F) for 45 minutes.

Casting waxes are used for thin sections of certain removable and fixed partial denture patterns. They are particularly convenient in the preparation of copings or clasps requiring uniformly thin regions. Casting waxes are supplied in sheets and rods and in bulk, and preformed patterns are available for partial denture applications.

Base plate wax, which is supplied in sheets, is used in the construction of full denture patterns and for occlusal rims, although an occlusal rim wax is also available. Setup wax may be used instead of base plate wax to set denture teeth.

The ANSI/ADA has established a specification that includes three types of base plate wax: type I is a soft base plate wax for veneers and contours; type II is a medium-hardness base plate wax designed for use in temperate climates; and type III is the hardest base plate wax and is for use in tropical climates. The hardness is based on the amount of flow the wax shows at 45°C (113°F).

Base plate wax is also used as a mold for the construction of provisional fixed partial dentures, as a bite registration wax, and for some applications in orthodontics.

Processing waxes

Boxing wax is a processing wax used to form containers for pouring casts and to fabricate replacement pontics for provisional fixed partial dentures. Sticky wax (Kerr Group) is used to join materials temporarily, while carding wax is used for attaching parts and in some soldering techniques. Blockout wax is used to fill voids and undercuts for removable partial denture fabrication, and white wax is used for making patterns to simulate a veneer facing. Finally, in miscellaneous applications for various laboratory procedures, utility wax (Heraeus Kulzer) is used.

Impression waxes

Waxes used for impressions (bite wax, Mizzy) exhibit high flow and distort on withdrawal from undercuts. Waxes used specifically for denture impressions are limited to use in edentulous regions of the mouth. Corrective waxes are used as wax washes to record detail and displace selected regions of soft tissue in edentulous impressions.

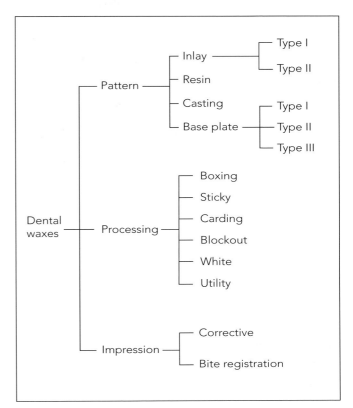

Fig 20-1 A classification of dental waxes.

Bite waxes are used in certain prosthetic techniques; a typical use would be bite registration. These waxes are supplied in a variety of forms and shapes.

● Properties

Waxes may consist of both crystalline and amorphous components, each with a distribution of molecular weights. Therefore, waxes melt over a range of 5°C to 30°C (41°F to 86°F) rather than at one temperature. Waxes have the highest coefficients of thermal expansion of any dental material. Resultant dimensional changes may produce poor-fitting castings if not balanced by compensating factors of mold expansion. The total wax shrinkage on cooling from liquid to solid at room temperature may be as great as 0.4%, with solidification shrinkage plus contraction on cooling to room temperature after solidification.

Flow is a measure of a wax's ability to deform under light forces and is analogous to creep. Flow increases with increasing temperature and force. At a temperature

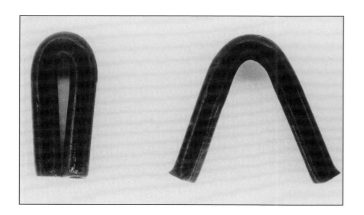

Fig 20-2 The wax rod on the right was originally bent to the shape of the wax rod on the left. After floating in room-temperature water for 24 hours, the rod opened as a result of the memory effect.

close to its softening range, a wax may flow under its own weight. In liquids, flow is measured by viscosity, and in solids is measured by the degree of plastic deformation over a fixed period of time. Type I direct inlay technique waxes need to flow well to reproduce details of the cavity preparation.[2] However, when the wax is cooled to oral temperature, flow must be minimized to reduce distortion when the pattern is removed.

■ Wax Distortion

Waxes are partly elastic in behavior and tend to return to their original shape after deformation. A straight bar of wax bent into a horseshoe shape will slowly straighten out at room temperature (Fig 20-2). This behavior is called the *memory effect*. **Residual stresses** as a result of nonuniform heating also contribute to later distortion. There are four ways of minimizing pattern distortion. First, wax used in the direct technique should be heated uniformly at 50°C (122°F) for 15 minutes before use. Next, the pattern should be invested quickly; the rigid walls of the set investment constrain the pattern and reduce distortion due to **recovery** and residual stress. Third, storage in a refrigerator is preferred if there will be a delay in investing, as elastic recovery is slower at low temperatures. If a pattern is refrigerated, however, it should be allowed to warm to room temperature before investing. Finally, it is essential that no wax residues are left in the mold after burnout in the lost wax process. Residues will result in poor castings because of inclusions or incomplete margins.

■ Glossary

fats Substances similar to wax but characterized as being soft and greasy to the touch. An example of a fat used in dental waxes is stearic acid.

flow Continued deformation resulting from application of a static force.

gums Viscous substances from plant or animal sources that harden in air. Gums combine with water to form sticky, viscous liquids. An example of a gum is gum arabic.

natural resins Mixtures of high-molecular-weight organic substances obtained directly from plants or trees as exudates. An example of a natural resin used in dental waxes is dammar.

natural wax A hydrocarbon or hydrocarbon-derivative polymer with an approximate molecular weight of 400 to 4,000; of mineral, plant, insect, or animal origin. Examples of natural wax are paraffin, beeswax, carnauba, spermaceti, and ceresin.

pattern A form used to make a mold.

recovery Change in shape resulting from the release of internal stresses.

residual stress Internal stress independent of applied force.

synthetic wax A man-made wax synthesized from appropriate monomers.

Discussion Questions

1. Waxes have the highest thermal expansion values of any dental material. What problems can result from this property, especially in casting accuracy?

2. Which type of inlay wax (I or II) should be used for the indirect die technique? How do the different flow properties of the two types make them suitable for their applications?

3. If a wax inlay pattern cannot be invested right away, it is recommended that it be stored in a refrigerator. Why and what phenomena will this storage affect?

4. Why are polymer cements recommended for use with computer-aided design/computer-assisted manufacture inlays with poor marginal fits?

Study Questions

(See appendix E for answers.)

1. List several common natural waxes used in dentistry.

2. Why must natural waxes be carefully monitored for properties?

3. Name three types of pattern waxes and their applications.

4. Wax pattern contraction arises from two sources. What are they?

5. List two means of increasing wax flow.

6. Describe three steps to minimize wax pattern distortion.

7. Type I pattern wax must have two types of flow behavior. Why?

8. What is the memory or recovery effect in waxes, and what does it lead to?

9. Why is complete burnout of wax patterns critical in the lost wax casting technique?

References

1. International Organization for Standardization. ISO 15854:2005. Dentistry—Casting and Baseplate Waxes. Geneva: International Organization for Standardization, 2005.
2. Warth AH. The Chemistry and Technology of Waxes. New York: Van Nostrand Reinhold, 1956.

Recommended Reading

American Dental Association. Dentists' Desk Reference: Materials, Instruments and Equipment, ed 2. Chicago: American Dental Association, 1983.

Mc Millan IC, Darvell BW. Rheology of dental waxes. Dent Mater 2000;16(5):337–350.

Powers JM, Craiig RG, Peyton FA. Calorimetric analysis of commercial and dental waxes. J Dent Res 1969;48):1165–1170.

Smith DC, Earnshaw R, McCrorie JW. Some properties of modeling and baseplate waxes. Br Dent J 1965;118:437–442.

Orthodontic Wires

There is a bewildering array of metallic wires available for orthodontic use, including the older stainless steel and cobalt-chromium-nickel wires, nickel-titanium and β-titanium wires, superelastic and shape-memory nickel-titanium wires, and ion-implanted nickel-titanium and β-titanium wires. Esthetic nonmetallic orthodontic wires are under investigation, although none are currently being marketed.

The principal objective of this chapter is to assist the clinician in selecting the most appropriate product among the wide variety of orthodontic wires available. The second objective is to provide a comprehensive list of references to research in this exciting field. A general classification of the alloy systems used for the metallic orthodontic wires is provided in Fig 21-1.

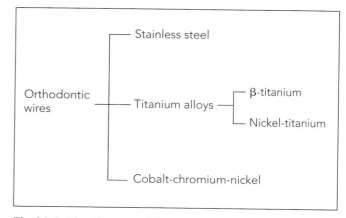

Fig 21-1 Classification of the alloy systems used for metallic orthodontic wires.

◖ Mechanical Properties

Manufacturing of orthodontic wires

Metallic orthodontic wires are manufactured by a series of proprietary steps, typically involving more than one company. Initially, the wire alloy is cast in the form of an ingot, which must be subjected to successive deformation stages until the cross section becomes sufficiently small for wire drawing. Several deformation stages and intermediate heat treatments are required because considerable work hardening of the alloy occurs during wire manufacturing. Important proprietary details include the rate of drawing, the amount of cross-section reduction per pass, the nature of intermediate heat treatments, the die material and lubricant in contact with the wires, and

the ambient atmosphere, which would be important for reactive titanium-containing wire alloys. In general, the casting of the starting ingot and the initial mechanical deformation stages are not performed by the orthodontic materials companies that market the wires.

Whereas round orthodontic wires are manufactured by drawing through dies, rectangular and square cross-section wires are fabricated from round wires by a rolling process using a Turk's head, which contains pairs of rolls. The resulting rectangular or square cross-section wires will necessarily have some degree of rounding at the corners, which varies with the specific wire type and the manufacturer. This edge bevel can be of clinical significance for the actual torque delivered by the archwire-bracket combination. Moreover, the surface roughness of the wire, which has a clinically significant effect on the archwire-bracket sliding friction, varies considerably among the various products and is generally greater for the β-titanium and nickel-titanium wires.

As a result of the wire-drawing sequence, orthodontic wires have a characteristic wrought microstructure. The original equiaxed grain structure of the starting cast ingot is completely eliminated, and when a polished and etched wire specimen is viewed through the optical microscope or the scanning electron microscope, the wrought grain structure appears as a series of closely spaced lines parallel to the original direction of drawing. It is well-known that this microstructure is essential for an orthodontic wire to maintain the desired **temper** (springiness) or optimal mechanical properties for clinical use. For example, heat treatment of stainless steel wires at temperatures of 700°C (1,300°F) and higher causes rapid softening and loss of the wrought microstructure as a result of recrystallization. Optimum heat treatments involve only the recovery stage of annealing. In practice, clinicians perform heat treatments using an electric resistance (spot) welding apparatus, and the stainless steel, cobalt-chromium-nickel, and some nickel-titanium wires may be advantageously heat treated.

There are four general wire alloys in significant current use: austenitic stainless steel, cobalt-chromium-nickel, β-titanium, and nickel-titanium. When selecting a wire based on the desired properties for a given patient, it is important to consider the basic alloy composition and the effect that processes, such as drawing, rolling, and heat treatments that are applied by the manufacturer and the clinician, will have on the specific wire properties and archwire-bracket torque delivery characteristics.

In general, an orthodontist should consider the following aspects in the selection of wires: force delivery, elastic working range, ease of joining individual segments to fabricate more complex appliances, and corrosion resistance and biocompatibility in the oral environment. Cost also represents a significant concern for the clinician, and there is a considerable difference between stainless steel archwires and β-titanium and nickel-titanium archwires. However, these more expensive alloys offer unique properties that should be carefully considered when selecting orthodontic wires.

Bending tests and mechanics principles

To understand the mechanical properties of primary importance when comparing different wire types and sizes, it is first necessary to review the underlying principles and terminology. Typically, the mechanical properties of or-

thodontic wires are determined from some type of bending test, because this mode of deformation is more representative of clinical conditions than the tension test conventionally used for metals. The cantilever bending test in the original form of American National Standards Institute/American Dental Association (ANSI/ADA) specification[1] for orthodontic wires not containing precious metals was strongly criticized. The revised specification[2] contains a three-point bending test that better simulates clinical interbracket distances and is more suitable for nickel-titanium wires with very low elastic modulus than the previous test, which used the Olsen stiffness tester.

All bending tests involve the measurement of angular or linear deflection of an archwire segment resulting from a bending moment or an applied force. The *bending moment* or force and the deflection are represented on the vertical and horizontal axes, respectively, of a graphic plot that is generally a straight line at the force levels for elastic deformation of clinical interest. The exception is when very short test spans are used. Although orthodontists typically activate wires somewhat into the permanent deformation range, the bending properties are based on elastic deformation. Although clinical interest is obviously in the unloading characteristics of activated archwires, investigators have generally determined mechanical properties during the initial loading stage. The elastic loading and unloading plots differ for the nickel-titanium wires, although they do not differ for the other alloy types.

There are several basic mechanical properties of orthodontic wires that are determined from the bending test plot:

1. The elastic **force delivery** is the slope of the initial straight line and is the amount of force required for unit **activation**. This property determines the stiffness of the wire and is the inverse of the property of flexibility. For those test plots in which bending moment is portrayed as a function of linear or angular deflection, the elastic force delivery is proportional to the slope of the initial straight line.

2. The *proportional limit* is the highest point on the bending plot at which the force or bending moment remains proportional to the deflection for a wire alloy that exhibits linear elasticity (stainless steel, cobalt-chromium-nickel, and β-titanium wires). Nickel-titanium wires typically exhibit nonlinear elastic behavior.

3. A force or moment at yielding occurs in response to a designated small amount of permanent bending deflection, and is analogous to the yield strength (*YS*) for the conventional tension test used to evaluate the mechanical properties of metals.

4. A maximum force or moment will be observed during the bending test, but will not have clinical relevance when substantial permanent deformation has taken place, since only elastic deformation is involved for tooth movement.

5. The maximum elastic activation before the onset of permanent deformation is the value of linear or angular deflection corresponding to the maximum elastic force or moment at the proportional limit. This property is known as the *elastic range* or **working range** (sometimes simply termed the *range*) of the wire.

Wire stiffness or elastic force delivery is dependent on two fundamental factors: *(1)* the composition and structure of the wire alloy, reflecting both the basic metallurgy and the manufacturing sequence, and *(2)* the wire segment geometry, that is, the cross-section shape and size and the segment length. The basic metallurgy contribution of the wire alloy is given by the modulus of elasticity (*E*), or the *Young modulus*, which relates tensile and compressive elastic stress and strain independent of the specimen cross-section area and length. The elastic modulus values determined from bending and tension tests should be the same, provided that the bending deformation is properly analyzed.

The resistance of a cross-section shape to elastic bending is related to the **moment of inertia** (*I*). For a round wire of diameter (*d*), the moment of inertia is given by:

$$I = \frac{\pi d^4}{64}$$

whereas for a rectangular wire of width (*w*) and thickness (*t*) in the plane of bending:

$$I = \frac{wt^3}{12}$$

The stiffness of an archwire is inversely proportional to the segment length (*l*), so that if the length is doubled, the wire flexibility or elastic deflection will be doubled for the same applied force or bending moment. Summarizing these contributions, the elastic stiffness or force delivery characteristics are given by the following expressions:

Round wire: $\dfrac{Ed^4}{l}$

Rectangular wire: $\dfrac{Ewt^3}{l}$

Many studies in the orthodontic literature use the property of flexural rigidity, given by the product of elastic modulus and moment of inertia, to compare the bending deflections for different wire segments having the same length.

There are two additional useful mechanical properties for orthodontic wires, which are obtained by combining the basic mechanical properties previously discussed (Table 21-1):

1. The *modulus of resilience* is the area under the elastic force-activation plot and represents the total biomechanical energy per unit volume available for tooth movement when the wire is loaded to the maximum elastic stress or bending moment or, equivalently, unloaded from this level. The modulus of resilience for an orthodontic wire is usually written as $(YS)^2/2E$. The yield strength is generally used to represent the onset of permanent deformation because of the difficulty in precisely locating the proportional limit (*PL*) on a bending test plot. The formal expression in materials science for the modulus of resilience is $(PL)^2/2E$. It follows that the resilience is much more strongly affected by changes in yield strength or proportional limit than elastic modulus, which is important for the heat-treatment response of cobalt-chromium-nickel and stainless steel wires.

2. The **springback** for an archwire after unloading is expressed as *YS/E*, which is approximately equal to the maximum elastic strain or working range of the wire. (The formal expression from materials science for springback would be *PL/E*.) Since the unloading curve from the permanent deformation range for linearly elastic orthodontic wire alloys (ie, other than nickel-titanium wires) is parallel to the elastic loading curve, the value of *YS/E* represents the approximate amount of elastic strain released by the archwire on unloading.

Numerous articles listed in the recommended readings have discussed the mechanics of bending tests for orthodontic wires.

Table 21-1 Summary of conventional terminology for important mechanical properties of orthodontic wires*

BASIC PROPERTY	LOCATION ON BENDING PLOT	EQUIVALENT TERMS[†]
Rate of force delivery (stiffness)	Slope of elastic loading curve or unloading curve	$\dfrac{EI}{l}$
Moment at yielding or flexural yield strength	Bending moment for designated small amount of permanent deformation (vertical axis of graph)	YS
Working range	Maximum value of purely elastic deformation (horizontal axis)	—
Modulus of resilience (resilience)	Area under elastic loading curve or unloading curve	$\dfrac{(YS)^2}{2E}$
Springback	Elastic strain recovered on unloading from permanent deformation range	$\dfrac{YS}{E}$

*The expressions are applicable to tension tests and bending tests for wire alloys exhibiting linear elasticity and sufficiently long specimens.[3,4] In these cases, the elastic unloading curve of clinical interest is essentially the same as the initial linear plot for elastic loading. For short loading spans and the nonsuperelastic nickel-titanium alloys, the unloading curves are nonlinear, and it is difficult to define a modulus of elasticity.

[†]For the idealized definitions, the yield strength (YS) should be replaced in the expressions for modulus of resilience (resilience) and springback by the proportional limit (PL). Other symbols have their usual meanings: E = modulus of elasticity, I = moment of inertia (proportional to d^4 for round wire and wt^3 for rectangular wire), l = segment length, d = diameter, w = width, t = thickness in plane of bending.

Orthodontic Wire Alloys

Stainless steel

Stainless steel wires continue to be popular in clinical orthodontics because of their adequate mechanical properties, good corrosion resistance in the oral environment, and low cost. However, these wires have relatively high values of elastic modulus and thus do not provide the light force delivery that is optimum for orthodontic tooth movement. The wires used in orthodontics are generally American Iron and Steel Institute (AISI) types 302 and 304 austenitic stainless steels, with similar nominal compositions, although the use of 17-7 precipitation-hardening stainless steel was explored. Type 302 is composed of 17% to 19% chromium, 8% to 10% nickel, and 0.15% maximum carbon. Type 304 contains 18% to 20% chromium, 8% to 12% nickel, and 0.08% maximum carbon. The balance of the alloy composition (Table 21-2) is essentially iron (approximately 70%). These are the well-known "18-8" stainless steels, so designated because of the percentages of chromium and nickel in the alloys.

Research has shown that the modulus of elasticity in tension for stainless steel orthodontic wires, where values are more reliable than for bending tests, ranges from about 160 to 180 GPa. These values depend on the man-

ufacturer and temper, and are indicative of differences in alloy compositions, wire drawing procedures, and heat-treatment conditions. For many years, it was not appreciated that the elastic modulus for stainless steel orthodontic wires can be significantly decreased below the 190 to 210 GPa range given in standard physical metallurgy textbooks for annealed stainless steel, although this reduction in elastic modulus was well-known more than five decades ago for heavily cold-worked industrial austenitic stainless steel alloys.

X-ray diffraction has shown that austenitic stainless steel archwires do not necessarily have the single-phase austenitic structure in the as-received condition from the manufacturers. The microstructural phases in these stainless steel wires depend on the manufacturer, temper, and cross-section size; the fundamental factors are the AISI type (particularly carbon content) and thermomechanical processing during manufacturing.

The yield strength for the stainless steel archwires shows a much wider variation than the elastic modulus and has been found to range from approximately 1,100 to 1,500 MPa. After heat treatment, the yield strength can increase to about 1,700 MPa for several wire sizes. Heat treatment also causes significant decreases in residual stress and modest increases (~10%) in resilience. The range in values of mechanical properties in tension for as-received stainless steel wires of clinically important

Table 21-2 General compositions for four major classes of orthodontic wire alloys

WIRE ALLOY	WEIGHT % OF ELEMENTS
Austenitic stainless steel[5]	17%–20% Cr, 8%–12% Ni, 0.15% C maximum, balance principally Fe (~ 70%)
Cobalt-chromium-nickel[6] (Elgiloy)	40% Co, 20% Cr, 15% Ni, 15.8% Fe, 7% Mo, 2% Mn, 0.16% C, 0.04% Be
β-titanium (TMA)[7]	77.8% Ti, 11.3% Mo, 6.6% Zr, 4.3% Sn
Nickel-titanium[8–10] (Nitinol)	55% Ni, 45% Ti (may contain small amounts of Cu or other elements)

Table 21-3 Range of mechanical properties in tension of principal clinical importance for four major orthodontic alloys and as-received wires*

WIRE ALLOY	MODULUS OF ELASTICITY (GPa)†	YIELD STRENGTH (MPa)†
Stainless steel (resilient temper)	160–180	1,100–1,500
Cobalt-chromium-nickel (Elgiloy Blue)	160–190	830–1,000
β-titanium (TMA)	62–69	690–970
Nickel-titanium (Nitinol)	34	210–410

*The data for modulus of elasticity and yield strength are for round wires with diameters from 0.016 to 0.020 inch and for rectangular wires having cross-section dimensions from 0.017 inch × 0.025 inch to 0.019 inch × 0.025 inch.[11,12]
†1 MPa = 145 psi and 1 GPa = 145,000 psi.

sizes is summarized in Table 21-3. Springback (YS/E) was found to range from 0.0060 to 0.0094 for eight different sizes of as-received stainless steel wires and from 0.0065 to 0.0099 after heat treatment.

The use of heat treatment to eliminate residual stresses that might cause fracture during manipulation of stainless steel appliances can be important under clinical conditions. However, austenitic stainless steel alloys can be rendered susceptible to intergranular corrosion when heated to temperatures between 400°C and 900°C, due to the formation of chromium carbides at the grain boundaries. These precipitates deplete the amount of chromium near the grain boundaries in the bulk stainless steel below that needed for corrosion resistance. Since the stainless steel alloys must be heated within this temperature range for soldering, clinicians are cautioned to minimize the time required for this process.

Cobalt-chromium-nickel

Cobalt-chromium-nickel orthodontic wires are similar to stainless steel wires in appearance, mechanical properties (see Table 21-3), and joining characteristics, but have a much different composition and considerably greater heat treatment response. Table 21-2 shows that the most commonly used alloy, Elgiloy (Rocky Mountain Ortho-

dontics) has a complex composition of 40% cobalt, 20% chromium, 15% nickel, 15.8% iron, 7% molybdenum, 2% manganese, 0.15% carbon, and 0.04% beryllium, which is similar to that of some base metal casting alloys for removable partial dentures.

The Elgiloy wires are available in four color-coded tempers: soft, ductile, semi-resilient, and resilient. The differences in mechanical properties arise from proprietary variations in the wire manufacturing process. The soft-temper wires (Elgiloy Blue) are popular because they are easily deformed and shaped into appliances, then heat treated to provide substantially increased values of yield strength and resilience. Increases of 20% to 30% in the yield strength of Elgiloy Blue wires after heat treatment have been reported, and similar heat-treatment responses appear to occur for the soft, ductile, and semi-resilient tempers. The large increases in modulus of resilience arise from the dependence on $(YS)^2$ (see Table 21-1). The effect of heat treatment on mechanical properties has been attributed to complex precipitation processes. Springback for the Elgiloy Blue alloy was found to range from 0.0045 to 0.0065 for five different sizes of as-received wires and from 0.0054 to 0.0074 after heat treatment.

The other Elgiloy tempers are less popular than the soft temper because wires made from these tempers have lower formability and are higher in cost than stainless steel. For Elgiloy Blue, the elastic modulus in tension ranges from about 160 to 190 GPa for as-received wires (see Table 21-3), and from about 180 to 210 GPa after heat treatment. The corresponding ranges in yield strength are approximately 830 to 1,000 MPa in the as-received condition, and 1,100 to 1,400 MPa after heat treatment. It is important to emphasize that the elastic force delivery is nearly the same for stainless steel and Elgiloy Blue archwire segments of the same size and length, as indicated in Table 21-3. A common misconception is that the elastic force delivery is much less for Elgiloy Blue wires compared with stainless steel wires because of the "feel" of the former. It is the yield strength and elastic range that are diminished relative to the more resilient stainless steel wires.

β-titanium

A β-titanium orthodontic alloy, TMA (Ormco/Sybron), was introduced to the orthodontic profession about 25 years ago. The nominal composition of TMA, which is derived from the two major component elements (titanium-molybdenum alloy), is similar to the 77.8% titanium, 11.3% molybdenum, 6.6% zirconium, and 4.3% tin composition of an industrial Beta III titanium alloy (see Table 21-2). The presence of molybdenum (a β-stabilizing element) causes the elevated-temperature body-centered cubic β phase of titanium, rather than the lower-temperature hexagonal close-packed α phase, to be metastable at room temperature. Cold work at ambient temperature or heating to slightly elevated temperature can cause partial transformation of metastable β-titanium alloys to the α phase. The presence of numerous slip systems for dislocation movement in the β phase results in excellent formability or capability for permanent deformation. Zirconium and tin contribute increased strength and hardness and hinder formation of an embrittling ω phase during wire processing at elevated temperatures. The TMA alloy has somewhat less than half the elastic force delivery (E ranging from about 62 to 69 GPa) of stainless steel wires, with the yield strength ranging from approximately 690 to 970 MPa (see Table 21-3). Springback for four different sizes of as-received TMA wires was found to range from 0.0094 to 0.011.

Another noteworthy characteristic is that the TMA alloy possesses true **weldability**. (Welded joints that are fabricated from stainless steel and cobalt-chromium-nickel alloys must be built up with the use of solders to maintain adequate strength.) Optimum conditions for welding TMA with commercial apparatus have been published by Nelson and colleagues.[13] Heat treatment by the clinician is not recommended for TMA, although this alloy does respond to a precipitation-hardening procedure. Solution heat treatment between approximately 700°C and 730°C, followed by water quenching, then aging at approximately 480°C, results in precipitation of the α-titanium phase and a peak value for the YS/E ratio.

Research by Kusy and colleagues[14] has shown that TMA wires have high surface roughness, which leads to high values of archwire-bracket friction. Ion-implanted TMA wires that have substantially reduced archwire-bracket friction are available from Ormco/Sybron.

With the expiration of the original patent for TMA, new β-titanium orthodontic wires have been introduced, such as Resolve (Dentsply International) and Beta III Titanium (3M Unitek). Transmission electron microscopic observations of microstructural precipitates in the TMA and Resolve β-titanium wires suggest that different processing procedures (wire drawing parameters and heat-treatment conditions) are used by the two manufacturers. These differences in processing procedures may have practical significance for the clinically important mechanical properties of β-titanium wire products. The metallurgy of the β-titanium wires and other recently introduced titanium alloy wires for orthodontics can be complex, and the interested reader should consult the appropriate textbook references listed at the end of the chapter.

The joining of β-titanium wires has recently been of substantial research interest. Research by Iijima and colleagues[15] using a new technique of micro–x-ray diffraction, which is capable of analyzing regions much smaller (50 μm in diameter) than conventional x-ray diffraction, has shown that brazed or soldered wires largely retained the original β-titanium structure and should be acceptable for clinical use. Further evaluation of mechanical properties and corrosion behavior for the β-titanium joints is needed.

Development of new β-titanium alloys and other titanium alloys has been an area of considerable activity by manufacturers in recent years, in part because of the biocompatibility of these nickel-free wires. However, the susceptibility of β-titanium wires to attack in acidulated fluoride solutions used for mouthwashes and the concomitant degradation of wire properties suggest that future research is needed to address clinical concerns about this potential problem. The susceptibility of β-titanium wires to hydrogen embrittlement with the possibility of delayed fracture in these acidulated solutions also warrants further investigation.

Nickel-titanium

The fourth wire alloy, nickel-titanium, has also remained a strong focus of materials research as well as considerable marketing activity by manufacturers. The name *nitinol*, which is a generic name for all of these nickel-titanium alloys, is derived from the words *nickel* and *titanium* that make up the composition, along with the acronym for Naval Ordnance Laboratory, which is where these alloys were originally developed by Buehler and associates. The use of nickel-titanium wires for orthodontics originated from work by Andreasen and colleagues in the early 1970s.[16,17]

Nickel-titanium orthodontic alloys are based on the intermetallic compound NiTi, which has weight percentages of 55% nickel and 45% titanium (see Table 21-2). X-ray energy-dispersive spectroscopic analyses of several nickel-titanium wire products suggest that the compositions are slightly titanium-rich (between 50 and 51 atomic percent titanium).

Although the **shape-memory effect** associated with engineering nickel-titanium alloys was not available in the original Nitinol wire (3M Unitek), there were two features of considerable importance for clinical orthodontics:

1. The very low elastic modulus (*E* about 34 GPa in tension) for Nitinol corresponds to about one-fifth of the force delivery for stainless steel archwires and half the force delivery for TMA wires having the same cross-section dimensions and length.
2. Because of the extremely wide elastic working range, 12.5-mm segments in the clinically important size ranges retained a permanent set of not more than 5 degrees after 90-degree cantilever bending by the original ANSI/ADA specification test procedure and release of the applied moment.

The yield strength for the original Nitinol orthodontic wires generally ranges from about 210 to 410 MPa. Springback for six different sizes of as-received wires was found to range from 0.0058 to 0.016.

Chinese NiTi orthodontic wire (Ni-Ti, Ormco/Sybron) was subsequently introduced and compared with the original Nitinol alloy and stainless steel wires, using a cantilever bending test and 5-mm span lengths appropriate to clinical interbracket distances. The nonlinear activation characteristics of clinical interest were evident. However, whereas the average unloading stiffness (ratio of bending moment to amount of deactivation in degrees) was the same for all activations of Nitinol, the unloading curves for Chinese NiTi wires were dependent on the level of activation (amount of bending deflection). These latter unloading curves have relatively high values of unloading stiffness for the initial and final stages (under 10 degrees) of deactivation; through the middle range of deactivation, the unloading stiffness is much smaller and approaches constant force delivery. The average stiffness of Chinese NiTi wire from these unloading curves was found to increase considerably from the largest to smallest activations. With the 5-mm test spans, the springback of Chinese NiTi wire was more than 4 times that for stainless steel and more than 50% greater than that for Nitinol wire.

Japanese NiTi wire (Sentalloy, Dentsply International) was introduced at about the same time as Chinese NiTi wire. The stress-strain curves in tension and the load-deflection curves for three-point bending of 14-mm test spans were compared for 0.016-inch diameter wires of this alloy, Nitinol, stainless steel, and Elgiloy. Tension and bending tests confirmed the existence of **superelastic** behavior in the Japanese NiTi wires. After a certain level of elastic tensile strain or bending deflection, further deformation (up to about 10% tensile strain or 2-mm deflection for a 0.016-inch diameter wire) takes place at nearly constant tensile stress or bending force (upper superelastic plateau). The unloading characteristics exhibit initial and final regions of relatively steep slope, along with an extensive intermediate region (lower superelastic plateau) where there is little change in stress or force. The superelastic plateaus are evident as horizontal regions on tension test plots, since stress is uniform over the wire cross-section. These plateaus are less well-defined on bending test plots, since stress varies over the wire cross section.

When Japanese NiTi wire was heat treated at 500°C from 5 minutes to 2 hours, the bending force remaining during the superelastic region of the deactivation curve could be varied over a wide range. This behavior was exploited to develop commercial nickel-titanium wires that can deliver low, medium, or high levels of force. A highly convenient electric resistance method has been devel-

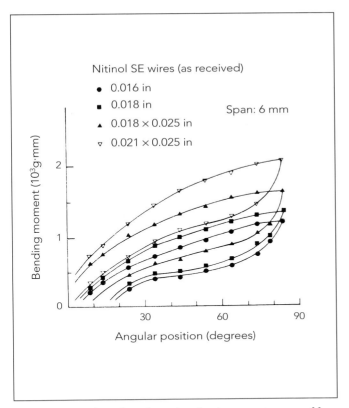

Fig 21-2 Cantilever bending plots for 6-mm test spans of four different sizes of as-received Nitinol SE (3M Unitek), a superelastic wire. (Reprinted with permission from Khier et al.[18])

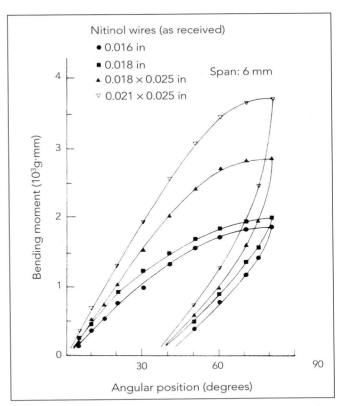

Fig 21-3 Cantilever bending plots for 6-mm test spans of four different sizes of as-received Nitinol (3M Unitek), a nonsuperelastic wire. (Reprinted with permission from Khier et al.[18])

oped for the heat treatment of Japanese NiTi wires. Dentsply International offers a superelastic nickel-titanium archwire (BioForce) that is body-heat–activated with force varying from about 100 gm in the anterior region to about 300 gm in the posterior region.

The bending properties of several nickel-titanium wire products with both round and rectangular cross-sections were subsequently compared, using cantilever specimens with 6-mm test spans. The bending test plots indicated that the Chinese NiTi and Nitinol SE (3M Unitek) wires possessed superelastic behavior (Fig 21-2) similar to that of Japanese NiTi wire and that the original Nitinol wire (Fig 21-3) should be classified as *nonsuperelastic*. The three superelastic wire products evaluated exhibited responses to vacuum heat treatment for 10 minutes and 2 hours at 500°C and 600°C (Fig 21-4), similar to those originally reported for Japanese NiTi wire. The constant bending moment in the superelastic deactivation range was decreased after heat treatment at 500°C, and loss of superelastic behavior occurred after heat treatment at 600°C. In contrast, the bending properties of the three

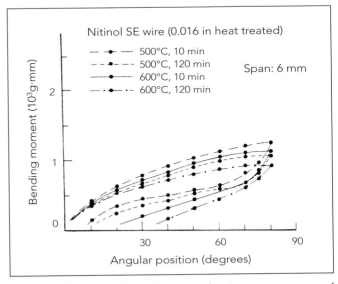

Fig 21-4 Cantilever bending plots for 6-mm test spans of 0.016-inch diameter Nitinol SE wires subjected to heat treatments of 10 minutes and 2 hours at 500°C and 600°C. (Reprinted with permission from Khier et al.[18])

nonsuperelastic wire products were unaffected by heat treatment. The amount of springback on unloading is considerably different for superelastic and nonsuperelastic wires, and can be used to easily distinguish between these two general types of nickel-titanium wires.

The shape-memory characteristics of the nickel-titanium alloys are associated with a reversible transformation between the austenitic and martensitic NiTi phases, which occurs by a twinning process. The **martensitic phase**, which has a distorted monoclinic, triclinic, or hexagonal structure, forms at lower temperatures than the **austenitic phase**, which has an ordered body-centered cubic CsCl structure, over a certain transformation temperature range (TTR) or when the stress is increased above some appropriate level. The austenitic phase forms at higher temperatures than the martensitic phase over a different TTR, or when the stress is decreased below the appropriate level. The difference in the temperature ranges for the forward transformation from the martensitic phase to the austenitic phase and for the reverse transformation is termed *hysteresis*. An intermediate phase, called *R-phase* because of its rhombohedral structure, forms during the forward and reverse transformations between martensite and austenite. Recent studies using the new technique of temperature-modulated differential scanning calorimetry (TMDSC), which has superior resolution to conventional DSC, found that the R-phase always formed during the forward and reverse transformations in the NiTi orthodontic wires. This result is to be expected, because formation of the R-phase is favored by the presence of dislocations and precipitates, which are abundant in these orthodontic wires.

For a nickel-titanium archwire to possess shape memory in vivo, the transformation from the martensitic NiTi structure to the austenitic NiTi structure must be completed at the temperature of the oral environment. The shape-memory characteristics of several commercial nickel-titanium wires have been evaluated by measuring the final length of segments that were permanently deformed approximately 7% in tension below the TTR reported by the manufacturers for the transformation to austenite, and then heated above the TTR to 150°C. The deformed alloys that were evaluated exhibited excellent shape (length) recovery, ranging from 89% to 94%.

Nickel-titanium alloys with shape-memory behavior activated at body temperature have been introduced by many manufacturers. A notable example is the three variants of the Copper Ni-Ti (Ormco/Sybron) wires that achieve shape memory at temperatures of 27°C, 35°C, and 40°C. The 27°C Copper Ni-Ti wire is useful for patients who are mouth-breathers, whereas the 40°C Copper Ni-Ti wire achieves shape memory only when exposed to hot fluids in the oral environment. It has been reported that Copper Ni-Ti contains nominally 5% to 6% by weight copper and 0.2% to 0.5% by weight chromium. The 27°C variant contains 0.5% chromium to compensate for the effect of copper in raising the austenite-finish temperature required to complete the transformation to austenitic NiTi, and the 40°C variant contains 0.2% chromium.

Decreases in the mechanical properties of nickel-titanium wires after long-term deflection have been reported by Hudgins and colleagues,[19] and time-dependent relaxation of bending deformation in Nitinol also has been reported by Lopez and colleagues.[20] In recent years, nickel-titanium orthodontic wires have been investigated under different conditions of temperature and stress and in a simulated oral environment, using micro–x-ray diffraction. Another recent study by Iijima and colleagues[21] has shown that the phase transformations in nickel-titanium wires found over a range of temperatures by TMDSC are also detected by x-ray diffraction, showing that these two complimentary analytic techniques yield consistent results. A low-temperature peak found by TMDSC, which corresponds to twinning within the martensitic NiTi, is detectable by transmission electron microscopy but appears to be less evident with x-ray diffraction. The clinical significance of the low-temperature twinning requires further study. There has been extensive study of the corrosion behavior and nickel release from the nickel-titanium wires. Hydrogen embrittlement has also been observed for nickel-titanium wires, as well as stress corrosion cracking. Evaluation of the mechanical properties of the nickel-titanium wires and their clinical relevance continues to be an area of active research.

Nickel-titanium archwires with ion-implanted surfaces to obtain reduced bracket friction have been introduced (Dentsply International). The clinical efficacy of these wires requires further investigation. One study by Cobb and colleagues[22] has reported no clinical advantage for the initial alignment compared with nickel-titanium archwires without ion-implanted surfaces. Other surface coatings and surface treatments have been investigated for nickel-titanium wires, and the interested reader should refer to the recently published articles at the end of this chapter.

Considerations for Selection

Although the stainless steel archwires are still widely used in orthodontics and cobalt-chromium-nickel wires are selected by many clinicians, the nickel-titanium and β-titanium wires are very popular, despite their higher cost. The expensive gold alloy wires now have minimal clinical use, and the former ADA specification no. 7 for these wires has been withdrawn. Each of the four major orthodontic wire alloys has distinct advantages for selection by the clinician, as well as some areas or potential areas of concern, as summarized in Box 21-1.

The stainless steel and cobalt-chromium-nickel wires offer the advantages of relatively low cost, known biocompatibility from extensive clinical use, and excellent formability for the fabrication of orthodontic appliances. However, these wires have much higher force delivery (elastic modulus) than the β-titanium and nickel-titanium wires, and the force delivery is increased after heat treatment by the clinician to increase resilience (particularly Elgiloy Blue) and relieve residual stresses.

The relatively high cost of the β-titanium orthodontic wires is offset by the intermediate force delivery, excellent formability, and true weldability of this alloy. The clinician may select β-titanium archwires because they fill more of the bracket slots because of their lower elastic modulus compared with the wire sizes of stainless steel alloys. The formability or ductility of b-titanium provides the orthodontist with the capability of fabricating arches or segments with complicated loop configurations that are not possible with the nickel-titanium alloys. Clinical examples include the alignment of teeth in an arch during finishing, the rotation and changing of the axial orientation of teeth, the use of specialized springs or auxiliaries such as an intrusive arch or a canine root spring, and the fabrication of closing loops that may contain helices. The direct welding of auxiliaries to archwires enables hooks, tie backs, and finger springs to be easily prepared with a commercial welding apparatus.

A clinical study by Kula and colleagues[23] has reported that the rate of orthodontic sliding space closure was not significantly different for ion-implanted and conventional (not ion-implanted) TMA wires, and that the rate of closure was similar to that reported for stainless steel wires. Manufacturing of the β-titanium wires is difficult because of the reactivity of titanium, and anecdotal reports have described the susceptibility of some batches of TMA

wires to undergo fracture during clinical manipulation. Further studies are needed to compare the clinical manipulation and performance of the currently available β-titanium wires and other recently introduced titanium alloy wires.

It is well-known from histologic studies on tooth movement that light, continuous, nearly constant forces represent optimum biomechanical conditions. The Chinese and Japanese NiTi wires, along with numerous more recently introduced superelastic and shape-memory nickel-titanium wires, have excellent springback (range of elastic action), low stiffness, and nearly constant force delivery during deactivation, and provide these desirable mechanical properties better than the stainless steel, cobalt-chromium-nickel, β-titanium, and original Nitinol wire alloys. However, the original nonsuperelastic Nitinol remains popular for clinical use, and no studies have demonstrated clinical superiority of the superelastic or shape-memory wires compared with the nonsuperelastic nickel-titanium wires. It is possible that under some clinical conditions the superelastic nickel-titanium wires are not sufficiently deformed for this property to be manifested during initial alignment of the teeth. A clinical study has found that there was no difference among multistrand stainless steel, superelastic nickel-titanium, and ion-implanted nickel-titanium archwires for tooth alignment.[22]

Another interesting feature is the increase in force delivery that occurs when an appliance is removed and then retied (ligated) with Chinese NiTi wire. These results would be anticipated with the other superelastic alloys. Superelastic nickel-titanium alloy coil springs developed for orthodontics have found wide applicability as optimal appliances for tooth movement under certain clinical conditions.

Corrosion resistance of the orthodontic wires is provided by a chromium oxide film for the stainless steel and cobalt-chromium-nickel alloys, and a titanium oxide film for the β-titanium and nickel-titanium alloys. Clinical experience is that corrosion of orthodontic wires is generally of minimal concern, although there have been a large number of recent studies of the in vitro corrosion behavior of nickel-titanium wires in a variety of media because of the concern about nickel release under clinical conditions. Corrosion of these alloys can become more pronounced when there is galvanic coupling with metallic brackets. It has been found that the corrosion and release of nickel ions is dependent on the composition and

---

Box 21-1 Advantages and disadvantages for each of the four major orthodontic wire alloys

---

Stainless steel

Advantages

Lowest cost of the wire alloys

Proven biocompatibility from extensive clinical use

Excellent formability for fabrication into orthodontic appliances

Can be soldered and welded, although welded joints may require solder reinforcement

Disadvantages

High force delivery

Relatively low springback in bending compared to β-titanium and nickel-titanium

Susceptible to intergranular corrosion after heating to temperatures required for joining

Elgiloy (soft temper)

Advantages

Relatively low cost, although greater than stainless steel

Proven biocompatibility from extensive clinical use

Outstanding formability in as-received condition (heat treated to increase YS and resilience)

Can be soldered and welded, with joining characteristics similar to stainless steel

Disadvantages

High elastic force delivery, similar to that for stainless steel

Lower springback than stainless steel (using YS/E values from tension test)

β-titanium

Advantages

Intermediate force delivery between stainless steel or Elgiloy and nickel-titanium

Excellent formability; the only orthodontic wire alloy with true weldability

Excellent springback characteristics (using YS/E values from tension test)

Excellent biocompatibility from high titanium content demonstrated by clinical use

Disadvantages

Expensive

High arch wire-bracket friction with original TMA (decreased for ion-implanted TMA)

Nickel-Titanium

Advantages

Lowest force delivery of the four orthodontic wire alloys

Excellent springback in bending, particularly for superelastic and shape-memory alloys

Superelastic alloys can be heat-treated by clinician to vary force delivery characteristics

Disadvantages

Expensive, particularly for newest products

Second highest arch wire-bracket friction after TMA (lower for ion-implanted product)

Difficult to place permanent bends and cannot bend over sharp edge or into complete loop

Wires cannot be soldered and must be joined by mechanical crimping process

Lowest in vitro corrosion resistance of wire alloys (may be concern about in vivo nickel release)

---

thickness of the surface oxide layer on the nickel-titanium alloys.

Research has shown that nickel dissolution occurs at sites of surface damage in nickel-titanium wires. Nickel hypersensitivity reactions to nickel-titanium wires have been reported in numerous studies. Although such cases do not appear to be common, this remains an area of active research with conflicting conclusions in recent publications about hazards to patients caused by nickel release from these wires. Several studies suggest that sterilization and clinical recycling only have small effects on the mechanical properties of the nickel-titanium wires. In recent years, studies have investigated the cytotoxicity of nickel-titanium alloys, and research is continuing to assess the incidence of localized corrosion at surface defects that arise during the manufacture of nickel-titanium wires.

Given the concerns about biocompatibility of the nickel-containing orthodontic wire alloys, there has been substantial interest in the development of biocompatible nonmetallic wires that would also provide a better color match to tooth structure. A transparent nonmetallic orthodontic archwire (Optiflex), developed for patient treatment by Ormco/Sybron, had a silica core, a silicon resin middle layer, and a stain-resistant outer layer. However, this product had problems with brittleness and fatigue, and is no longer marketed (private communication, Ormco/Sybron, 2006). No major US orthodontic manufacturer is currently marketing transparent orthodontic wires, although there continues to be research activity on fiber-reinforced composite archwires. A recent review article by Eliades[24] has noted that shape-memory polymer wires may eventually become important for clinical orthodontics.

Clinical Decision Scenario

This section presents an approach for choosing materials and a system for a specific clinical situation. It uses the same format as that presented in chapter 7. Advantages and disadvantages of each material/system are prioritized using the following codes: • of minor importance, •• important, and ••• very important.

Materials Superelastic NiTi wire vs stainless steel wires*

Critical Factors Good esthetics, speed of completion

SUPERELASTIC NICKEL-TITANIUM WIRES	STAINLESS STEEL WIRES
ADVANTAGES	ADVANTAGES

••• Produce lower moments and forces
••• Constant force over wide range of deflection
••• Low stiffness
•• High springback
•• High stored energy
• More effective in initial tooth alignment
   Shape memory
••• Less patient discomfort
	••• Less expensive
	   Good formability
	   High resilience
	• Can be soldered or welded
	•• Good in final detailing
	•• Great for arch coordination
	••• Good torque control
	   Relatively predictable biomechanical properties

DISADVANTAGES	DISADVANTAGES

• Cannot be soldered or welded
•• Cannot be easily formed or bent
••• Tendency for dentoalveolar expansion
••• High cost
   Poor torque control
••• Patient discomfort with larger activation
	•• More chair time
	   Resilience depends on diameter
	   No shape memory or superelasticity
	•• Poor deflection range

Decision Wire selection depends on the nature of teeth malpositions, treatment time with alternative wires, as well as patient age, availability, and acceptance of discomfort.

---

*Prepared by Dr David E. Wacker.

■ Glossary

activation Bending a wire that will produce an elastic force for tooth movement.

austenitic phase The face-centered cubic solid solution structure of iron, chromium, nickel, and carbon for stainless steels, or the body-centered cubic structure of NiTi for the nickel-titanium alloys.

force delivery The force produced by an orthodontic wire against a tooth.

martensitic phase A body-centered cubic phase in austenitic stainless steels or a phase (reported as monoclinic, triclinic, or hexagonal) in nickel-titanium alloys that forms at low temperatures or as a result of cold working the austenitic phase.

moment of inertia A geometric parameter dependent on cross-section shape and dimensions that expresses the relative resistance of an orthodontic wire to bending. The stiffness in bending is directly proportional to the moment of inertia of the cross section and the elastic modulus of the wire alloy, and inversely proportional to the length.

shape-memory effect A property of certain nickel-titanium wires that will permit shaping at a higher temperature, followed by deformation at a lower temperature, and a return to the original shape by reheating.

springback The elastic deformation or strain recovered when an orthodontic wire is unloaded, typically in bending deformation. For a wire that exhibits linear elasticity, the expression for springback in the orthodontic materials literature (YS/E) is equivalent to the elastic strain at the yield strength.

superelasticity A property of certain nickel-titanium wires characterized by an extensive region of elastic activation and deactivation at nearly constant bending moment or force, arising from reversible transformation between the austenitic and martensitic NiTi phases.

temper The spring character of an orthodontic wire that is related to the mechanical properties of yield strength and elastic modulus.

weldability Having the capability of being joined by the passage of a strong electric current.

working range The maximum deflection of a wire within the elastic range.

■ Discussion Questions

1. What phenomenon is responsible for the force delivery to teeth by deformed wires?

2. How is it possible to obtain different mechanical properties from the same wire?

3. Which type of orthodontic wire is most easily joined by welding?

4. What is shape memory, and which wires have it?

5. What factors would be important for the development and clinical use of composite ceramic-polymer orthodontic wires?

■ Study Questions

(See appendix E for answers.)

1. What are the types of orthodontic wires in current use?

2. What are the main criteria for the selection of an orthodontic wire?

3. What determines wire stiffness or elastic force delivery?

4. What are the advantages of stainless steel wires?

5. What is Elgiloy?

6. What is the composition of β-titanium wires?

7. What are the advantages of β-titanium orthodontic wires?

8. What are the disadvantages of nickel-titanium wires?

9. How do manufacturers obtain shape memory or superelastic characteristics for some nickel-titanium wires?

■ References

1. American Dental Association. Specification no. 32 for orthodontic wires not containing precious metals. J Am Dent Assoc 1977;95:1169–1171.

2. American National Standards Institute/American Dental Association ANSI/ADA Specification No. 32-2006. Orthodontic Wires. Chicago: American Dental Association, 2006.

3. Thurow RC. Edgewise Orthodontics, ed 4. St Louis: Mosby, 1982:chapter 3–5, 17.

4. Popov EP. Introduction to Mechanics of Solids. Englewood Cliffs, NJ: Prentice-Hall, 1968.

5. ASM Committee on Wrought Stainless Steels. Wrought stainless steels. In: Metals Handbook, vol 1, ed 8. Metals Park, OH: American Society for Metals, 1961.

6. Brantley WA. Wrought alloys. In: Anusavice KJ (ed). Phillips' Science of Dental Materials, ed 11. St Louis: Elsevier Science/Saunders, 2003.

7. Burstone CJ, Goldberg AJ. Beta titanium: A new orthodontic alloy. Am J Orthod 1980;77:121–132.

8. Civjan S, Huget EF, DeSimon LB. Potential applications of certain nickel-titanium (Nitinol) alloys. J Dent Res 1975;54:89–96.

9. Khier SE. Structural Characterization, Biomechanical Properties, and Potentiodynamic Polarization Behavior of Nickel-Titanium Orthodontic Wire Alloys [dissertation]. Milwaukee, WI: Marquette University, 1988.

10. Quo SD, Marshall SJ, Marshall GW. Chemical and phase contents analysis of Ni-Ti wires. J Dent Res 1994;73(IADR Abstracts):413.

11. Asgharnia MK, Brantley WA. Comparison of bending and tension tests for orthodontic wires. Am J Orthod 1986;89:228–236.

12. Drake SR, Wayne DM, Powers JM, Asgar K. Mechanical properties of orthodontic wires in tension, bending and torsion. Am J Orthod 1982;82:206–210.

13. Nelson KR, Burstone CJ, Goldberg AJ. Optimal welding of beta titanium orthodontic wires. Am J Orthod Dentofacial Orthop 1987;92:213–219.

14. Kusy RP, Whitley JQ, Prewitt MJ. Comparison of the frictional coefficients for selected archwire-bracket slot combinations in the dry and wet states. Angle Orthod 1991;61:293–302.

15. Iijima M, Brantley WA, Kawashima I, et al. Micro-X-ray diffraction observation of nickel-titanium orthodontic wires in simulated oral environment. Biomaterials 2004;25:171–176.

16. Andreasen GF, Brady PR. A use hypothesis for 55 nitinol wire for orthodontics. Angle Orthod 1972;42:172–177.

17. Andreasen GF, Hilleman TB. An evaluation of 55 cobalt substituted nitinol wire for use in orthodontics. J Am Dent Assoc 1971;82:1373–1375.

18. Khier SE, Brantley WA, Fournelle RA. Bending properties of superelastic and nonsuperelastic nickel-titanium orthodontic wires. Am J Orthod Dentofacial Orthop 1991;99:310–318.

19. Hudgins JJ, Bagby MD, Erickson LC. The effect of long-term deflection on permanent deformation of nickel-titanium archwires. Angle Orthod 1990;60:283–288.

20. Lopez I, Goldberg J, Burstone CJ. Bending characteristics of nitinol wire. Am J Orthod 1979;75:569–575.

21. Iijima M, Brantley WA, Guo W, Clark WAT, Yuasa T, Mizoguchi I. X-ray diffraction study of low-temperature phase transformations in nickel-titanium orthodontic wires. Dent Mater (accepted for publication).

22. Cobb NW III, Kula KS, Phillips C, Proffit WR. Efficiency of multistrand steel, superelastic Ni-Ti and ion-implanted Ni-Ti archwires for initial alignment. Clin Orthod Res 1998;1:12–19.

23. Kula K, Phillips C, Gibilaro A, Proffit WR. Effect of ion implantation of TMA archwires on the rate of orthodontic sliding space closure. Am J Orthod Dentofacial Orthop 1998;114:577–580.

24. Eliades T. Orthodontic materials research and applications: Part 2. Current status and projected future developments in materials and biocompatibility. Am J Orthod Dentofacial Orthop 2007;131:253–262.

Recommended Reading

Anotated textbook references

Brantley WA. Wrought alloys. In: Anusavice KJ (ed). Phillips' Science of Dental Materials, ed 11. St Louis: Elsevier Science/Saunders, 2003:621–654.

An extensive description of the compositions and properties of orthodontic wires, along with other wrought alloys used in dentistry.

Brantley WA, Eliades T (eds). Orthodontic Materials: Scientific and Clinical Aspects. Stuttgart, Germany: Thieme, 2001.

A lengthy presentation of the materials science aspects for orthodontic wires is provided in chapter 4, and biocompatibility aspects are discussed in chapters 14 and 15. Chapters 1 through 3 provide important background information. An extensive list of references is presented.

Brick RM, Pense AW, Gordon RB. Structure and Properties of Engineering Materials, ed 4. New York: McGraw-Hill, 1977.

The classification, composition and property information presented for stainless steel alloys is relevant for orthodontic wires. The chapter on titanium alloys is concise and highly readable. See chapters 10 and 14.

Dieter GE. Mechanical Metallurgy, ed 3. New York: McGraw-Hill, 1986.

This well-known engineering materials textbook provides a lucid account of the mechanical behavior, mechanical testing, and plastic forming of metals. See chapters 8, 9, and 19.

Donache MJ Jr. Titanium: A Technical Guide, ed 2. Metals Park, OH: ASM International, 2000.

This engineering materials book provides an excellent introduction to titanium, its alloys, and their properties. See chapters 1 to 3, 12, 13, and appendices A and B.

Duerig TW, Melton KN, Stöckel D, Wayman CM (eds). Engineering Aspects of Shape Memory Alloys. London: Butterworth-Heinemann, 1990:3–45, 369–413, 452–469.

A lucid description is given of shape memory and superelastic behavior, along with properties of nickel-titanium and other shape memory alloys for numerous applications.

Popov EP. Introduction to Mechanics of Solids. Englewood Cliffs, NJ: Prentice-Hall, 1968.

The forces, moments, stresses and strains in solids subjected to a wide variety of loading conditions are discussed in a highly understandable manner. Chapter 6 on bending stresses in beams is recommended.

Thurow RC. Edgewise Orthodontics, ed 4. St Louis: Mosby, 1982.

This classic textbook presents the terminology for mechanical properties for orthodontic wires that is frequently used in the orthodontic literature. See chapters 3, 5, and 7.

Zapffe CA. Stainless Steels. Cleveland: American Society for Metals, 1949.

This publication presents ample evidence of the effect of cold work on reducing the elastic modulus of stainless steels. See chapter 6.

Recent publications

Ahn HS, Kim MJ, Seol HJ, Lee JH, Kim HI, Kwon YH. Effect of pH and temperature on orthodontic NiTi wires immersed in acidic fluoride solution. J Biomed Mater Res B Appl Biomater 2006;79:7–15.

Amini F, Borzabadi Farahani A, Jafari A, Rabbani M. In vivo study of metal content of oral mucosa cells in patients with and without fixed orthodontic appliances. Orthod Craniofac Res 2008;11:51–56.

Bokas J, Woods M. A clinical comparison between nickel titanium springs and elastomeric chains. Aust Orthod J 2006;22:39–46.

Brantley WA, Guo W, Clark WAT, Iijima M. Microstructural studies of 35°C Copper Ni-Ti orthodontic wire and TEM confirmation of low-temperature martensite transformation. Dent Mater 2008;24:204–210.

Brantley WA, Iijima M, Grentzer TH. Temperature-modulated DSC study of phase transformations in nickel-titanium orthodontic wires. Thermochimica Acta 2002;392–393:329–337.

Brantley WA, Iijima M, Grentzer TH. Temperature-modulated DSC provides new insight about nickel-titanium wire transformations. Am J Orthod Dentofacial Orthop 2003;124:387–394.

Cioffi M, Gilliland D, Ceccone G, Chiesa R, Cigada A. Electrochemical release testing of nickel-titanium orthodontic wires in artificial saliva using thin layer activation. Acta Biomater 2005;1:717–724.

Clarke B, Carroll W, Rochev Y, Hynes M, Bradley D, Plumley D. Influence of Nitinol wire surface treatment on oxide thickness and composition and its subsequent effect on corrosion resistance and nickel ion release. J Biomed Mater Res A 2006;79:61–70.

Dalstra M, Melsen B. Does the transition temperature of Cu-NiTi arch-wires affect the amount of tooth movement during alignment? Orthod Craniofac Res 2004;7:21–25.

David A, Lobner D. In vitro cytotoxicity of orthodontic archwires in cortical cell cultures. Eur J Orthod 2004;26:421–426.

Eliades T, Pratsinis H, Kletsas D, Eliades G, Makou M. Characterization and cytotoxicity of ions released from stainless steel and nickel-titanium orthodontic alloys. Am J Orthod Dentofacial Orthop 2004;125:24–29.

Eliades T, Zinelis S, Papadopoulos MA, Eliades G, Athanasiou AE. Nickel content of as-received and retrieved NiTi and stainless steel archwires: assessing the nickel release hypothesis. Angle Orthod 2004;74:151–154.

Es-Souni M, Es-Souni M, Fischer-Brandies H. On the properties of two binary NiTi shape memory alloys. Effects of surface finish on the corrosion behaviour and in vitro biocompatibility. Biomaterials 2002;23:2887–2894.

Es-Souni M, Fischer-Brandies H, Es-Souni M. On the in vitro biocompatibility of Elgiloy, a Co-based alloy, compared to two titanium alloys. J Orofac Orthop 2003;64:16–26.

Fischer-Brandies H, Es-Souni M, Kock N, Raetzke K, Bock O. Transformation behavior, chemical composition, surface topography and bending properties of five selected 0.016″ x 0.022″ NiTi arch-wires. J Orofac Orthop 2003;64:88–99.

Fors R, Persson M. Nickel in dental plaque and saliva in patients with and without orthodontic appliances. Eur J Orthod 2006;28:292–297.

Fukushima O, Yoneyama T, Doi H, Hanawa T. Corrosion resistance and surface characterization of electrolyzed Ti-Ni alloy. Dent Mater J 2006;25:151–160.

Garrec P, Tavernier B, Jordan L. Evolution of flexural rigidity according to the cross-sectional dimension of a superelastic nickel titanium orthodontic wire. Eur J Orthod 2005;27:402–407.

Guo W, Brantley WA, Clark WAT, Iijima M. Transmission electron microscopic study of beta-titanium orthodontic wires. J Dent Res 2001;80(AADR Abstracts):52.

Huang HH. Corrosion resistance of stressed NiTi and stainless steel orthodontic wires in acid artificial saliva. J Biomed Mater Res A 2003;66:829–839.

Huang HH. Variation in corrosion resistance of nickel-titanium wires from different manufacturers. Angle Orthod 2005;75:661–665.

Huang HH. Surface characterizations and corrosion resistance of nickel-titanium orthodontic archwires in artificial saliva of various degrees of acidity. J Biomed Mater Res A 2005;74:629–639.

Huang HH, Chiu YH, Lee TH, Wu SC, Yang HW, Su KH, Hsu CC. Ion release from NiTi orthodontic wires in artificial saliva with various acidities. Biomaterials 2003;24:3585–3592.

Huang ZM, Gopal R, Fujihara K, et al. Fabrication of a new composite orthodontic archwire and validation by a bridging micromechanics model. Biomaterials 2003;24:2941–2953.

Iijima M, Brantley WA, Baba N, et al. Micro-XRD study of beta-titanium wires and infrared soldered joints. Dent Mater 2007;23:1051–1056.

Iijima M, Brantley WA, Kawashima I, et al. Microstructures of beta-titanium orthodontic wires joined by infrared brazing. J Biomed Mater Res B Appl Biomater 2006;79:137–141.

Iijima M, Brantley WA, Mitchell JC, Wade AB, Frankmann JG. Bending performance, microstructures and x-ray diffraction of two beta-titanium wires. J Dent Res 2001;80(AADR Abstracts):51.

Iijima M, Endo K, Yuasa T, et al. Galvanic corrosion behavior of orthodontic archwire alloys coupled to bracket alloys. Angle Orthod 2006;76:705–711.

Iijima M, Endo K, Ohno H, Yonekura Y, Mizoguchi I. Corrosion behavior and surface structure of orthodontic Ni-Ti alloy wires. Dent Mater J 2001;20:103–113.

Iijima M, Ohno H, Kawashima I, Endo K, Brantley WA, Mizoguchi I. Micro x-ray diffraction study of superelastic nickel-titanium orthodontic wires at different temperatures and stresses. Biomaterials 2002;23:1769–1774.

Johnson E. Relative stiffness of beta titanium archwires. Angle Orthod 2003;73:259–269.

Kaneko K, Yokoyama K, Moriyama K, Asaoka K, Sakai J. Degradation in performance of orthodontic wires caused by hydrogen absorption during short-term immersion in 2.0% acidulated phosphate fluoride solution. Angle Orthod 2004;74:487–495.

Kaneko K, Yokoyama K, Moriyama K, Asaoka K, Sakai J, Nagumo M. Delayed fracture of beta titanium orthodontic wire in fluoride aqueous solutions. Biomaterials 2003;24:2113–2120.

Kao CT, Ding SJ, He H, Chou MY, Huang TH. Cytotoxicity of orthodontic wire corroded in fluoride solution in vitro. Angle Orthod 2007;77:349–354.

Klocke A, Kahl-Nieke B, Adam G, Kemper J. Magnetic forces on orthodontic wires in high field magnetic resonance imaging (MRI) at 3 Tesla. J Orofac Orthop 2006;67:424–429.

Krishnan V, Kumar KJ. Weld characteristics of orthodontic archwire materials. Angle Orthod 2004;74:533–538.

Krishnan V, Kumar KJ. Mechanical properties and surface characteristics of three archwire alloys. Angle Orthod 2004;74:825–831.

Kusy RP, Whitley JQ. Thermal and mechanical characteristics of stainless steel, titanium-molybdenum, and nickel-titanium archwires. Am J Orthod Dentofacial Orthop 2007;131:229–237.

Kusy RP, Whitley JQ, de Araujo Gurgel J. Comparisons of surface roughnesses and sliding resistances of 6 titanium-based or TMA-type archwires. Am J Orthod Dentofacial Orthop 2004;126:589–603.

Kusy RP, Mims L, Whitley JQ. Mechanical characteristics of various tempers of as-received cobalt-chromium archwires. Am J Orthod Dentofacial Orthop 2001;119:274–291.

Laheurte P, Eberhardt A, Philippe M, Deblock L. Improvement of pseudoelasticity and ductility of Beta III titanium alloy application to orthodontic wires. Eur J Orthod 2007;29:8–13.

Lee SH, Kim HW, Kong YM, Kim HE, Lee SH, Chang YI. Fluoride coatings on orthodontic wire for controlled release of fluorine ion. J Biomed Mater Res B Appl Biomater 2005;75:200–204.

Levrini L, Lusvardi G, Gentile D. Nickel ions release in patients with fixed orthodontic appliances. Minerva Stomatol 2006;55:115–121.

Mallory DC, English JD, Brantley WA, Bussa H, Hutchins M, Kerr S, Powers J. Force-deflection comparisons of superelastic nickel-titanium archwires. Am J Orthod Dentofacial Orthop 2004;126:110–112.

Meling TR, Odegaard J. The effect of short-term temperature changes on superelastic nickel-titanium archwires activated in orthodontic bending. Am J Orthod Dentofacial Orthop 2001;119:263–273.

Neumann P, Bourauel C, Jager A. Corrosion and permanent fracture resistance of coated and conventional orthodontic wires. J Mater Sci Mater Med 2002;13:141–147.

Ogawa T, Yokoyama K, Asaoka K, Sakai J. Hydrogen absorption behavior of beta titanium alloy in acid fluoride solutions. Biomaterials 2004;25:2419–2425.

Oh KT, Kim KN. Ion release and cytotoxicity of stainless steel wires. Eur J Orthod 2005;27:533–540.

Ozeki K, Yuhta T, Aoki H, Asaoka T, Daisaku T, Fukui Y. Deterioration in the superelasticity of Ti sputter coated on NiTi orthodontic wire. Biomed Mater Eng 2003;13:355–362.

Parvizi F, Rock WP. The load/deflection characteristics of thermally activated orthodontic archwires. Eur J Orthod 2003;25:417–421.

Peitsch T, Klocke A, Kahl-Nieke B, Prymak O, Epple M. The release of nickel from orthodontic NiTi wires is increased by dynamic mechanical loading but not constrained by surface nitridation. J Biomed Mater Res A 2007;82:731–739.

Rucker BK, Kusy RP. Resistance to sliding of stainless steel multi-stranded archwires and comparison with single-stranded leveling wires. Am J Orthod Dentofacial Orthop 2002;122:73–83.

Rucker BK, Kusy RP. Elastic properties of alternative versus single-stranded leveling archwires. Am J Orthod Dentofacial Orthop 2002;122:528–541.

Sakima MT, Dalstra M, Melsen B. How does temperature influence the properties of rectangular nickel-titanium wires? Eur J Orthod 2006;28:282–291.

Schiff N, Boinet M, Morgon L, Lissac M, Dalard F, Grosgogeat B. Galvanic corrosion between orthodontic wires and brackets in fluoride mouthwashes. Eur J Orthod 2006;28:298–304.

Schiff N, Grosgogeat B, Lissac M, Dalard F. Influence of fluoridated mouthwashes on corrosion resistance of orthodontics wires. Biomaterials 2004;25:4535–4342.

Sestini S, Notarantonio L, Cerboni B, et al. In vitro toxicity evaluation of silver soldering, electrical resistance, and laser welding of orthodontic wires. Eur J Orthod 2006;28:567–572.

Suwa N, Watari F, Yamagata S, Iida J, Kobayashi M. Static-dynamic friction transition of FRP esthetic orthodontic wires on various brackets by suspension-type friction test. J Biomed Mater Res B Appl Biomater 2003;67:765–771.

Suzuki A, Kanetaka H, Shimizu Y, et al. Orthodontic buccal tooth movement by nickel-free titanium-based shape memory and superelastic alloy wire. Angle Orthod 2006;76:1041–1046.

Vande Vannet B, Mohebbian N, Wehrbein H. Toxicity of used orthodontic archwires assessed by three-dimensional cell culture. Eur J Orthod 2006;28:426–432.

Verstrynge A, Van Humbeeck J, Willems G. In-vitro evaluation of the material characteristics of stainless steel and beta-titanium orthodontic wires. Am J Orthod Dentofacial Orthop 2006;130:460–470.

Wang J, Li N, Rao G, Han EH, Ke W. Stress corrosion cracking of NiTi in artificial saliva. Dent Mater 2007;23:133–137.

Wilkinson PD, Dysart PS, Hood JA, Herbison GP. Load-deflection characteristics of superelastic nickel-titanium orthodontic wires. Am J Orthod Dentofacial Orthop 2002;121:483–495.

Yanaru K, Yamaguchi K, Kakigawa H, Kozono Y. Temperature- and deflection-dependences of orthodontic force with Ni-Ti wires. Dent Mater J 2003;22:146–159.

Yokoyama K, Hamada K, Moriyama K, Asaoka K. Degradation and fracture of Ni-Ti superelastic wire in an oral cavity. Biomaterials 2001;22:2257–2262.

Yokoyama K, Kaneko K, Ogawa T, Moriyama K, Asaoka K, Sakai J. Hydrogen embrittlement of work-hardened Ni-Ti alloy in fluoride solutions. Biomaterials 2005;26:101–108.

Yonekura Y, Endo K, Iijima M, Ohno H, Mizoguchi I. In vitro corrosion characteristics of commercially available orthodontic wires. Dent Mater J 2004;23:197–202.

Publications on metallic orthodontic wires

Abujudom DN, Thoma PE, Fariabi S. The effect of cold work and heat treatment on the phase transformations of near equiatomic NiTi shape memory alloy. Mater Sci Forum 1990;56–58:565–570.

Andreasen GF, Morrow RE. Laboratory and clinical analyses of nitinol wire. Am J Orthod 1978;73:142–151.

Bass JK, Fine H, Cisneros GJ. Nickel hypersensitivity in the orthodontic patient. Am J Orthod Dentofacial Orthop 1993;103:280–285.

Bradley TG, Brantley WA, Culbertson BM. Differential scanning calorimetry (DSC) analyses of superelastic and nonsuperelastic nickel-titanium orthodontic wires. Am J Orthod Dentofac Orthop 1996;109:589–597.

Buehler WJ, Gilfrich JV, Riley RC. Effect of low-temperature phase changes on the mechanical properties of alloys near the composition of TiNi. J Appl Phys 1963;34:1475–1477.

Buehler WJ, Wang FE. A summary of recent research on the nitinol alloys and their potential application in ocean engineering. Ocean Eng 1968;1:105–120.

Buckthal JE, Kusy RP. Effects of cold disinfectants on the mechanical properties and the surface topography of nickel-titanium arch wires. Am J Orthod Dentofacial Orthop 1988;94:117–122.

Burstone CJ. Variable-modulus orthodontics. Am J Orthod 1981;80:1–16.

Burstone CJ, Qin B, Morton JY. Chinese NiTi wire—a new orthodontic alloy. Am J Orthod 1985;87:445–452.

Chen R, Zhi YF, Arvystas MG. Advanced Chinese NiTi alloy wire and clinical observations. Angle Orthod 1992;62:59–66.

Chen RS, Vijayaraghavan TV, Schulman A. Electric spot welding of NiTi wires. J Dent Res 1990;69(IADR Abstracts):312.

Di Giovanni J, Staley RN, Jakobsen JR. Effect of electric heat treatment on martensitic-active nickel titanium. J Dent Res 1994;73(IADR Abstracts):413.

Donovan MT, Lin JJ, Brantley WA, Conover JP. Weldability of beta-titanium arch wires. Am J Orthod 1984;85:207–216.

Evans TJW, Jones ML, Newcombe RG. Clinical comparison and performance perspective of three aligning arch wires. Am J Orthod Dentofacial Orthop 1998;114:32–39.

Filleul MP, Jordan L. Torsional properties of Ni-Ti and Copper Ni-Ti wires: The effect of temperature on physical properties. Eur J Orthod 1997;19:637–646.

Fukuyo S, Nakazato H, Masukawa T, Sachdeva R, Fukuyo S. Cytotoxicity studies on TiNi alloy using tissue culture agar overlay test (AOT). J Dent Res 1991;70(IADR Abstracts):398.

Goldberg AJ, Vanderby R Jr, Burstone CJ. Reduction in the modulus of elasticity in orthodontic wires. J Dent Res 1977;56:1227–1231.

Goldberg J, Burstone CJ. An evaluation of beta titanium alloys for use in orthodontic appliances. J Dent Res 1979;58:593–599.

Greppi L, Smith DC, Woodside DG, Varrela T, Lugowski S. Nickel hypersensitivity reactions in orthodontic patients. J Dent Res 1991;70(IADR Abstracts):361.

Grímsdóttir MR, Hensten-Pettersen A. Surface analysis of nickel-titanium archwire used in vivo. Dent Mater 1997;13:163–167.

Harris EF, Newman SM, Nicholson JA. Nitinol arch wire in a simulated oral environment: changes in mechanical properties. Am J Orthod Dentofacial Orthop 1988;93:508–513.

Hurst CL, Duncanson MG Jr, Nanda RS, Angolkar PV. An evaluation of the shape-memory phenomenon of nickel-titanium orthodontic wires. Am J Orthod Dentofacial Orthop 1990;98:72–76.

Iijima M, Endo K, Ohno H, Mizoguchi I. Effect of Cr and Cu addition on corrosion behavior of Ni-Ti alloys. Dent Mater J 1998;17:31-40.

Kapila S, Angolkar PV, Duncanson MG Jr, Nanda RS. Evaluation of friction between edgewise stainless steel brackets and orthodontic wires of four alloys. Am J Orthod Dentofacial Orthop 1990;98:117–126.

Kapila S, Haugen JW, Watanabe LG. Load-deflection characteristics of nickel-titanium alloy wires after clinical recycling and dry heat sterilization. Am J Orthod Dentofacial Orthop 1992;102:120–126.

Khier SE, Brantley WA, Fournelle RA. Structure and mechanical properties of as-received and heat-treated stainless steel orthodontic wires. Am J Orthod Dentofacial Orthop 1988;93:206–212.

Kusy RP. On the use of nomograms to determine the elastic property ratios of orthodontic arch wires. Am J Orthod 1983;83:374–381.

Kusy RP. Nitinol alloys: So, who's on first? [letter]. Am J Orthod Dentofacial Orthop 1991;100:25A–26A.

Kusy RP. A review of contemporary archwires: Their properties and characteristics. Angle Orthod 1997;67:197–207.

Kusy RP. The future of orthodontic materials: The long-term view. Am J Orthod Dentofacial Orthop 1998;113:91–95.

Kusy RP, Tobin EJ, Whitley JQ, Sioshansi P. Frictional coefficients of ion-implanted alumina against ion-implanted beta-titanium in the low load, low velocity, single pass regime. Dent Mater 1992;8:167–172.

Mayhew MJ, Kusy RP. Effects of sterilization on the mechanical properties and the surface topography of nickel-titanium arch wires. Am J Orthod Dentofacial Orthop 1988;93:232–236.

McCoy BP. Comparison of Compositions and Differential Scanning Calorimetric Analyses of the New Copper-Nickel-Titanium Wires with Existing Nickel-Titanium Orthodontic Wires [Thesis]. Columbus, OH: Ohio State University 1996.

McCoy BP, Brantley WA, Culbertson BM, Mitchell JC. DSC and EDS analyses of new Copper Ni-Ti orthodontic wires. J Dent Res 1997;76(IADR Abstracts):400.

Mitchell JC, Bradley TG, Brantley WA. Elemental analyses of six commercial nickel-titanium orthodontic wires. J Dent Res 1996;75(IADR Abstracts):168.

Miura F, Mogi M, Ohura Y. Japanese NiTi alloy wire: use of the direct electric resistance heat treatment method. Eur J Orthod 1988;10:187–191.

Miura F, Mogi M, Ohura Y, Hamanaka H. The super-elastic property of the Japanese NiTi alloy wire for use in orthodontics. Am J Orthod Dentofacial Orthop 1986;90:1–10.

Miura F, Mogi M, Ohura Y, Karibe M. The super-elastic Japanese NiTi alloy wire for use in orthodontics. Part III. Studies on the Japanese NiTi alloy coil springs. Am J Orthod Dentofacial Orthop 1988; 94:89–96.

Mullins WS, Bagby MD, Norman TL. Mechanical behavior of thermo-responsive orthodontic archwires. Dent Mater 1996;12:308–314.

Nakazato H, Fukuyo S, Masukawa T, Sachdeva R, Fukuyo S. Cytotoxicity studies on shape memory TiNi alloy. J Dent Res 1991;70 (IADR Abstracts):397.

Oshida Y, Miyazaki S, Sachdeva R. Microanalytical studies of orthodontic NiTi archwire. J Dent Res 1990;69(IADR Abstracts):313.

Sarkar NK, Redmond W, Schwaninger B, Goldberg AJ. The chloride corrosion behaviour of four orthodontic wires. J Oral Rehabil 1983;10:121–128.

Sebanc J, Brantley WA, Pincsak JJ, Conover JP. Variability of effective root torque as a function of edge bevel on orthodontic arch wires. Am J Orthod 1984;86:43–51.

Sonis AL. Comparison of NiTi coil springs vs. elastics in canine retraction. J Clin Orthod 1994;28:293–295.

Thayer TA, Bagby MD, Moore RN, De Angelis RJ. X-ray diffraction of nitinol orthodontic arch wires. Am J Orthod Dentofacial Orthop 1995;107:604–612.

Todoroki T, Tamura H. Effect of heat treatment after cold working on the phase transformation in TiNi alloy. Trans Japan Inst Metals 1987;28:83–94.

Wilson DF, Goldberg AJ. Alternative beta-titanium alloys for orthodontic wires. Dent Mater 1987;3:337–341.

Yoneyama T, Doi H, Hamanaka H, Okamoto Y, Mogi M, Miura F. Super-elasticity and thermal behavior of Ni-Ti alloy orthodontic arch wires. Dent Mater J 1992;11:1–10.

Yoshikawa DK, Burstone CJ, Goldberg AJ, Morton J. Flexure modulus of orthodontic stainless steel wires. J Dent Res 1981;60:139–145.

Publications on nonmetallic orthodontic wires

Imai T, Watari F, Yamagata S, Kobayashi M, Nagayama K, Nakamura S. Effects of water immersion on mechanical properties of new esthetic orthodontic wire. Am J Orthod Dentofacial Orthop 1999; 116:533–538.

Imai T, Watari F, Yamagata S, et al. Mechanical properties and aesthetics of FRP orthodontic wire fabricated by hot drawing. Biomaterials 1998;19:2195–2200.

Imai T, Yamagata S, Watari F, et al. Temperature-dependence of the mechanical properties of FRP orthodontic wire. Dent Mater J 1999;18:167–175.

McKamey RP, Kusy RP. Stress-relaxing composite ligature wires: Formulations and characteristics. Angle Orthod 1999;69:441–449.

Nakasima A, Hu JR, Ichinose M, Shimada H. Potential application of shape memory plastic as elastic material in clinical orthodontics. Eur J Orthod 1991;13:179–186.

Talass MF. Optiflex archwire treatment of a skeletal Class III open bite. J Clin Orthod 1992;26:245–252.

Watanabe M, Nakata S, Morishita T. Organic polymer wire for esthetic maxillary retainers. J Clin Orthod 1996;30:266–271.

Zufall SW, Kusy RP. Sliding mechanics of coated composite wires and the development of an engineering model for binding. Angle Orthod 2000;70:34–47.

Zufall SW, Kusy RP. Stress relaxation and recovery behaviour of composite orthodontic archwires in bending. Eur J Orthod 2000;22:1–12.

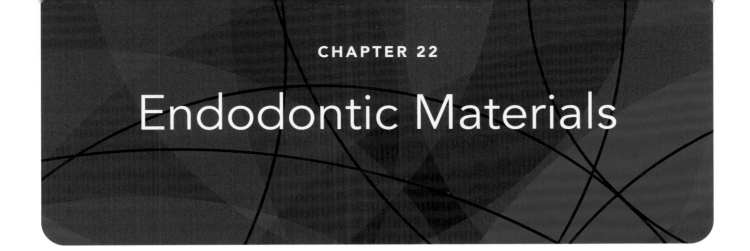

CHAPTER 22

Endodontic Materials

Endodontics is the branch of dentistry concerned with the morphology, physiology, and pathology of human dental pulp and periradicular tissues. Its study and practice encompass the biology of normal pulp and the etiology, diagnosis, prevention, and treatment of diseases and injuries of the pulp and associated periradicular conditions.

The scope of endodontics includes the differential diagnosis and treatment of oral pain of pulpal and/or periradicular origin; vital pulp therapy, including **pulp capping** and **pulpotomy**; nonsurgical treatment of root canal systems and the **obturation** of these systems; selective surgical removal of pathologic tissues resulting from pulpal pathosis; repair procedures related to surgical removal of pathologic tissues; intentional replantation and replantation of avulsed teeth; root-end resection, hemisection, and root resection; root-end obturation; bleaching of discolored teeth; re-treatment of teeth previously treated endodontically; and treatment with posts and/or cores for coronal restorations.

The success of basic nonsurgical endodontic treatment is highly dependent on the triad of access cavity preparation, proper cleaning and shaping of the root canals, and the quality of the obturation of the root canal system. The long-term prognosis is determined by the quality and integrity of the coronal seal. It is therefore imperative that further ingress of oral fluids (microleakage) through restorative and endodontic materials be kept to a minimum.

■ Endodontic Access

Rubber dam materials

First and foremost in endodontic treatment, rubber dam must be placed around the tooth or teeth to be treated. The use of rubber dam is mandatory as a standard of care in nonsurgical root canal treatment. It facilitates treatment by isolating the tooth, preventing aspiration of small endodontic instruments and endodontic irrigants, reducing salivary and bacterial contamination during treatment, protecting and retracting the oral soft tissues, and improving the visibility and efficiency of the clinician. The rubber dam system consists of a thin, flat sheet of latex in various colors and thicknesses (thin, medium, heavy, extra heavy). The medium thickness is generally preferred because it resists tear, retracts soft tissue better than the thin materials, and is easier to place than heavy rubber dam. Dark-colored rubber dam allows for better visual contrast, thus reducing eyestrain, but light-colored rubber dam naturally illuminates the operating field and provides easier film placement underneath the latex. Sheets of rubber dam are typically 5 × 5 or 6 × 6 in, and they are available in latex-free materials (eg, nitrile, synthetic) for persons with latex allergies.

For application, a rubber dam punch is used to place a hole in the rubber dam so that it will fit over the tooth. A rubber dam clamp, which is a plastic or metal retainer, is available in a number of anatomic shapes. A rubber dam forceps is used to secure the clamp around the cervical portion of the tooth, thus stabilizing the rubber dam and aiding in retraction of soft tissue adjacent to the isolated tooth. A pronged rubber dam frame, made of plastic or metal, is then placed on the rubber dam extraorally to retract and stabilize it over the patient's mouth.

Access cavity preparation

Access to the pulp chamber and canal system is achieved through the use of rotary high-speed burs in a dental handpiece to bore an opening in the affected tooth, typically on the lingual surface of anterior teeth and the occlusal surface of posterior teeth. A variety of bur types can be used depending on the preference of the operator and the status of the clinical crown. Long-shanked tungsten-carbide burs and size 2, 4, or 6 round burs can be used to make the access cavity. After the pulp chamber is located with a sharp, stainless steel endodontic explorer, safe-ended diamond burs or Endo-Z (Dentsply International) burs are used to unroof the chamber and refine the axial walls of the cavity preparation. Enhanced illumination and magnification with head lamps, loupes, or a surgical operating endodontic microscope with magnifications up to ×26 can aid the clinician in locating calcified canals and identifying fractures.

● Biomechanical Instrumentation

The second component of the endodontic triad involves cleaning and shaping of the canals. Removal of the coronal portion of the pulp is usually performed with a metallic spoon excavator or a rotary bur on a slow-speed handpiece. For the initial **debridement** of the canals, root canal broaches or rotary orifice-shaping instruments can be used. Manufactured in a number of sizes, the root canal broach is a very narrow, flexible, round stainless steel instrument with barbs along its shaft. Prone to breakage, the broach must be used passively in the canal and should not engage dentin. It is designed to remove gross amounts of pulpal tissue in large canals by locking remnants of pulp with its sharp barbs. Broaches can also be used to remove cotton products that have been placed in the chamber between appointments.

Newer on the market are rotary orifice shapers, which are made of flexible nickel-titanium. These variably tapered instruments are used in special controlled-speed, high-torque handpieces. Their use in the canal is typically limited to the coronal half of the canal. Because of their larger tapers, they facilitate straight-line access to the root apex by removing restrictive coronal dentin early in the cleaning and shaping process.

Gates-Glidden instruments are commonly used to enlarge canal orifices and shape the coronal portion of the canal. Used in a slow-speed handpiece, they consist of flexible, stainless steel, noncutting shafts with flame-shaped burs at their tips. They are available in a variety of lengths and sizes (Fig 22-1).

Specially designed hand instruments known as files and reamers are necessary for biomechanical instrumentation of the various anatomic forms of root canals (Fig 22-2). K-files are tapered metallic instruments made from rectangular, triangular, or rhomboidal cross-sectional wires. They are available in stainless steel or nickel-titanium and are manufactured by twisting or grinding the metal blank. Various cutting angles on the wires are created to plane or scrape the walls of the canal. Depending on the file design and canal size and curvature, these files may be used in a push-pull, twisting, watch-winding, or circumferential motion. The nature of the metal (nickel-titanium being five times more flexible than stainless steel), the size of the instrument, and the cross-sectional configuration determine the relative flexibility of each instrument (Fig 22-3). To accommodate different root lengths, these instruments are manufactured in lengths ranging from 21 to 31 mm. Moveable silicone rubber stops on the instruments can be adjusted to correspond to the exact length of each canal.

Many newer file designs incorporate a noncutting tip, which can be used instead of a cutting tip to help guide the file. Cutting tips can create deviations in canal anatomy during instrumentation. Examples of K-type files include Flex-R files (Miltex) (triangular cross section), Flexo-Files (Dentsply International) (triangular cross section), and K-Flex files (Kerr Dental) (rhomboidal cross section).

The size of the file is determined by the diameter of the shaft 1 mm from the tip and is recorded in millimeters. For example, a no. 25 K-file measures 0.25 mm in diameter 1 mm from its tip. The standard taper for these instruments is a 0.02-mm increase for every 1 mm up the shaft from its tip (the length of the working blades). For instance, the width of a no. 25 K-file at 16 mm above its tip is 0.57 mm (0.25 mm + 16 × 0.02 mm). Most traditional instrument designs adhere to this standard of sizing and tapering.

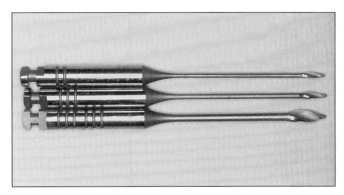

Fig 22-1 Gates-Glidden instruments. Rings on handle indicate sizing.

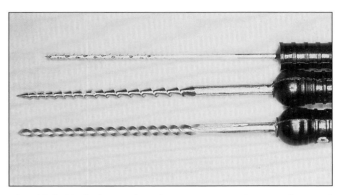

Fig 22-2 Endodontic hand instruments. *(top to bottom)* Barbed broach, Hedstrom file, reamer.

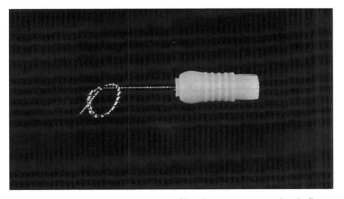

Fig 22-3 Nickel-titanium hand file demonstrating high flexibility.

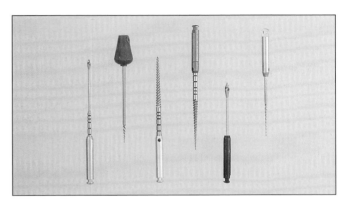

Fig 22-4 Specially designed nickel-titanium hand and rotary instruments with varying tapers.

Another type of file is the Hedstrom file. These files are long, thin, and tapered like K-files but are composed of round cross-sectional wires. Generally made from stainless steel or nickel-titanium, these aggressive files have cutting angles that are ground into the shaft and can only be used in a scraping or rasping motion as the file moves out of the canal. Rotation of Hedstrom files is contraindicated because they tend to self-thread and have a strong predilection toward fracture when used in this manner. Like the K-files, Hedstroms are manufactured in uniform sizes, tapers, and lengths. They are used primarily for removal of bulk amounts of dentin.

Classic hand root canal reamers are long, tapered, stainless steel instruments made from rectangular, triangular, or rhomboidal cross-sectional wires. They cut only during twisting and have fewer cutting edges than a typical K-file. Their use has diminished over time due to their lack of efficiency and their tendency to deviate from normal root canal anatomy during use. More tapered rotary reamers made of nickel-titanium have essentially replaced the stainless steel hand reamer. These instruments have radial land-cutting regions along their shafts and thus have been termed "U-bladed" in cross section. Like the orifice openers previously described, rotary reamers are used in a slow-speed, high-torque, gear-reduction, air-driven, or electric handpiece. Their tapers range from the standard 0.02-mm increase up to a 0.12-mm increase per millimeter. Examples include Profiles (Dentsply International), GT Rotaries (Dentsply International), Quantec 2000 (Tycom), and Lightspeed (Lightspeed) (Fig 22-4).

● Irrigants and Chelating Agents

Endodontic **irrigants** dissolve tissue and necrotic debris as well as destroy bacteria and disinfect the canal spaces. They also serve as lubricants for the metallic instruments used in the canal. Typically, they are delivered to the canal via an irrigating syringe with a nonbinding, blunt-tipped needle. The ideal irrigating solution in contemporary endodontics is sodium hypochlorite (NaOCl), used in percentages ranging from 1% to 5.25% (household bleach). Hydrogen peroxide has been used, but it is significantly less effective than NaOCl due to its inability to dissolve necrotic tissue.

Many practitioners use a **chelating agent** such as ethylenediaminetetraacetic acid (EDTA) in conjunction with sodium hypochlorite. EDTA has been shown to assist in smear layer removal and may facilitate the loosening of calcific obstructions in the root canal. It is often used in paste form with special additives, or it can be used in pure liquid form as an aqueous base of 17% EDTA. The paste form, such as RC-Prep (Premier Products) or Glyde (Dentsply International), enhances lubrication for rotary nickel-titanium instrumentation as well as traditional instrumentation techniques.

● Materials and Instruments for Root Canal Obturation

The goal of obturation is to seal off the root canal and its ramifications from oral fluids and bacteria. Although there is no ideal filling material, **gutta-percha** and **sealer cements** have proved to be the materials of choice in contemporary endodontics because they exhibit minimal toxicity and tissue irritability when confined to the root canal system.

Gutta-percha

Originating from trees in Africa and South America, pure gutta-percha is considered to be an isomer of natural rubber known as *trans-polyisoprene*, and is less elastic, more brittle, and harder than natural rubber. It can exist in both α and β crystalline forms; these forms are interchangeable depending on the temperature of the material. The α form is the natural state, is less subject to shrinkage, and is often used in obturating systems that use thermoplasticized, or heat-softened, gutta-percha.

The β form, which is typically found in gutta-percha cones or points, is used in cold compaction techniques such as lateral condensation. These cones or pellets contain approximately 19% to 22% gutta-percha, 59% to 75% zinc oxide, and a series of other additives, including waxes, coloring agents, antioxidants, and metallic salts.

The gutta-percha cone or pellet, in conjunction with a root canal sealer, must be compacted in the canal to conform to the prepared root canal system. Gutta-percha cones are available in standardized and nonstandardized forms (Fig 22-5). The standardized forms conform to the same dimensions and uniformity as those used for endodontic files; thus, a no. 40 gutta-percha cone should reasonably fit a canal that has been properly prepared with a no. 40 file. The nonstandardized forms, classified as medium, medium-fine, or fine-fine, have greater tapers than standardized cones and are often used in techniques that involve vertical compaction of heat-softened gutta-percha or filling of the coronal two-thirds of a canal after a standardized cone has been compacted in the apical third.

A number of obturating techniques and instruments can be used to compact gutta-percha into the root canal system (Fig 22-6). In lateral condensation, a long (17 to 30 mm), tapered, metallic instrument with a pointed tip known as a *spreader* is used to compact the gutta-percha cones and sealer laterally against the canal walls. Spreaders are available in both hand and finger forms and are made of stainless steel or nickel-titanium for greater flexibility. Root canal *pluggers*, which are long, slightly tapered, metallic instruments with flattened or blunt tips, are used in the vertical condensation method. Available in both hand and finger types, pluggers are designed to compact gutta-percha and sealer vertically after the gutta-percha has been thermosoftened with a heating device.

Root canal sealers

Root canal sealers are used to cement the gutta-percha in place, to fill voids and the intricate ramifications of the canal system, and to lubricate the cones during lateral compaction of the relatively nonrigid gutta-percha points. They should be biocompatible with and well tolerated by periradicular tissues.

The most commonly used sealers are zinc oxide–eugenol (ZOE) and calcium hydroxide–based cements because of their good working properties, sealability, biocompatibility, and ease of removal. Resin-, glass-

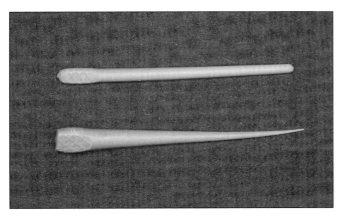

Fig 22-5 Gutta-percha cones or points. *(top)* Standardized cone; *(bottom)* nonstandardized cone.

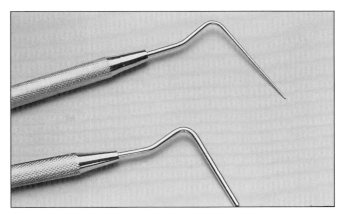

Fig 22-6 Endodontic hand condensers for compacting gutta-percha. *(top)* Spreader; *(bottom)* plugger.

Fig 22-7 Properly mixed endodontic sealer.

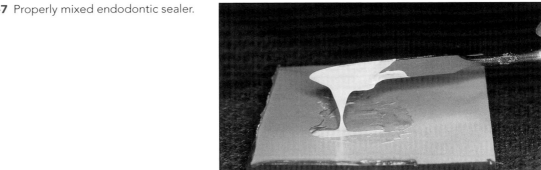

ionomer–, and silicone-based sealers are also available but are more technique sensitive, difficult to remove, and more variable in their sealing properties.

When mixed into a thick, creamy consistency (Fig 22-7), sealers are placed inside the root canal via paper points or a lentulo spiral, or are deposited in a light layer through the counter-clockwise rotation of an endodontic file. Examples of endodontic sealers include the 801 (ZOE-based, Roth Drug), pulp canal sealer (ZOE-based, Kerr Dental), Sealapex (calcium hydroxide–based, Kerr Dental), ThermaSeal Plus (resin-based, Dentsply International), and Ketac-Endo (glass ionomer–based, 3M ESPE).

■ Adjunct Materials

Calcium hydroxide

Calcium hydroxide has been used in dentistry for many years, both as an intracanal medication and as a pulp-capping agent. It is available in a variety of forms, ranging from pure chemical grade to proprietary compounds (Calasept, JS Dental; TempCanal, Pulpdent). For intracanal use, calcium hydroxide has been proven to be antibacterial and may aid in the dissolution of necrotic pulp tissue. Its high pH is responsible for the destruction of bacterial cell membranes and protein structures. When pulp is exposed during routine cavity preparation, a pulp-capping calcium hydroxide agent (Dycal, Dentsply International) or mineral trioxide aggregate can be placed as a "bandage" over the bleeding tissue in an attempt to promote dentinal bridge formation over time, thus preserving the vitality of the pulp.

Mineral trioxide aggregate

Mineral trioxide aggregate (ProRoot, Dentsply International) is a relatively recent material in the realm of endodontics, and certainly one of the most promising. This root canal repair material is a grayish powder consisting of fine, hydrophilic particles that set in the presence of

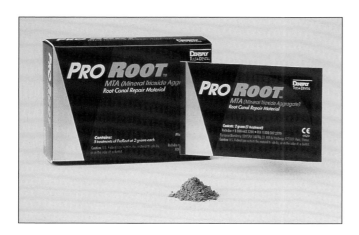

Fig 22-8 Mineral trioxide aggregate (ProRoot).

moisture (Fig 22-8). The hydration of the powder, composed of tricalcium silicate, tricalcium phosphate, tricalcium oxide, and other mineral oxides, creates a colloidal gel that solidifies to form a strong impermeable barrier. The material sets within 3 to 4 hours and has a working time of 5 minutes; it has been shown to be biocompatible and its seal is superior to that of amalgam. Although the material is costly and difficult to work with, primarily due to its naturally sandy consistency when hydrated, the indications for its use include clinical situations that often have no other viable options, such as perforation repair. Indications for ProRoot include pulp capping, internal repair of perforations (noncommunicative), apexification, and root-end filling in endodontic surgery.

■ Glossary

chelating agents Chemicals used for the removal of inorganic ions, usually the disodium salt of EDTA, from tooth structure.

debridement Elimination of organic and inorganic substances as well as microorganisms from the root canal by mechanical and/or chemical means.

gutta-percha The purified coagulated exudate from the mazer wood tree. It is a high-molecular-weight stereoisomer of polyisoprene. Since the 1950s, material compounded in the United States for "gutta-percha" points has been made from balata, a nearly identical latex from a tree in South America.

irrigants Liquids used to dissolve and flush out root canal debris; examples include sodium hypochlorite, saline, and hydrogen peroxide.

obturation The complete filling and closing of a cleaned and shaped root canal with a root canal sealer and core filling material.

pulp capping The procedure of placing a dental material over an exposed or nearly exposed pulp to encourage the formation of irritation dentin at the site of injury.

pulpotomy The surgical removal of the coronal portion of a vital pulp as a means of preserving the vitality of the remaining radicular portion.

sealer cements Radiopaque dental cements used, usually in combination with a solid or semisolid core material, to fill voids and seal root canals during obturation.

■ Discussion Questions

1. List all of the materials necessary for the proper placement of rubber dam on a tooth requiring endodontic therapy.

2. Discuss the types and properties of the materials used in obturating a cleaned and properly shaped root canal.

3. Discuss the various types of instruments that can be used to biomechanically prepare the root canal.

4. Why are irrigants necessary in endodontic therapy?

5. What are the roles of calcium hydroxide and mineral trioxide aggregate in endodontic therapy?

▣ Study Questions

(See appendix E for answers.)

1. All of the following endodontic instruments are designed to remove dentin except which one? (*a*) K-file; (*b*) reamer; (*c*) broach; (*d*) Hedstrom

2. The endodontic "triad" consists of which of the following? (*a*) access, biomechanical instrumentation, and obturation; (*b*) rubber dam placement, access, and obturation; (*c*) biomechanical instrumentation, obturation, and restoration; (*d*) access, obturation, and restoration

3. All of the following are true about Hedstrom files except which one? (*a*) they work best by rotation; (*b*) they are made from a circular wire; (*c*) they are manufactured in uniform sizes; (*d*) they are made from either stainless steel or nickel titanium metal

4. Which of the following is a chelating agent, helping to loosen calcific obstructions in the root canal? (*a*) gutta-percha; (*b*) Roth 801; (*c*) sodium hypochlorite; (*d*) EDTA

5. Which of the following instruments is used in the lateral condensation of gutta-percha? (*a*) plugger; (*b*) spreader; (*c*) explorer; (*d*) broach

▣ Recommended Reading

American Association of Endodontists. Glossary: Contemporary Terminology for Endodontics, ed 6. Chicago: American Association of Endodontists, 1998.

American National Standards Institute. Revised American National Standards Institute/American Dental Association Specification No. 28 for Root Canal Files and Reamers, Type K. New York: American National Standards Institute, 1988.

Dumsha TC, Gutmann JL. Clinician's Endodontic Handbook. Cleveland, OH: Lexi-Comp, 2000.

Foreman PC, Barnes IE. Review of calcium hydroxide. Int Endod J 1990;23:283–297.

Glickman GN, Pileggi R. Preparation for treatment. In: Cohen S, Burns RC (eds). Pathways of the Pulp, ed 8. St Louis: Mosby, 2002.

Glickman GN, Koch KA. 21st-century endodontics. J Am Dent Assoc 2000;131(suppl):39S–46S.

Gutmann JL, Witherspoon DE. Obturation of the cleaned and shaped root canal system. In: Cohen S, Burns RC (eds). Pathways of the Pulp, ed 8. St Louis: Mosby, 2002.

Kim S. Color Atlas of Microsurgery in Endodontics. Philadelphia: Saunders, 2001.

Spangberg L. Instruments, materials, and devices. In: Cohen S, Burns RC (eds). Pathways of the Pulp, ed 7. St Louis: Mosby, 1998.

Torabinejad M, Chivian N. Clinical applications of mineral trioxide aggregate. J Endod 1999;25:197–205.

Walia HM, Brantley WA, Gerstein H. An initial investigation of the bending and torsional properties of Nitinol root canal files. J Endod 1988;14:346–351.

CHAPTER 23

Implant and Bone Augmentation Materials

A critical problem in dentistry is treating the edentulous patient. According to a survey by the World Health Organization, 26% of the US population older than 65 years is totally edentulous, and a substantial number of other patients are partially edentulous, missing an average of 10 teeth.[1,2] Although removable dentures and fixed partial dentures offer effective treatments for many edentulous patients, those who have lost substantial tooth-bearing portions of bone and cannot manage prostheses or masticate properly can improve their oral function through the use of dental implants.

The use of implants as a means of treating these patients has accelerated in the last two decades, and there are now more than 1 million dental implants in use in the United States. Dental implants are effective in providing long-term total and partial support for restorations. Despite the expanded use of implants, however, they are largely evaluated only on a qualitative level. To better understand and quantify the clinical effectiveness of dental implants, a greater understanding of the parameters governing the long-term success of this complex material/tissue aggregate is needed.

In this chapter, design considerations important to implant dentistry are presented. Following an overview of general concepts and indications for implant use, osseointegration is defined and discussed, methods of achieving osseointegration are presented, and parameters important to achieving implant success are reviewed, with a primary focus on biomaterials and biomechanical factors.

● Indications for Dental Implant Use

The general requirement for dental implants is adequate bone to support the implant with the physiologic parameters of width, height, length, contour, and density. Note that the importance of these parameters varies, depending on the specific implant type (Table 23-1). Despite the "glamour" of implant dentistry, a conservative treatment protocol must be stressed. Dental implants should not be the first treatment option considered. Unsatisfactory treatment with removable dentures or fixed partial dentures is often an important indication for implant use. A number of contraindications for implant use also exist (Box 23-1).

Box 23-1 Contraindications for dental implant use[1]

Unattainable prosthodontic reconstruction

Patient sensitivity to implant component(s)

Debilitating or uncontrolled disease

Pregnancy

Inadequate practitioner training

Conditions, diseases, or treatments that may compromise healing (ie, radiation therapy)

Poor patient motivation/hygiene

Perceived poor patient compliance

Unrealistic patient expectations

Table 23-1 Summary of dental implant types and indications for each[1]

IMPLANT TYPE	INDICATIONS
Endosseous	
Cylindric	Adequate bone to support implant—width and height of primary concern Maxillary and mandibular arch locations Completely or partially edentulous patients
Blade	Adequate bone to support implant—width and length of primary concern Maxillary and mandibular arch locations Completely or partially edentulous patients
Ramus frame	Adequate anterior bone to support implant—width and height of primary concern Mandibular arch location Completely edentulous patients
Subperiosteal	
Complete	Atrophy of bone, but adequate and stable bone to support implant
Unilateral	Maxillary and mandibular arch locations
Circumferential	Completely and partially edentulous patients
Transosseous	
Staple	Adequate anterior bone to support implant—width and height of primary concern
Single pin	Anterior mandibular arch location
Multiple pin	Completely and partially edentulous patients

Types of Implants

Dental implants are classified into three categories (see Table 23-1, Fig 23-1).

1. *Endosseous implants* are embedded in mandibular or maxillary bone and project through the oral mucosa covering the edentulous ridge.
2. *Subperiosteal implants* rest on the surface of the bone beneath the periosteum.
3. *Transosseous implants* penetrate the inferior mandibular border and also project through the oral mucosa covering the edentulous ridge.

Root-form endosseous screw-threaded implants are the most common implants in clinical practice. This subclass of implants is the only one for which good long-term (eg, 10- to 15-year) clinical tracking of large patient populations is available. Success rates for implants placed in the mandible are approximately 95% at 5 years and greater than 85% at 15 years. For maxillary implants, success rates are approximately 85% to 90% at 5 years and

80% at 15 years. The clinician's expertise and surgical technique are more important than the specific implant and are the primary factors dictating clinical outcome.

Osseointegration

Unlike many biomaterials, which serve to replace as much of a tissue's natural structure and function as possible, dental implants do not restore function by mimicking the natural function of the periodontal ligament (Fig 23-2). Instead, **osseointegration**, or the direct structural and functional connection between ordered, living bone and the surface of a load-carrying implant, is what should occur with a well-functioning implant. This definition was originally based on retrospective radiographic and light microscopic observations and has since been modified based on scanning and transmission electron microscopic observations. However, the general working definition of osseointegration is fundamentally the same—the host bone responds in a safe, predictable, and versatile manner, to surgical placement of an implant in a sterile wound, with a healing cascade leading to interfacial os-

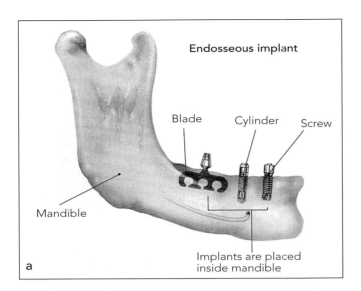

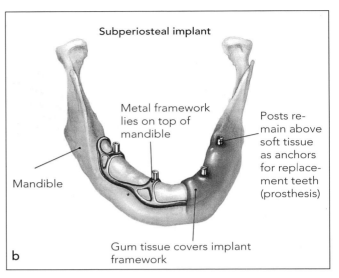

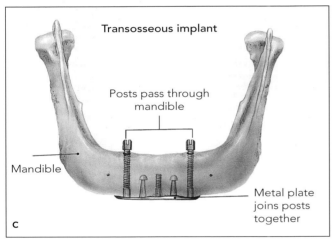

Fig 23-1 Three main classes of dental implants: (*a*) endosseous, (*b*) subperiosteal, (*c*) transosseous. (Reprinted with permission from Taylor.[3])

teogenesis and mechanical stability of the implant (Fig 23-3). In a well-functioning implant, interfacial osteogenesis and clinical stability are achieved (Fig 23-4a), and a stable marginal bone level is maintained. In comparison, poorly differentiated connective tissue adjacent to an implant can lead to clinical mobility and implant failure (Fig 23-4b).

There are a multitude of interrelated clinical, biologic, and engineering factors that control the oral cavity's response and dictate the success of osseointegration.

Achieving and enhancing implant-tissue attachment

An implant must be capable of carrying occlusal stresses. In addition, stresses must be transferred to the adjacent bone. Not only must stresses be transferred across the implant-tissue interface, but they must be of a "correct"

orientation and magnitude so that they mimic the normal physiologic stresses and allow tissue viability to be maintained. The ability to transmit stress from the implant to the adjacent bone is largely dependent on attaining interfacial fixation. Thus, the interface must stabilize in as short a time postoperatively as possible and remain stable for as long a time as possible.

Developing an "optimal" implant that meets all of these objectives requires the integration of material, physical, chemical, mechanical, biologic, and economic factors. While all of these properties are important, they cannot all be optimized in a given design. Optimization of one property often detracts from another. Thus, in designing a dental implant and in choosing an implant for a specific clinical scenario, a ranking of requirements and objectives is necessary.

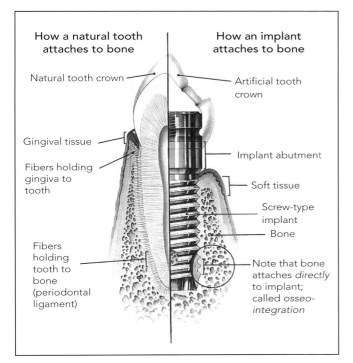

Fig 23-2 Schematic of natural tooth vs implant attachment to bone. (Reprinted with permission from Taylor.[3])

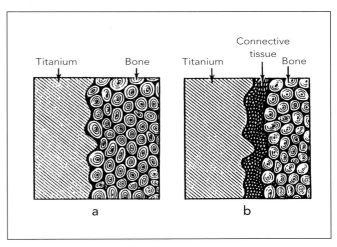

Fig 23-3 Schematic of localized sections of interfacial zone, showing (a) osseointegrated and (b) fibrous-integrated tissue adjacent to implant surface. Osseointegration is more likely to be achieved with a greater implant stability, as excess tissue-implant–relative motion may result in fibrous-integrated tissue. (Reprinted with permission from Brånemark et al.[4])

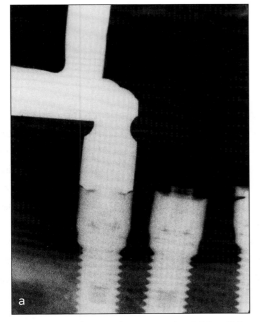

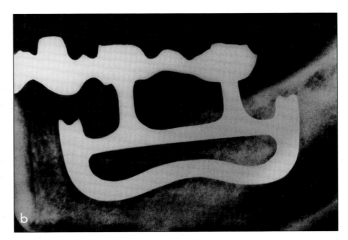

Fig 23-4 Radiographic example of (a) well-functioning and (b) failing dental implants. (a) A well-osseointegrated interfacial zone provides interfacial stability, whereas (b) a poorly differentiated interfacial connective tissue can lead to mobility and implant failure.

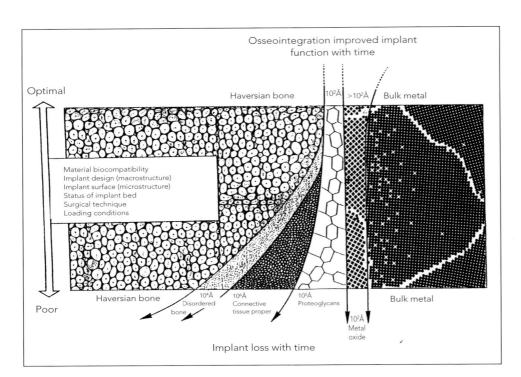

Fig 23-5 Schematic of interfacial zone, showing constituents: bulk metal, metal oxide, proteoglycans, connective tissue, disordered and ordered bone, and relative proportions of each for good and poor osseointegration. (Reprinted with permission from Brånemark et al.[4])

In an ideal situation, such as that achieved with commercially pure titanium (CPTi), calcified tissue can be observed within several hundred Angstroms of the implant surface. In Fig 23-5, a layer of proteoglycans 200 to 400 Å thick lies adjacent to the metal oxide, and collagen filaments can be observed about 200 Å from the surface. Less-than-optimal surgical techniques or implant surface chemistry and relative motion between the implant and tissue can lead to a thicker zone of proteoglycans, soft connective tissue, and disordered bone.

Because a stable interface must be developed before loading, it is desirable to accelerate tissue apposition to dental implant surfaces. Material developments that have been implemented in clinical practice include the use of surface-roughened implants and bioactive ceramic coatings. Other techniques include electric stimulation, bone grafting, and recombinant growth factors.

A variety of implant surface configurations can improve the cohesiveness of the implant-tissue interface, leading to increased transfer of occlusal loads to the adjacent tissue that minimizes relative motion between implant and tissue, fibrous integration, and ultimately loosening, thereby lengthening the service life of the implant. Metal implant surfaces may be smooth, textured, screw threaded, plasma sprayed, or porous coated. By far, the most common surface configuration is the screw-threaded dental implant. Osseointegration around screw-threaded implants occurs through tissue ongrowth, or direct apposition between tissue and the implant surface. Alternative methods of implant-tissue attachment, based on tissue ingrowth into roughened or three-dimensional surface layers, yield higher bone-metal shear strength than other types of fixation. Increased interfacial shear strength results in a better stress transfer from the implant to the surrounding bone, a more uniform stress distribution between the implant and bone, and lower stresses in the implant. In principle, the result of a stronger interfacial bond is decreased implant loosening.

A progression of surfaces from the lowest implant-tissue shear strength to the highest is as follows: smooth, textured, screw threaded, plasma sprayed, and porous. Two factors must be stressed, though. First, different surface structures necessitate different osseointegration times. Second, surface roughening, particularly of titanium-based materials, results in reduced fatigue strength. Thus, improvements in implant-tissue attachment strength are often countered by a loss of structural strength and must be met with design compromises to avoid material failure.

Fig 23-6 Schematic of interdependent engineering factors that affect the success of dental implants. (Reprinted with permission from Kohn.[5])

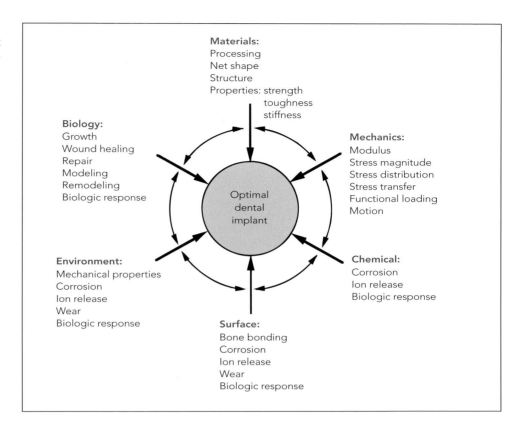

◼ Criteria for Successful Implant Placement

Three aspects of an implant-tissue system are important in determining clinical success: *(1)* the implant material(s) and adjacent tissue(s), *(2)* the **interfacial zone** between the implant and tissue, and *(3)* the effect of the implant and its breakdown products on the local and systemic tissues. Although the interfacial zone is composed of a relatively thin (< 100 μm) layer consisting of heterogeneous metallic oxide, proteins, and connective tissue, it has an effect on the maintenance of interfacial integrity. The integrity of the implant-tissue interface is also dependent on material, mechanical, chemical, surface, biologic, and local environmental factors, all of which change as functions of time in vivo. In addition, implant "success" is dependent on the patient's overall medical and dental status, the surgical techniques used, and the extent and time course of tissue healing. The focus of this section is on the biomaterial and biomechanical factors, summarized in Fig 23-6.

Surgical parameters

Adequate preparation of bone is critical for bone-cell survival, well-ordered connective tissue apposition close to an implant surface, the establishment of a reliable bone anchor, and long-term implant and tissue viability. Poor surgical technique or premature functional loading may result in an inability to achieve osseointegration, a fibrous adaptation, and an early implant failure. The standard clinical protocol therefore calls for a two-stage implant procedure. The first stage involves the careful preparation of the implant site in a manner that minimizes trauma and optimizes healing and interfacial osteogenesis. Certain thermal limits should not be exceeded during surgery. If these temperatures are exceeded, thermal necrosis can occur, resulting in a thicker layer of soft tissue directly apposing the implant surface and jeopardizing osseointegration. Following the initial surgery, the implants undergo a submerged healing in situ for 3 to 6 months. During this period, ordered, living bone, with the potential for ultimately carrying occlusal loads, develops within the interfacial zone.

Surface chemistry and biologic response

Implant materials may corrode and/or wear, leading to the generation of micron- or submicron-sized debris that may elicit both local and systemic biologic responses. Metals are more susceptible to electrochemical degradation than ceramics. Therefore, a fundamental criterion for choosing a metallic implant material is that it elicits a minimal biologic response. **Titanium**-based materials are well tolerated by the body because of their passive oxide layers. The main elemental constituents as well as the minor alloying constituents can be tolerated by the body in trace amounts. However, larger amounts of metals usually cannot be tolerated. Therefore, minimizing mechanical and chemical breakdown of implant materials is a primary objective.

Local accumulation of material around an implant may include membrane-bound ions released due to wear or fatigue processes or insoluble reaction products. Excessive metal ion accumulation can lead to metallosis or tissue discoloration and also to reduced phagocytosis and cytoxicity.

Understanding implant surface chemistry is important to ensure that (1) implant materials must not adversely affect local tissues, organ systems, and organ functions; and (2) the in vivo environment must not degrade the implant and compromise its long-term function. The interfacial zone between an implant and the surrounding tissue is therefore the most important entity in defining the biologic response to the implant and the response of the implant to the body.

The success of any implant depends on its bulk and surface properties, the site of implantation, tissue trauma during surgery, and motion at the implant-tissue interface. The surface of a material is almost always different in chemical composition and morphology than the bulk material. These differences arise from the molecular arrangement, surface reactions, and contamination. Interface chemistry is therefore determined primarily by the properties of the metal oxide and not as much by the metal itself.

Metallic oxides dictate the type of cellular and protein binding at the implant surface. Surface oxides are continually altered by the indiffusion of oxygen, hydroxide formation, and the outdiffusion of metallic ions. Thus, a single oxide stoichiometry does not exist. The surface potential may also play an important role in osseointe-gration. For example, oxides with high dielectric constants may inhibit the movement of cells to an implant surface. Last, the type and orientation of cells attaching to metal surfaces is influenced by the microscopic geometry of the substrate surface.

Mechanical parameters

Mechanical properties important in designing implant materials include stiffness, yield and ultimate strengths, fracture toughness, and fatigue strength. Stiffness, or modulus of elasticity, dictates, to a large extent, the ability of the implant to transmit stresses to the adjacent tissue and maintain tissue viability over time. Static and fatigue strengths obviously are important in minimizing material failures. Fracture toughness is a gauge of the energy needed to cause failure in the presence of a defect, and is a critical parameter in evaluating implants with surface contours that could serve as stress raisers.

Implants are subjected to axial, shear, bending, and torsional loads, so in addition to the magnitude of the loading, directionality must also be considered. With the above-mentioned considerations and only a qualitative knowledge of "*stability*"—the maximum allowable displacement at an implant-tissue interface that will still result in osseointegration and bone maintenance—it must be stressed that the time at which an implant can begin to undergo loading is most likely implant- and location-specific and generally unknown.

Although rare, material failure of implants, generally by fatigue, does occur. Failure of implant structures or abutments should be not disregarded or viewed as isolated instances. Fatigue of implant materials is clinically important for several reasons. First, fatigue properties of implant materials should be accurately quantified so improvements in implant design may be achieved. Second, the stress distribution between an implant and surrounding bone tissue depends on the section size of the implant as well as the elastic moduli of both the implant and tissue. Therefore, use of a larger, stiffer implant to avoid mechanical failure may result in less stress transfer to the adjacent bone. Third, coated implants may undergo local fracture processes that do not necessarily compromise the integrity of the implant but do compromise its functionality and ability to transmit stress to tissue.

Implant design

The design of dental implants is based on many interrelated factors, including the geometry of the implant, how this geometry affects mechanical properties, and the initial and long-term stability of the implant-tissue interface. There is no singularly agreed-on design criterion. Implants can be designed to maximize strength, interfacial stability, or load transfer, with each of these criteria requiring different material and interface properties. Two goals of any implant design are to maximize initial stability (ie, through implant design and surgical precision, create as tight a fit as possible at the time of surgery and accomplish osseointegration in as short a time as possible following implant placement) and minimize loosening (ie, maintain osseointegration for as long a time as possible following achievement of stability).

To ensure osseointegration and achieve the potential benefits of biologic fixation, the interface must be stable (ie, relative motion must be minimized) before loading and throughout the service life of the implant. However, there is no quantitative definition of stability, only the qualitative understanding that excessive relative motion at the implant-tissue interface leads to bone atrophy and the formation of a fibrous tissue layer, further increasing motion (Fig 23-7).

Quantifying stresses and strains in implants, tissues, and implant-tissue interfaces is important for understanding mechanically mediated response mechanisms and for implant design. Implant and tissue geometry, elastic properties, loading, boundary conditions, interface conditions, and local stresses and strains are all important.

Biologic parameters and properties of tissue

Perhaps more important than the definition of osseointegration is the corollary that the creation and maintenance of osseointegration depends on the understanding of the tissue's healing, repair, and remodeling capacities. Dental implant design and function, therefore, are not only based on material considerations but also on the properties of the surrounding tissue.

The microstructure of the mandible and maxilla is complex. For example, the basilar and alveolar bone of the mandible are composed of secondary Haversian bone, regular and irregular primary lamellar bone, and plexiform lamellae of varying orientations. The basilar bone forms the body of the mandible. Alveolar bone, formed in conjunction with tooth eruption, is a thin lamella that surrounds the tooth roots, attaches to the periodontal ligament fibers, and is surrounded by another layer of bone that supports the tooth sockets.

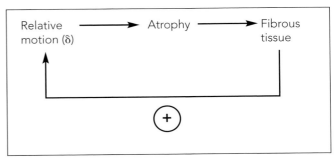

Fig 23-7 Schematic of positive feedback mechanisms leading to implant loosening. (Reprinted with permission from Kohn.[5])

The material and mechanical properties of the mandible and maxilla are nonuniform and vary as functions of anatomic location, age, sex, and metabolic state. Variations in these properties are functions of variations in composition, microstructure, and cellular and molecular signaling. An understanding of regional properties will provide a better understanding of localized bone regeneration, repair, modeling, remodeling, and disease states and possibly facilitate the design of site-specific dental implants and bone augmentation materials.

Materials Used in Dental Implants

Two classes of materials—metals and ceramics—are used in dental implants, either alone or in hybrid fashion (Fig 23-8). Metallic implant materials are largely titanium based, either CPTi or Ti-6Al-4V alloy. However, the synergistic relationship among processing, composition, structure, and properties of both the bulk metals and their surface oxides effectively leaves more than two metals. Processing conditions, such as casting, forging, and machining of metal implants, densification of ceramics, deposition of ceramic and metal coatings onto metal implants, as well as cleaning and sterilization procedures, can all alter the microstructure, surface chemistry, and properties, primarily through temperature and pressure effects.

Metals

Metallic dental implants are almost exclusively titanium based. A good deal of the knowledge about titanium stems from the extensive aerospace and metallurgy literature. Many requirements of an aerospace component, primarily high strength and corrosion resistance, are char-

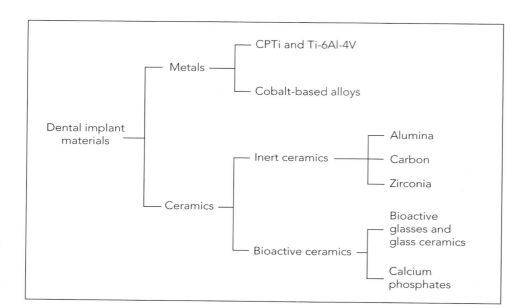

Fig 23-8 Classification of dental implant materials.

acteristic properties needed in a dental implant. Thus, titanium has been called the "material of choice" in dentistry because of its strength and the minimal biologic response it elicits. The strength of titanium is due to its hexagonal close-packed crystal lattice and crystallographic orientation, whereas its biocompatibility (corrosion resistance) is attributed to its stable, passive oxide layer.

Titanium-based implants are in their passive state (ie, their oxide is stable) under typical physiologic conditions, and breakdown of passivity should not occur. Both CPTi and Ti-6Al-4V alloy possess excellent corrosion resistance for a full range of oxide states and pH levels. It is the coherent oxide layer and the fact that titanium repassivates almost instantaneously that renders titanium so corrosion resistant. However, even in its passive condition, titanium is not "inert." The release of titanium ions that does occur results from chemical dissolution of titanium oxide. However, the low dissolution rate and relative nonreactivity of titanium dissolution products allow bone to thrive and therefore osseointegrate with titanium.

The Ti-6Al-4V alloy has a 60% greater strength than pure titanium, but it is more expensive. Both CPTi and Ti-6Al-4V alloy have complex, heterogeneous surface oxides. There may be differences in cell adhesion, and tissues may be in closer proximity to pure titanium surfaces than to alloy surfaces. However, there does not seem to be any difference in implant function between the two types of titanium.

The mechanical properties of titanium-based materials are well established. Microstructures with small ($<$ 20 μm) grain sizes have the highest fatigue strength (approximately 500 to 700 MPa). Surface roughening, whether through screw threading or deposition of coatings, results in a reduced fatigue strength compared with smooth-surfaced implants.

Ceramics

The initial rationale for using ceramics in dentistry was based on the relative biologic inertness of ceramics compared with metals. Ceramics are fully oxidized materials and therefore chemically stable. Thus, ceramics are less likely to elicit an adverse biologic response than metals, which only oxidize at their surface. Ceramics promote osseointegration by nature of their excellent osteoconductivity of host cells.

Three types of "inert" ceramics of interest are carbon, alumina (Al_2O_3), and zirconia (ZrO_2). Recently, a greater emphasis has been placed on bioactive and bioresorbable ceramics, materials that not only elicit normal tissue formation but may also form an intimate bond with bone tissue and even be replaced by tissue over time. While "inert" ceramics elicit a minimal tissue response, bioactive ceramics are partially soluble, enabling ion transfer and the formation of a direct bond between implant and bone. Bioresorbable or biodegradable ceramics have a higher degree of solubility than bioactive ceramics, gradually resorb and integrate into the surrounding tissue, and are used as bone augmentation materials. Bioactive ceramics are primarily used as scaffold materials or as coatings on more structurally sound metal substrates.

The concept of bioactivity was originally introduced with respect to bioactive glasses via the following hypothesis: The biocompatibility of an implant material is optimal if the material elicits the formation of normal tissues at its surface, and, in addition, if it establishes a contiguous interface capable of supporting the loads that normally occur at the site of implantation. Examples of these materials are bioactive glasses, glass ceramics, and **calcium phosphate ceramics**. Bioactive glasses and glass ceramics include bioglass, which is a synthesis of several glasses containing mixtures of silica, phosphate, calcia, and soda; Ceravital (E. Leitz Wetzlar), which has a different alkali oxide concentration from that of bioglass; and apatite-wollastonite glass ceramic, a glass ceramic containing crystalline oxyapatite and fluorapatite $[Ca_{10}(PO_4)6(O,F_2)]$ and β-wollastonite $(SiO_2\text{-}CaO)$ in a $MgO\text{-}CaO\text{-}SiO_2$ glassy matrix. The calcium phosphate ceramics can have varying calcium-to-phosphate ratios, depending on processing-induced physical and chemical changes. Among them, the apatite ceramics, one of which is **hydroxyapatite**, have been studied most and are the focus of this section.

The impetus for using synthetic hydroxyapatite as a biomaterial stems from the perceived advantage of using a material similar to the mineral phase in bone and teeth for replacing these materials. As such, better tissue bonding is expected. Additional advantages of bioactive ceramics include low thermal and electric conductivity, elastic properties similar to those of bone, control of degradation rates through control of material properties, and the possibility of the ceramic functioning as a barrier to metallic corrosion products when it is coated onto a metal substrate.

However, processing-induced phase transformations provoke changes in dissolution rates and the different structures and compositions alter the biologic response. Given the range of chemical compositions available in bioactive ceramics and the fact that pure hydroxyapatite is rarely used, the broader term *calcium phosphate ceramics* (CPC) should be used in lieu of the more specific *hydroxyapatite*. Each CPC is defined by a unique set of chemical and physical properties.

Mixtures of hydroxyapatite, tricalcium phosphate, and tetracalcium phosphate may evolve as a result of plasma spraying and other processes used to coat ceramics onto metal implants. Physical properties of importance to the clinical function of calcium phosphate ceramics include:

1. Powder particle size and shape
2. Pore size, shape, and distribution
3. Specific surface area
4. Phases present
5. Crystal structure and size
6. Grain size
7. Density
8. Coating thickness, hardness, and surface roughness

Problems and Future Directions

Although there is no consensus regarding methods of evaluating dental implants and what parameters are most important, clinical evaluations have generally shown that dental implants are successful 5 years after placement in at least 75% of cases. Despite advances in materials synthesis and processing, surgical technique, and clinical protocols, clinical failures occur at rates of approximately 2% to 5% per year. Causes of failure and current problems with dental implants include:

1. Early loosening, stemming from a lack of initial osseointegration
2. Late loosening, or loss of osseointegration
3. Bone resorption
4. Infection
5. Fracture of the implant and/or abutment
6. Delamination of the coating from the bulk implant

The most common failure mechanism with endosseous implants is alveolar crest resorption, leading to progressive periodontal lesions, decreased areas of supporting tissues, and ultimately implant loosening. Aseptic failures are most often the cumulative result of more than one of the above-mentioned factors.

As a result of these clinical problems, basic and clinical research should focus on the complete characterization of materials, including bulk and surface properties, development of new materials, more engineering-based designs for both existing and new materials, quantification of stresses and stress transfer between implant and tissue, mechanical and biologic responses of tissues, and host response to implants.

Future materials

Although titanium and, to a lesser extent, ceramic and ceramic-coated implants have an excellent clinical record

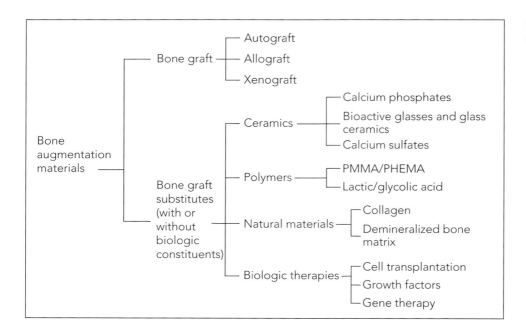

Fig 23-9 Classification of bone augmentation materials.

in implant dentistry, these materials are not necessarily end-stage materials. Continuing developments in the materials and biomedical fields can be expected in the next decade.

Because one of the long-term problems with dental implants is stress shielding, or mechanically mediated bone resorption, which is due in part to the elastic mismatch between metal and bone, polymer and composite implants that offer reduced moduli are being considered. The motivation for using composite materials for implants is based on several concepts. Composite materials can be very strong, because materials in fiber form exhibit strengths near the theoretical values. As a result, advanced composites can be as strong as metals and, in some cases, more flexible. The properties of composites can be more easily tailored than those of metals. A specific example is that of the modulus of composites, which can be tailored to be near that of bone.

● Augmentation Materials and Tissue Engineering

Persistent skeletal defects arising from trauma, infection, tumor resection, congenital malformations, and progressively deforming skeletal diseases are of significant clinical concern. The standard approach to repair skeletal defects is a bone graft, either an *autogenous bone graft* (graft from a patient's own body) or an *allogeneic bone*

graft (graft from another person). While bone grafts are widely used and clinically successful, they have limitations and, in some cases, lack clinical predictability. For example, autogenous bone grafts can have failure rates as high as 30%, and there is concern about transmission of viruses with allogeneic bone grafts. Therefore, increased research into alternative substitute materials, such as ceramics, polymers, composites, bone derivatives, and natural materials is underway (Fig 23-9). Examples of dense and porous calcium phosphate ceramics are shown in Figs 23-10 and 23-11. Many of these synthetic materials are designed to be permanently implanted. Most problems with synthetic materials manifest themselves at the biomaterial/tissue interface, in part because the tissue has the ability to functionally adapt, whereas the synthetic material does not. Therefore, despite the success of current treatments for skeletal defects, and the significant impact that man-made biomaterials have had on dentistry, combinations of synthetic materials and biologic constituents (eg, cells or growth factors), as well as more biologically interactive materials are being investigated.

The three primary application areas for augmentation materials in dentistry are intramucosal, endodontic, and bone-substitute materials. An ideal bone-substitute material for these clinical applications should be:

1. Biocompatible
2. Easy to fabricate, sterilize, and shape intraoperatively
3. **Osteoinductive**

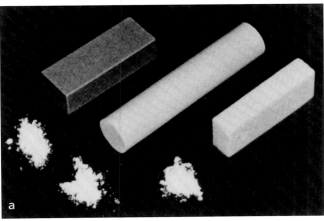 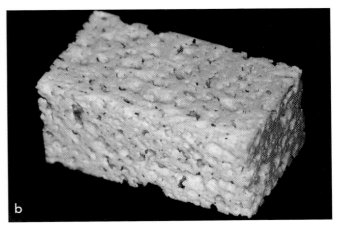

Fig 23-10 (a) Dense hydroxyapatite ceramic augmentation material with starting powders. (Reprinted with permission from Denissen et al.[6]) (b) Porous hydroxyapatite augmentation material, 44 × 18 × 16 mm; porosity = 45%. (Reprinted with permission from Osborn.[7])

4. **Osteoconductive**
5. Of sufficient mechanical integrity to support loads encountered at the implant site over a lengthy service life
6. Inexpensive

Regeneration of bone defects can be pursued by one or a combination of three general strategies: conduction, induction, and/or cell transplantation. In a conductive approach, a biomaterial provides an appropriate microenvironment for host cells to attach, grow, and function, ultimately leading to the formation of new bone within the material. Currently such materials are the most clinically prevalent. An inductive approach is more proactive in that biologic agents, typically growth factors, are introduced to induce the host cells to form new bone. Cell-based therapies may include not only the transplantation of differentiated and uncommitted cells, but also genetically manipulated cells, and can be used in combination with a supporting biomaterial (conductive) and also with inductive agents.

Stem cells from a number of sites, including bone marrow, periosteum and muscle, have been pursued as sources of cells capable of differentiating into bone, ultimately leading to bone regeneration. When transplanted under appropriate conditions, ex vivo expanded cells are capable of regenerating bone. This capacity has obvious clinical and commercial applications. However, results demonstrate large variability, implying that the nature of the microenvironment that cells are exposed to, including the biomaterial used for transplanting the cells, is a critical parameter.

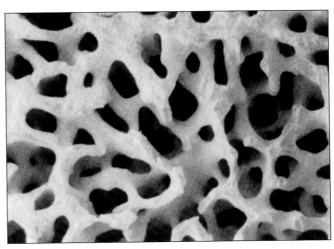

Fig 23-11 Porous coralline hydroxyapatite ceramic augmentation material (Pro Osteon Implant 500, Interpore Cross International).

◼ Glossary

calcium phosphate ceramics A class of ceramics with varying calcium-to-phosphate ratios, which can form a direct bond with bone.

hydroxyapatite A specific form of calcium phosphate with a stoichiometry $Ca_{10}(PO_4)6(OH)_2$ and a Ca/P ratio of 1.67. Bone is a nonstoichiometric form of hydroxyapatite.

interfacial zone The thin zone at the surface of an implant, which includes the surface oxides, protein layers, and connective tissue.

osseointegration A direct structural and functional connection between ordered, living bone and the surface of a load-carrying implant.

osteoconductive material A material that acts as a scaffold for new bone formation by providing an appropriate environment for attachment, proliferation, and function of osteoblasts or their progenitors, leading to formation of new bone matrix.

osteoinductive material A material and/or biologic agent that causes the conversion of nonlineage committed cells preferentially to bone progenitor cells.

titanium The "material of choice" in dentistry, primarily because of its excellent biocompatibility (as a result of its stable oxide layer), mechanical properties, and its proven ability to achieve osseointegration in implant dentistry.

● Discussion Questions

1. What are the properties (bulk and surface) of titanium that make it attractive for use as a dental implant?

2. What is/are the rationale(s) for using bioactive ceramics (eg, hydroxyapatite) as coatings on dental implants?

3. What is the importance of implant-tissue interfacial stability, and what are current methods of accelerating osseointegration such that the time between stage-one and stage-two implant placement may be reduced?

4. What are the physical, mechanical, and biologic parameters affecting the clinical success of dental implants?

● Study Questions

(See appendix E for answers.)

1. What is osseointegration?

2. What materials are used for osseointegrated implants?

3. What factors dictate the effectiveness of osseointegration?

4. What parameters influence implant success?

● References

1. National Institutes of Health. Consensus Development Conference statement on dental implants, 13–15 June, 1988. J Dent Ed 1988; 52:824–827.
2. Petersen PE, Yamamoto T. Improving the oral health of older people: The approach of the WHO Global Oral Health Programme. Community Dent Oral Epidemiol 2005;33:81–92.
3. Taylor TD. Dental Implants: Are They for Me? Chicago: Quintessence, 1990.
4. Brånemark PI, Zarb GA, Albrektsson T. Tissue-Integrated Prostheses—Osseointegration in Clinical Dentistry. Chicago: Quintessence, 1985.
5. Kohn DH. Overview of factors important in implant design. J Oral Implantol 1992;18:204–219.
6. Denissen H, Mangano C, Venini G. Hydroxylapatite Implants. Padua, Italy: Piccin, 1985.
7. Osborn JF. Implantatwerkstoff Hydroxylapatitkeramik. Berlin: Quintessence, 1985.

● Recommended Reading

Adell R, Lekholm U, Rockler B, Brånemark PI. A 15-year study of osseointegrated implants in the treatment of the edentulous jaw. Int J Oral Surg 1981;10:387–416.

Albrektsson T, Brånemark PI, Hansson HA, et al. The interface zone of inorganic implants in vivo: Titanium implants in bone. Ann Biomed Eng 1983;11:1–27.

Kasemo B. Biocompatibility of titanium implants: Surface science aspects. J Prosthet Dent 1983;49:832–837.

Kohn DH. Bioceramics. In: Kutz M (ed). Biomedical Engineers Handbook. New York: McGraw-Hill, 2002:13.1–13.24.

Kohn DH, Ducheyne P. Materials for bone, joint and cartilage replacement. In: Cahn RW, Haasen P, Kramer EJ (eds). Materials Science and Technology—A Comprehensive Treatment. Weinheim, Germany: VCH Verlagsgesellschaft, 1992:29–109. Medical and Dental Materials; vol 14.

Lemons JE. Biomaterials, biomechanics, tissue healing, and immediate-function dental implants. J Oral Implantol 2004;30:318–24.

Lynch SE, Genco RJ, Marx RE (eds). Tissue Engineering: Applications in Maxillofacial Surgery and Prosthodontics. Chicago: Quintessence, 1999.

Moradian-Oldak J, Wen HB, Schneider GB, Stanford CM. Tissue engineering strategies for the future generation of dental implants. Periodontol 2000 2006;41:157–176.

Nakashima M, Reddi AH. The application of bone morphogenetic proteins to dental tissue engineering. Nat Biotechnol. 2003;21:1025–1032.

Ong JL, Chan DC. Hydroxyapatite and their use as coatings in dental implants: A review. Crit Rev Biomed Eng 2000;28:667–707.

Petersen PE, Yamamota T. Improving the oral health of older people: The approach of the WHO Global Oral Health Programme. Community Dent Oral Epidemiol 2005;33:81–92.

Puleo DA, Thomas MV. Implant surfaces. Dent Clin N Am 2006;50:

Ratner BD. Replacing and renewing: Synthetic materials, biomimetics, and tissue engineering in implant dentistry. J Dent Ed 2001;65:1340–1347.

Schwartz Z, Nasazky E, Boyan BD. Surface microtopography regulates osteointegration: The role of implant surface microtopography in osteointegration. Alpha Omegan 2005;98:9–19.

Williams DF (ed). Biocompatibility of Clinical Implant Materials, vol I. Boca Raton, FL: CRC Press, 1981:9–44.

Tabulated Values of Physical and Mechanical Properties

Bond Strengths Between Restorative Materials and Tooth Structures

Adhesion of restorative materials to tooth structures has been studied since 1955. The bond strength is the load required to fracture the bond divided by the cross-sectional area of the bond. Bond strengths are measured either in shear or tension. Many factors, including the dentinal substrate, the storage conditions, and the test method, affect the bond strength values.

Substrate[1]	Adhesive	Adherend	Shear bond strength	
			psi × 10³	MPa
Dentin	Dentin bonding system	Composite	3.2–5.1	22–35
Dentin	No smear layer	Light-cured hybrid glass ionomer	1.5–1.7	10–12
Enamel	Enamel bonding system	Composite	2.6–3.2	18–22
Enamel	Amalgam bonding system	Composite	1.5–1.7	10–12
Enamel	Amalgam bonding system	Amalgam	0.3–0.9	2–6
Enamel	No smear layer	Traditional glass ionomer	1.2–1.7	8–12
Enamel	Enamel bonding system	Orthodontic bracket	2.6–2.9	18–20

Substrate[2]	Adhesive	Adherend	Tensile bond strength	
			psi × 10³	MPa
Dentin	Polyurethane	Composite	0.1–0.9	1–6
Dentin	Polyacrylic acid	Composite	0.3–0.6	2–4
Dentin	Organic phosphonates	Composite	0.4–1.4	3–10
Dentin	4-META*	Composite	0.4–1.0	3–7
Dentin	HEMA + GA[†]	Composite	1.6–2.4	11–17
Dentin	NPG-GMA/PMDM[‡]	Composite	0.6–1.8	4–12
Dentin		Glass ionomer	0.6	4
Dentin		Zinc polycarboxylate	0.4–0.6	3–4
Dentin		Adhesive resin cement	0.6	4.1
Dentin		Conventional resin cement	0.0	0.0
Etched enamel		Fine composite	2.4–2.8	17–20
Etched enamel		Microfine composite	1.4	10
Enamel		Glass ionomer	0.7	5
Etched enamel		Adhesive resin cement	2.2	15
Etched enamel		Conventional resin cement	1.5	10

*4-META = 4-methacryloxyethyl trimellitate anhydride.
[†]HEMA = hydroxyethyl methacrylate; GA = glutaraldehyde.
[‡]NPG-GMA = N-phenylglycine—glycidyl methacrylate; PMDM = pyromellitic acid dimethacrylate.

Brinell Hardness Number, *BHN*

The *Brinell hardness test* depends upon the resistance offered to the penetration of a steel ball (1.6-mm diameter) when subjected to a weight of 12.6 kg. The resulting hardness value is computed as the ratio of the applied load to the area of the indentation produced.

Material	Product	BHN (kg/mm^2)
Cobalt-chromium alloy[3]	Genesis II	265
Gold (condensed)[4]		
Foil		69
Mat		40
Powdered	Goldent	46
Gold alloys		
Type I[5]	Ney-Oro A	45
Type II[5]	Ney-Oro A-1	95
Type III, soft[5]	Ney-Oro B-2	110
Type III, hard[5]	Ney-Oro B-2	120
Type IV, soft[5]	Ney-Oro G-3	140
Type IV, hard[5]	Ney-Oro G-3	220
40% Au-Ag-Cu, soft[3]	Forticast	175
40% Au-Ag-Cu, hard[3]	Forticast	265
10–15% Au-Ag-Pd, soft[5]	Paliney No. 4	150
10–15% Au-Ag-Pd, hard[5]	Paliney No. 4	205
Au-Pd[3]	Olympia	200
Porcelain-fused-to-metal[3]	Jelenko O	165
Palladium-based dental alloy[3]	Microstar	240
Silver-palladium alloys[3]		
Fixed partial denture, soft	Albacast	130
Fixed partial denture, hard	Albacast	140
Porcelain-fused-to-metal	Jel-5	170

Coefficient of Friction, μ

The *coefficient of friction* is defined as the ratio of tangential force to normal load during a sliding process.

Material couples	μ	
	Dry	Wet
Amalgam[6] on:		
Amalgam	0.19–0.35	
Bovine enamel		0.12–0.28
Gold alloy		0.10–0.35
Resin composite		0.10–0.18
Porcelain	0.06–0.12	0.07–0.15
Bone[7] on:		
Metal (bead-coated)	0.50	
Metal (fiber mesh–coated)	0.60	
Metal (smooth)	0.42	
Bovine enamel[6] on:		
Acrylic resin	0.19–0.65	
Amalgam	0.18–0.22	
Bovine dentin	0.35–0.40	0.45–0.55
Bovine enamel	0.22–0.60	0.50–0.60
Chromium-nickel alloy	0.10–0.12	
Gold	0.12–0.20	
Porcelain	0.10–0.12	0.50–0.90
Gold alloy[6] on:		
Acrylic	0.6–0.8	
Amalgam	0.15–0.25	
Gold alloy	0.2–0.6	
Porcelain	0.22–0.25	0.16–0.17
Hydrogel-coated latex[8] on:		
Hydrogel		0.054
Latex[8] on:		
Glass		0.470
Hydrogel		0.095
Metal (bead-coated)[7] on:		
Bone	0.54	
Metal (fiber mesh–coated)[7] on:		
Bone	0.58	
Metal (smooth)[7] on:		
Bone	0.43	
Prosthetic tooth materials[9]:		
Acrylic on acrylic	0.21	0.37
Acrylic on porcelain	0.23	0.30
Porcelain on acrylic	0.34	0.32
Porcelain on porcelain	0.14	0.51
Resin composite[6] on:		
Amalgam	0.13–0.25	0.22–0.34
Bovine enamel		0.30–0.75

Coefficient of Thermal Expansion (Linear), α

The *coefficient of thermal expansion (linear)* is the change in length per unit length of material for a 1°C change in temperature.

Material	Product	α ([°C^{-1}] $\times$ 10^6)	Temperature range (°C)
Alumina (recrystallized)[10]		6.2	0–200
Amalgam[2]		22.1–28.0	20–50
Cement, unmodified ZOE[11]		35	25–60
Cobalt-chromium alloys	Master Tec[12]	14.7	25–500
	Novarex[13]	14.1	25–500
Denture resins			
Acrylic[14]		76	5–37
Polystyrene[15]	Jectron	67.3	20–37
Polyvinylacrylic[15]	Luxene 44	69.2	20–37
Gold alloys			
Au-Pd[3]	Olympia	14.1	25–500
Au-Pt-Pd[16]	TPW	15.48	200–700
Porcelain-fused-to-metal[17]	Jelenko O	14.71	40–500
	SMG-2	15.73	40–500
	Williams-Y	14.83	40–500
Gutta-percha[18]		54.9	23–38
Impression materials[19]			
Silicone, addition	Exaflex		
	Light	142	22–40
	Medium	128	22–40
	Permagum		
	Light	184	22–40
	Medium	158	22–40
	Heavy	147	22–40
	Putty	132	22–40
	President		
	Light	156	22–40
	Medium	144	22–40
	Heavy	120	22–40
	Putty	109	22–40
	Reflect	152	22–40
	Reprosil		
	Light	154	22–40
	Medium	152	22–40
	Heavy	136	22–40
	Putty	109	22–40
	Xantogum	160	22–40
Mercury[2]		60.6	20–50
Nickel-chromium alloys	Biobond C & B[17]	14.27	40–500
	Ceramalloy II[17]	14.63	40–500
	NP-2[17]	15.28	40–500
	Pentillium[17]	14.14	40–500
	Unimetal[16]	15.68	200–700

(continued)

Coefficient of Thermal Expansion (Linear), α (continued)

Material	Product	α ([°C⁻¹] × 10⁶)	Temperature range (°C)
Palladium-based dental alloys	Microstar[3]	14.3	25–500
	Spartan[12]	14.2	25–500
	W-1[12]	15.2	25–500
Pit and fissure sealants[20]			
Self-cured	Delton	90.3–97.1	0–60
	Kerr	70.9–78.2	0–60
	White	93.7–99.1	0–60
Light-cured	Nuva Seal	78–80	0–60
Porcelains			
Feldspathic[10]		6.4–7.8	0–200
Body[17]	Biobond	13.59–14.82*	40–500
	Ceramco	12.93–13.07*	40–500
	Microbond	14.59–15.28*	40–500
	Neydium	14.04–15.93*	40–500
	Vita (VMK-68)	12.73–14.45*	40–500
	Will-Ceram	15.94–16.23*	40–500
Opaque[17]	Biobond	13.10–14.35*	40–500
	Ceramco	12.70–14.23*	40–500
	Microbond	12.38–14.80*	40–500
	Neydium	13.25–14.23*	40–500
	Vita (VMK-68)	14.29–16.03*	40–500
	Will-Ceram	14.68–15.45*	40–500
Pure metals			
Gold[2]		14.4	20–50
Platinum[21]		8.9	Near 20
Silver[2]		19.2	20–50
Titanium[22]		11.9	23
Restorative materials			
Acrylic[23]	Sevriton[23]	92.0	24–88
Resin composite	Adaptic[20,23]	39.4	24–88
		35.8–40.1	0–60
	Adaptic (radiopaque)[20]	32.2–39.0	0–60
	Concise[20]	39.6–43.4	0–60
	Nuva Fil[20]	28.3–30.2	0–60
	Simulate[20]	28.2–31.6	0–60
	Vytol[16,20]	26.5–27.8	0–60
Ti-6Al-4V alloy		12.43	200–700
Tooth structures			
Crown[2]		11.4	20–50
Root[24]		8.3	20–50
Vitreous carbon[25]		2.2	0–100
Waxes[26]			
Inlay casting, hard	Kerr blue hard	320	22–37
Inlay casting, soft	Kerr blue regular	260	22–37

*Range is for 1–7 firing cycles. Values of the coefficients are not necessarily related to the specific firing cycle.

Colors of Dental Shade Guides

The colors of shade guide teeth were determined using a methodology developed for a reflectance spectro-photometer.[27] The spectral reflectance of each shade tab was measured using a dual-beam spectrophotometer equipped with an integrating sphere and a beam-reducing accessory. Relative reflectance measurements were converted to absolute reflectance. Tristimulus coordinates were determined for each sample by use of the CIE standard observer function and standard illuminant source C. The tristimulus coordinates were then converted to the CIE L*a*b* and Munsell Color Systems.

Bioform shade-guide colors[27]

Shade	Munsell notation			Chromaticity coordinates			CIE L* a* b*		
	H	V	C	Y	x	y	L*	a*	b*
B-59	3.5Y	7.80/2.0		55.72	0.3407	0.3502	79.49	−1.10	15.26
B-51	3.2Y	7.80/2.2		55.24	0.3432	0.3525	79.21	−0.99	16.31
B-91	2.4Y	7.45/1.9		49.57	0.3406	0.3484	75.84	−0.42	14.14
B-62	3.1Y	7.45/2.3		49.92	0.3454	0.3539	76.05	−0.64	16.53
B-66	2.8Y	7.55/2.8		51.21	0.3534	0.3615	76.84	−0.42	20.18
B-52	3.6Y	7.50/2.1		50.42	0.3451	0.3553	76.36	−1.28	16.94
B-53	2.1Y	7.40/2.5		49.39	0.3499	0.3559	75.72	0.33	17.76
B-92	3.0Y	7.35/2.0		48.67	0.3429	0.3514	75.28	−0.66	15.27
B-63	1.7Y	7.45/2.8		50.00	0.3548	0.3594	76.10	0.87	19.64
B-54	2.0Y	7.40/2.7		49.15	0.3532	0.3589	75.58	0.46	19.13
B-65	1.1Y	7.30/3.1		49.14	0.3606	0.3629	75.57	1.73	21.48
B-93	2.2Y	7.15/2.6		45.01	0.3526	0.3584	72.93	0.40	18.34
B-55	2.9Y	7.30/2.9		47.10	0.3558	0.3639	74.28	−0.39	20.69
B-69	2.6Y	6.95/2.6		42.49	0.3545	0.3614	71.24	0.03	19.11
B-94	3.0Y	6.95/2.7		42.30	0.3548	0.3627	71.11	−0.32	19.48
B-95	2.6Y	6.85/2.4		41.22	0.3502	0.3570	70.36	0.03	17.07
B-67	2.5Y	7.20/3.2		46.26	0.3614	0.3681	73.74	0.14	22.66
B-56	2.0Y	7.30/2.9		47.80	0.3581	0.3633	74.73	0.66	21.00
B-77	2.3Y	7.05/2.8		44.09	0.3572	0.3628	72.32	0.50	20.16
B-81	1.5Y	6.60/2.8		38.82	0.3588	0.3616	68.65	1.43	19.24
B-96	1.9Y	6.55/2.9		37.05	0.3610	0.3641	67.34	1.31	19.93
B-83	1.3Y	7.00/3.6		43.25	0.3693	0.3701	71.52	2.25	23.94
B-84	0.9Y	6.65/3.2		37.98	0.3663	0.3653	68.01	2.74	21.21
B-85	1.8Y	6.65/4.1		38.24	0.3811	0.3794	68.23	2.91	27.38

H = hue; V = value; C = chroma; Y = lightness; x and y = hue and chroma; L* = lightness; a* = hue and chroma on a red-green scale; b* = hue and chroma on a yellow-blue scale.

Vita shade-guide colors

Shade	Munsell notation[28]			Chromaticity coordinates[29]			CIE L*a*b*[28]		
	H	V	C	Y	x	y	L*	a*	b*
A1	4.5Y	7.80/1.7		55.92	0.3352	0.3459	79.57	−1.61	13.05
A2	2.4Y	7.45/2.3		49.95	0.3468	0.3539	76.04	−0.08	16.73
A3	1.3Y	7.40/2.9		48.85	0.3559	0.3593	75.36	1.36	19.61
A3.5	1.6Y	7.05/3.2		44.12	0.3627	0.3657	72.31	1.48	21.81
A4	1.6Y	6.70/3.1		38.74	0.3633	0.3658	68.56	1.58	21.00
B1	5.1Y	7.75/1.6		54.76	0.3336	0.3447	78.90	−1.76	12.33
B2	4.3Y	7.50/2.2		50.97	0.3437	0.3549	76.66	−1.62	16.62
B3	2.3Y	7.25/3.2		46.91	0.3611	0.3669	74.13	0.47	22.34
B4	2.4Y	7.00/3.2		43.38	0.3620	0.3678	71.81	0.50	22.15
C1	4.3Y	7.30/1.6		47.16	0.3361	0.3462	74.29	−1.26	12.56
C2	2.8Y	6.95/2.3		42.12	0.3487	0.3563	70.95	−0.22	16.72
C3	2.6Y	6.70/2.3		39.11	0.3499	0.3569	68.83	−0.01	16.68
C4	1.6Y	6.30/2.7		33.77	0.3600	0.3622	64.78	1.59	18.66
D2	3.0Y	7.35/1.8		48.71	0.3391	0.3473	75.27	−0.54	13.47
D3	1.8Y	7.10/2.3		44.48	0.3482	0.3534	72.55	0.62	16.14
D4	3.7Y	7.05/2.4		43.45	0.3492	0.3591	71.86	−1.03	17.77

H = hue; V = value; C = chroma; Y = lightness; x and y = hue and chroma; L* = lightness; a* = hue and chroma on a red-green scale; b* = hue and chroma on a yellow-blue scale.

Contact Angle (Liquid Phase), θ

The *angle of contact* between a liquid and a solid is a measure of the tendency for the liquid to spread over or wet the solid surface. The lower the contact angle, the greater the tendency for the liquid to wet the solid, until complete wetting occurs at an angle of zero degrees.

Material	Product	Liquid phase	θ (degrees)
Amalgam[30]	New True Dentalloy	Water	77
Bacteria[31]			
A odontolyticus A7-1		Water	41
A viscosus C7-4		Water	35
S mutans C7-3		Water	12
S salivarius B3-4		Water	24
S sanguis C7-2		Water	48
Cement[32]			
Orthodontic	Concise	Water	30
Denture resins			
Acrylic[33]		Alcohol	0
		Saliva	73
		Water	75
Acrylic (modified)[34]	Hydrocryl	Water	78
Polystyrene[30,35]		Saliva	79
		Water	86
Glass		Water	14
Gold alloy[36]			
Porcelain-fused-to-metal	Ceramco No. 1	Porcelain	40*
Impression materials			
Polyether	Impregum[37]		
	Untreated[38]	Dental stone mix	55–58
			40.4
	30 min in Clorox	Dental stone mix	59–60
	30 min in Sporicidin	Dental stone mix	81–93
	Impregum F[39]	Water	42.6
	Permadyne[39]		
	Light	Water	43.1
	Heavy	Water	43.9
Polysulfide	Permlastic[37]		
	Untreated[39]	Water	42.1
		Dental stone mix	76–82
	30 min in Clorox	Dental stone mix	78–82
	30 min in Sporicidin	Dental stone mix	43–47†
Silicone, addition	Examix[37]		
	Untreated	Dental stone mix	71–74
	30 min in Clorox	Dental stone mix	90–92
	30 min in Sporicidin	Dental stone mix	94–95
	Express[39]		
	Light	Water	104.9
	Putty	Water	101.7

*Measured at 1038°C.
†"The polysulfide appeared to have reacted with the 0.5% sodium hypochlorite."[37]

(continued)

Contact Angle (Liquid Phase), θ (continued)

Material	Product	Liquid phase	θ (degrees)
Impression materials			
Silicone, addition (continued)	Express Hydrophilic[39]		
	Light	Water	19.7
	Medium[38]	Water	78.3
		Dental stone mix	64.4
	Putty	Water	63.8
	Imprint Hydrophilic[39]		
	Medium	Water	46.3
	Mirror 3 Extrude[39]		
	Light	Water	33.9
	Medium	Water	57.7
	Putty	Water	98.4
	President[37]		
	Untreated	Dental stone mix	92–96
	30 min in Clorox	Dental stone mix	98–99
	30 min in Sporicidin	Dental stone mix	94–98
	Unosil[38]	Dental stone mix	75.0
Silicone, addition[40]	Aquasil		
	Rigid fast	Water	32
	Rigid regular	Water	33
	Monophase	Water	35
	XLV regular	Water	34
	XLV fast	Water	31
	LV regular	Water	35
	LV fast	Water	34
	Examix		
	Heavy	Water	42
	Putty	Water	100
	Regular	Water	43.5
	Injection	Water	37
	Express		
	Putty	Water	101
	Regular body	Water	35.5
	Light body	Water	24
	Extrude		
	Extra	Water	34.5
	XP	Water	110
	Medium	Water	31
	Wash	Water	34.5
	Impregum	Water	42
	Imprint 2		
	Tray	Water	77
	Regular	Water	22
	Low	Water	25

See page 321 for footnotes.

(continued)

Contact Angle (Liquid Phase), θ (continued)

Material	Product	Liquid phase	θ (degrees)
Impression materials			
Silicone, addition (continued)[40]	Polygel	Water	50
	President		
	Putty, soft	Water	99
	Regular body	Water	34
	Light body	Water	41
	Reprosil		
	Putty	Water	100
	Heavy	Water	45
	Medium	Water	38
	Light	Water	58
	Splash		
	Heavy	Water	27
	Regular	Water	29
	Light	Water	24
	Extra light	Water	24
	Splash Half-time		
	Heavy	Water	64
	Light	Water	36
	Take 1		
	Regular set	Water	30
	Fast set	Water	31
Silicone, condensation	Citricon[39]		
	Light	Water	81.7
	Putty	Water	90.7
	Rapid[39]		
	Light	Water	95.2
	Putty	Water	102.6
	Xantopren[38]	Dental stone mix	89.1
Polymers			
Poly(butylcyanoacrylate)[41]		Water	69
Poly(etherurethane)[42]		Water	80
Poly(ethylcyanoacrylate)[41]		Water	65
Poly(2-hydroxyethyl methacrylate)[41]			
Atactic		Water	17
Isotactic		Water	13
Poly(2-hydroxyethyl methacrylate-methoxyethyl methacrylate) (1:1)[41]		Water	22

See page 321 for footnotes.

(continued)

Contact Angle (Liquid Phase), θ (continued)

Material	Product	Liquid phase	θ (degrees)
Polymers (continued)			
Poly(methoxyethyl methacrylate)[41]		Water	46
Poly(methyl cyanoacrylate)[41]		Water	57
Polymethyl methacrylate[41]		Water	62–73
Polystyrene[41]		Water	66
Poly(tetrafluoroethylene)[30]	Teflon	Water	110
Poly(vinyl chloride)[42]		Water	69
Silicone[42]		Water	110
Restorative materials[30]			
Acrylic	Bonfil	Water	38
Resin composite	Addent	Water	51
Silicate[30]	Improved Filling Porcelain	Water	12
Wax, paraffin[35]		Water	109

Contact Angle (Solid Surface), θ

Material	Product	Solid surface	θ (degrees)
Bonding agents[43]	Adaptic Bonding Agent	Enamel	0
	Concise Enamel Bond	Enamel	0
Fluoride gels[44]	Flura-Gel	Enamel	30
	Luride	Enamel	31
	Predent	Enamel	36
	Rafluor	Enamel	38
Fluoride solutions[44]	Rafluor	Enamel	0
	NaF Rinse	Enamel	0
Glaze[43]	Adaptic Glaze	Enamel	0
Pit and fissure sealants[43]			
Light-cured	Nuva-Seal	Enamel	28
Self-cured	Delton	Enamel	0

Creep of Amalgam

Creep is a measure of the viscoelastic properties of a material. In the *dynamic* creep method, a compressive load is applied to a specimen to produce a fluctuating stress that is cycled from 500 to 10,000 psi (3.45 to 69.0 MPa) at a rate of 1,800 times/minute. In the *static* creep method, a constant compressive stress of 5,250 psi (36.2 MPa) is applied to the specimen. In the American National Standards Institute/American Dental Association's *flow* method,[45] the specimen is subjected to a compressive stress of 1,450 psi (10.0 MPa). In each method the change in length of the specimen is measured and divided by the original length.

		Method		
Material	Product	Dynamic creep (%)	Static creep (%)	ADA flow (%)
Amalgams				
Admixed	Dispersalloy[46–48]	0.86	0.76	0.50
			0.67	
			0.3	
	Dispersalloy			
	Fast set[49]		0.41*	
			0.32†	
	Regular set[49]		0.46*	
			0.37†	
	Non zinc[47]		1.01	
	Optaloy II[47,49]		1.77	
			1.47*	
			1.08†	
	Valiant PhD[50]		0.21	
Lathe-cut	ANA 68 Dental Alloy[48]		2.1	
	ANA 2000 Nongamma 2[48]		0.15	
	Aristoloy[47]		3.77	
	Caulk Fine Cut[49]		1.56*	
			1.57†	
	New True Dentalloy[46,47]	1.85	2.36	0.65
			1.53	
	Revalloy[48]		1.2	
	20th Century Micro[46]	8.76	8.37	3.91
Spherical	Cupralloy Esp[49]		0.37*	
			0.25†	
	Indiloy[49]		0.34*	
			0.15†	
	Sybraloy[47,49]		0.10	
			0.10*	
			0.05†	
	Tytin[47,50]		0.20	
			0.08	
	Valiant[50]		0.06	

*Hand triturated.
†Mechanically triturated.

Critical Surface Tension, γ_c

The *critical surface tension* is the surface tension of a liquid that would completely wet the solid of interest.

Material	Product	γ_c (dynes/cm)
Amalgam[51]	Argos Alloy	48.1
Co-Cr-Mo, as polished[52]	Vitallium*	22.3
Co-Cr-Mo, plasma cleaned[52]	Vitallium*	>72
Glass[53]	Pyrex	170
Gold[51]	AB Adelmetall	57.4
Impression materials[54]		
Polyether	Impregum	27.9
Silicone, addition	Express Hydrophilic	53.8
	Imprint Hydrophilic	52.4
	President	21.2
	Provil	20.2
Silicone, condensation	Xantopren	14.4
Paraffin[53]		22–26
Polymers[55]		
Polyetherurethane	Pellethane 80A	19.3
	Pellethane 55D	22.1
	Pellethane 75D	35.7
Polyetherurethane urea[53]	Biomer	23.0
Polyethylene[53]		31–33
Polymethyl methacrylate[53]		39.0
Polystyrene[53]		33–43
Poly(tetrafluoroethylene)[56]	Teflon	18
Tooth structure, enamel[56]		38.5–40[†]
		31.5[‡]

*Surgical.
[†]23°C, 50% relative humidity.
[‡]37°C, 100% relative humidity.

Density, ρ

Density is the concentration of matter as measured by the mass per unit volume. The *specific gravity* of a substance is the ratio of the density of the substance to that of water.

Material	Product	ρ (g/cm³)
Amalgam[57]		11.6
Bonding agent[58]	Silux Enamel Bond	1.20
Bones[59]		
Cancellous		1.3
Cortical		1.3
Cements		
Calcium hydroxide[60]	Dycal	1.91
	Life	1.88
Glass ionomer[61]	Base cement	2.13*
	Dentin cement	2.02*
	Ketac-cem	2.16*
Polymer-modified ZOE[62]	IRM	2.29†
Resin[63]	CBA 9080	2.02
Unmodified ZOE[60]	Cavitec	2.05
Zinc phosphate[62]	Tenacin	2.59‡
Zinc polycarboxylate[64]		2.19
Cobalt-chromium alloys	Genesis II[3]	8.8
	Master Tec[12]	8.1
	Novarex[13]	8.75§
	Vitallium[57]	8.5
Denture resin, acrylic[14]		1.19
Fluoroapatite, mineral[65]	Durango, Mexico	3.215
Gold (condensed)[4]		
Foil		17.22
Mat		16.44
Powdered	Goldent	17.36
Gold alloys		
Type II[66]		16.4
Type III[57]		15.5
40% Au-Ag-Cu[3]	Forticast	12.5
10%–15% Au-Ag-Pd[5]	Paliney No. 4	12.3
Au-Pd[3]	Olympia	13.7
Porcelain-fused-to-metal[3]	Jelenko O	18.2
Gypsum[67]	Moldablaster	1.9–2.0
Hydroxyapatite[59]		3.1
Impression materials (polymerized)[68]		
Polyether	Impregum	1.06
Silicone, addition	Baysilex	1.37
	Provil	
Medium		1.40
High		1.43

*Powder/liquid ratio 1.0.
†Powder/liquid ratio, 5.0 g/mL.
‡Powder/liquid ratio, 2.5 g/mL.
§Specific gravity.
¶Powder/liquid ratio, 3.0 g/mL.

(continued)

Density, ρ *(continued)*

Material	Product	ρ (g/cm^3)
Mercury[21]		13.55
Monomers (fixed partial denture resins)		
Methyl methacrylate[69]		0.9374
Ethylene glycol dimethacrylate[70]		1.055
1,3-butylene glycol dimethacrylate[70]		1.02
Triethylene glycol dimethacrylate[70]		1.072
Nickel-chromium alloys		
Fixed partial denture[71]	Howmedica III	7.9
Porcelain-fused-to-metal[72]	Ultratek	8.0
Palladium-based dental alloys	Microstar[3]	10.8
	Spartan[12]	10.6
	W-1[12]	11.1
Pit and fissure sealant[73]	Delton	1.23
Porcelain, feldspathic[10]		2.4
Pure metals[21]		
Chromium		7.19
Copper		8.96
Gold		19.3
Nickel		8.9
Palladium		12.02
Platinum		21.45
Silver		10.49
Titanium		4.51
Zinc		7.13
Resin composite[58]		
All-purpose	Heliomolar Radiopaque	1.84
	Herculite XR	2.09
Anterior	Silux Plus	1.61
Posterior	Ful Fil	2.14
	Visiomolar	2.38
Silicate[62]	Improved Filling Porcelain¶	2.01¶
Silver-palladium alloys[3]		
Fixed partial denture	Albacast	10.6
Porcelain-fused-to-metal	Jel-5	10.9
Ti-6Al-4V alloy[57]		4.5
Tooth structures		
Cementum[74]		2.03
Dentin (primary)[75]		2.18
Dentin (permanent)[74]		2.14
Enamel (primary)[75]		2.95
Enamel (permanent)[74]		2.97
Vitreous carbon[25]		1.47
Water (4°C)[76]		1.00

See page 327 for footnotes.

Dynamic Modulus

The *dynamic modulus* is defined as the ratio of stress to strain for small cyclic deformations at a given frequency and at a particular point on the stress-strain curve.

Material	Product	Dynamic modulus	
		psi $\times$ 10^3	MPa
Maxillofacial materials[77]			
Polyurethane	Dermathane 100	0.444*	3.06*
Polyvinyl chloride	Sartomer Resins	0.364*	2.51*
Silicone rubber	Silastic 382	0.435*	3.00*
	Silastic 399	0.554*	3.82*
Mouth protector material[78]			
Polyvinyl acetate-polyethylene	Proform	3.07*	21.2*
	Sta-Guard	1.36*	9.39*
Restorative materials[79]			
Resin composite			
Anterior	Silar	372.6†	2569†
	Silux	374.5†	2582†
Posterior	P10	1218†	8396†
	P50	1399†	9645†
	Profile	1147†	7911†
	Profile TLC	1274†	8786†

*Measured at 37°C.
†Dynamic shear modulus, measured wet at 40°C.

Elastic Modulus, *E*

The *elastic modulus* of a material represents the relative stiffness of the material within the elastic range and can be determined from a stress-strain curve by calculating the ratio of stress to strain. Unless indicated otherwise, values were determined in tension.

Material	Product	E psi × 10⁶	E GPa
Alumina[80]	De Trey	60.6*	418*
Amalgams (7 d)[81]			
Admixed	Dispersalloy	7.60*	52.4*
	Valiant PhD	8.05*	55.5*
Spherical	Indiloy	7.56*	52.1*
	Logic	7.82*	53.9*
	Sybraloy	8.72*	60.1*
	Tytin	7.64*	52.7*
	Valiant	8.54*	58.9*
Bones			
Cancellous[59]		0.071	0.49
Cortical[59]		2.1	14.7
Long bones[82]			
Femur		2.49	17.2
Humerus		2.49	17.2
Radius		2.70	18.6
Tibia		2.63	18.1
Vertebrae[82]			
Cervical		0.033	0.23
Lumbar		0.023	0.16
Cements (base consistency, 24 h)[83]			
Polymer-modified ZOE	B & T	0.310†	2.14†
Zinc phosphate	Zinc Cement Improved	3.25†	22.4†
Zinc polycarboxylate	Durelon	0.718†	4.95†
Cements (luting consistency, 24 h)			
EBA-alumina ZOE[83,84]	Opotow	0.787†	5.43†
		0.45‡	3.1‡
Glass ionomer	ASPA[84]	1.4‡	9.8‡
	Fuji[84]	0.58‡	4.0‡
	Ketac-cem[85]	0.91*	6.3*
Noneugenol zinc oxide[83]	Nogenol	0.0257†	0.177†
Polymer-modified ZOE[83,84]	Fynal	0.441†	3.04†
		0.17‡	1.2‡
Zinc phosphate[83]	Zinc Cement Improved	1.99†	13.7†
Zinc polycarboxylate	Carboxylon[84]	0.35‡	2.4‡
	Durelon[83,84]	0.638†	4.40†
		0.46‡	3.2‡
	Durelon (thin liquid)[84]	0.44‡	3.0‡

*Measured in bending.
†Measured in compression with optical strain gauge.
‡Measured in compression.
§As cast.
¶Heat treated.
#Cord modulus in tension at 5% strain.
**Measured with Shearheometer at setting time.
††Measured in tensile stress with Dentsply/Caulk elastic modulus technique.

(continued)

Elastic Modulus, *E* (continued)

Material	Product	E psi × 10⁶	E GPa
Cements (liners, 24 h)			
Calcium hydroxide[85]			
Light-cured	VLC Dycal	0.087*	0.6*
Self-cured	Dycal	0.32*	2.2*
	Life	0.29*	2.0*
Glass ionomer			
Light-cured[86]	Vitrabond	0.16*	1.1*
	XR Ionomer	0.35*	2.4*
Self-cured[85]	GC Lining Cement	0.42*	2.9*
	Ketac Bond	0.68*	4.7*
Resin[86]	Cavalite	0.38*	2.6*
	Timeline	0.25*	1.7*
Unmodified ZOE[83]	Cavitec	0.0406†	0.280†
Cobalt-chromium alloys[87]	Advantage§	18.2	125
	Advantage¶	21.6	149
	Cobond§	21.8	150
	Cobond¶	23.0	159
	Genesis II§	30.6	211
	Genesis II¶	22.8	157
	Master Tec§	21.2	146
	Master Tec¶	22.8	157
	Novarex§	22.4	154
	Novarex¶	26.3	181
	Novarex II§	23.8	164
	Novarex II¶	21.8	150
	Vi-Comp§	21.6	149
	Vi-Comp¶	22.8	157
	Vitallium[88]	31.6	218
Compomers[89]	Dyract AP	2.36	16.3
	Elan	1.73	11.9
	F2000	3.02	20.8
	Hytac	1.81	12.5
Denture resins			
Cold-cured[90]	PERform	0.236	1.63
Heat-cured	Lucitone 199[90]	0.154	1.06
	Paragon[91]	0.426	2.94
	Perma-cryl 20[90]	0.193	1.33
Light-cured	Triad[90]	0.306	2.11
Duplicating material[92]			
Agar	Nobiloid	70 × 10⁻⁶	0.48 × 10⁻³
Fixed partial denture[93]			
Acrylic	Biotone	0.327†	2.26†
Polyester	Mer-Don 7	0.267†	1.84†
Polyvinyl acrylic	Luxene	0.410†	2.83†
Fluoroapatite, mineral[65]	Durango, Mexico	21.4	148

See page 330 for footnotes.

(continued)

Elastic Modulus, *E* (continued)

Material	Product	E psi x 10^6	GPa
Gold alloys			
Type I[94]	Special Inlay	11.2[†]	77.2[†]
Type III[95]	Sjoding C-3	14.5	100
Type IV	Ney-Oro G-3[94]	14.4[†]	99.3[†]
	Sjoding D[95]	13.8	95
64% Au-Ag-Cu[95]	Begolloyd	11.5	79
48% Au-Ag-Cu[95]	Midigold	14.5	100
Au-Ag-Pd[59]		11.4	78
Au-Pd[96]	Olympia[§]	14.9	103
	Olympia[¶]	15.7	108
Porcelain-fused-to-metal[72]	Ceramco O	12.5	86.2
Gutta-percha[97]	Indian Head	0.027	0.186
	Mynol	0.022	0.152
Gypsum[98]			
Improved stone	Velmix	2.1*	14.5*
Hydroxyapatite[59]		5.0	34
Impression materials			
Agar[92]	Surgident	200×10^{-6}[†]	1.38×10^{-3}[†]
Alginate, 6 min[99]	Jeltrate	38×10^{-6}[#]	0.26×10^{-3}[#]
Polyether[100]	Impregum F	51×10^{-6}**	0.35×10^{-3}**
	Permadyne	59×10^{-6}**	0.41×10^{-3}**
Polysulfide[100]	Permlastic		
	Light	2×10^{-6}**	0.013×10^{-3}**
	Heavy	17×10^{-6}**	0.12×10^{-3}**
Silicone, addition	Aquasil[40]		
	Rigid fast	1183×10^{-6}[††]	8.2×10^{-3}[††]
	Rigid regular	1111×10^{-6}[††]	7.7×10^{-3}[††]
	Monophase	672×10^{-6}[††]	4.6×10^{-3}[††]
	XLV regular	336×10^{-6}[††]	2.3×10^{-3}[††]
	XLV fast	338×10^{-6}[††]	2.3×10^{-3}[††]
	LV regular	672×10^{-6}[††]	4.6×10^{-3}[††]
	LV fast	672×10^{-6}[††]	4.6×10^{-3}[††]
	Examix[40]		
	Heavy	672×10^{-6}[††]	4.6×10^{-3}[††]
	Putty	1887×10^{-6}[††]	13×10^{-3}[††]
	Regular	383×10^{-6}[††]	2.6×10^{-3}[††]
	Injection	383×10^{-6}[††]	2.6×10^{-3}[††]
	Express[40]		
	Putty	961×10^{-6}[††]	6.6×10^{-3}[††]
	Regular body	382×10^{-6}[††]	2.6×10^{-3}[††]
	Light body	382×10^{-6}[††]	2.6×10^{-3}[††]
	Extrude[40]		
	Extra	672×10^{-6}[††]	4.6×10^{-3}[††]
	XP	623×10^{-6}[††]	4.3×10^{-3}[††]
	Medium	381×10^{-6}[††]	2.6×10^{-3}[††]
	Wash	383×10^{-6}[††]	2.6×10^{-3}[††]

See page 330 for footnotes.

(continued)

Elastic Modulus, *E* (continued)

Material	Product	E psi $\times 10^6$	E GPa
Silicone, addition (continued)	Impregum[40]	$374 \times 10^{-6\dagger\dagger}$	$2.6 \times 10^{-3\dagger\dagger}$
	Imprint 2[40]		
	Tray	$672 \times 10^{-6\dagger\dagger}$	$4.6 \times 10^{-3\dagger\dagger}$
	Regular wash	$380 \times 10^{-6\dagger\dagger}$	$2.6 \times 10^{-3\dagger\dagger}$
	Low wash	$381 \times 10^{-6\dagger\dagger}$	$2.6 \times 10^{-3\dagger\dagger}$
	Polygel[40]	$336 \times 10^{-6\dagger\dagger}$	$2.3 \times 10^{-3\dagger\dagger}$
	President[40]		
	Putty, soft	$721 \times 10^{-6\dagger\dagger}$	$5 \times 10^{-3\dagger\dagger}$
	Regular body	$547 \times 10^{-6\dagger\dagger}$	$3.8 \times 10^{-3\dagger\dagger}$
	Light body	$382 \times 10^{-6\dagger\dagger}$	$2.6 \times 10^{-3\dagger\dagger}$
	Provil[100]		
	Light	$45 \times 10^{-6\ast\ast}$	$0.31 \times 10^{-3\ast\ast}$
	Putty	$51 \times 10^{-6\ast\ast}$	$0.35 \times 10^{-3\ast\ast}$
	Reprosil[40]		
	Putty	$381 \times 10^{-6\dagger\dagger}$	$2.6 \times 10^{-3\dagger\dagger}$
	Heavy	$692 \times 10^{-6\dagger\dagger}$	$4.8 \times 10^{-3\dagger\dagger}$
	Medium	$381 \times 10^{-6\dagger\dagger}$	$2.6 \times 10^{-3\dagger\dagger}$
	Light	$381 \times 10^{-6\dagger\dagger}$	$2.6 \times 10^{-3\dagger\dagger}$
	Splash[40]		
	Heavy	$114 \times 10^{-6\dagger\dagger}$	$7.9 \times 10^{-3\dagger\dagger}$
	Regular	$730 \times 10^{-6\dagger\dagger}$	$5.0 \times 10^{-3\dagger\dagger}$
	Light	$363 \times 10^{-6\dagger\dagger}$	$2.5 \times 10^{-3\dagger\dagger}$
	Extra light	$309 \times 10^{-6\dagger\dagger}$	$2.1 \times 10^{-3\dagger\dagger}$
	Putty, soft	$97 \times 10^{-6\dagger\dagger}$	$6.7 \times 10^{-3\dagger\dagger}$
	Putty, regular	$1214 \times 10^{-6\dagger\dagger}$	$8.4 \times 10^{-3\dagger\dagger}$
	Splash (Half-time)[40]		
	Heavy	$114.7 \times 10^{-6\dagger\dagger}$	$7.9 \times 10^{-3\dagger\dagger}$
	Regular	$73.9 \times 10^{-6\dagger\dagger}$	$5.1 \times 10^{-3\dagger\dagger}$
	Light	$52.5 \times 10^{-6\dagger\dagger}$	$3.6 \times 10^{-3\dagger\dagger}$
	Extra light	$27.2 \times 10^{-6\dagger\dagger}$	$1.9 \times 10^{-3\dagger\dagger}$
	Putty, soft	$137.1 \times 10^{-6\dagger\dagger}$	$9.5 \times 10^{-3\dagger\dagger}$
	Putty, regular	$130.7 \times 10^{-6\dagger\dagger}$	$9.0 \times 10^{-3\dagger\dagger}$
	Take 1 (Monophase)[40]		
	Regular set	$376 \times 10^{-6\dagger\dagger}$	$2.6 \times 10^{-3\dagger\dagger}$
	Fast set	$336 \times 10^{-6\dagger\dagger}$	$2.3 \times 10^{-3\dagger\dagger}$
Silicone, condensation	Rapid[100]		
	Light	$13 \times 10^{-6\ast\ast}$	$0.088 \times 10^{-3\ast\ast}$
	Putty	$38 \times 10^{-6\ast\ast}$	$0.26 \times 10^{-3\ast\ast}$
Iron-chromium alloys[88]			
Fixed partial denture	Dentillium C-B	25.7	177
Removable partial denture	Dentillium P-D	29.3	202
Maxillofacial material[101]			
Silicone rubber	Silastic 382	297×10^{-6}	2.05×10^{-3}

See page 330 for footnotes.

(continued)

Elastic Modulus, *E* (continued)

Material	Product	E psi × 10⁶	E GPa
Nickel-chromium alloys[96]	Ceramalloy II[§]	27.2	188
	Ceramalloy II[¶]	23.1	159
	Micro-Bond N-P2[§]	21.1	145
	Micro-Bond N-P2[¶]	21.1	145
	Pentillium[102]	24.9	172
	Ticon[§]	25.6	177
	Ticon[¶]	24.8	171
Fixed partial denture[112]	Howmedica III	26.0	179
Porcelain-fused-to-metal[72]	Ultratek	29.4	203
Palladium-based dental alloys[96]	Microstar[§]	19.5	134
	Microstar[¶]	17.9	123
	Spartan[§]	15.8	109
	Spartan[¶]	15.0	103
	W-1[§]	16.9	117
	W-1[¶]	16.8	116
Polymers			
Polyetherurethane[104]	Pellethane 2363-80A	0.0023	0.016
Polyetherurethane urea[104]	Biomer	0.0016	0.011
Polymethyl methacrylate[105]		0.345	2.38
Porcelains[106]			
Alumina-reinforced	Vitadur-N(Core)	15.5	107
Castable ceramic	Dicor	10.7	74
Ceramic-whisker-reinforced	Mirage II	10.0	69
Feldspathic	Excelco	8.7	60
	Vita VMK 68	10.2	70
	Vita VMK 68-N	10.0	69
	Will-Ceram	9.1	63
Leucite-reinforced	Optec HSP	9.1	63
Restorative materials			
Resin composite			
All-purpose	Brilliant[107]	2.41	16.6
	Charisma[107]	2.04	14.1
	Conquest DFC[107]	2.54	17.5
	Heliomolar Radiopaque[107]	1.41	9.8
	Herculite XR[107]	2.33	16.0
	Herculite XRV[108]	1.38	9.5
	Marathon[107]	2.95	20.3
	P-50 APC[107]	3.63	25.0
	Pertac Hybrid[107]	2.18	15.1
	Prisma APH[107]	1.98	13.6
	True Vitality[108]	0.78	5.4
	Z100[107]	3.05	21.0

See page 330 for footnotes.

(continued)

Elastic Modulus, *E* (continued)

Material	Product	E psi × 10⁶	E GPa
Resin composite (continued)			
Anterior[107]	Durafill	0.88	6.1
	Helio Progress	1.32	9.1
	Multifil VS	1.14	7.8
	Prisma Fil	2.07	14.3
	Prisma Microfine	0.83	5.7
	Silar	1.32	9.1
	Silux	1.36	9.4
	Silux Plus	1.37	9.5
	Valux	2.86	19.7
	Visio Dispers	1.56	10.8
	Visio Fil	3.15	21.7
Hybrid[109]	Prodigy[89]	1.78	12.25
	Z100	2.74	18.9
Packable[109]	Alert	3.28	22.6
	Solitaire	0.75	5.2
	SureFil	2.44	16.8
Posterior[107]	Clearfil Photo Posterior	3.68	25.3
	Ful Fil	2.10	14.5
	Heliomolar	1.54	10.6
	Occlusin	3.45	23.8
	P-10	3.64	25.1
	Post Comp II LC	2.33	16.1
Glass ionomer[110]	Ketac-fil	1.57	10.8
Metal-reinforced glass ionomer[85]	Ketac-Silver	0.62*	4.3*
Silicate[94]	Improved Filling Porcelain	3.25†	22.4†
Silver-palladium alloys[95]	Alborium	14.4	99
	Hvitstøp	15.2	105
	Palliag H	15.8	109
Titanium[22]		17.0	117
Tooth structures			
Dentin (bovine)[111]			
Demineralized		0.036	0.25
Mineralized		1.99	13.7
Dentin (human)[111]			
Demineralized		0.038	0.26
Mineralized		2.13	14.7
Enamel[59,94]		12.2†	84.1†
		18.9	130
Periodontal membrane (young calf)[112]		172 × 10⁻⁶	1.18 × 10⁻³
Vitreous carbon[25]		3.5	24.1
Waxes[113]			
Inlay casting, hard	Kerr blue hard	0.092†	0.634†
Inlay casting, soft	Kerr blue regular	0.101†	0.696†

See page 330 for footnotes.

Flexural Strength, *MOR*

The *flexural strength*, also known as *transverse strength* or *modulus of rupture*, is obtained by supporting a bar or beam at each end, and loading it in the middle. This test is called a *three pointing bending (3PB) test*.

Material	Product	MOR	
		psi × 10³	MPa
Alumina (recrystallized)[10]		55.0	379
Amalgams (7 d)[81]			
Admixed	Dispersalloy	17.7	122
	Valiant PhD	20.6	142
Spherical	Indiloy	19.5	134
	Lojic	17.2	118
	Sybraloy	17.3	119
	Tytin	21.4	148
	Valiant	21.1	146
Cements (luting consistency, 24 h)[114]			
Glass ionomer	Fuji I	0.39	2.7
	Ketac-cem Radiopaque	0.42	2.9
Cements (liners, 24 h)			
Calcium hydroxide[85]	Dycal	0.61	4.2
	Life	0.38	2.6
Glass ionomer			
Light-cured[86]	Vitrabond	3.51	24.2
	XR Ionomer	2.55	17.6
Self-cured[114]	Baseline	1.68	11.6
	Baseline in Caps	1.71	11.8
	GC lining cement	0.20	1.4
	Ketac-bond	0.45	3.1
	Ketac-bond Capsule	0.96	6.6
	3M Glass ionomer liner	0.45	3.1
Resin[86]	Cavalite	8.41	58.0
	Timeline	9.27	63.9
Denture resins[90]			
Cold-cured	PERform	12	84
Heat-cured	Lucitone 199	11	78
	Perma-cryl 20	12	86
Light-cured	Triad	12	80
Gold (condensed)[115]			
Foil	Morgan, Hastings & Co.	42.3	292
Mat	Williams	23.0	159
Powdered	Goldent	23.6	163
Gypsum[98]			
Improved stone	Velmix	2.40	16.6
Investment[116]			
Ethyl silicate, 23°C–1000°C	Hartex	0.071	0.49
Gypsum-bonded, 23°C	Kerr Model	0.355	2.45
Gypsum-bonded, 600°C	Kerr Model	0.014	0.10
Phosphate-bonded, 23°C		0.384	2.65
Phosphate-bonded, 1000°C		1.10	7.64

(continued)

Flexural Strength, *MOR* (continued)

Material	Product	MOR psi × 10³	MOR MPa
Porcelains			
Alumina-reinforced[117]	HiCeram (core)	20.2	139
	Vitadur-N (core)	17.9	123
Castable ceramic[117]	Dicor	18.1	125
Ceramic-whisker-reinforced[117]	Mirage	10	70
Feldspathic[117]	Ceramco II	8.9	61
	Excelco	8.0	55
	Vitadur-N (dentin)	9.1	62
	Vita VMK 68	9.5	66
Leucite-reinforced[117]	Optec HSP	15	104
Magnesia core[118]			
Glazed		39	270
Untreated		19	130
Restorative materials			
Compomer	Compoglass[119–121]	5.7–15.9	39.0–110.0
	Dyract[119,121,122]	6.4–17.1	43.8–118.0
	Dyract AP[122]	16.7	115.0
	Elan[122]	17.7	122.0
	F2000[109,122]	7.7–15.1	53.0–104.0
	Hytac[120,122]	8.6–19.1	59.1–132.0
Glass ionomer	Chelon-fil[114]	1.09	7.5
	Chelon-silver[114]	1.65	11.4
	Chemfil II[114]	1.35	9.3
	Chemfil II in caps[114]	3.63	25.0
	Fuji II[114]	0.51	3.5
	Fuji II[119]	0.58–2.9	4.0–20.0
	Fuji IX[123]	2.2–3.3	15.4–22.6
	Ketac-fil Capsule[114]	1.49	10.3
	Ketac-silver Capsule[114,124]	1.00	6.9
		4.76	31.8
Resin composite	Herculite XRV[125]	14.5	99.8
	P-50[125]	12.3	85.1
	Silux Plus[125]	8.9	61.4
	Z100[124]	20.2	139.4
Flowable[126]	AeliteFlo	16.4	112.8
	Flo Restore	21.5	148.4
	Revolution	13.6	94.1
	Ultra Seal XT Plus	20.1	138.5
Hybrid	Herculite[122]	17.0	117.0
	Prodigy[126–128]	19.7–26.5	136.0–182.5
	Tetric Ceram[129]	15.5	107.0
	TPH Spectrum[127]	19.7	136.0
	Z100[120,126]	13.4–26.3	92.3–181.4

(continued)

Flexural Strength, *MOR* (continued)

Material	Product	MOR	
		psi × 10³	MPa
Restorative materials			
Resin composite (continued)			
Microfilled	Durafil[127]	12.0	83.0
	Heliomolar[129,130]	12.7	87.8
	Silux Plus[127]	11.5	79.0
Packable	Alert[128,129,131]	19.4	133.7
	Exp Condensable[131]	14.6	101.0
	Pyramid[128]	21.6	148.9
	Solitaire[123,128–131]	3.5–17.7	24.4–122.3
	SureFil[128,129,131]	17.5	120.9
Resin-modifed glass ionomer	Fuji II LC[119]	2.3–7.8	16.9–54.0
	Photac-Fil[123]	3.9–6.1	26.7–41.8
	Vitremer[120]	3.6	24.9
Vitreous carbon[25]		22	152

Flow

Flow is defined as the permanent strain of an elastic impression material when it is loaded in compression at a fixed stress (100 g on 12.7 × 19 mm cylinder) for 15 minutes at 1 hour after mixing. The method of testing is described in American National Standards Institute/American Dental Association Specification No. 19.[45]

Material	Product	Flow (%)
Bite registration material[132]	Correct-Bite	0.00
Impression materials		
Alginate[99]		
Normal consistency	Jeltrate	3.6*
Thin consistency	Jeltrate	6.3*
Thick consistency	Jeltrate	2.7*
Polyether[133]	Impregum F	0.02
	Permadyne	
	Light	0.03
	Heavy	0.02
	Polyjel NF	0.02
Polysulfide[133]	Coeflex	
	Light	0.45
	Medium	0.45
	Heavy	0.42
Silicone, addition	Absolute[133]	
	Light	0.03
	Medium	0.02
	Heavy	0.02
	Putty	0.03
	Baysilex[133]	0.04
	Exaflex Hydrophilic[133]	
	Light	0.05
	Medium	0.03
	Examix Hydrophilic	
	Light[133]	0.03
	Medium[133]	0.01
	Monophase[132]	0.00
	Express Hydrophilic[133]	
	Light	0.03
	Medium	0.02
	Putty	0.09
	Hydrosil[133]	0.02
	Imprint[133]	0.03
	Mirror 3 Extrude[133]	
	Light	0.03
	Medium	0.02
	Putty	0.03
	Omnisil[133]	
	Light	0.02
	Medium	0.02
	Putty	0.07

*Measured at 6 min.

(continued)

Flow (continued)

Material	Product	Flow (%)
Impression materials		
Silicone, addition (continued)	Permagum[132]	
	Light	0.00
	Medium	0.00
	Heavy	0.02
	President[133]	
	Light	0.01
	Heavy	0.01
	Putty	0.01
	Reprosil Hydrophilic[133]	
	Light	0.02
	Medium	0.02
	Heavy	0.02
	Putty	0.02
Silicone, condensation	Coltex[133]	
	Light	0.11
	Medium	0.15
	Coltoflax[133]	0.08
	Cuttersil[132]	
	Light	0.02
	Medium	0.04
	Elasticon[132]	
	Light	0.03
	Heavy	0.00
	Rapid[132]	
	Light	0.01
	Putty	0.01

Heat of Fusion

The *heat of fusion* is the heat in calories required to convert 1 g of a material from the solid to the liquid state at the melting temperature. The equation for the calculation of heat of fusion is $L = Q/m$, where Q is the total heat absorbed and m is the mass of the substance.

Material	Product	L (cal/g)	Temperature (°C)
Gutta-percha (pure)[134]		45.2	74
Ice[76]		79.7	0
Mercury[21]		2.8	−38
Pure metals[21]			
Chromium		96	1875
Copper		50.6	1083
Gold		16.1	1063
Nickel		73.8	1453
Palladium		34.2	1552
Platinum		26.9	1769
Silver		25	961
Zinc		24.09	420
Waxes[135]			
Beeswax	Ross Co.	42.8	62.8
Carnauba	Ross Co.	45.5	82.8
Inlay casting	Kerr blue hard	45.9	60.0
Paraffin	Ross Co.	42.4	52.0

Heat of Reaction, ΔH

The *heat of reaction* represents the difference in the enthalpies of the reaction products and reactants at constant pressure and at a definite temperature, with every substance in a definite physical state. If heat is liberated in the reaction, the process is said to be exothermic and ΔH is a negative number. If heat is absorbed, the process is endothermic and ΔH is a positive number.

Material	Reaction	ΔH (kcal/g-mol)
Denture resin, acrylic[136]	$n\ CH_2{=}C \Rightarrow {-}({-}CH_2{-}C{-}){-}$ (methacrylate polymerization)	−13.9
Gypsum[137]	$CaSO_4 \cdot \tfrac{1}{2}H_2O + 1\tfrac{1}{2}H_2O \Rightarrow CaSO_4 \cdot 2H_2O$	−3.9

Impact Strength, *IZOD*

Impact strength is a measure of the energy required to cause a material to fracture when struck by a sudden blow (high rate of deformation).

Material	Product	IZOD (J/m)
Denture resins[90]		
Cold-cured	PERform	15
Heat-cured	Lucitone 199	27–31
	Perma-cryl 20	14
Light-cured	Triad	13

Index of Refraction, χ

The *index of refraction* for any substance is the ratio of the velocity of light in a vacuum to its velocity in the substance. The extraordinary and ordinary indices of refraction are denoted as χ_e and χ_o, respectively.

Material	χ_e	χ_o
Filler particles for dental composites[106]		
Barium borosilicate		1.554
Quartz		1.540
Strontium glass		1.550
Ytterbium trifluoride		1.530
Zirconium glass		1.520
Fluoroapatite, synthetic[138]	1.630	1.633
Hydroxyapatite, synthetic[139]	1.643	1.649
Monomers[140]		
Bisphenol-A-glycidyl dimethacrylate		1.545
2-Hydroxyethyl methacrylate		1.448
Triethyleneglycol dimethacrylate		1.457
Urethane dimethacrylate		1.481
Porcelain, feldspathic[2]		1.504
Quartz[2]		1.544
Tooth structure, enamel[141]		1.655
Water[76]		1.333

Knoop Hardness Number, *KHN*

The *Knoop hardness test* is a micro-indentation method. A load is applied to a diamond indenting tool and the dimensions of the resulting indentation are measured. The *Knoop hardness number* is the ratio of the applied load to the area of the indentation.

Material	Product	KHN (kg/mm^2)
Abrasives[142]		
Aluminum oxide	E.C. Moore	2100
Flint (quartz)	E.C. Moore	820
Garnet	E.C. Moore	1360
Silicon carbide	E.C. Moore	2480
Cements (luting consistency)[143]		
Resin	C&B Metabond	12
	Panavia EX	53
Cements (liners)[144]		
Calcium hydroxide		
Light-cured	VLC Dycal	2.4
Glass ionomer		
Light-cured	Vitrabond	1.7
	XR Ionomer	0.1
	Zionomer	14–16
Self-cured	GC Lining Cement	2.8
Resin	Cavalite	15
	TimeLine	7.3
Cobalt-chromium alloys[87]	Advantage*	356
	Advantage†	360
	Cobond*	406
	Cobond†	424
	Genesis II*	329
	Genesis II†	345
	Master Tec*	345
	Master Tec†	363
	Niranium N/N[88]	391
	Novarex*	349
	Novarex†	375
	Novarex II*	352
	Novarex II†	368
	Vi-Comp*	386
	Vi-Comp†	399
	Vitallium[88]	415
Denture resins[90]		
Cold-cured	PERform	16.2
Heat-cured	Lucitone 199	14.0
	Perma-cryl 20	16.5
Light-cured	Triad	17.6
Denture teeth[145]		
Acrylic	Dura-Blend	19.9
Gold (condensed)[114]		
Foil	Morgan, Hastings & Co.	69
Mat	Williams	52
Powdered	Goldent	55
Gold-alloy[96]		
Au-Pd alloy	Olympia*	206
	Olympia†	226

*As cast.
†Heat treated.

(continued)

Knoop Hardness Number, *KHN* (continued)

Material	Product	KHN (kg/mm²)
Iron-chromium alloys[88]		
Fixed partial denture	Dentillium C-B	331
Removable partial denture	Dentillium P-D	335
Nickel-chromium alloys[96]	Ceramalloy II*	314
	Ceramalloy II†	270
	Micro-Bond N-P2*	207
	Micro-Bond N-P2†	153
	Ticon*	328
	Ticon†	256
Palladium-based dental alloys[96]	Microstar*	259
	Microstar†	247
	Spartan*	371
	Spartan†	362
	W-1*	232
	W-1†	228
Pit and fissure sealants (24 h)[146]		
Light-cured	Delton LC	18
	Helioseal	21
	Pentra-Seal	19
	Visioseal	16
Self-cured	Delton	14
Porcelain[147]		
Feldspathic	B.F. Vacuum	591
Restorative materials		
Resin composite		
All-purpose	Brilliant[107]	57
	Charisma[107]	43
	Conquest DFC[107]	63
	Herculite XRV[148]	69–71
	Pertac Hybrid[107]	60
	Prisma APH[149]	26
	True Vitality[107]	28
Anterior	Helio Progress[148]	46–48
	Prisma Microfine[149]	25
	Silux Plus[150]	28
	Valux[150]	46
	Visio Dispers[150]	27
	Visio Fil[150]	45
Hybrid[151]	Herculite	18.7–57.6
Microfilled[151]	Heliomolar	11.1–26.8
Packable[151]	Alert	17.3–64.8
	Solitaire	24.2–42.7
	Surefil	31.1–56.4
Posterior	Clearfil Photo Posterior[107]	45
	P 50[150]	60
	Visio Molar[150]	64
Glass ionomer[152]	Chelon-Fil	31
	Chemfil II	18
	Fuji Ionomer II	18
Metal-reinforced glass ionomer[153]	Chelon Silver	24
	Miracle Mix	14

See page 343 for footnotes.

(continued)

Knoop Hardness Number, *KHN* (continued)

Material	Product	KHN (kg/mm²)
Tooth structures		
Calculus (on teeth)[154]		86
Cementum[154]		40
Dentin[155]		68
Enamel (bovine)[156]		
Etched		60–161
Softened		79–145
Sound		339–418
Enamel (human)[156]		
Etched		88–171
Softened		149–179
Sound		355–431
Vitreous carbon[25]		820

See page 343 for footnotes.

Melting Temperatures and Ranges

The temperature at which a single element or compound transforms from a solid to a liquid is the *melting temperature*. Materials that are mixtures or alloys generally do not melt at a single temperature but possess a melting range. The lower temperature of the range is the *solidus temperature*, below which the material is solid. The higher temperature is the *liquidus*, above which the material is liquid. Within the melting range, both solid and liquid are present.

Material	Product	°F	°C
Cobalt-chromium alloys	Genesis II[3]	2415–2550	1325–1400
	Master Tec[12]	2215–2380	1215–1300
	Novarex[13]	2425–2475	1330–1357
Gold alloys			
Type I[5]	Ney-Oro A	1825–1900	996–1038
Type II[5]	Ney-Oro A-1	1650–1775	899–968
Type III[5]	Ney-Oro B-2	1650–1775	899–968
Type IV[5]	Ney-Oro G-3	1630–1740	888–949
40% Au-Ag-Cu[3]	Forticast	1555–1665	846–907
10%–15% Au-Ag-Pd[5]	Paliney No. 4	1670–1810	910–988
Au-Pd[3]	Olympia	2213–2380	1210–1304
Au-Pt-Pd[16]	TPW	2012–2282	1100–1250
Porcelain-fused-to-metal[3]	Jelenko O	2034–2206	1112–1208
Mercury[21]		–37	–38
Nickel-chromium alloy[16]	Unimetal	2098–2282	1148–1250
Palladium-based dental alloys	Athenium[157]	2120–2330	1160–1277
	Legacy[157]	2020–2360	1104–1293
	Liberty[157]	2020–2280	1104–1249
	Microstar[3]	2156–2336	1180–1280
	PTM-88[157]	2120–2340	1160–1282
	Protocol[157]	2320–2390	1271–1310
	Spartan[157]	2040–2120	1116–1160
	W1[12]	2165–2320	1185–1270
Pure metals[21]			
Chromium		3407	1875
Copper		1981	1083
Gold		1945	1063
Nickel		2647	1453
Palladium		2826	1552
Platinum		3217	1769
Silver		1761	961
Titanium		3035	1668
Zinc		787	420
Silver-palladium alloys[3]			
Fixed partial denture	Albacast	1870–2010	1021–1099
Porcelain-fused-to-metal	Jel-5	2116–2341	1158–1283
Ti-6Al-4V alloy[16]		3002	1650
Waxes[158]			
Beeswax	Ross	93–158	34–70
Carnauba	Ross	127–189	53–87
Inlay casting	Kerr blue hard	122–176	50–80
Paraffin	Ross	111–140	44–60

Mohs Hardness

A material's *Mohs hardness* value indicates the material's resistance to scratching. Diamond has a maximum Mohs hardness of 10.

Material	Mohs hardness
Abrasives	
Aluminum oxide[76]	9
Boron carbide[76]	9–10
Chalk (CaCO$_3$)[76]	3
Cuttlebone[1]	7
Diamond[76]	10
Garnet[76]	6.5–7
Gypsum[76]	2
Pumice[76]	6
Quartz[76]	7
Silicon carbide[76]	9–10
Talc[76]	1
Tungsten carbide[76]	9
Zirconium silicate[76]	7.5
Amalgam[1]	4–5
Gold[76]	2.5–3
Porcelain, feldspathic[1]	6–7
Resin composite[1]	5–7
Tooth structures[1]	
Dentin	3–4
Enamel	5

Penetration Coefficient, *PC*

The *penetration coefficient* is the rate at which a liquid penetrates into a capillary space. Units are cm/s.

$$PC = \frac{\gamma \cos \theta}{2\,\eta}$$

where γ is the surface tension of the liquid, η is the viscosity, and θ is the contact angle.

Material	Product	PC
Fluoride gels[45]	Flura-Gel	0.0508
	Luride	0.217
	Predent	0.0870
	Rafluor	0.115
Fluoride solutions[45]	NaF Rinse	2,350
Pit and fissure sealants[146]		
Light-cured	Delton	5.18
	Helioseal	1.72
	Pentra-Seal	2.67
	Visioseal	2.21
Self-cured	Delton	4.90

Percent Elongation (Ductility), n

Elongation is the deformation that results from the application of a tensile force and is calculated as the change in length divided by the original length. It is usually measured over a 5-cm gauge length.

Material	Product	n (% in 5-cm gauge length)
Cobalt-chromium alloys[87]	Advantage*	3
	Advantage†	4
	Cobond*	4
	Cobond†	3
	Genesis II*	7
	Genesis II†	6
	Master Tec*	2
	Master Tec†	3
	Novarex*	2
	Novarex†	1
	Novarex II^v	2
	Novarex II†	2
	Vi-Comp*	5
	Vi-Comp†	4
	Vitallium[88]	1.5‡
Denture liners (resilient)[159]		
Polyphosphazene fluoroelastomer	Novus	240
Silicone	Molloplast-B	325
Gold (999.9 fine)[160]	Wilkinson Co.	60.1§
Gold alloys		
Type I[5]	Ney-Oro A	29.5
Type II[5]	Ney-Oro A-1	32
Type III, soft[5]	Ney-Oro B-2	35
Type III, hard[5]	Ney-Oro B-2	34
Type IV, soft[5]	Ney-Oro G-3	24
Type IV, hard[5]	Ney-Oro G-3	6.5
40% Au-Ag-Cu, soft[3]	Forticast	18
40% Au-Ag-Cu, hard[3]	Forticast	3
10%–15% Au-Ag-Pd, soft[5]	Paliney No. 4	17
10%–15% Au-Ag-Pd, hard[5]	Paliney No. 4	7
Au-Pd[96]	Olympia*	8
	Olympia†	12
Au-Pt-Pd[96]	TPW	9.2
Porcelain-fused-to-metal[3]	Jelenko O	5
Impression material		
Alginate[161]	Krompan	38
Silicone, addition rxn[40]	Aquasil	
	Rigid fast	28
	Rigid regular	30
	Monophase	83
	XLV regular	71
	XLV fast	70
	LV regular	65
	LV fast	68

*As cast.
†Heat treated.
‡Measured on 2.5-cm gauge length.
§Measured on 0.64-cm gauge length.
#Measured on 1.5-cm gauge length.

(continued)

Percent Elongation (Ductility), *n (continued)*

Material	Product	*n* (% in 5-cm gauge length)
Impression material	Examix	
Silicone, addition rxn (continued)[40]	Heavy	72
	Putty	25
	Regular	91
	Injection	94
	Express	
	Putty	41
	Regular body	88
	Light body	94
	Extrude	
	Extra	47
	XP	56
	Medium	92
	Wash	92
	Impregum	105
	Imprint 2	
	Tray	46
	Regular wash	71
	Low wash	68
	Polygel	93
	President	
	Putty soft	61
	Regular body	69
	Light body	83
	Reprosil	
	Putty	92
	Heavy	39
	Medium	96
	Light	97
	Splash	
	Heavy	23
	Regular	30
	Light	65
	Extra light	91
	Splash Half-time	
	Heavy	37
	Regular	45
	Light	64
	Extra light	81
	Putty	
	Soft	40
	Half-time, soft	37
	Regular	38
	Half-time, regular	40
	Take 1 Monophase	
	Regular set	94
	Fast set	98

See page 348 for footnotes.

(continued)

Percent Elongation (Ductility), *n (continued)*

Material	Product	*n* (% in 5-cm gauge length)
Iron-chromium alloys[88]		
Fixed partial denture	Dentillium C-B	8.5‡
Removable partial denture	Dentillium P-D	9.0‡
Maxillofacial materials		
Polyurethane[162]	Epithane-3	224‡
Silicone rubber	A 102[162]	130‡
	A-2186[163]	480
	Cosmesil[163]	588
	MDX 4-4210[163]	438
	Medical Adhesive A[162]	304‡
	Silastic 4-4515[162]	476‡
Mouth protector materials[164]		
Polyvinyl acetate-polyethylene	Proform	1000
	Sta-Guard	1150
Nickel-chromium alloys[96]	Ceramalloy II*	6
	Ceramalloy II†	11
	Micro-Bond N-P2*	29
	Micro-Bond N-P2†	35
	Ticon*	4
	Ticon†	12
	Unimetal[16]	12.2
Palladium-based dental alloys[96]	Athenium[157]	25#
	Liberty[157]	20#
	Legacy[157]	20#
	Microstar*	6
	Microstar†	18
	Protocol[157]	34#
	PTM-88[157]	25#
	Spartan*	2
	Spartan†	9
	W-1*	6
	W-1†	10
Silver-palladium alloys[3]		
Fixed partial denture, soft	Albacast	10
Fixed partial denture, hard	Albacast	8
Porcelain-fused-to-metal	Jel-5	25
Titanium[165]		13
Ti-6Al-4V alloy[165]		5

See page 348 for footnotes.

Permanent Deformation

Permanent deformation is the lack of recovery from deformation of an elastic impression or duplicating material compressed at a fixed strain, usually for 30 seconds. The method of testing is described in American National Standards Institute/American Dental Association Specification Nos. 11, 18, 19, and 20.[45] The trend is to report percent recovery rather than permanent deformation. Therefore a material with a permanent deformation of 1% has a 99% recovery.

Material	Product	Permanent deformation (%)*
Bite registration material[132]	Correct-Bite	0.7
Duplicating material[92]		
Agar	Nobiloid	2.4†
Impression materials		
Agar[92]	Sugident	1.8†
Alginate, 6 min[99]	Jeltrate	2.2
Polyether[133]	Impregum F	1.10
	Permadyne	
	Light	1.52
	Heavy	1.70
	Polyjel NF	0.99
Polysulfide	Coeflex[133]	
	Light	4.13
	Medium	4.39
	Heavy	5.55
	Permlastic[166]	
	Light	2.90
	Medium	2.28
	Heavy	2.81
Silicone, addition	Absolute[133]	
	Light	0.26
	Medium	0.22
	Heavy	0.27
	Putty	0.40
	Aquasil[40]	
	Rigid fast	0.5
	Rigid regular	0.6
	Monophase (cartridge)	0.8
	Monophase (tube)	0.3
	XLV regular	0.7
	XLV fast	0.5
	LV regular	0.6
	LV fast	0.9
	Baysilex	0.17
	Exaflex Hydrophilic[133]	
	Light	0.29
	Medium	0.43
	Examix Hydrophilic	
	Light[133]	1.23
	Medium[133]	0.63
	Monophase[132]	0.14

*Fixed strain, 12%, for 30 s.
†Tested for 1 min.

(continued)

Permanent Deformation (continued)

Material	Product	Permanent deformation (%)*
Impression materials		
Silicone, addition (continued)	Express Hydrophilic[133]	
	Light	0.42
	Medium	0.25
	Putty	0.51
	Hydrosil[133]	0.50
	Impregum[40]	1.10
	Imprint[133]	0.41
	Imprint 2[40]	
	Tray	0.4
	Wash, regular	0.25
	Wash, low	0.20
	Mirror 3 Extrude[133]	
	Light	0.23
	Medium	0.18
	Putty	0.30
	Omnisil[133]	
	Light	0.17
	Medium	0.26
	Putty	0.35
	Permagum[132]	
	Light	0.13
	Medium	0.11
	Heavy	0.12
	Polygel[40]	1.10
	President[133]	
	Light	0.05
	Medium	0.04
	Heavy	0.01
	Putty	0.24
	Reprosil Hydrophilic[133]	
	Light	0.18
	Medium	0.16
	Heavy	0.15
	Putty	0.15
	Splash[40]	
	Heavy	0.45
	Regular	0.85
	Light	1.4
	Extra light	1.45
	Splash Half-time[40]	
	Heavy	0.45
	Regular	0.55
	Light	0.6
	Extra light	0.45

See page 351 for footnotes.

(continued)

Permanent Deformation *(continued)*

Material	Product	Permanent deformation (%)*
Impression materials		
Silicone, addition (continued)	Take 1 Monophase[40]	
	Regular set	0.25
	Fast set	0.35
Silicone, condensation	Coltex[133]	
	Light	1.18
	Medium	1.50
	Coltoflax[133]	1.41
	CutterSil[132]	
	Light	1.20
	Medium	1.39
	Elasticon[132]	
	Light	0.84
	Heavy	0.47
	Rapid[132]	
	Light	1.73
	Putty	1.09

See page 351 for footnotes.

Poisson Ratio, v

Poisson ratio is a measure of the simultaneous change in elongation and in cross-sectional area within the elastic range during a tensile or compressive test. During a tensile test, the reduction in cross-sectional area is proportional to the increase in length in the elastic range by the dimensionless factor, v.

Material	Product	v
Amalgam[167,168]		0.35*
		0.334*
Cements[169]		
Zinc phosphate	Tenacin	0.35*
Zinc silicophosphate	Dorcate	0.30*
Fluoroapatite (mineral)[170]		0.28*
Gold alloys		
Au-Ag-Pd[59]		0.33
Au-Pd[171]		0.33
Hydroxyapatite (synthetic)[170]		0.28*
Impression materials[172]		
Polyether	Impregum	0.13†
Silicones, addition	Baysilex Monophase	0.41†
	Provil	
	Medium	0.19‡
	Heavy	0.44‡
Nickel-chromium alloys[102]	Ceramalloy	0.27
	Micro-Bond N-P2	0.24
	Pentillium	0.32
Polymers[173]		
Acrylic		0.37–0.45‡
Polycarbonate		0.41–0.44‡
Polyethylene		0.54–0.61‡
Porcelain[174]	Ceramco	0.19
	Vita	0.19
Restorative materials[175]		
Acrylic	Sevriton	0.35*
Resin composite	Adaptic	0.24*
Silicate[169]	Syntrex	0.30*
Titanium[59]		0.33
Tooth and supporting structures[176]		
Bone		
Cancellous		0.30
Cortical		0.30
Cementum		0.31
Dentin		0.31
Enamel		0.33
Periodontal ligament		0.45

*Measured by ultrasonic method.
†Measured by dynamic method.
‡Measured in tension with transverse strain gauge extensometers.

Proportional Limit, *PL*

The *proportional limit* is defined as the greatest stress that a material will sustain without a deviation from the law of proportionality of stress to strain. Unless indicated otherwise, values are for tests in tension.

Material	Product	PL	
		psi $\times 10^3$	MPa
Duplicating material[92]			
Agar	Nobiloid	0.051*	0.35*
Fixed partial denture resins[93]			
Acrylic	Biotone	6.9†	47.6†
Polyester	Mer-Don 7	4.95†	34.1†
Polyvinyl acrylic	Luxene	8.12†	56.0†
Gold alloys[5]			
Type I	Ney-Oro A	10	69
Type II	Ney-Oro A-1	27.5	190
Type III, soft	Ney-Oro B-2	32.0	221
Type III, hard	Ney-Oro B-2	38.0	262
Type IV, soft	Ney-Oro G-3	41.5	286
Type IV, hard	Ney-Oro G-3	83.0	572
10%–15% Au-Ag-Pd, soft	Paliney No. 4	63.5	438
10%–15% Au-Ag-Pd, hard	Paliney No. 4	84.5	583
Porcelain-fused-to-metal[72]	Ceramco O	60.8	419
Impression materials[92]			
Agar	Surgident	0.095*	0.66*
Nickel-chromium alloys			
Fixed partial denture[103]	Howmedica III	28.0	193
Porcelain-fused-to-metal[72]	Ultratek	9.0	545
Silicate[94]	Improved Filling Porcelain	19.6‡	135‡
Tooth structures[94]			
Dentin		24.2§	167§
Enamel (cusp)		51.2§	353§
Waxes[113]			
Inlay casting, hard	Kerr blue hard	0.501¶	3.46¶
Inlay casting, soft	Kerr blue regular	0.634¶	4.37¶

*Tested in compression, head speed 25 cm/min.
†Tested in compression, head speed 0.05 cm/min.
‡Tested in compression, head speed 0.04 cm/min.
§Tested in compression.
¶Tested in compression, head speed 0.50 cm/min.

Shear Strength, S

The *shear strength* is defined as the maximum stress that a material can withstand before failure in shear. Calculation of shear strength depends upon the test method.

Material	Product	S* psi × 10³	S* MPa
Amalgam[177]	New True Dentalloy	27.3	188
Cement (base consistency)[178]			
Polymer-modified ZOE	B & T	1.85	12.7
Cements (luting consistency)			
Polymer-modified ZOE[178]	Fynal	1.85	12.7
Unmodified ZOE[11]		0.60	4.1
Zinc phosphate[11,179]		1.90	13.1
		9.17	63.4
Zinc polycarboxylate[179]	Durelon	3.96	27.4
	Poly F	4.44	30.7
Denture resins			
Acrylic	Kallodent	17.8	122
Porcelains[180]			
Aluminous	Vita Aluminous	24	165
Feldspathic	Ceramco Opaque	18	128
Tooth structures			
Dentin[177,181]		20.0	138
Vital		17.1	118
Vital, constrained		19.4	134
Nonvital (endodontically treated)		14.8	102
Enamel[177]		13.1	90.2

*Tested by punch method.

Shore A Hardness

The relative hardness of elastic materials, such as rubber or soft plastics, can be determined with an instrument called a *Shore A durometer*. If the indenter completely penetrates the sample, a reading of 0 is obtained, and if no penetration occurs, a reading of 100 results. The reading is dimensionless.

Material	Product	Shore A hardness
Denture liners (resilient)[159]		
Polyphosphazene fluoroelastomer	Novus	50
Silicone	Molloplast-B	43
Impression materials[182]		
Polyether	Impregum	58.0*
Polysulfide	Permlastic	
	Light	13.0*
	Medium	24.2*
	Heavy	34.2*
Silicone, addition	Aquasil[40]	
	Rigid fast	76
	Rigid regular	77
	Monophase (cartridge)	61
	Monophase (tube)	63
	XLV regular	53
	XLV fast	53
	LV regular	62
	LV fast	60.5
	Examix[40]	
	Heavy	56
	Putty	63
	Regular	47
	Injection	41
	Express[40]	
	Putty	67
	Regular body	58
	Light body	54
	Extrude[40]	
	Extra	61
	XP	64
	Medium	40
	Wash	36
	Impregum[40]	55
	Imprint 2[40]	
	Tray	68
	Wash, regular	57
	Wash, low	55
	Polygel[40]	59
	President[182]	
	Medium	62.5*
	Putty	77.4*
	Provil[182]	
	Light	43.7*
	Heavy	59.3*

*Measured at 24 h.

(continued)

Shore A Hardness (continued)

Material	Product	Shore A hardness
Impression materials		
Silicone, addition (continued)	Reprosil[40]	
	Putty	60
	Heavy	72
	Medium	46
	Light	42
	Splash[40]	
	Heavy	67
	Regular	68
	Light	57
	Extra light	50
	Putty, soft	68
	Putty, regular	65
	Splash Half-time[40]	
	Heavy	70
	Regular	70
	Light	57
	Extra light	50
	Putty, soft	55
	Putty, regular	71
	Take 1 Monophase[40]	
	Regular set	46
	Fast set	47
Silicone, condensation[182]	Optosil Plus	66.0*
	Xantopren blue	43.9*
Maxillofacial materials		
Polyurethane[162]	Epithane-3	46.6*
Silicone rubber	A-102[162]	38.3*
	A-2186[163]	24.6*
	Cosmesil[163]	30.4*
	MDX 4-4210[163]	24.0*
	Medical Adhesive A[162]	29.4*
	Silastic 4-4515[162]	50.2*
Mouth protector materials[78]		
Polyvinyl acetate-polyethylene	Proform	82
	Sta-Guard	67

See page 357 for footnote.

Solubility and Disintegration in Water

Solubility and *disintegration* are measured by suspending two disks 20 mm in diameter, representing approximately 1,260 mm^2 of exposed surface, in distilled water at 37°C.

Material	Product	Mass loss (%)	Solubility (mg/cm^2)
Denture liners (resilient)			
Polyphosphazene[183]			
Fluoroelastomer	Novus		0.03*
Silicone[183]	Molloplast-B		0.13*
Cement (base consistency)[178]			
Polymer-modified ZOE	B & T	0.06†	
Cements (luting consistency)			
EBA-alumina ZOE[184]		0.05†	
Glass ionomer[185]	Fuji I	0.08†	
	Ketac-Cem	0.40†	
Polymer-modified ZOE[178]	Fynal	0.08†	
Resin[186]	Comspan	0.017†	
Unmodified ZOE	Temporary Cement[184]	0.10†	
	Temporary Cement[187]		0.39†
Zinc hydrophosphate[188]	New Calmix	0.4†	
Zinc phosphate	Flecks Cement[186]	0.025†	
	Flecks Cement[189]		0.82‡
Zinc polycarboxylate	Durelon[190]	<0.04†	
	Durelon[189]		0.81‡
Zinc silicophosphate	Kryptex Improved[191]	1.0*	
Cements (liners)			
Glass ionomer			
Light-cured[192]	Vitrebond	3.6†	
	XR Ionomer	1.5†	
Self-cured	GC Lining Cement[185]		0.50†
	Ketac-cem[13]	0.023†	
Periodontal dressings[193]	Barricaid	0.54	
	COEpak	1.5	
	PerioCare	2.7	
Pit and fissure sealants[194]			
Light-cured	Nuva-Seal		0.5*
Self-cured	9075		0.2*
Restorative materials[185]			
Glass ionomer	Fuji II		0.07†
	Ketac-Fil		0.10†
Metal-reinforced glass ionomer	Ketac-Silver		0.12†
Silicate[186]	New Improved Filling Porcelain		2.09†

*Stored for 7 days.
†Stored for 1 day.
‡Stored for 5 days.

Specific Heat, C_p

The *specific heat* of a substance is the quantity of heat needed to raise the temperature of a unit mass of the substance 1°C. Water usually is chosen as a standard substance and 1 g as a standard mass.

Material	Product	C_p (cal/[g°C])
Bones[59]		
Cancellous		0.44
Cortical		0.44
Cements		
Calcium hydroxide[60]	Dycal	0.429
	Life	0.346
Glass ionomer[61]	Base cement	0.273*
	Dentin cement	0.275*
	Ketac-Cem	0.293*
Polymer-modified ZOE[62]	IRM	0.178†
Unmodified ZOE[62]		0.138‡
	Cavitec[60]	0.421
Zinc phosphate[62]	Tenacin	0.122§
Gold alloy[59]		
Au-Ag-Pd alloy		0.03
Hydroxyapatite[59]		0.21
Impression materials (polymerized)[68]		
Polyether	Impregum	0.502
Silicone, addition	Baysilex	0.229
	Provil	
	Medium	0.256
	High	0.227
Mercury[21]		0.033
Pure metals[21]		
Chromium		0.11¶
Copper		0.092¶
Gold		0.0312#
Nickel		0.105¶
Palladium		0.0584**
Platinum		0.0314**
Silver		0.0559**
Titanium		0.124¶
Zinc		0.0915¶
Restorative materials[62]		
Acrylic	Bonfil	0.280
Resin composite	Adaptic	0.197
Silicate[62]	Improved Filling Porcelain	0.167‡
Tooth structures		
Dentin[60,195,196]		0.28
		0.31
		0.38
Enamel[195]		0.18
Vitreous carbon[25]		0.30
Water[76]		1.00
Zinc oxide[62]	USP grade	0.095

*Powder/liquid ratio, 1.0 g/mL.
†Powder/liquid ratio, 5.0 g/mL.
‡Powder/liquid ratio, 3.0 g/mL.
§Powder/liquid ratio, 2.5 g/mL.
¶At 20°C.
#At 18°C.
**At 0°C.

Strain in Compression

Strain in compression (or flexibility) of an elastomeric impression or duplicating material is measured between stresses of 100 and 1000 g/cm^2 (ca. 0.01 and 0.1 MPa). The method of testing is described in American National Standards Institute/American Dental Association Specification Nos. 11, 18, 19, and 20.[45]

Material	Product	Strain in compression (%)
Bite registration material[132]	Correct-Bite	0.9–1.3
Duplicating materials[132]		
Agar	Multi-Gel	14.580
Impression materials		
Alginate[99]		
Normal consistency	Jeltrate	13.4
Thin consistency	Jeltrate	18.5
Thick consistency	Jeltrate	10.1
Polyether[133]	Impregum F	1.93
	Permadyne	
	Light	3.31
	Heavy	2.91
	Polyjel NF	2.65
Polysulfide	Coeflex[133]	
	Light	13.5
	Medium	13.9
	Heavy	11.1
	Permlastic[166]	
	Light	11.8
	Medium	10.2
	Heavy	6.2
Silicone, addition	Absolute[133]	
	Light	3.59
	Medium	2.42
	Heavy	2.64
	Putty	1.55
	Aquasil[40]	
	Rigid fast	1.5
	Rigid regular	1.5
	Monophase (cartridge)	3.2
	Monophase (tube)	3.0
	XLV regular	4.9
	XLV fast	4.7
	LV regular	3.6
	LV fast	4.1
	Baysilex[133]	4.60
	Exaflex Hydrophilic[133]	
	Light	5.17
	Medium	4.65
	Examix Hydrophilic[133]	
	Light	5.77
	Medium	5.25
	Monophase	2.81

(continued)

Strain in Compression *(continued)*

Material	Product	Strain in compression (%)
Impression materials		
Silicone, addition (continued)	Express Hydrophilic[133]	
	Light	5.32
	Medium	4.64
	Putty	5.90
	Extrude[40]	
	Extra	3.15
	XP	2.10
	Medium	5.65
	Wash	12.95
	Hydrosil[133]	1.88
	Impregum[40]	2.10
	Imprint[133]	2.71
	Imprint 2[40]	
	Tray	1.80
	Wash, regular	2.30
	Wash, low	2.50
	Mirror 3 Extrude[133]	
	Light	5.76
	Medium	4.0
	Putty	2.53
	Omnisil[133]	
	Light	4.95
	Medium	4.72
	Putty	1.62
	Permagum[132]	
	Light	2.94
	Medium	2.06
	Heavy	2.44
	Polygel[40]	1.65
	President[133]	
	Light	3.5
	Medium	2.6
	Heavy	2.2
	Putty	1.7
	Reprosil Hydrophilic[133]	
	Light	4.1
	Medium	3.6
	Heavy	2.6
	Putty	1.7
	Splash[40]	
	Heavy	1.90
	Regular	2.70
	Light	3.50
	Extra light	4.30
	Putty, soft	2.40
	Putty, regular	1.90

(continued)

Strain in Compression *(continued)*

Material	Product	Strain in compression (%)
Impression materials		
Silicone, addition (continued)	Splash Half-time[40]	
	Heavy	2.10
	Regular	2.20
	Light	3.30
	Extra light	4.30
	Putty, soft	2.90
	Putty, regular	1.80
	Take 1 (Monophase)[40]	
	Regular set	3.80
	Fast set	3.60
Silicone, condensation	Coltex[133]	
	Light	11.1
	Medium	5.66
	Coltoflax[133]	2.13
	CutterSil[132]	
	Light	3.66
	Medium	6.29
	Elasticon[132]	
	Light	6.37
	Heavy	7.77
	Rapid[132]	
	Light	4.98
	Putty	1.66

Surface Free Energy, γ_s

The *surface free energy* is defined as the work required to increase the area of a substance by 1 cm^2.

Material	Product	γ_s (ergs/cm^2)
Bacteria[31]		
A odontolyticus A7-1		106
A viscosus C7-4		111
S mutans C7-3		128
S salivarius B3-4		113
S sanguis C7-2		99
Polymers[53]		
Polyethylene		33.5
Polymethyl methacrylate		36.5
Polystyrene		38.0
Poly(tetrafluoroethylene)	Teflon	24.0
Tooth structures[31]		
Dentin		92
Enamel		87
Wax[53]		
Paraffin		25.0

Surface Tension, γ

Surface tension is a measure of the surface free energy of a liquid and is defined as the force acting along the surface of a liquid at right angles to any line 1 cm in length.

Material	Product	γ (dynes/cm)	Temperature (°C)
Blood[197]		55.5–61.2	
Mercury[198]		483.5	25
Polymers[55]			
Polyetherurethane	Pellethane 80A	24.0	
	Pellethane 55D	24.8	
	Pellethane 75D	32.3	
Polyetherurethaneurea	Biomer	33.9	
Porcelain[199]	Ceramco Undercoat A	366	1038
Saliva[200]		53	37
Water[35]		72.3	25

Tear Energy

The *tear energy* is a measure of the energy per unit area of newly torn surface and is calculated from the load required to propagate a tear in a trouser-shaped specimen.

Material	Product	Tear energy (M ergs/cm^2)
Denture liners (resilient)[159]		
Polyphosphazene fluoroelastomer	Novus	23*
Silicone	Molloplast-B	1.4*
Impression materials		
Alginate[201,202]	Tissutex	0.4
		0.066
Polyether[203]	Impregum F†	0.81*
	Permadyne‡	0.45*
	Polyjel NF†	0.85*
Polysulfide[203]	Coe-flex	1.89*
	Permlastic‡	0.71*
Silicone, addition[203]	Absolute‡	0.52*
	Baysilex§	1.50*
	Express‡	0.65*
	Extrude‡	0.78*
	Hydrosil†	0.63*
	Panapren†	0.81*
	Permagum‡	0.64*
	Reprosil‡	0.60*
	Unosil†	0.47*
Maxillofacial materials[204]		
Polyurethane	Dermathane 100	1.8¶
Polyvinyl chloride	Sartomer Resins	11¶
Silicone rubber	Silastic 382	0.66¶
	Silastic 399	0.61¶

*Head speed, 5 cm/min.
†Medium viscosity, monophase.
‡Low viscosity.
§High viscosity, monophase.
¶Head speed, 2 cm/min.

Tear Strength

The *tear strength* is a measure of the resistance of a material to tear forces. The tear strength of a notched specimen is calculated by dividing the maximum load by the thickness of the specimen. A specimen suitable for measuring tear strength is described in American National Standards Institute/American Dental Association Specification No. 20.[45]

Material	Product	Tear strength	
		lb/in	kg/cm
Denture liners (resilient)[159]			
Polyphosphazene fluoroelastomer	Novus	54*	9.7*
Silicone	Molloplast-B	33*	5.9*
Duplicating material[92]			
Agar	Nobiloid	1.3†	0.232†
Impression materials			
Agar, tray[99]	Surgident	5.68†	1.01†
Alginate[99]	Jeltrate	3.0†	0.536†
Polyether[133]	Impregum F	26.8‡	4.80‡
	Permadyne		
	Light	10.1‡	1.80‡
	Heavy	16.8‡	3.00‡
	Polyjel NF	19.6‡	3.50‡
Polysulfide[133]	Coeflex		
	Light	18.4‡	3.29‡
	Medium	19.9‡	3.56‡
Silicone, addition	Absolute[133]		
	Light	15.7‡	2.80‡
	Medium	19.6‡	3.50‡
	Aquasil[205]		
	LV fast	30.2	5.4
	Baysilex[133]	21.6‡	3.86‡
	Correct Quick[205]	17.9	3.2
	Exaflex Hydrophilic[133]		
	Light	15.9‡	2.84‡
	Medium	16.2‡	2.90‡
	Examix Hydrophilic[133]		
	Light	15.7‡	2.80‡
	Medium	16.2‡	2.90‡
	Monophase	18.8‡	3.36‡
	Express Hydrophilic[133]		
	Light	18.5‡	3.30‡
	Medium	18.5‡	3.30‡
	Hydrosil[133]	13.4‡	2.40‡
	Imprint[133]	21.8‡	3.90‡
	Imprint 2[205]		
	Low	29.1	5.2
	Regular	25.8	4.6

*Head speed, 50 cm/min.
†Head speed, 25 cm/min.
‡Head speed, 30 cm/min.

(continued)

Tear Strength *(continued)*

Material	Product	Tear strength	
		lb/in	kg/cm
Impression materials			
Silicone, addition (continued)	Imprint 2 Quick Step[205]		
	Low	23.5	4.2
	Regular	26.9	4.8
	Mirror 3 Extrude[133]		
	Light	12.3‡	2.20‡
	Medium	26.3‡	4.70‡
	Omnisil[133]		
	Light	14.6‡	2.60‡
	Medium	10.4‡	1.85‡
	Permagum[132]		
	Light	10.4‡	1.85‡
	Medium	28.4‡	5.07‡
	Heavy	29.5‡	5.26‡
	President[133]		
	Light	15.1‡	2.70‡
	Medium	30.8‡	5.50‡
	Reprosil Hydrophilic[133]		
	Light	14.3‡	2.56‡
	Medium	17.4‡	3.10‡
	Splash Half-time, light body[205]	29.7	5.3
	Take 1[205]		
	Wash, fast	23.0	4.1
Silicone, condensation	Coltex[133]		
	Light	8.96‡	1.60‡
	Medium	14.6‡	2.61‡
	Cuttersil[132]		
	Light	15.1‡	2.70‡
	Medium	13.0‡	2.33‡
	Elasticon[132]		
	Light	15.5‡	2.76‡
	Heavy	24.5‡	4.37‡
	Rapid[132]		
	Light	18.3‡	3.26‡
Maxillofacial materials			
Polyurethane[162]	Epithane-3	45*	8.1*
Silicone rubber	A-102[162]	23*	4.1*
	A-2186[162,163]	203*	36.2*
		40*	7.1*
	Cosmesil[163]	44*	7.8*
	MDX 4-4210[163]	23*	4.1*
	Medical Adhesive A[162]	70*	12.4*
	Silastic 4-4515[162]	104*	18.6*
Mouth protector materials[164]			
Polyvinyl acetate-polyethylene	Proform	160†	28.6†
	Sta-Guard	120†	21.4†

See page 366 for footnotes.

Thermal Conductivity, K

The *thermal conductivity* of a substance is the quantity of heat in cal/s passing through a body 1 cm thick with a cross section of 1 cm^2 when the temperature difference between the hot and cold sides of the body is 1°C.

Material	Product	K mcal/s(cm^2)(°C/cm)
Amalgam[206]		54.0
Alumina (recrystallized)[10]		38.7
Bones[59]		
Cancellous		1.4
Cortical		1.4
Cement (base consistency)[206]		
Zinc phosphate	Tenacin	3.1
Cements (luting consistency)		
Glass ionomer[61]	Ketac-cem	1.5*
Zinc phosphate[206]	Tenacin	2.5
Cements (liners)		
Calcium hydroxide[60]	Dycal	1.5
	Life	1.2
Glass ionomer[61]	Base cement	1.6*
	Dentin cement	1.3*
Unmodified ZOE[62]		1.4†
	Cavitec[57]	0.7
Denture resins[207]		
Acrylic		0.37
Polystyrene		0.22
Gold alloy (Au-Ag-Pd)[59]		300
Gypsum[2]		3.1
Hydroxyapatite[58]		3.0
Impression materials (polymerized)[68]		
Polyether	Impregum	2.3
Silicone, addition	Baysilex	1.0
	Provil	
	Medium	1.4
	High	0.72
Mercury[21]		19.6‡
Porcelain (feldspathic)[10]		2.39
Pure metals[21]		
Chromium		160§
Copper		941§
Gold		710§
Nickel		220¶
Palladium		1680#
Platinum		165**
Silver		1000‡
Titanium[59]		10.0
Zinc		270¶

*Powder/liquid ratio, 1.0 g/mL.
†Powder/liquid ratio, 3.0 g/mL.
‡At 0°C.
§Near 20°C.
¶At 25°C.
#At 18°C.
**At 17°C.

(continued)

Thermal Conductivity, *K* (continued)

Material	Product	K mcal/s(cm²)(°C/cm)
Restorative materials		
Acrylic[62]	Bonfil	0.38
Resin composite[62,63]	Adaptic	2.61
		3.27
Silicate[62,206]	Improved Filling Porcelain	1.78–1.86
		0.82[†]
Tooth structures[196]		
Dentin		1.36
Enamel		2.23
Vitreous carbon[25]		15
Water[76]		1.42**

See page 368 for footnotes.

Thermal Diffusivity, ∅

The *thermal diffusivity* is a measure of transient heat flow and is defined as the thermal conductivity divided by the product of specific heat times density.

Material	Product	$\varnothing$(mm^2/s)
Amalgam[208]	Caulk Fine Cut	9.6
Cements		
Calcium hydroxide[60,209]	Dycal	0.187
		0.240
	Life	0.186
Glass ionomer		
Light-cured[210]	Vitrabond	0.184
	XR Ionomer	0.194
	Zionomer	0.290
Self-cured	Base cement[61]	0.266*
	Dentin cement[61]	0.232*
	Fuji[179]	0.262
	Ketac-bond[210]	0.205
	Ketac-cem[61]	0.239*
Resin[210]	Time Line	0.174
Unmodified ZOE[62,209]		0.389†
		0.471‡
	Cavitec[60]	0.086
Zinc phosphate	Tenacin[62]	0.290‡
	Stratford Cookson[209]	0.308§
Zinc polycarboxylate[209]	Poly-C	0.332
Gold (pure)[208]		118
Impression materials		
Dental compound[211]	Kerr	0.226
Polyether[68]	Impregum	0.43
Silicone, addition[68]	Baysilex	0.32
	Provil	
	Medium	0.38
	High	0.22
Polymethyl methacrylate[209]	Lucite	0.124
Restorative materials		
Acrylic	Bonfil[62]	0.123
	Sevriton[209]	0.125
Glass ionomer[210]	Fuji Type II	0.216
	Improved Fuji Type II	0.228
Metal-reinforced glass ionomer[210]	Ketac-Silver	0.516
	Miracle Mix	0.407
Resin composite	Adaptic[62,209]	0.675
		0.655
	Adaptic Radiopaque[179]	0.725
	Concise[179]	0.338

*Powder/liquid ratio, 1.0 g/mL.
†Powder/liquid ratio, 3.0 g/mL.
‡Powder/liquid ratio, 2.5 g/mL.
§Powder/liquid ratio, 1.85 g/mL.

(continued)

Thermal Diffusivity, $\varnothing$ (continued)

Material	Product	$\varnothing$(mm^2/s)
Restorative materials		
Resin composite (continued)[179]	Cosmic	0.310
	Isopast	0.191
	Profile	0.283
Silicate	Improved Filling Porcelain[62]	0.243†
	Silicap[208]	0.275
Tooth structures[60,196]		
Dentin		0.183
		0.258
Enamel		0.469

See page 370 for footnotes.

Ultimate Compressive Strength, *C*

The *ultimate compressive strength* is defined as the maximum stress that a material can withstand before failure in compression. It is determined by dividing the maximum load in compression by the original cross-sectional area of the test specimen.

Material	Product	C psi × 10³	C MPa
Alumina (recrystallized)[10]		316	2180
Amalgams (1 h)[50]			
Admixed	Valiant PhD	29.2	201
Spherical	Tytin	29.7	205
	Valiant	42.1	290
Amalgams (24 h)			
Admixed	Dispersalloy[212]	61.3*	423*
	Fast set[49]	56.1†	387†
		64.5‡	445‡
	Regular set[49]	51.2†	353†
		62.8‡	433‡
	Optaloy II[49]	46.8†	323†
		50.9‡	351‡
Lathe-cut	Caulk Fine Cut[49]	45.0†	310†
		49.0‡	338‡
	New True Dentalloy[212]	46.1*	318*
Spherical[49]	Indiloy	59.0†	407†
		60.3‡	416‡
	Sybraloy	52.3†	361†
		57.4‡	396‡
Bones (human)[82]			
Long bones			
Femur		24.2	167
Humerus		19.1	132
Radius		16.5	114
Tibia		23.1	159
Vertebrae			
Cervical		1.5	10
Lumbar		0.73	5
Cements (base consistency, 24 h)			
Polymer-modified ZOE[82]	B & T	5.52*	38.1*
Zinc phosphate[82]	Zinc Cement Improved	23.3*	161*
Zinc polycarboxylate	Durelon[82]	11.5*	79.6*
	PCA[64]	9.93§	68.5§
Cements (luting consistency, 24 h)[82]			
EBA-alumina ZOE	Opotow	9.32*	64.3*
		9.53	65.7

*Head speed 0.02 cm/min.
†Head speed 0.025 cm/min hand triturated.
‡Head speed 0.025 cm/min mechanically triturated.
§Head speed 0.5 cm/min.
¶Head speed 0.05 cm/min.
#Head speed 0.01 cm/min.

**Head speed 0.1 cm/min.
††Head speed 25 cm/min.
‡‡Head speed 0.15 cm/min.
§§Head speed 0.12 cm/min.

(continued)

Ultimate Compressive Strength, *C* (continued)

Material	Product	C	
		psi × 10³	MPa
Cements (luting consistency, 24 h)			
EBA-alumina ZOE (continued)[84]		6.5[¶]	45[¶]
Glass ionomer[113]	Fuji I	17.4[#]	120[#]
	Ketac-cem Radiopaque	17.7[#]	122[#]
Noneugenol zinc oxide[83]	Nogenol	0.587*	4.05*
Polymer-modified ZOE[83,84]	Fynal	7.31*	50.4*
		5.1[¶]	35[¶]
Resin[213]	Panavia EX	25.9[#]	178[#]
Unmodified ZOE[187]	Temporary Cement	1.20*	8.28*
Zinc hydrophosphate[188]	New Calmix	9.56[#]	66.0[#]
Zinc phosphate[213]	Flecks	9.01[#]	62.1[#]
	Modern Tenacin	11.2[#]	77.5[#]
Zinc polycarboxylate[213]	Durelon	9.78[#]	67.4[#]
	Shofu	7.98[#]	55.0[#]
Zinc silicophosphate[191]	Kryptex Improved	24.8	171
Cements (liners, 24 h)			
Calcium hydroxide			
Light-cured[214]	VLC Dycal	20.0**	138**
Self-cured	Dycal[214]	2.10**	14.5**
	Life[85]	5.50	37.9
Glass ionomer			
Light-cured	Fuji lining[215]	24.7**	170.3**
	Vitrabond[214,215]	19.0**	130.9**
		8.24**	56.8**
	XR Ionomer[214,215]	9.28**	64.0**
		2.9**	20.0**
	Zionomer[85]	6.67	46.0
Self-cured[113]	Baseline	9.64[#]	66.5[#]
	Baseline in caps	20.0[#]	138[#]
	GC lining cement	8.44[#]	58.2[#]
	Ketac-bond	17.0[#]	117[#]
	Ketac-bond Capsule	20.6[#]	142[#]
	3M Glass ionomer liner	9.51[#]	65.6[#]
Resin[214]	Timeline	22.2**	153**
Unmodified ZOE[83]	Cavitec	0.798*	5.50*
Duplicating material[92]			
Agar	Nobiloid	0.052[††]	0.36[††]
Fixed partal denture resins[93]			
Acrylic	Biotone	11.8[#]	81.4[#]
Polyester	Mer-Don 7	8.65[#]	59.6[#]
Polyvinyl acrylic	Luxene	12.0[#]	82.8[#]
Gypsum (dried)[216]			
Improved stone	Velmix	11.7[‡‡]	80.7[‡‡]
Plaster	Calspar	3.40[‡‡]	23.4[‡‡]
Stone	Calestone	8.70[‡‡]	60.0[‡‡]

See page 372 for footnotes.

(continued)

Ultimate Compressive Strength, *C* (continued)

Material	Product	C psi × 10³	MPa
Impression materials			
Agar[92]	Surgident	0.11[††]	0.76[††]
Alginate (6 min)[99]	Jeltrate	0.12[††]	0.82[††]
Polysulfide (8 min)[99]	Rubberjel	0.28[††]	1.93[††]
Porcelains[217]			
Feldspathic	Trubyte Bioform 2100	21.6[§§]	149[§§]
Fused to metal	Ceramco Opaque	21.7[§§]	150[§§]
Restorative materials			
Compomers	Compoglass[120,121]	33.1–41.3	228.0–285.0
	Dyract[122,218]	29.9	206.0
	Dyract AP[122]	36.5	252.0
	Elan[122]	43.9	303.0
	F2000[122]	37.3	257.0
	Hytac[120,122]	36.3	250.5
Glass ionomer[114]	Chelon-fil	22.4[#]	155[#]
	Chemfil II	28.6[#]	198[#]
	Chemfil II in caps	19.7[#]	136[#]
	Fuji II	23.0[#]	159[#]
	Ketac-fil Capsule	22.1[#]	152[#]
Metal-reinforced glass ionomer	Chelon-silver[114]	18.1[#]	125[#]
	Ketac-silver Capsule[114]	16.3[#]	113[#]
	Miracle mix[219]	18.7[#]	129[#]
Resin composite			
All-purpose	Brilliant[108]	40.6[#]	280[#]
	Charisma[108]	42.5[#]	293[#]
	Conquest DFC[108]	42.9[#]	296[#]
	Heliomolar Radiopaque[107]	49.3	340
	Herculite XR[107]	57.6	397
	Herculite XRV[108]	35.7[#]	246[#]
	Marathon[107]	43.4	299
	P-50 APC[107]	57.3	395
	Pertac Hybrid[108]	47.9[#]	330[#]
	Prisma APH[107]	55.5	383
	True Vitality[108]	27.4[#]	189[#]
	Z100[107]	65.0	448
Anterior[107]	Durafill	67.2	463
	Helio Progress	47.9	330
	Prisma Microfine	38.0	262
	Silar	41.0	283
	Silux	49.9	344
	Valux	62.4	430
	Visio Dispers	66.0	455
	Visio Fil	50.8	350

See page 372 for footnotes.

(continued)

Ultimate Compressive Strength, *C* (continued)

Material	Product	C psi × 10³	C MPa
Restorative materials			
Resin composite (continued)			
Flowable[126]	AeliteFlo	29.4	202.9
	Flow-It	35.9	247.7
	Florestore	30.4	209.6
	Revolution	28.4	195.9
	Ultra Seal XT Plus	23.5	161.7
Hybrid	Herculite[122]	34.2	236.0
	Prodigy[126,128]	34.6	238.5
	Z100[120,126]	45.0	310.1
Microfilled[129]	Heliomolar	34.4	236.91
Packable	Alert[128,129,131]	37.3	256.9
	Exp Condensable[131]	29.3	202.0
	Pyramid[128]	32.4	223.3
	Solitaire[128,129,131]	36.0	248.4
	Surefil[129,131]	37.1–51.7	256.0–356.8
Posterior	Clearfil Photoposterior[108]	42.6[#]	294[#]
	Heliomolar[107]	47.1	325
	Occlusin[107]	50.5	348
	P10[107]	56.6	390
	Post Comp II LC[107]	50.0	345
Resin-modified glass ionomers[220]	Fuji II LC	23.2	159.7
	Photac-Fil	18.6	128.2
	Vitremer[120]	23.1	159.1
Tooth structures			
Dentin[221]		43.1	297
Enamel (cusp)[94]		55.7	384
Vitreous carbon[25]		100	690
Waxes[113]			
Inlay casting, hard	Kerr blue hard	0.94[#]	6.48[#]
Inlay casting, soft	Kerr blue regular	1.13[#]	7.79[#]

See page 372 for footnotes.

Ultimate Tensile Strength, *UTS*

The *ultimate tensile strength* is defined as the maximum stress that a material can withstand before failure in tension. Unless indicated otherwise, values were determined by an extension test.

Material	Product	UTS	
		psi $\times 10^3$	MPa
Alumina (recrystallized)[10]		17.2*	119*
Amalgams (7d)			
Admixed	Dispersalloy[46]	6.94*	47.9*
	Phasealloy[222]	3.96*	27.3*
	Valiant PhD[222]	4.68*	32.2*
Lathe-cut[46]	New True Dentalloy	7.93*	54.7*
Bones (human)[82]			
Long bones			
Femur		17.5	121
Humerus		18.9	130
Radius		21.6	149
Tibia		20.3	140
Vertebrae			
Cervical		0.45	3.1
Lumbar		0.54	3.7
Cements (base consistency, 24 h)			
Polymer-modified ZOE[83]	B & T	0.500*	3.45*
Zinc phosphate[83]	Zinc Cement Improved	1.20*	8.3*
Zinc polyacrylate	Durelon[83]	2.25*	15.5*
	PCA[64]	1.00*	6.92*
Cements (luting consistency, 24 h)			
EBA-alumina ZOE[83]	Opotow	1.03*	7.12*
Glass ionomer[114]	Fuji I	0.80*	5.5*
	Ketac-cem Radiopaque	0.65*	4.5*
Noneugenol zinc oxide[83]	Nogenol	0.157*	1.08*
Polymer-modified ZOE[83]	Fynal	0.603*	4.16*
Resin[213]	Panavia EX	6.54*	45.1*
Zinc phosphate[213]	Flecks	1.35*	9.3*
	Modern Tenacin	1.38*	9.5*
Zinc polycarboxylate[213]	Durelon	2.19*	15.1*
	Shofu	1.57*	10.8*
Cements (liners, 24 h)[85]			
Calcium hydroxide	Dycal	0.33*	2.3*
	Life	0.35*	2.4*
Glass ionomer			
Light-cured	Fuji Lining LC[215]	2.06*	14.2*
	Vitrabond[86]	1.83*	12.6*
	XR Ionomer[86,215]	1.07*	7.4*
		0.32*	2.2*
	Zionomer[85]	0.55*	3.8*

*Values determined from diametral compression test.
†As cast.
‡Head speed, 0.05 cm/min.
§Heat treated.
¶Head speed, 50 cm/min.
#Head speed, 5 cm/min.
**Head speed, 25 cm/min.
††Head speed, 0.85 cm/min.
‡‡Head speed, 1.27 cm/min.
§§Head speed, 0.1 cm/min.
¶¶Head speed, 0.005 cm/min.

(continued)

Ultimate Tensile Strength, *UTS* (continued)

Material	Product	UTS	
		psi × 10³	MPa
Cements (liners, 24 h)			
Glass ionomer (continued)[114]			
Self-cured	Baseline	0.90*	6.2*
	Baseline in caps	1.52*	10.5*
	GC lining cement	0.57*	3.9*
	Ketac-bond	0.84*	5.8*
	Ketac-bond Capsule	1.60*	11.0*
	3M Glass ionomer liner	0.33*	2.3*
Resin[86]	Cavalite	3.33*	23.0*
	Timeline	2.04*	14.1*
Unmodified ZOE[83]	Cavitec	0.062*	0.43*
Cobalt-chromium alloys[87]	Advantage†	99.4‡	685‡
	Advantage§	95.7‡	660‡
	Cobond†	111.9‡	772‡
	Cobond§	113.9‡	785‡
	Genesis II†	93.9‡	647‡
	Genesis II§	86.9‡	599‡
	Master Tec†	103.0‡	710‡
	Master Tec§	108.9‡	751‡
	Novarex†	97.7‡	674‡
	Novarex§	101.8‡	702‡
	Novarex II†	93.4‡	644‡
	Novarex II§	95.4‡	658‡
	ViComp†	98.8‡	681‡
	ViComp§	104.2‡	718‡
	Vitallium[88]	126	869
Denture liners (resilient)[159]			
Polyphosphazene fluoroelastomer	Novus	0.534¶	3.68¶
Silicone	Molloplast-B	0.634¶	4.37¶
Denture resins[223]			
Acrylic	Kallodent 333	11.6#	80.4#
Polyvinylacrylic	Luxene T75	12.2#	84.3#
Gold (999.9 fine)[160]	Wilkinson Co.	15.6	108
Gold (condensed)[4]			
Foil		7.35	50.7
Mat		3.60	24.8
Powdered	Goldent	6.76	46.6
Gold alloys			
Type I[5]	Ney-Oro A	32.0	221
Type II[5]	Ney-Oro A-1	55.0	379
Type III, soft[5]	Ney-Oro B-2	61.0	421
Type III, hard	Ney-Oro B-2[5]	65.0	448
	Sjoding C-3[95]	66.3	457
Type IV, soft[5]	Ney-Oro G-3	68.0	469
Type IV, hard	Ney-Oro G-3[5]	110	759
	Sjoding D[95]	101	699

Ultimate Tensile Strength, *UTS* (continued)

Material	Product	UTS psi × 10³	MPa
Gold alloys (continued)			
64% Au-Ag-Cu, hard[95]	Begolloyd G	80.5	555
48% Au-Ag-Cu, hard[95]	Midigold	90.8	626
40% Au-Ag-Cu, soft[3]	Forticast	85	586
40% Au-Ag-Cu, hard[3]	Forticast	129	890
10%–15% Au-Ag-Pd, soft[5]	Paliney No. 4	81.0	559
10%–15% Au-Ag-Pd, hard[5]	Paliney No. 4	106	731
Au-Pd[96]	Olympia†	88.6‡	611‡
	Olympia§	97.5‡	672‡
Au-Pt-Pd[16]	TPW	38.1	263
Porcelain-fused-to-metal[3]	Jelenko O	73	503
Gutta-percha[97]	Indian Head	2.80	19.3
	Mynol	2.40	16.6
Gypsum (dried)[216]			
Improved stone	Velmix	1.11*	7.66*
Plaster	Calspar	0.600*	4.14*
Stone	Calestone	0.820*	5.66*
Impression materials			
Alginate	Krompan	0.034¶	0.24¶
Polyether	Impregum[224]	0.300¶	2.07¶
	Reprosil[224]		
Medium		0.287¶	1.98¶
	Permadyne[225]		
Light		0.122**	0.841**
Heavy		0.180**	1.24**
Polysulfide[224]			
Copper hydroxide cured	Omniflex	0.135¶	0.929¶
Lead dioxide cured	Coeflex	0.165¶	1.14¶
Silicone, addition[225]	Express		
Light		0.174**	1.20**
Medium		0.269**	1.85**
Putty		0.092**	0.634**
	Mirror 3 Extrude		
Light		0.193**	1.33**
Medium		0.232**	1.60**
Putty		0.330**	2.28**
Silicone, condensation[225]	Citricon		
Light		0.142**	0.979**
Putty		0.348**	2.40**
	Rapid		
Light		0.222**	1.53**
Putty		0.191**	1.32**
Iron-chromium alloys[88]			
Fixed partial denture	Dentillium C-B	134	924
Removable partial denture	Dentillium P-D	122	841

See page 376 for footnotes.

(continued)

Ultimate Tensile Strength, *UTS* (continued)

Material	Product	UTS	
		psi × 10³	MPa
Maxillofacial materials			
Polyurethane[162]	Epithane-3	0.12[††]	0.83[††]
Silicone rubber	A-102[162]	0.28[††]	1.9[††]
	A-2186[163]	0.73[¶]	5.0[¶]
	Cosmesil[163]	0.73[¶]	5.0[¶]
	MDX 4-4210[163]	0.57[¶]	4.0[¶]
	Medical Adhesive A[162]	0.16[††]	1.1[††]
	Silastic 4-4515[162]	1.38[††]	9.5[††]
Mouth protector materials			
Polyvinyl acetate-polyethylene[164]	Proform	1.06[**]	7.31[**]
	Sta-guard	0.46[**]	3.17[**]
Nickel-chromium alloys[96]	Ceramalloy II[†]	114.6[‡]	790[‡]
	Ceramalloy II[§]	103.0[‡]	710[‡]
	Micro-Bond N-P2[†]	73.3[‡]	505[‡]
	Micro-Bond N-P2[§]	71.5[‡]	493[‡]
	Ticon[†]	116.4[‡]	803[‡]
	Ticon[§]	96.7[‡]	667[‡]
	Unimetal[16]	119.9	827
Fixed partial denture[103]	Howmedica III	61.0	421
Porcelain-fused-to-metal[72]	Ultratek	133	917
Removable partial denture[226]	Ticonium 100	117	807
Palladium-based dental alloys[96]	Microstar[†]	100.8[‡]	695[‡]
	Microstar[§]	106.7[‡]	736[‡]
	Spartan[†]	165.5[‡]	1141[‡]
	Spartan[§]	163.2[‡]	1125[‡]
	W-1[†]	103.6[‡]	714[‡]
	W-1[§]	105.0[‡]	724[‡]
Polymers			
Polyetherurethane[104]	Pellethane 2363-80A	7.21[‡‡]	49.7[‡‡]
Polyetherurethane urea[104]	Biomer	7.28[‡‡]	50.2[‡‡]
Polymethyl methacrylate[105]		8.48[§§]	58.5[§§]
Porcelains[227]			
Feldspathic	Trubyte Bioform 2100	3.60	24.8
Fused to metal	Ceramco Opaque	5.40	37.2
Restorative materials			
Compomers	Compoglass[119]	4.9–6.4	34.0–44.0
	Dyract[119,122]	4.6–5.9	32.0–41.0
	Dyract AP[89,122]	5.4	37.5
	Elan[89,122]	7.1	48.8
	F2000[122,123]	4.4–5.2	30.5–35.6
	Hytac[89,122]	9.0	62.1
Glass ionomer[114]	Chelon-fil	1.46[*]	10.1[*]
	Chemfil II	1.80[*]	12.2[*]
	Chemfil II in caps	1.87[*]	12.9[*]
	Fuji II	1.26[*]	8.7[*]

See page 376 for footnotes.

(continued)

Ultimate Tensile Strength, *UTS* (continued)

Material	Product	UTS psi × 10³	UTS MPa
Restorative materials			
Glass ionomer (continued)	Fuji II[119]	1.0–1.3	7.0–9.0
	Fuji IX[123]	1.1	7.5
	Ketac-fil Capsule[114]	2.03*	14.0*[114]
Metal-reinforced glass ionomer	Chelon-silver[114]	1.60*	11.0*
	Ketac-silver Capsule[114]	1.87*	12.9*
	Miracle Mix[219]	1.33*	9.2*
Resin-modified glass ionomer	Fuji II LC[123,227]	1.4–4.5	9.5–31.0
	Photac-Fil[123]	3.0–3.7	20.4–25.3
Resin composite			
All-purpose	Brilliant[108]	5.80*	40*
	Charisma[108]	5.95*	41*
	Conquest DFC[108]	7.54*	52*
	Herculite XRV[228]	5.66*	39.0*
	Pertac Hybrid[108]	6.24*	43*
	True Vitality[108]	4.64*	32*
	Z100[228]	7.89*	54.4*
Anterior[229]	Multifil VS	6.16*	42.5*
	Prisma Fil	8.47*	58.4*
	Silux Plus	5.86*	40.4*
Hybrid	Herculite[122]	5.7	39.0
	Prodigy[89,109,128]	6.5	44.8
	Z100[109]	5.8	40.2
Microfilled[129]	Heliomolar	6.6	45.4
Packable	Alert[109,128–130]	5.1–9.9	35.0–68.4
	Exp Condensable[131]	4.6	32.0
	Pyramid[128]	6.9	47.75
	Solitaire[109,128]	6.8	47.0
	SureFil[109]	6.6	45.3
Posterior	Clearfil Photo Posterior[108]	6.53*	45*
	Coltene D1[229]	6.54*	45.1*
	Ful Fil[229]	8.67*	59.8*
	Heliomolar[229]	5.99*	41.3*
	Marathon One[228]	5.41*	37.3*
	P10[229]	9.25*	63.8*
Silicate[230]		0.630	4.34
Silver-palladium alloys[95]	Alborium	88.6	611
	Hvitstøp	76.3	526
	Palliag M	59.6	411
Fixed partial denture, soft[3]	Albacast	63.0	434
Fixed partial denture, hard[3]	Albacast	68.0	469
Porcelain-fused-to-metal[3]	Jel-5	105.0	724

See page 376 for footnotes.

(continued)

Ultimate Tensile Strength, *UTS* (continued)

Material	Product	UTS	
		psi $\times$ 10^3	MPa
Titanium[165]		79.8	550
Ti-6Al-4V alloy[165]		134.9	930
Tooth structures			
Dentin (bovine)[111]			
Demineralized		3.77[§§]	26.0[§§]
Mineralized		13.1[§§]	90.6[§§]
Dentin (human)[111]			
Demineralized		4.29[§§]	29.6[§§]
Mineralized		15.3[§§]	105.5[§§]
Enamel (bovine)[230]		3.00[¶¶]	20.7[¶¶]
Enamel (human)[230]		1.50[¶¶]	10.3[¶¶]

See page 376 for footnotes.

Vapor Pressure, *P*

Vapor pressure is the pressure exerted when a solid or liquid is in equilibrium with its own vapor.

Material	P (mm Hg)	Temperature (°C)
Mercury[231]	0.0014	22
	0.0050	38
	0.26	100
Mercury (in dental amalgam)[232]	10^{-8}	37
Monomers (fixed partial denture resins)[233]		
Methyl methacrylate	125	50
	760	100
Ethylene glycol dimethacrylate	8	100
1,3-butylene glycol dimethacrylate	1	100
Triethylene glycol dimethacrylate	0.01	100
Water[76]	19.8	22
	47.1	37

Vickers Hardness, *VHN*

The *Vickers hardness test,* or the 136° diamond pyramid hardness test, is a micro-indentation method. The indenter produces a square indentation, the diagonals of which are measured. The diamond pyramid hardness is calculated by dividing the applied load by the surface area of the indentation.

Material	Product	VHN (kg/mm^2)
Alumina (recrystallized)[10]		1200
Amalgam[234]		
Ag-Hg phase		120
Sn-Hg phase		15
Cements (liners)		
Glass ionomer[215]		
Light-cured	Fuji Lining LC	57
	Vitrabond	62
	XR Ionomer	38
Cobalt-chromium alloys	Genesis II[3]	350
	Master Tec[12]	390
	Novarex[13]	350
Gold alloys		
Type I[5]	Ney-Oro A	55
Type II[5]	Ney-Oro A-1	105
Type III, soft[5]	Ney-Oro B-2	125
Type III, hard[5]	Ney-Oro B-2	135
Type IV, soft[5]	Ney-Oro G-3	160
Type IV, hard[5]	Ney-Oro G-3	250
40% Au-Ag-Cu, soft[3]	Forticast	193
40% Au-Ag-Cu, hard[3]	Forticast	292
10%–15% Au-Ag-Pd, soft[5]	Paliney No. 4	170
10%–15% Au-Ag-Pd, hard[5]	Paliney No. 4	230
Au-Pd[3]	Olympia	220
Au-Pt-Pd alloy[16]	TPW	104
Porcelain-fused-to-metal[3]	Jelenko O	182
Gypsum[66]	Moldablaster	12
Nickel-chromium alloys	Unimetal[16]	395
Fixed partial denture[112]	Howmedica III	330
Porcelain-fused-to-metal[72]	Ultratek	270
Palladium-based dental alloys[3,12,158]	Athenium*	270
	Legacy*	270
	Liberty*	340
	Microstar	265
	Protocol*	235
	PTM-88*	235
	Spartan*	360
	W1*	240
	W1†	285
Porcelains[106]		
Alumina-reinforced	Vitadur-N (core)	775
Castable ceramic	Dicor	449
Ceramic-whisker-reinforced	Mirage II	663
Feldspathic	Excelco	663
	Vita VMK 68	703

*Specimens subjected to the porcelain firing cycles.
†Oven hardened.

(continued)

Vickers Hardness, *VHN* (continued)

Material	Product	VHN (kg/mm^2)
Porcelains[106]		
Feldspathic (continued)	Vita VMK 68-N	703
	Will-Ceram	611
Leucite-reinforced	Optec HSP	703
Restorative materials		
Compomers	Compoglass[120]	33.0
	Dyract[120,121]	31.0–60.0
	Dyract AP[122]	63.0
	Elan[122]	86.0
	F2000[122]	119.0
	Hytac[120]	65.0
Glass ionomer[235]	Chemfil II	51
	Fujicap II	74
	Ketac-Fil	90
Metal-reinforced glass ionomer[235]	Ketac-Silver	40
Resin composite		
All-purpose[107]	Charisma	81
	Conquest DFC	95
	Heliomolar Radiopaque	56
	Herculite XR	74
	Marathon	100
	P-50 APC	159
	Pertac Hybrid	126
	Prisma APH	77
	Z100	120
Anterior[107]	Durafill	48
	Helio Progress	50
	Multifil VS	55
	Prisma Fil	83
	Prisma Microfine	39
	Silux Plus[235]	59
		41
	Valux	107
	Visio Dispers	63
	Visio Fil	160
Hybrid	Herculite[122]	71.0
	Tetric Ceram[236]	54.8
	Z100[120]	97.0
Packable[131,236]	Alert	88.5
	Exp Condensable	67.0
	Solitaire	45.3
	Surefil	83.2

See page 382 for footnotes.

(continued)

Vickers Hardness, *VHN (continued)*

Material	Product	VHN (kg/mm²)
Restorative materials		
Resin composite (continued)[107]		
Posterior	Clearfil Photo Posterior	159
	Ful Fil	97
	Heliomolar	61
	P-10	174
	Post Comp II LC	97
Resin-modified glass ionomers	Fuji II LC[220]	36.2
	Photac-Fil[220]	37.4
	Vitremer[120]	41.0
Silver-palladium alloys[3]		
Fixed partial denture, soft	Albacast	143
Fixed partial denture, hard	Albacast	154
Porcelain-fused-to-metal	Jel-5	187
Titanium[165]		210
Ti-6Al-4V alloy[165]		320
Tooth structures		
Dentin[107,235]		60
		57
Enamel[108,235]		408
		294

See page 382 for footnotes.

Viscosity, η

Viscosity is defined as the resistance of a substance to flow under stress. Units are g/(cm s) or *poise*. *Centipoise* (cp) is 10^{-2} poise.

Material	Product	η (cp)	Temperature (°C)
Cements[237]			
Zinc phosphate	Modern Tenacin	43,200*	18
		94,700*	25
Zinc polycarboxylate	Durelon	101,000*	18
		109,800*	25
Impression materials			
Agar[238]		281,000	45
Alginate[239]	Jeltrate	252,000†	37
Impression plaster[239]	Plastogum	23,800†	37
Polysulfide, light[238,239]		109,000‡	36
	Permlastic	57,200†	37
Polysulfide, heavy[238]		1,360,000‡	36
Silicone, addition[240]			
Medium	Hydrosil	1,294,000§	37
	Imprint	797,000§	37
	Omnisil	1,025,000§	37
Heavy	Baysilex	689,000§	37
Silicone, condensation[238,239]			
Light		63,400‡	36
	Elasticon	95,000†	37
Medium		420,000‡	36
Zinc oxide–eugenol[239]	Luralite	99,600†	37
Mercury[241]		1.554	20
Monomers (fixed partial denture resins)			
Methyl methacrylate[69]		0.52	25
Ethylene glycol dimethacrylate[71]		3.40	25
1,3-butylene glycol dimethacrylate[71]		3.5	25
Triethylene glycol dimethacrylate[71]		7.5	25
Water[77]		1.000	20

*Measured at 45 s after completion of mix and 5 rpm.
†Measured at 1.5 min from start of mix and 5 rpm.
‡Measured at 2 min from start of mix.
§Measured at 1 min from start of mix and 2.5 rpm.

Water Sorption

Water sorption of a material represents the amount of water adsorbed on the surface and absorbed into the body of the material. The method of testing is described in American National Standards Institute/American Dental Association Specification Nos. 12 and 27.[45]

Material	Product	Water sorption (mg/cm^2)
Denture liners (resilient)[183]		
Polyphosphazene fluoroelastomer	Novus	4.01*
Silicone	Molloplast-B	0.23*
Denture resins[242]		
Acrylic	Hy-Pro Lucitone	0.69†
Polystyrene	Jectron	0.36†
Polyvinylacrylic	Luxene 44	0.26†
Pit and fissure sealants		
Light-cured	Nuva-Seal[194]	0.9*
Self-cured	Delton[73]	1.29‡
	9075[194]	1.8*
Restorative materials[243]		
Resin composite, posterior	Occlusin	0.71*
	P-50	0.52*

*Stored for 7 days.
†Stored for 1 day.
‡Stored for 30 days.

Yield Strength, YS

The *yield strength* is defined as the stress at which a material exhibits a specified limiting deviation from proportionality of stress to strain. The amount of permanent strain arbitrarily selected is referred to as the *percent offset* and is commonly 0.1%.

Material	Product	YS psi × 10³	YS MPa
Cements (liners)[86]			
Glass ionomer			
Light-cured	Vitrabond	1.60	11.0
	XR Ionomer	3.15	21.7
Resin	Cavalite	8.99	62.0
	Timeline	4.31	29.7
Cobalt-chromium alloys[87]	Advantage*	69.8[†]	481[†]
	Advantage[‡]	67.7[†]	467[†]
	Cobond*	71.8[†]	495[†]
	Cobond[‡]	66.0[†]	455[†]
	Genesis II*	68.4[†]	472[†]
	Genesis II[‡]	71.9[†]	496[†]
	Master Tec*	70.1[†]	483[†]
	Master Tec[‡]	73.8[†]	509[†]
	Novarex*	68.9[†]	475[†]
	Novarex[‡]	81.4[†]	561[†]
	Novarex II*	70.9[†]	489[†]
	Novarex II[‡]	75.5[†]	521[†]
	Vi-Comp*	77.3[†]	533[†]
	Vi-Comp[‡]	73.8[†]	509[†]
	Vitallium[88]	93.4	644
Gold alloys			
40% Au-Ag-Cu, soft[3]	Forticast	68[†]	469[†]
40% Au-Ag-Cu, hard[3]	Forticast	125[†]	862[†]
Au-Pd[96]	Olympia*	63.3[†]	436[†]
	Olympia[‡]	77.9[†]	537[†]
Porcelain-fused-to-metal[3]	Jelenko O	72.5[†]	500[†]
Gutta-percha[97]	Indian Head	1.70	11.7
	Mynol	1.20	8.28
Iron-chromium alloy[88]			
Removable partial denture	Dentillium P-D	94.4	651
Nickel-chromium alloys[96]	Ceramalloy II*	71.3[†]	492[†]
	Ceramalloy II[‡]	49.6[†]	342[†]
	Micro-Bond N-P2*	44.6[†]	308[†]
	Micro-Bond N-P2[‡]	34.0[†]	234[†]
	Ticon*	103.0[†]	710[†]
	Ticon[‡]	71.9[†]	496[†]
Palladium-based dental alloys[157]	Athenium	76.1	525
	Legacy	95.5	658
	Liberty	115.5	796

*As cast.
[†]Percent offset of 0.2%.
[‡]Heat treated.

(continued)

Yield Strength, *YS* (continued)

Material	Product	YS psi × 10³	YS MPa
Palladium-based dental alloys (continued)[96]	Microstar*	76.8[†]	530[†]
	Microstar[‡]	70.7[†]	487[†]
	Protocol[157]	68.7	474
	PTM-88[157]	83.0	572
	Spartan*	153.7[†]	1060[†]
	Spartan[‡]	138.6[†]	956[†]
	W-1*	76.1[†]	525[†]
	W-1[‡]	80.5[†]	555[†]
Restorative materials[23]			
Acrylic	Sevriton	7.50	51.7
Resin composite	Adaptic	23.4	161
Silver-palladium alloys[3]			
Fixed partial denture	Albacast	42[†]	290[†]
Porcelain-fused-to-metal	Jel-5	70[†]	483[†]

See page 387 for footnotes.

Zeta Potential, ζ

A charged particle suspended in an electrolytic solution attracts ions of opposite charge to those at its surface, where they form the Stern layer. To maintain the electric balance of the suspending fluid, ions of opposite charge are attracted to the Stern layer. The potential at the surface of that part of this diffuse double layer of ions that can move with the particle when subjected to a voltage gradient is the *zeta potential*. This potential measured is very dependent upon the ionic concentration, pH, viscosity, and dielectric constant of the solution being analyzed.

Material	ζ, mV
Bacteria	
A odontolyticus A7-1[31]	−16.0*
A viscosus C7-4[31]	−11.1*
S mutans	
C7-3[31]	−7.1*
M4S[244]	−13.7†
S salivarius B3-4[31]	−4.8*
S sanguis C7-2[31]	−12.4*
Bone[245]	−7.01‡
Hydroxyapatite, synthetic[244,246]	−10.9§
	−9.0†
Polymers[42]	
Polyetherurethane	−17.3
Silicone	−98.5
Tooth structures[247]	
Calculus	−15.3¶
Cementum, exposed	−6.96¶
Cementum, unexposed	−9.34¶
Dentin[31]	−6.23¶
	+0.4*
Enamel[31]	−10.3¶
	+0.9*

*Measured at 25°C in a physiologic ionic strength ($\mu = 0.057$) medium, pH 7.0.
†Measured in distilled water.
‡Measured in 0.145 M NaCl solution, pH 7.3.
§Measured at 25°C at a solid/solution ratio of 0.1.
¶Measured at 30°C in Hanks' balanced salt solution.

■ References

1. Sturdevant CM, Roberson TM, Heymann HO, Sturdevant JR (eds). The Art and Science of Operative Dentistry. St Louis: Mosby, 1995.

2. Craig RG (ed). Restorative Dental Materials, ed 9. St Louis: Mosby-Year Book, 1993.

3. JF Jelenko & Co. Product information sheet. Armonk, NY: JF Jelenko & Co.

4. Mahan J, Charbeneau GT. A study of certain mechanical properties and the density of condensed specimens made from various forms of pure gold. Am Acad Gold Foil Operators J 1965;8:6–12.

5. JM Ney Co. Product information sheet. Bloomfield, Conn: JM Ney Co.

6. Tillitson EW, Craig RG, Peyton FA. Friction and wear of restorative dental materials. J Dent Res 1971;50:149–154.

7. Shirazi-Adl A, Dammak M, Paiement G. Experimental determination of friction characteristics at the trabecular bone/porous-coated metal interface in cementless implants. J Biomed Mater Res 1993;27:167–175.

8. Graiver D, Durall RL, Okada T. Surface morphology and friction coefficient of various types of Foley catheter. Biomaterials 1993;14:465–469.

9. Koran A, Craig RG, Tillitson EW. Coefficient of friction of prosthetic tooth materials. J Prosthet Dent 1972;27:269–274.

10. McLean JW, Hughes TH. The reinforcement of dental porcelain with the ceramic oxides. Br Dent J 1965;119:251–267.

11. Civjan S, Brauer GM. Physical properties of cements, based on zinc oxide, hydrogenated rosin, o-ethoxybenzoic acid, and eugenol. J Dent Res 1964;43:281–299.

12. Ivoclar Williams. Product information sheet. Amherst, NY: Ivoclar Williams.

13. Jeneric/Pentron. Product information sheet. Wallingford, Conn: Jeneric/Pentron.

14. Chandler HH, Bowen RL, Paffenbarger GC. Physical properties of a radiopaque denture base material. J Biomed Mater Res 1971;5:335–357.

15. Woelfel JB, Paffenbarger GC, Sweeney WT. Some physical properties of organic denture-base materials. J Am Dent Assoc 1963;67:489–504.

16. Akagi K, Okamoto Y, Matsuura T, Horibe T. Properties of test metal ceramic titanium alloys. J Prosthet Dent 1992;68: 462–467.

17. Whitlock RP, Tesk JA, Widera GEO, Holmes A, Parry EE. Consideration of some factors influencing compatibility of dental porcelains and alloys. Part I. Thermo-physical properties. In: Proceedings of the 4th International Precious Metals Conference, Toronto, ON, June 1980. Willowdale, Ontario: Pergamon Press, 1981:273–282.

18. Price WA. Report of laboratory investigations on the physical properties of root filling materials and the efficiency of root fillings for blocking infection from sterile tooth structures. Natl Dent Assoc J 1918;5:1260–1280.

19. Jørgensen KD. Thermal expansion of addition polymerization (Type II) silicone impression materials. Aust Dent J 1982; 27:377–381.

20. Powers JM, Hostetler RW, Dennison JB. Thermal expansion of composite resins and sealants. J Dent Res 1979;58:584–587.

21. Boyer HE, Gall TL (eds). Metals Handbook Desk Edition. Metals Park, Ohio: American Society for Metals, 1985.

22. Bever MB (ed). Encyclopedia of Materials Science and Engineering. New York: Pergamon Press, 1986:1059.

23. Dennison JB, Craig RG. Physical properties and finished surface texture of composite restorative resins. J Am Dent Assoc 1972;85:101–108.

24. Souder WH, Paffenbarger GC. Physical properties of dental materials. National Bureau Standards Circular no. C433. Washington, DC: US Government Printing Office, 1942.

25. Benson J. Elemental carbon as a biomaterial. J Biomed Mater Res 1971;5(6):41–47.

26. Craig RG, Eick JD, Peyton FA. Properties of natural waxes used in dentistry. J Dent Res 1965;44:1308–1316.

27. O'Brien WJ, Groh CL, Boenke KM. A one-dimensional color order system for dental shade guides. Dent Mater 1989; 5:371–374.

28. O'Brien WJ, Groh CL, Boenke KM. A new, small-color-difference equation for dental shades. J Dent Res 1990;69:1762–1764.

29. O'Brien WJ, Groh CL, Boenke KM. Unpublished data. Ann Arbor: Univ of Michigan School of Dentistry, 1990.

30. O'Brien WJ. Capillary penetration of liquids between dissimilar solids [doctoral dissertation]. Microfilm no. 6715666. Ann Arbor: Univ of Michigan, 1967.

31. Weerkamp AH, Uyen HM, Busscher HJ. Effect of zeta potential and surface energy on bacterial adhesion to uncoated and saliva-coated human enamel and dentin. J Dent Res 1988; 67:1483–1487.

32. O'Kane C, Oliver RG, Blunden RE. Surface roughness and droplet contact angle measurement of various orthodontic bonding cements. Br J Orthod 1993;20:297–305.

33. O'Brien WJ, Ryge G. Wettability of poly(methyl methacrylate) treated with silicon tetrachloride. J Prosthet Dent 1965;15: 304–308.

34. Winkler S, Ortman HR, Ryczek MT. Improving the retention of complete dentures. J Prosthet Dent 1975;34:11–15.

35. Craig RG, Berry GC, Peyton FA. Wetting of poly(methyl methacrylate) and polystyrene by water and saliva. J Phys Chem 1960;64:541–543.

36. O'Brien WJ, Ryge G. Contact angles of drops of enamels on metals. J Prosthet Dent 1965;15:1094–1100.

37. DeWald JP, Nakajima H, Schneiderman E, Okabe T. Wettability of impression materials treated with disinfectants. Am J Dent 1992;5:103–108.

38. Chong YH, Soh G, Setchell DJ, Wickens JL. The relationship between contact angles of die stone on elastomeric impression materials and voids in stone casts. Dent Mater 1990;6: 162–166.

39. Cullen DR, Mikesell JW, Sandrik JL. Stability of elastomeric impression materials and voids in gypsum casts. J Prosthet Dent 1991;66:261–265.

40. Dentsply/Caulk Laboratories. Product information sheet. Milford, DE: Dentsply/Caulk Laboratories, 1999.

41. Arshady R. Microspheres for biomedical applications: Preparation of reactive and labelled microspheres. Biomaterials 1993; 14:5–15.

42. Fujimoto K, Minato M, Tadokoro H, Ikada Y. Platelet deposition onto polymeric surfaces during shunting. J Biomed Mater Res 1993;27:335–343.

43. Fan PL, O'Brien WJ, Craig RG. Wetting properties of sealants and glazes. Oper Dent 1979;4:100–103.

44. Strach EP, Fan PL, O'Brien WJ. Penetrativity and wetting of topical fluoride preparations: An in vitro study. J Clin Prev Dent 1979;1(6):11–13.

45. Council on Dental Materials, Instruments, and Equipment. Certification programs of the Council on Dental Materials, Instruments and Equipment: ANSI/ADA specifications. Chicago: Council on Dental Materials, Instruments and Equipment, 1990.

46. Mahler DB, Terkla LG, Van Eysden J, Reisbick MH. Marginal fracture vs mechanical properties of amalgam. J Dent Res 1970;49:1452–1457.

47. Mahler DB, Adey JD. Factors influencing the creep of dental amalgam. J Dent Res 1991;70:1394–1400.

48. Holland RI, Jørgensen RB, Ekstrand J. Strength and creep of dental amalgam: the effects of deviation from recommended procedure. J Prosthet Dent 1985;54:189–194.

49. Iglesias AM, Sorensen SE, Carter JM, Wilko RA. Some properties of high-copper amalgam alloys comparing hand and mechanical trituration. J Prosthet Dent 1984;52:194–198.

50. Chung K. Effects of palladium addition on properties of dental amalgams. Dent Mater 1992;8:190–192.

51. Glantz P-O. On wettability and adhesiveness. A study of enamel, dentin, some restorative materials, and dental plaque. Odontol Revy 1969;20(suppl 17):1–132.

52. Carter JM, Flynn HE, Meenaghan MA, Natiella JR, Akers CK, Baier RE. Organic surface film contamination of Vitallium implants. J Biomed Mater Res 1981;15:843–851.

53. Lyman DJ, Muir WM, Lee IJ. The effect of chemical structure and surface properties of polymers on the coagulation of blood. I. Surface free energy effects. Trans Am Soc Artif Int Organs 1965;11:301–306.

54. Vassilakos N, Fernandes CP. Effect of salivary films on the surface properties of elastomeric impression materials. Eur J Prosthodont Restorative Dent 1993;2(1):29–33.

55. Bordenave L, Baquey Ch, Bareille R, et al. Endothelial cell compatibility testing of three different Pellethanes. J Biomed Mater Res 1993;27:1367–1381.

56. Uy KC, Chang R. An approach to the study of the mechanism of adhesion to teeth. In: Austin RH, Wilsdorf HGF, Phillips RW (eds). Adhesive Restorative Dental Materials. II: Proceedings of a workshop of the Bio-Materials Research Advisory Committee. Public Health Service Publication. no. 1494. Washington, DC: US Government Printing Office, 1966:103–131.

57. Lautenschlager EP, Monaghan P. Titanium and titanium alloys as dental materials. Int Dent J 1993;43:245–253.

58. de Gee AJ, Feilzer AJ, Davidson CL. True linear polymerization shrinkage of unfilled resins and composites determined with a linometer. Dent Mater 1993;9:11–14.

59. Moroi HH, Okimoto K, Moroi R, Terada Y. Numeric approach to the biomechanical analysis of thermal effects in coated implants. Int J Prosthodont 1993;6:564–572.

60. Fukase Y, Saitoh M, Kaketani M, Ohashi M, Nishiyama M. Thermal coefficients of paste-paste type pulp capping cements. Dent Mater J 1992;11:189–196.

61. Inoue T, Saitoh M, Nishiyama M. Thermal properties of glass ionomer cement. J Nihon Univ Sch Dent 1993;35:252–257.

62. Civjan S, Barone JJ, Reinke PE, Selting WJ. Thermal properties of nonmetallic restorative materials. J Dent Res 1972;51:1030–1037.

63. Brady AP, Lee H, Orlowski JA. Thermal conductivity studies of composite dental restorative materials. J Biomed Mater Res 1974;8:471–485.

64. Barton JA Jr, Brauer GM, Antonucci JM, Raney MJ. Reinforced polycarboxylate cements. J Dent Res 1975;54:310–323.

65. Yoon HS, Newnham RE. Elastic properties of fluorapatite. Am Mineralogist 1969;54:1193–1197.

66. Shell JS. Some factors influencing specific gravity determinations on gold cast alloys. J Dent Res 1966;45:337–342.

67. Li J, Alatli-Kut I, Hermansson L. High-strength dental gypsum prepared by cold isostatic pressing. Biomaterials 1993;14:1186–1187.

68. Pamenius M, Ohlson NG. Determination of thermal properties of impression materials. Dent Mater 1992;8:140–144.

69. Riddle EH. Monomeric Acrylic Esters. New York: Van Nostrand Reinhold, 1954:13.

70. Sartomer Monomer Product Information Chart. 19380. West Chester, PA: Sartomer.

71. Austenal Dental. Product information sheet. Chicago, IL: Austenal Dental.

72. Moffa JP, Lugassy AA, Guckes AD, Gettleman L. An evaluation of nonprecious alloys for use with porcelain veneers. Part I. Physical properties. J Prosthet Dent 1973;30:424–431.

73. Fan PL, Edahl A, Leung RL, Stanford JW. Alternative interpretations of water sorption values of composite resins. J Dent Res 1985;64:78–80.

74. Manly RS, Hodge HC, Ange LE. Density and refractive index studies of dental hard tissues. II. Density distribution curves. J Dent Res 1939;18:203–211.

75. Berghash SR, Hodge HC. Density and refractive index studies of dental hard tissues. III. Density distribution of deciduous enamel and dentin. J Dent Res 1940;19:487–495.

76. Lide DR (ed). CRC Handbook of Chemistry and Physics, ed 73. Boca Raton, FL: CRC Press, 1992–1993.

77. Koran A, Craig RG. Dynamic mechanical properties of maxillofacial materials. J Dent Res 1975;54:1216–1221.

78. Godwin WC, Koran A, Craig RG. Evaluation of the dynamic and static physical properties of mouth protectors. Presented at the annual meeting of the International Association for Dental Research, Dental Materials Group, Atlanta, Ga, 21–24 Mar 1974.

79. Papadogiannis Y, Lakes RS, Petrou-Americanos A, Theothoridou-Pahini S. Temperature dependence of the dynamic viscoelastic behavior of chemical- and light-cured composites. Dent Mater 1993;9:118–122.

80. Jones DW, Jones PA, Wilson HJ. The modulus of elasticity of dental ceramics. Dent Pract Dent Rec 1972;22:170–173.

81. Bryant RW, Mahler DB. Modulus of elasticity in bending of composites and amalgams. J Prosthet Dent 1986;56:243–248.

82. Boeree NR, Dove J, Cooper JJ, Knowles J, Hastings GW. Development of a degradable composite for orthopaedic use: Mechanical evaluation of an hydroxyapatite-polyhydroxybutyrate composite material. Biomaterials 1993;14:793–796.

83. Powers JM, Farah JW, Craig RG. Modulus of elasticity and strength properties of dental cements. J Am Dent Assoc 1976;92:588–591.

84. Øilo G, Espevik S. Compressive strength and deformation of dental cements [in Norweigen]. Nor Tannlaegeforen Tid 1978;88:500–503.

85. Tam LE, Pulver E, McComb D, Smith DC. Physical properties of calcium hydroxide and glass-ionomer base and lining materials. Dent Mater 1989;5:145–149.

86. Tam LE, McComb D, Pulver F. Physical properties of proprietary light-cured lining materials. Oper Dent 1991;16:210–217.

87. Morris HF. Properties of cobalt-chromium metal ceramic alloys after heat treatment. J Prosthet Dent 1989;62:426–433.

88. Morris HF, Asgar K. Physical properties and microstructure of four new commercial partial denture alloys. J Prosthet Dent 1975;33:36–46.

89. Latta MA, Randall CJ. Physical properties of compomer restorative materials [abstract 412]. J Dent Res 1999;78:157.

90. Smith LT, Powers JM, Ladd D. Mechanical properties of new denture resins polymerized by visible light, heat, and microwave energy. Int J Prosthodont 1992;5:315–320.

91. Scherrer SS, de Rijk WG. The fracture resistance of all-ceramic crowns on supporting structures with different elastic moduli. Int J Prosthodont 1993;6:462–467.

92. Craig RG, Peyton FA. Physical properties of elastic duplicating materials. J Dent Res 1960;39:391–404.

93. Peyton FA, Craig RG. Current evaluation of plastics in crown and bridge prosthesis. J Prosthet Dent 1963;13:743–753.

94. Craig RG, Peyton FA, Johnson DW. Compressive properties of enamel, dental cements, and gold. J Dent Res 1961;40:936–945.

95. Øilo G, Gjerdet NR. Dental casting alloys with a low content of noble metals: Physical properties. Acta Odontol Scand 1983;41:111–116.

96. Morris HF. Veterans Administration Cooperative Studies Project No. 147/242. Part VII: The mechanical properties of metal ceramic alloys as cast and after simulated porcelain firing. J Prosthet Dent 1989;61:160–169.

97. Friedman CE. The chemical composition and mechanical properties of gutta-percha endodontic filling materials [thesis]. Chicago: Loyola Univ Medical Center, l972.

98. Combe EC, Smith DC. Some properties of gypsum plasters. Br Dent J 1964;117:237–245.

99. MacPherson GW, Craig RG, Peyton FA. Mechanical properties of hydrocolloid and rubber impression materials. J Dent Res 1967;46:714–721.

100. Jamani KD, Harrington E, Wilson HJ. Rigidity of elastomeric impression materials. J Oral Rehabil 1989;16:241–248.

101. Lontz JF, Schweiger JW, Burger AW. Modifying stress-strain profiles of polysiloxane elastomers for improved maxillofacial conformity. Presented at the annual meeting of the International Association for Dental Research, Dental Materials Group, Atlanta, Ga, 21–24 Mar 1974.

102. Kase HR, Tesk JA. Elastic constants of nonprecious alloys at room and elevated temperatures. Presented at the annual meeting of the International Association for Dental Research, Dental Materials Group, Dallas, TX, 15–18 Mar 1984.

103. Caputo AA, Reisbick MH. Mechanical properties of a nonprecious type III alloy. J Dent Res 1975;54:428.

104. Hergenrother RW, Wabers HD, Cooper SL. Effect of hard segment chemistry and strain on the stability of polyurethanes: In vivo biostability. Biomaterials 1993;14:449–458.

105. Caycik S, Jagger RG. The effect of cross-linking chain length on mechanical properties of a dough-molded poly(methylmethacrylate) resin. Dent Mater 1992;8:153–157.

106. Seghi RR, Denry I, Brajevic F. Effects of ion exchange on hardness and fracture toughness of dental ceramics. Int J Prosthodont 1992;5:309–314.

107. Willems G, Lambrechts P, Braem M, Celis JP, Vanherle G. A classification of dental composites according to their morphological and mechanical characteristics. Dent Mater 1992;8:310–319.

108. Eldiwany M, Powers JM, George LA. Mechanical properties of direct and post-cured composites. Am J Dent 1993;6:222–224.

109. Kelsey WP, Latta MA, Barkmeier WW. Physical properties of high density, composite restorative materials [abstract 810]. J Dent Res 1999;78:207.

110. Beatty MW, Pidaparti RMV. Elastic and fracture properties of dental direct filling materials. Biomaterials 1993;14:999–1002.

111. Sano H, Ciucchi B, Matthews WG, Pashley DH. Tensile properties of mineralized and demineralized human and bovine dentin. J Dent Res 1994;73:1205–1211.

112. Dyment MI, Synge JL. The elasticity of the periodontal membrane. Oral Health 1935;25:105–109.

113. Craig RG, Eick JD, Peyton FA. Strength properties of waxes at various temperatures and their practical application. J Dent Res 1967;46:300–305.

114. Cattani-Lorente M-A, Godin C, Meyer JM. Early strength of glass ionomer cements. Dent Mater 1993;9:57–62.

115. Richter WA, Mahler DB. Physical properties vs clinical performance of pure gold restorations. J Prosthet Dent 1973;29:434–438.

116. Jones DW. The high temperature strength and thermal expansion of investment mould refractories. In: Proceedings of the 11th International Ceramic Congress, Madrid, 1968:343–381.

117. Seghi RR, Daher T, Caputo A. Relative flexural strength of dental restorative ceramics. Dent Mater 1990;6:181–184.

118. O'Brien WJ. Magnesia ceramic jacket crowns. Dent Clin North Am 1985;29:719–723.

119. Meyer JM, Cattani-Lorente MA, Dupuis V. Compomer: Between glass-ionomer cements and composites. Biomaterials 1998;19:529–539.

120. El-Kalla IH, Garcia-Godoy F. Mechanical properties of compomer restorative materials. Oper Dent 1999;24:2–8.

121. Compoglass F physical properties [product information sheet]. Amherst, NY: Ivoclar Vivadent.

122. Thompson JY, Ruddle DE, Stamatiades PJ, Ward JC, Bayne SC, Shellard ER. Mechanical properties and wear behavior of new compomer materials [abstract 406]. J Dent Res 1999;78:156.

123. Iazetti G, Burgess JO, Tavares C. Mechanical properties of fluoride releasing materials [abstract 417]. J Dent Res 1999;78:158.

124. Dhummarungrong S, Moore BK, Avery DR. Properties related to strength and resistance to abrasion of VariGlass VLC, Fuji II LC, Ketac-Silver, and Z-100 composite resin. ASDC J Dent Child 1994;61:17–20.

125. Swift EJ Jr, LeValley BD, Boyer DB. Evaluation of new methods for composite repair. Dent Mater 1992;8:362–365.

126. Bayne SC, Thompson JY, Swift EJ Jr, Stamatiades P, Wilkerson M. A characterization of first-generation flowable composites. J Am Dent Assoc 1998;129:567–577.

127. Nguyen D, Angeletakis C, Shellard E. A new high polish retention microhybrid composite [abstract 1081]. J Dent Res 2000;79:279.

128. MacGregor KM, Cobb DS, Denehy GE. Physical properties of new packable composites vs. a conventional hybrid [abstract 1777]. 2000;J Dent Res 79:366.

129. MacGregor KM, Cobb DS, Vargas MA. Physical proprties of condensable versus conventional composites [abstract 411]. J Dent Res 1999;78:157.

130. Lohbauer U, Schoch M, Frankenburger R, Braem MJA, Kramer N. Flexural strength characterization of resin composites by Weibull analysis [abstract 805]. J Dent Res 1999;78:206.

131. Ruddle DE, Thompson JY, Stamatiades PJ, Ward JC, Bayne SC, Shellard ER. Mechanical properties and wear behavior of condensable composites [abstract 407]. J Dent Res 1999;78:156.

132. Craig RG, Sun Z. Trends in elastomeric impression materials. Oper Dent 1994;19:138–145.

133. Craig RG, Urquiola NJ, Liu CC. Comparison of commercial elastomeric impression materials. Oper Dent 1990;15:94–104.

134. Mandelkern L, Quinn FA Jr, Roberts DE. Thermodynamics of crystallization in high polymers: Gutta percha. Am Chem Soc J 1956;78:926–932.

135. Powers JM, Craig RG, Peyton FA. Calorimetric analysis of commercial and dental waxes. J Dent Res 1969;48:1165–1170.

136. Ekegren S, Ohrn O, Granath D, Kinell P-O. Heat of polymerization of chloroprene. Acta Chem Scand 1950;4:126–139.

137. Neville HA. Adsorption and reaction. I. The setting of plaster of Paris. J Phys Chem 1926;30:1037–1042.

138. Carlstrom D. Polarization microscopy of dental enamel with reference to incipient carious lesions. In: Staple PH (ed). Advances in Oral Biology. London: Academic Press, 1964:277.

139. Perloff A, Posner AS. Preparation of pure hydroxyapatite crystals. Science 1956;124:583–584.

140. Asmussen E, Uno S. Solubility parameters, fractional polarities, and bond strengths of some intermediary resins used in dentin bonding. J Dent Res 1993;72:558–565.

141. Houwink B. The index of refraction of dental enamel apatite. Br Dent J 1974;137:472–475.

142. Craig RG, O'Brien WJ, Powers JM. Dental Materials-Properties and Manipulation. St Louis: Mosby, 1992.

143. White SN, Yu Z. Physical properties of fixed prosthodontic, resin composite luting agents. Int J Prosthodont 1993;6:384–389.

144. Murchison DF, Moore BK. Influence of curing time and distance on microhardness of eight light-cured liners. Oper Dent 1992;17:135–141.

145. Martins EA, Peyton FA, Kingery RH. Properties of custom-made plastic teeth formed by different techniques. J Prosthet Dent 1962;12:1059–1065.

146. Lekka MP, Papagiannoulis L, Eliades GC, Caputo AA. A comparative in vitro study of visible light-cured sealants. J Oral Rehabil 1989;16:287–299.

147. Miller GR, Powers JM, Ludema KC. Frictional behavior and surface failure of dental feldspathic porcelain. Wear 1975;31:307–316.

148. Natho SA, Chmielewski MB, Kirkup RE. Effects of Colgate Platinum Professional Toothwhitening System™ on microhardness of enamel, dentin, and composite resins. Compend Contin Educ Dent 1994;15(suppl 17):S627–S630.

149. Pagniano RP, Johnston WM. The effect of unfilled resin dilution on composite resin hardness and abrasion resistance. J Prosthet Dent 1993;70:214–218.

150. Pilo R, Cardash HS. Post-irradiation polymerization of different anterior and posterior visible light–activated resin composites. Dent Mater 1992;8:299–304.

151. Kirby R, Lee J, Knobloch L, Seghi R. Hardness and degree of conversion of posterior condensable composite resin [abstract 414]. J Dent Res 1999;78:157.

152. Hotta M, Hirukawa H. Abrasion resistance of restorative glass-ionomer cements with a light-cured surface coating. Oper Dent 1994;19:42–46.

153. Miyawaki H, Taira M, Toyooka H, Wakasa K, Yamaki M. Hardness and fracture toughness of commercial core composite resins. Dent Mater J 1993;12:62–68.

154. Rautiola CA, Craig RG. The microhardness of cementum and underlying dentin of normal teeth and teeth exposed to periodontal disease. J Periodontol 1961;32:113–123.

155. Craig RG, Peyton FA. The microhardness of enamel and dentin. J Dent Res 1958;37:661–668.

156. Collys K, Slop D, Cleymaet R, Coomans D, Michotte Y. Load dependency and reliability of microhardness measurements on acid-etched enamel surfaces. Dent Mater 1992;8:332–335.

157. Carr AB, Brantley WA. New high-palladium casting alloys: Part 1. Overview and initial studies. Int J Prosthodont 1991;4:265–275.

158. Craig RG, Powers JM, Peyton FA. Differential thermal analysis of commercial and dental waxes. J Dent Res 1967;46:1090–1097.

159. Dootz ER, Koran A, Craig RG. Comparison of the physical properties of 11 soft denture liners. J Prosthet Dent 1992;67:707–712.

160. Shell JS, Hollenback GM. Tensile strength and elongation of pure gold. J South Calif State Dent Assoc 1966;34:219–221.

161. Wilson HJ. Some properties of alginate impression materials relevant to clinical practice. Br Dent J 1966;121:463–467.

162. Haug SP, Andres CJ, Munoz CA, Okamura M. Effects of environmental factors on maxillofacial elastomers: Part III—Physical properties. J Prosthet Dent 1992;68:644–651.

163. Dootz ER, Koran A, Craig RG. Physical properties of three maxillofacial materials as a function of accelerated aging. J Prosthet Dent 1994;71:379–383.

164. Going RE, Loehman RE, Chan MS. Mouthguard materials: Their physical and mechanical properties. J Am Dent Assoc 1974;89:132–138.

165. Ida K, Togaya T, Tsutsumi S, Takeuchi M. Effect of magnesia investments in the dental casting of pure titanium or titanium alloys. Dent Mater J 1982;1:8–22.

166. Rueggeberg FA, Paschal S. Proportioning effect on physical and chemical properties of polysulfide impression material. J Prosthet Dent 1994;72:406–413.

167. Grenoble DE, Katz JL. The pressure dependence of the elastic constants of dental amalgam. J Biomed Mater Res 1971;5:489–502.

168. Dickson G, Oglesby PL. Elastic constants of dental amalgam. J Dent Res 1967;46:1475.

169. Hall DR, Nakayama WT, Grenoble DE, Katz JL. Elastic constants of three representative dental cements. J Dent Res 1973;52:390.

170. Grenoble DE, Katz JL, Dunn KL, Gilmore RS, Murty KL. The elastic properties of hard tissues and apatites. J Biomed Mater Res 1972;6:221–223.

171. Anusavice KJ, Hojjatie B, Dehoff PH. Influence of metal thickness on stress distribution in metal-ceramic crowns. J Dent Res 1986;65:1173–1178.

172. Pamenius M, Ohlson NG. The determination of elastic constants by dynamic experiments. Dent Mater 1986;2:246–250.

173. Powers JM, Caddell RM. The macroscopic volume changes of selected polymers subjected to uniform tensile deformation. Polym Eng Sci 1972;12:432–436.

174. Kase HR, Tesk JA, Case ED. Elastic constants of two dental porcelains. J Mater Sci 1985;20:524–531.

175. Nakayama WT, Hall DR, Grenoble DE, Katz JL. Elastic properties of dental resin restorative materials. J Dent Res 1974;53(5):1121–1126.

176. Farah JW, Craig RG, Meroueh KA. Finite element analysis of three- and four-unit bridges. J Oral Rehabil 1989;16:603–611.

177. Smith DC, Cooper WEG. The determination of shear strength—A method using a micro-punch apparatus. Br Dent J 1971;130:333–337.

178. Civjan S, Huget EF, Wolfhard G, Waddell LS. Characterization of zinc oxide–eugenol cements reinforced with acrylic resin. J Dent Res 1972;51:107–114.

179. Carter JM. Unpublished data. State Univ of New York at Buffalo, School of Dental Medicine.

180. Johnston WM, O'Brien WJ. Shear strength of dental porcelain. J Dent Res 1980;59:1409–1411.

181. Carter JM, Sorensen SE, Johnson RR, Teitelbaum RL, Levine MS. Punch shear testing of extracted vital and endodontically treated teeth. J Biomech 1983;16:841–848.

182. Finger W, Komatsu M. Elastic and plastic properties of elastic dental impression materials. Dent Mater 1985;1:129–134.

183. Kawano F, Dootz ER, Koran A, Craig RG. Sorption and solubility of 12 soft denture liners. J Prosthet Dent 1994;72:393–398.

184. Brauer GM, McLaughlin R, Huget EF. Aluminum oxide as a reinforcing agent for zinc oxide–eugenol-o-ethoxybenzoic acid cements. J Dent Res 1968;47(4):622–628.

185. Onose H. Properties and characteristics. Section 1: Physical and mechanical properties. In: Katsuyama S, Ishikawa T, Fujii B (eds). Glass Ionomer Dental Cement—The Materials and Their Clinical Use. St Louis: I Shiyaku EuroAmerica, 1993.

186. Gorodovsky S, Zidan O. Retentive strength, disintegration, and marginal quality of luting cements. J Prosthet Dent 1992;68:269–274.

187. Norman RD, Swartz ML, Phillips RW, Virmini R. A comparison of the intraoral disintegration of three dental cements. J Am Dent Assoc 1969;78:777–782.

188. Simmons FF, D'Anton EW, Hudson DC. Property studies of a hydrophosphate cement. J Am Dent Assoc 1968;76:337–339.

189. Phillips RW, Swartz ML, Rhodes B. An evaluation of a carboxylate adhesive cement. J Am Dent Assoc 1970;81:1353–1359.

190. Smith DC. A review of the zinc polycarboxylate cements. J Can Dent Assoc 1971;37:22–29.

191. Anderson JN, Paffenbarger GC. Properties of silico-phosphate cements. Dent Progress 1962;2:72–75.

192. Nicholson JW, Anstice HM, McLean JW. A preliminary report on the effect of storage in water on the properties of commercial light-cured glass-ionomer cements. Br Dent J 1992;173:98–101.

193. von Fraunhofer JA, Argyropoulos DC. Properties of periodontal dressings. Dent Mater 1990;6:51–55.

194. Dennison JB, Thompson WH. Unpublished data. Ann Arbor: Univ of Michigan School of Dentistry.

195. Peyton FA, Simeral WG. The specific heat of tooth structure. In: Alumni Bull. Ann Arbor, MI: Univ of Michigan School of Dentistry, 1954:33.

196. Brown WS, Dewey WA, Jacobs HR. Thermal properties of teeth. J Dent Res 1970;49:752–755.

197. Altman PL, Dittmer DS. Blood and Other Body Fluids. FASEB J 1961:12.

198. Nicholas ME, Joyner PA, Tessem BM, Olson MD. The effect of various gases and vapors on the surface tension of mercury. J Phys Chem 1961;65:1373–1375.

199. O'Brien WJ, Ryge G. Relation between molecular force calculations and observed strengths of enamel-metal interfaces. J Am Ceram Soc 1964;47:5–8.

200. Glantz P-O. The surface tension of saliva. Odontol Revy 1970;21:119–127.

201. Braden M. Characterization of the rupture properties of impression materials. Dent Pract Dent Rec 1963;14:67–71.

202. Webber RL, Ryge G. The determination of tear energy of extensible materials of dental interest. J Biomed Mater Res 1968;2:281–296.

203. Tam LE, Brown JW. The tear resistance of various impression materials with and without modifiers. J Prosthet Dent 1990;63:282–285.

204. Powers JM, Koran A. Unpublished data. Ann Arbor: Univ of Michigan School of Dentistry, 1975.

205. 3M Dental Products. Product information sheet. St Paul, MN: 3M Dental, 1999.

206. Craig RG, Peyton FA. Thermal conductivity of tooth structure, dental cements, and amalgam. J Dent Res 1961;40:411–418.

207. Chen RYS, Barker RE Jr. Effect of pressure on heat transport in polymers used in dentistry. J Biomed Mater Res 1972;6:147–154.

208. Carter JM. Thermal properties of dental restoratives. Presented at the annual meeting of the International Association for Dental Research, Dental Materials Group, Las Vegas, 23–26 Mar 1972.

209. Doctors M, Carter JM. Thermal properties of non-metallic dental restoratives. Presented at the annual meeting of the International Association for Dental Research, Dental Materials Group, Chicago, 18–21 Mar 1972.

210. Brantley WA, Kerby RE. Thermal diffusivity of glass ionomer cement systems. J Oral Rehabil 1993;20:61–68.

211. Braden M. Thermal properties of dental composition. J Dent Res 1966;45:1453–1457.

212. Powers JM, Farah JW. Apparent modulus of elasticity of dental amalgams. J Dent Res 1975;54:902.

213. White SN, Yu Z. Compressive and diametral tensile strengths of current adhesive luting agents. J Prosthet Dent 1993;69:568–572.

214. Lewis BA, Burgess JO, Gray SE. Mechanical properties of dental base materials. Am J Dent 1992;5:69–72.

215. Eliades G, Palaghias G. In vitro characterization of visible light-cured glass ionomer liners. Dent Mater 1993;9:198–203.

216. Earnshaw R, Smith DC. The tensile and compressive strength of plaster and stone. Aust Dent J 1966;11:415–422.

217. Leone EF, Fairhurst CW. Bond strength and mechanical properties of dental porcelain enamels. J Prosthet Dent 1967;18:155–159.

218. Mitra SB. Adhesion to dentin and physical properties of a light-cured glass ionomer liner/base. J Dent Res 1991;70:72–74.

219. Roeder LB, Fulton RS, Powers JM. Bond strength of repaired glass ionomer core materials. Am J Dent 1991;24:15–18.

220. Attin T, Vataschki M, Hellwig E. Properties of resin-modified glass-ionomer restorative materials and two polyacid-modified resin composite materials. Quintessence Int 1996;27:203–209.

221. Craig RG, Peyton FA. Elastic and mechanical properties of human dentin. J Dent Res 1958;37:710–718.

222. Bapna MS, Mueller HJ. Fracture toughness, diametrical strength, and fractography of amalgam and of amalgam to amalgam bonds. Dent Mater 1993;9:51–56.

223. Stafford GD, Smith DC. Some studies of the properties of denture base polymers. Br Dent J 1968;125:337–342.

224. Klooster J, Logan GI, Tjan AHL. Effects of strain rate on the behavior of elastomeric impression. J Prosthet Dent 1991;66:292–298.

225. Cullen DR, Sandrik JL. Tensile strength of elastomeric impression materials, adhesive and cohesive bonding. J Prosthet Dent 1989;62:142–145.

226. Asgar K, Allan FC. Microstructure and physical properties of alloys for partial denture castings. J Dent Res 1968;47:189–197.

227. Skinner EW, Phillips RW (eds). Skinner's Science of Dental Materials, ed 8. Philadelphia: Saunders, 1982:224.

228. Lee SY, Greener EH. Effect of excitation energy on dentine bond strength and composite properties. J Dent 1994; 22:175–181.

229. Covey DA, Tahaney SR, Davenport JM. Mechanical properties of heat-treated composite resin restorative materials. J Prosthet Dent 1992;68:458–461.

230. Bowen RL, Rodriquez MS. Tensile strength and modulus of elasticity of tooth structure and several restorative materials. J Am Dent Assoc 1962;64:378–387.

231. Drake HJ. Mercury. In: Grayson M (ed). Kirk-Othmer Encyclopedia of Chemical Technology, vol 15, ed 3. New York: John Wiley & Sons, 1981;143–156.

232. Reynolds CL Jr. Determination of mercury vapor pressure over amalgams from weight loss data. J Biomed Mater Res 1974;8:369–373.

233. Cornell JA, inventor. Composite tooth and veneer gel composite formed of non-volatile dimethacrylate as the sole polymerizable constituent. HD Justi Co, Div. Williams Gold-Refining US Patent 3,265,202, 1966.

234. Wing G. Phase identification in dental amalgam. Aust Dent J 1966;11:105–113.

235. Forss H, Seppä L, Lappalainen R. In vitro abrasion resistance and hardness of glass-ionomer cements. Dent Mater 1991;7:36–39.

236. Manhart J, Chen HY, Draegert U, Kunzelmann KH, Hickel R. Vickers hardness and depth of cure of light-cured packable composite resins [abstract 1807]. J Dent Res 2000;79:369.

237. Vermilyea SG, Powers JM, Craig RG. Rotational viscometry of a zinc phosphate and a zinc polyacrylate cement. J Dent Res 1977;56:762–767.

238. Reisbick MH. Effect of viscosity on the accuracy and stability of elastic impression materials. J Dent Res 1973;52:407–417.

239. Koran A, Powers JM, Craig RG. Apparent viscosity of materials used for making edentulous impressions. J Am Dent Assoc 1977;95:75–79.

240. Kim KN, Craig RG, Koran A. Viscosity of monophase addition silicones as a function of shear rate. J Prosthet Dent 1992;67:794–798.

241. Aylett BJ. Group IIB. In: Trotman-Dickenson AF (ed). Comprehensive Inorganic Chemistry, vol 3. Oxford: Pergamon Press, 1973:187–328.

242. Chevitarese O, Craig RG, Peyton FA. Properties of various types of denture-base plastics. J Prosthet Dent 1962;12:711–719.

243. Tietge JD, Dixon DL, Breeding LC, Leary JM, Aquilino SA. In vitro investigation of the wear of resin composite materials and cast direct retainers during removable partial denture placement and removal. Int J Prosthodont 1992;5:145–153.

244. O'Brien WJ, Fan PL, Loesche WJ, Walker MC, Apostolides A. Adsorption of Streptococcus mutans on chemically treated hydroxyapatite. J Dent Res 1978;57:910–914.

245. Walsh WR, Guzelsu N. Ion concentration effects on bone streaming potentials and zeta potentials. Biomaterials 1993;14:331–336.

246. Leach SA. Electrophoresis of synthetic hydroxyapatite. Arch Oral Biol 1960;3:48–56.

247. Neiders ME, Weiss L, Cudney TL. An electrokinetic characterization of human tooth surfaces. Arch Oral Biol 1970;15:135–151.

APPENDIX B

Biocompatibility Tests

▣ Initial Tests

Cytotoxicity tests One of the primary criteria for bio-compatibility is that the material not be toxic to cells. The material must not affect the cell number or growth, the integrity of the cell membranes, the activity (primarily enzymatic) of the cells, the genetic integrity, or the genetic expression. These tests are designed to determine how a material sample affects a particular cell type. The results, however, yield little information on how the sample affects a whole organism.

Mutagenesis tests These tests assess how the sample affects (or mutates) the genetic material of the host cells, either directly or indirectly, through a degradation product of the sample. An example is the Ames test, in which histidine-dependent mutants are exposed to the sample, and the rate of reversion to nonhistidine-dependent strains is used as a measure of mutagenic potential.

Immune function These tests detect immune responses to the sample, including proliferation, differentiation, chemotaxis, cytokine production, and bioactivity changes of immune cells such as T-cells, macrophages, and lymphocytes. Immune function tests are not used as often as many of the other biocompatibility tests, possibly in part due to the difficulty in quantifying the results and interpreting their meaning/severity. Some researchers believe that a mild immune response is not a substantial problem and may even be beneficial as a method of programmed biodegradation.

Complement activation assay This test is primarily concerned with engineered blood vessels and other devices that are in contact with the blood. Specifically, it determines whether the sample activates complements that will initiate thrombosis or generate inflammation. This is less of an issue for dental materials, but is pertinent to a material's effect on the pulp and gingiva.

Hemolysis assay This test is concerned with a material's potential to damage red blood cell membranes, either directly by permeating the membrane or by lysis. Such damage may result in malfunction or death of the red blood cells. A material is screened for this effect by searching for cell components in the medium's solution that should be internalized in healthy cells. Conversely, it can be identified by using tracers that should be excluded from the cell but have been allowed to permeate due to membrane damage.

Oral and intraperitoneal median lethal dose assays Also known as the *lethal dose, 50%* (LD50), these tests determine acute lethal effects administered orally or intraperitoneally to the laboratory specimens, typically rats. The sample is mixed into a solution or suspension of water, propylene glycol, vegetable oil, etc, and then injected into the stomach or peritoneum. The standard LD50 is the minimum amount that will kill 50% of the animals in 2 weeks. If this amount is less than 1 g of sample per 1 kg of body weight, then it is considered to have acute systematic toxicity.

■ Secondary Tests

Mucous membrane irritation test This test determines whether there is an inflammatory response in the mucous membranes or abraded skin. The skin sample is usually taken from the oral tissue of hamsters or rabbits. After a period of weeks, the test samples are compared with controls to evaluate the inflammatory response. Photographs are taken, followed by biopsies for a more in-depth analysis.

Skin sensitization tests Materials are injected intradermally to test for hypersensitivity. The reaction can be augmented with the Freund adjuvant. Hypersensitivity is subsequently tested via adhesive patches containing the test substance. The frequency and severity of inflammation in test subjects is a measure of the allergenic sensitization of the material.

Implantation tests These tests are required for samples that will contact tissue or bone and evaluate a material's potential to cause chronic inflammation or tumor growth. After inflammation from surgery has subsided, the samples are implanted in plastic tubes at sites that correspond with its intended use. The response is then analyzed using histologic, histochemical, and/or immunohistochemical methods. Short-term tests last 1 to 11 weeks. Long-term tests last 1 to 2 years. Other methods of implantation are being developed due to the complicating tissue reactions caused by some plastic tubes.

■ Usage Tests

Dental pulp irritation tests For this test, the materials are placed into Class 5 cavity preparations in intact, non-carious teeth of monkeys or other suitable test subjects. The cavities are prepared in all types of teeth under sterile conditions with a water-spray coolant to minimize pulpal trauma and should be of uniform size and shape. Zinc oxide–eugenol and silicate cement are used as negative and positive controls, respectively. After a period of 1 to 8 weeks, the teeth are extracted and sectioned for microscopic evaluation, necrotic and inflammatory responses are analyzed, and the thicknesses of the remaining and reparative dentin are quantified. The pulpal response is classified as *slight*, *moderate*, or *severe* based on these data. These tests are presently under development, particularly in attempts to account for bacterial insults to the pulp.

Dental implants into bone There are three basic evaluations for the success of implants: the penetration of a periodontal probe along the side of an implant, the mobility of the implant, and the bone-implant integration. A successful implant should have no mobility, no peri-implant radiolucency, minimal vertical bone loss, minimal fibrous encapsulation (preferably none), and no soft tissue complications. Ideally, the bone will contact the implant with strong, healthy tissue without any fibrous encapsulation.

Mucosa and gingiva tests These tests are performed in cavity preparations with subgingival extensions. The effects are typically examined at 7 and 30 days. Based on the degree of inflammation and the reaction of the epithelium, the responses are categorized as *slight*, *moderate*, or *severe*. Complications include preexisting inflammation; inflammation due to preparation, bacterial effects, or surface properties (ie, roughness) of the implant; and poorly designed contours. Prophylaxis minimizes complications due to plaque but causes minor inflammatory complications of its own.

Periodic Chart of the Elements

GROUP	I	II	3	4	5	6	7	8	1	2	III	IV	V	VI	VII	O
VALENCES	+1	+2				VARIABLE					+3	−4 +4	−3 +5	−2 +6	−1 +7	0
PERIOD 1	1 **H** 1.00797 ±0.00001															2 **He** 4.0026 ±0.00005
2	3 **Li** 6.941 ±0.0005	4 **Be** 9.0122 ±0.00005									5 **B** 10.811 ±0.003	6 **C** 12.01115 ±0.00005	7 **N** 14.0067 ±0.00005	8 **O** 15.9994 ±0.0001	9 **F** 18.9984 ±0.00005	10 **Ne** 20.183 ±0.0005
3	11 **Na** 22.9898 ±0.0005	12 **Mg** 24.312 ±0.0005									13 **Al** 26.9815 ±0.00005	14 **Si** 28.086 ±0.001	15 **P** 30.9738 ±0.00005	16 **S** 32.064 ±0.003	17 **Cl** 35.453 ±0.001	18 **Ar** 39.948 ±0.0005
4	19 **K** 39.102 ±0.0005	20 **Ca** 40.08 ±0.005	21 **Sc** 44.956 ±0.0005	22 **Ti** 47.90 ±0.005	23 **V** 50.942 ±0.0005	24 **Cr** 51.996 ±0.001	25 **Mn** 54.9380 ±0.00005	26 **Fe** 55.847 ±0.003	27 **Co** 58.9332 ±0.0005	28 **Ni** 58.71 ±0.005 / 29 **Cu** 63.54 ±0.005	30 **Zn** 65.37 ±0.005	31 **Ga** 69.72 ±0.005	32 **Ge** 72.59 ±0.005	33 **As** 74.9216 ±0.00005	34 **Se** 78.96 ±0.005	35 **Br** 79.909 ±0.002 / 36 **Kr** 83.80 ±0.005
5	37 **Rb** 85.47 ±0.005	38 **Sr** 87.62 ±0.005	39 **Y** 88.905 ±0.0005	40 **Zr** 91.22 ±0.005	41 **Nb** 92.906 ±0.0005	42 **Mo** 95.94 ±0.005	43 **Tc** (99)	44 **Ru** 101.07 ±0.005	45 **Rh** 102.905 ±0.0005	46 **Pd** 106.4 ±0.05 / 47 **Ag** 107.870 ±0.003	48 **Cd** 112.40 ±0.005	49 **In** 114.82 ±0.005	50 **Sn** 118.69 ±0.005	51 **Sb** 121.75 ±0.005	52 **Te** 127.60 ±0.005	53 **I** 126.9044 ±0.00005 / 54 **Xe** 131.30 ±0.005
6	55 **Cs** 132.905 ±0.0005	56 **Ba** 137.34 ±0.005	57 **La** 138.91 ±0.005	72 **Hf** 178.49 ±0.005	73 **Ta** 180.948 ±0.0005	74 **W** 183.85 ±0.005	75 **Re** 186.2 ±0.05	76 **Os** 190.2 ±0.05	77 **Ir** 192.2 ±0.05	78 **Pt** 195.09 ±0.005 / 79 **Au** 196.987 ±0.0005	80 **Hg** 200.59 ±0.005	81 **Tl** 204.37 ±0.005	82 **Pb** 207.19 ±0.005	83 **Bi** 208.980 ±0.0005	84 **Po** (210)	85 **At** (210) / 86 **Rn** (222)
7	87 **Fr** (223)	88 **Ra** (226)	89 †**Ac** (227)	104 (257)												

Noble metals

Lanthanum Series

58 **Ce** 140.12 ±0.005	59 **Pr** 140.907 ±0.0005	60 **Nd** 144.24 ±0.005	61 **Pm** (147)	62 **Sm** 150.35 ±0.005	63 **Eu** 151.96 ±0.005	64 **Gd** 157.25 ±0.005	65 **Tb** 158.924 ±0.0005	66 **Dy** 162.50 ±0.005	67 **Ho** 164.930 ±0.0005	68 **Er** 167.26 ±0.005	69 **Tm** 168.934 ±0.0005	70 **Yb** 173.04 ±0.005	71 **Lu** 174.97 ±0.005

Actinium Series

90 **Th** 232.038 ±0.0005	91 **Pa** (231)	92 **U** 238.03 ±0.005	93 **Np** (237)	94 **Pu** (244)	95 **Am** (243)	96 **Cm** (245)	97 **Bk** (247)	98 **Cf** (249)	99 **Es** (254)	100 **Fm** (255)	101 **Md** (256)	102 **No** (253)	103 **Lw** (257)

Units and Conversion Factors

Unit	SI equivalent
angstrom (Å)	1×10^{-10} m
	1×10^{-1} nm
nanometer (nm)	1×10^{-9} m
micrometer (µm)	1×10^{-6} m
inch (in)	0.0254 m
	2.54 cm
pound (lb)	0.4536 kg
dyne (dyn)	1×10^{-5} N
pound force (lbf)	4.4482 N
erg	1×10^{-7} J
calorie (Cal)	4.1868 J
British thermal unit (Btu)	1055.06 J
dyn/cm2	1×10^{-1} N/m²
atmosphere (atm)	1.013×10^{5} N/m² (Pa)
pound per square	6.895×10^{3} N/m² (Pa)
inch (psi)	6.895×10^{-3} MN/m² (MPa)
kg/cm²	9.804×10^{4} MN/m² (Pa)
pennyweight (dwt)	1.555 g
(20 dwt = 1 ozt = 1.097 oz)	

Photomicrograph distance: $\mu m/cm = \dfrac{10{,}000}{\text{magnification}}$

Temperature: $(°C \times 1.8) + 32 = °F$

$$\frac{(°F - 32)}{1.8} = °C$$

Prefixes for SI units

Multiply by this factor	Symbol	Prefix
10^{12}	T	tera
10^{9}	G	giga
10^{6}	M	mega
10^{3}	k	kilo
10^{2}	h	hecto
10	da	deca
10^{-1}	d	deci
10^{-2}	c	centi
10^{-3}	m	milli
10^{-6}	µ	micro
10^{-9}	n	nano
10^{-12}	p	pico
10^{-15}	f	femto
10^{-18}	a	atto

Answers to Study Questions

Chapter 1 A Comparison of Metals, Ceramics, and Polymers

1. See Table 1-1.
2. The sharper the stress raiser, the greater the concentration of stress around it.
3. Ceramics—Stress concentration at surface scratches and other defects causes ceramics to fail at stresses far below their theoretical strengths.
   Metals—The ability of crystal defects called dislocations to move within the crystal structure of metals gives them their ability to bend without fracturing.
   Polymers—Strong bonds within the polymer chains and weak bonds between polymer chains are responsible for the low strengths and elastic moduli of polymers.

Chapter 2 Physical Properties and Biocompatibility

1. Knowledge and understanding of physical and mechanical properties help the clinician predict how a material will behave in vivo and how it should be manipulated.
2. Thermal diffusivity is a time-dependent property, and, since the temperature of the oral cavity changes dramatically within a few seconds (drinking hot coffee versus eating ice cream), it predicts the behavior of materials under more realistic conditions. Thermal conductivity, on the other hand, is a steady-state property, and the temperature of the mouth is not constant over time.
3. See Fig 2-4.
4. *Hardness* is the resistance of a material to permanent indentation in its surface. It involves complex stresses, so it cannot be directly related to any other physical property.
5. Material *a* is brittle, *b* is ductile; *a* is stiffer than *b*; *a* is stronger than *b*, *b* is tougher than *a*.
6. *Fracture toughness* is the resistance of a material to brittle fracture when a crack is present in (or at the surface of) the material. Two materials with equivalent strengths may have markedly different fracture toughness values. A material with low fracture toughness will behave in a brittle manner and is more prone to catastrophic failure.
7. Laboratory testing is necessary to screen out materials that could be obviously harmful before use with patients in a clinical trial. Both might be performed if initial screening tests are favorable.

Chapter 3 Color and Appearance

1. Hue, value, and chroma; X, Y, and Z tristimulus values; L*, a*, and b*.
2. A crown that appears gray and nonvital has a low value.
3. The green object absorbs the blue light. Since no light is reflected, the object appears black.
4. The source, the surroundings, and the observer.
5. A high translucency gives a lighter color appearance.
6. A high gloss lightens color appearance.
7. *Metamerism* is the change in color matching of two objects under different light sources.
8. Metamerism may cause a restoration to have a good color match under one lighting condition but a poor color match under another lighting condition.
9. Dental porcelains are fluorescent in some lighting environments.

Chapter 4 Gypsum Products

1. The major constituent is the same in all products—calcium sulfate hemihydrate. Minor differences in composition exist between stones and die stones because of the presence of accelerators, retarders, and coloring matter.
2. Plaster is produced by the dry calcination of ground gypsum (calcium sulfate dihydrate). Partial loss of water of crystallization is not accompanied by a change in shape or size of the individual particles, which are therefore irregular and porous, giving the powder a relatively low apparent density. Stone and die stone are produced by wet calcination, which allows formation of dense regular crystals of hemihydrate, producing powders that have a higher apparent

density than plaster. Grinding under controlled conditions increases the apparent density still further.

3. Typical W/P ratios: plaster, 0.50; stone, 0.30; die stone, 0.20. Lower W/P ratios can be used with stone and die stone, because the apparent densities of their powders are higher, so less water is needed to make a workable mix. Uncombined water in set mass: for plaster, 100 g powder + 50 g water = 150 g set mass. Only 18.6 g water combines chemically. Therefore, after the setting reaction is complete, uncombined water is 31.4 g in 150 g, approximately 20%. Similarly, for stone, uncombined water is approximately 9%; for die stone, approximately 1%. (Note: These are theoretical calculations. In actual practice, the setting reaction does not reach completion, even in relatively high W/P ratios.)

4. *Chemical change*—Hydration of calcium sulfate hemihydrate to form the dihydrate (gypsum): $2CaSO_4 \cdot \frac{1}{2}H_2O + 3H_2O \rightarrow 2CaSO_4 \cdot 2H_2O$.

 Physical changes: The mix is first a viscous liquid, then a plastic mass, and then a rigid solid, friable at first but increasing in strength until the reaction has ceased.

5. Set plaster has a higher proportion of inherent microporosity than set stone. The microporosity is caused by (a) residual unreacted water and (b) setting expansion. Both of these factors are greater in the case of plaster. Thus, set plaster is less dense and therefore weaker than set stone.

6. Setting is a continuous process. In practice, any figure given for setting time is arbitrary, unless it refers to the time when the setting reaction ceases. (a) Loss of surface gloss gives an indication of the time when the mix will not pour or flow under vibration. (b) and (c) Both the Gillmore and Vicat initial sets give an indication of the time when the solid material can be handled safely.

7. By the empirical addition of accelerators or retarders to the raw hemihydrate powder.

8. The setting rate is reduced, because increasing the W/P ratio increases the relative amount of aqueous phase present in the mix. Therefore, the physical changes associated with setting occur more slowly because interaction of growing gypsum crystals takes place later.

9. There is a decrease in the volume of the actual solid. However, the gypsum crystals formed are usually long and thin, and crystal growth creates microscopic voids that cause an increase in the total volume of the mass.

10. When setting occurs in water, there is a continuous aqueous phase present, and crystal growth is relatively unimpeded. When setting occurs in air, the water content of the mix decreases as the reaction proceeds. Residual liquid in the mix is drawn into voids created between growing gypsum crystals, over which it forms a film. Surface tension forces crowd the growing crystals together and restrain further expansion.

11. It affects the dimensional accuracy of the ultimate dental restoration.

12. Impression plaster, 0.15%; plaster, 0.30%; stone, 0.15%; low-expansion die stone, 0.10%; high-expansion die stone, 0.25%.

13. By the empirical addition of a blend of a suitable accelerator and retarder, both of which reduce setting expansion.

14. Accelerators and retarders also reduce the strength properties of the set material, so when strength is an important consideration the concentration that can be used is relatively low.

15. Setting expansion is reduced, because the relative amount of aqueous phase is increased and interaction of growing gypsum crystals is less effective.

16. Tensile strength is an indication of resistance to fracture; compressive strength is an indication of surface hardness.

17. It reduces both. With a higher W/P ratio there is more residual water remaining after setting is complete, and this causes increased microporosity which reduces strength properties.

18. Drying approximately doubles both tensile and compressive strengths, since the presence of free water in the cast material weakens it.

19. Calcium sulfate hemihydrate acts as a binder. Silica (quartz, cristobalite, or a mixture of both) offsets the contraction of the binder that occurs on heating and often provides a positive thermal expansion. Modifiers may be present in small concentrations to adjust the rate of setting, to give a reducing atmosphere when the mold is heated, or to give an increased thermal expansion.

20. (a) Rate of setting decreases; (b) setting expansion in air increases; (c) setting expansion in water increases; (d) thermal expansion increases; and (e) compressive strength decreases.

21. When the investment powder is mixed with water, the silica is unaffected. The calcium sulfate hemihydrate reacts with water to precipitate gypsum crystals, which bind the silica particles together.

22. The porosity is continuous and provides venting of the mold cavity when the molten alloy is cast.

23. The powder should have a uniform fine particle size (not more than 75 µm). A uniform particle size ensures adequate venting of the mold cavity, because the silica particles show least-dense packing. A fine particle size produces a smooth casting; surface roughness of the casting can interfere with its fit.

24. The particles of refractory filler remain unchanged during setting and have a major effect on the smoothness of the mold surface. The particles of binder are dissolved during setting, and gypsum crystals are precipitated that are much smaller than the refractory particles.

25. Expansion, provided by a summation of setting and thermal expansions, is most important. Mold expansion is used to offset the casting shrinkage of the alloy and thus produce an accurate casting.

26. A casting technique in which most of the mold expansion is gained by the increased setting expansion that occurs when the setting investment is exposed to additional water. The need for thermal expansion of the mold is small.

27. A casting technique in which thermal expansion contributes greatly to mold expansion. In most thermal expansion techniques, setting expansion also plays an important part.

28. At the relatively low burnout temperatures used, oxidation of carbon remaining from the wax pattern is slow. Most of it must be removed to allow adequate mold venting.

29. The refractory can be identified by studying the investment's thermal expansion curve, which should be provided by the manufacturer. Cristobalite investments show a large isothermal expansion at about 250°C. Quartz investments show a smaller isothermal expansion at about 570°C. The type of refractory filler in the investment affects the heating rate to be used and sometimes the burnout temperature.

30. Cristobalite investments undergo a large isothermal expansion at a relatively low temperature (250°C). If a large temperature difference, resulting from rapid heating, is present within the mold at this temperature, nonuniform expansion can cause cracking. This problem can be prevented by following a slow heating rate below 300°C. The problem does not arise with quartz investments, which have a more gradual thermal expansion. (Note: The need for slow heating during the inversion of cristobalite does not apply to rapid-heat investments.)

31. With quartz investments, the required thermal expansion is available only over restricted temperature ranges (hygroscopic expansion techniques, 350°C to 480°C; thermal expansion techniques, 600°C to 700°C). With cristobalite investments, the thermal expansion is reasonably constant over a wide temperature range (400°C to 700°C).

32. At temperatures above 700°C, the calcium sulfate binder decomposes in the presence of carbon, liberating corrosive gases that can adversely affect the casting.

33. It increases it.

34. (a) Setting expansion in air decreases; (b) setting expansion in water decreases; and (c) thermal expansion decreases.

35. By varying the W/P ratio, or by varying the length of time additional water is available to the setting investment. In the latter case this may be achieved by delaying the immersion of the investment, or by adding controlled amounts of excess water to the setting investment instead of immersing it.

36. By varying the W/P ratio.

37. At the casting temperature, the investment mold may be strong enough to restrain the thermal contraction of the solidified casting as it cools. The effect will vary in different directions, depending on the amount of interlocking of casting and mold. This can cause distortion of the casting shape.

    An investment with a low hot strength is more likely to allow uniform thermal contraction of the alloy and give an undistorted casting. A safe lower limit for compressive strength at the casting temperature is 1.8 MPa.

38. They should be stored in airtight containers, in a cool dry region of the laboratory. When hemihydrate powders are exposed to the atmosphere, particularly when the water vapor pressure is high, the particles adsorb water from the air. This can react with the hemihydrate to form gypsum crystals. Initially this increases the setting rate of the material increases, but if deterioration proceeds further, the setting rate is retarded, and eventually the strength properties of the set material are adversely affected.

Chapter 5 Surface Phenomena and Adhesion to Tooth Structure

1. The molecules at the surfaces of liquids exert a greater intermolecular force on each other than do interior molecules, due to their greater average separation. This attraction, or pull, results in a contractile surface stress.

2. The degree of capillary penetration decreases as the contact angle increases. Above a contact angle of 90 degrees, a liquid will not penetrate and depression occurs (eg, mercury in a glass tube).

3. Adsorption involves the uptake of one substance at the surface of another. Absorption involves the penetration of one substance into the interior of another.

4. Agar and alginate impression materials, colloidal gold, and detergents.

5. The penetration coefficient includes viscosity, surface tension, and contact angle as follows (PC in cm/sec):

$$PC = \frac{\gamma \cos \theta}{2\eta}$$

6. Major, since previously there was no way to bond materials to dentin.

Chapter 6 Polymers and Polymerization

1. Heat- and cold-cured acrylic resins; rubber- and fiber-reinforced acrylic; polycarbonate injection molded; nylon injection molded; and light-activated dimethacrylate.

2. Good appearance, high flexural strength, high impact resistance, high stiffness, long fatigue life, high craze resistance, high creep resistance, high radiopacity, low free-monomer content, good adhesion with teeth and liners, low solubility, low water uptake, dimensional stability, and dimensional accuracy.

3. *Advantages*: Good appearance, high glass-transition temperature, ease of fabrication, low capital costs, good surface finish
   Disadvantages: Free-monomer content or formaldehyde can cause sensitization, low impact strength, flexural strength low enough to penalize poor denture design, fatigue life too short, radiolucency

4. *Advantages*: Easy to deflask, dimensionally accurate, can have higher flexural strength than heat-cured materials
   Disadvantages: No cheaper over the long term, increased creep, increased free-monomer content, color instability, reduced stiffness, tooth adhesion failure

5. *Advantage*: Improved impact strength
   Disadvantage: Reduced stiffness

6. *Advantages*: High stiffness, very good impact strength, good fatigue life; polypropylene fibers: good translucency and good surface finish
   Disadvantage: Carbon and Kevlar fibers: poor color and poor surface

7. *Advantages*: Dimensional accuracy, low free-monomer content, good impact strength
   Disadvantages: High capital costs, difficult mold design problems, less craze resistance, less creep resistance

8. *Advantages*: No methyl methacrylate monomer, reduced polymerization shrinkage, time savings, possible better fit than conventional denture base materials, processing procedure requiring little equipment
Disadvantage: Somewhat increased elastic deformation during mastication

9. Acrylic, silicone (RTV), and heat-cured silicone.

10. *Advantage*: Resilient
Disadvantages: Low tear strength, low bond strength to dentures, attacked by cleansers, buckle in water, poor abrasion resistance

11. *Advantages*: Resilience, adequate bond strength to acrylic, more resistant to aqueous environment and cleansers than RTV
Disadvantages: Low tear strength, poor abrasion resistance

12. *Advantages*: High peel strength to acrylic denture base, high rupture strength, some can be polished if cooled, reasonable resistance to damage by denture cleansers
Disadvantages: Poor resilience, loses plasticizer in time, some buckle in water

13. Flow under constant force, resilience at high rates of deformation, remain viscous for several days, have high tack to aid retention to denture base.

Chapter 7 Impression Materials

1. Natural resins and waxes provide thermoplastic properties. Stearic acid acts as a lubricant and plasticizer. Inorganic fillers and pigments give control of flow and color, respectively.

2. Thermoplastic.

3. Impression compound has a higher flow. Tray material, with a lower flow, does not record fine detail.

4. Avoid burning in a direct flame or heating in a water bath for long periods.

5. Low thermal conductivity requires time for thorough cooling to prevent distortion during removal.

6. The amounts of filler and water incorporated during kneading control the flow properties.

7. Zinc oxide and eugenol.

8. ZnO + eugenol $\rightarrow$ Zn eugenolate, which forms a solid matrix holding unreacted ZnO.

9. Increases in temperature and/or humidity shorten the setting time.

10. Agar acts as a gelling agent. Borax improves strength. Potassium sulfate provides good surfaces on models or dies. Alkylbenzoates are preservatives.

11. The liquefaction and gelation temperatures are different.

12. Storage in air results in shrinkage; water, in expansion; 100% relative humidity, in shrinkage (synersis); and potassium sulfate solution, in shrinkage or expansion, depending on the ionic strength of the solution.

13. Sodium alginate and calcium sulfate are reactants to give calcium alginate. Sodium phosphate is a retarder; filler (eg, diatomaceous earth) controls stiffness; alkali zinc fluorides provide good surfaces on dies and models; and coloring and flavoring are for esthetics.

14. A low W/P ratio and/or high temperature shorten the setting time.

15. $CaSO_4 + Na_3PO_4 \rightarrow Na_2SO_4 + Ca_3(PO_4)_2$ provides working time. Na alginate + $CaSO_4$ $\rightarrow$ Ca alginate + Na_2SO_4, in the presence of water, provides setting time.

16. Alginates do not revert to a sol on heating or by chemical means.

17. A decreased W/P ratio increases strength, tear resistance, and consistency, but decreases working time, setting time, and flexibility.

18. Insufficient spatulation gives a grainy mix and poor recording of detail. Adequate spatulation yields a smooth, creamy mix with a minimum of voids.

19. Decreased water temperature increases the working and setting times of alginates.

20. Alginates and agars have similar properties.

21. Polysulfide cures by condensation of terminal mercaptan groups catalyzed by lead peroxide or other catalysts. Condensation silicones cure by condensation of terminal hydroxyl groups by orthoalkylsilicates to form polymer and alcohol. Addition silicones cure by free-radical polymerization with a platinum catalyst. Polyethers cure by ring opening of the ethylene-imine group.

22.

	Proportioning	Increased temperature
Polysulfide	Decreases with increased amount of catalyst	Decreases
Silicone	Minimal	Decreases
Polyether	Decreases with increased amount of accelerator	Decreases

23. Addition silicones.

24. Addition silicone $\geq$ condensation silicone $\geq$ polyether > polysulfide. A large elastic recovery value indicates smaller distortion of the impression on removal.

25. Polysulfide > condensation silicone $\geq$ addition silicone $\geq$ polyether.

26. Follow the instructions given by the manufacturer for the impression material used, because the recommended procedure depends on the material.

27. (a) Hydrophilic materials will wet the tooth surface more readily during impression taking and are more readily wet by dental stone. Therefore, they are less likely to entrap air. Also, their wetting characteristics make them easier to electroplate. (b) A single material can be used as both the low- and high-viscosity material for the syringe-tray impression technique. (c) This method of mixing is quick and produces bubble-free mixes.

Chapter 8 Polymeric Restorative Materials

1. Resin composites contain two major components: a polymer matrix and a ceramic filler. The polymer consists of a dimethacrylate oligomer (bis-GMA or UDMA). Larger filler particles may be quartz or any of a number of glasses. The colloidal-size particles of microfine composites are silica.

In addition, a silane coupling agent is attached to the filler surface to create a particle-matrix bond during polymerization.

2. Resin composites are commonly used for the restoration of Class 3 and Class 5 cavity preparations, for replacement of fractured incisal edges (Class 4), and for veneering of facial surfaces of natural teeth. Continued improvement has led to their use in selected, conservative posterior restorations. They are also used in the repair of porcelain and for the cosmetic recontour of anterior teeth.

3. Longevity of conventional resin composites varies. In general, composite restorations in anterior teeth provide adequate serviceability for up to 10 years. Class 3 restorations tend to last longer than those placed in cervical regions because they are exposed to less mechanical abrasion and stress due to tooth flexure. Posterior resin composites have a shorter service life, generally requiring replacement within 7 years. Reasons for replacement of any composite include deterioration of esthetics, wear, microleakage, and recurrent decay.

4. Fine-particle composites generally have superior physical and mechanical properties compared with microfine composites, which have a lower filler content.

5. Microfilled composites contain colloidal silica (0.01 to 0.12 μm) as filler. Because the diameter of the particles is less than 0.05 μm, they cannot be detected visually, giving the composite a translucent quality and allowing polishing to a high luster.

6. A hybrid composite contains colloidal silica in addition to larger filler particles. The colloidal silica is commonly added to improve certain handling characteristics, such as flow and packability. Hybrid composites can be used for both anterior and posterior restorations, because they combine the physical properties of fine-particle composites and the esthetics of microfills.

7. Polymerization of the polymer matrix after placement results in shrinkage of the matrix and places stresses on the bond at the tooth-composite interface. At present, the enamel-composite bond is more likely to withstand these stresses than is the dentin-composite bond. Loss of marginal integrity results in an influx of oral fluids and greatly increases the possibility of microleakage, postoperative sensitivity, and recurrent decay.

8. Glass ionomers, resin-modified glass ionomers, compomers, and fluoride-releasing composites. Additionally, the materials with higher fluoride release have higher fluoride recharge capacity.

9. The success of a cervical restoration may increase with increased flexibility. Current research suggests that restorative materials with higher flexibility (lower elastic modulus) may be desirable. Flowable composites and resin-modified glass ionomers are more flexible than most all-purpose composites or compomers, and are therefore the materials of choice.

Chapter 9 Dental Cements

1. About 55 MPa (8,000 psi).

2. A cored structure of unreacted zinc oxide particles in an amorphous zinc phosphate matrix.

3. The solubility in organic acid solutions, such as citric or lactic acid, is 20 to 30 times higher than in water.

4. These cements contain monomers with polar groups, such as phosphate or carboxyl, that improve wetting and are potentially adhesive to the tooth or restorative material surface. Adhesive cements may also utilize require a dentin bonding primer system before application of the cement.

5. They are combinations of glass ionomers with resin additions, providing easier handling, dual curing, and higher flexural strength.

6. Water, zinc salts such as acetate and sulfate, and other acidic materials.

7. The high solubility of zinc oxide–eugenol cements is due to hydrolytic breakdown of zinc eugenolate and the extraction of eugenol from the set cement.

8. Mineral fillers, such as silica or alumina; natural resins, such as pine rosin; and synthetic polymers, such as poly(methyl methacrylate), polystyrene, or polycarbonate.

9. Zinc oxide–eugenol cements inhibit the polymerization of resin restorative materials, resulting in softening and discoloration.

10. The powder of EBA cements contains more mineral filler, such as alumina, than does the powder of zinc oxide–eugenol cements, and in the liquid only about one third is eugenol; the remainder is ethoxybenzoic acid.

11. The powder/liquid ratio, the reactivity and particle size of the zinc oxide, the presence of additives, and the molecular weight and concentration of the polyacrylic acid.

12. The mild effect of polycarboxylate cements on pulp may be due to the relatively high pH of the setting cement; localization of the polyacrylic acid molecules; and/or the minimal osmotic effects on fluid in the dentinal tubules.

13. The components of the cement should be carefully proportioned and mixed on a cooled slab. All of the powder may be added to the liquid at one time so that the total mix time is no more than 30 to 40 seconds. The mix should be used while it is still glossy, before the onset of cobwebbing.

14. They set by both acid-base reaction and polymerization of monomer groups, giving higher early strength, improved physical properties, and water resistance.

15. High strength and stiffness, adhesion, translucency, leachable fluoride and potential cariostatic effect, and good resistance to dissolution in the mouth.

16. The two types of resin cement are acrylic resin cements, based on poly(methyl methacrylate) and methyl methacrylate monomer, and resin composite materials, based on a ceramic filler and a bis-GMA dimethacrylate monomer.

17. Short working time, viscous behavior of the mix, microleakage and pulpal irritation, and difficulty of removal of excess cement.

18. Long-term clinical studies were not performed on hybrid ionomers before marketing. Furthermore, the physical prop-

erties studies, including dimensional changes on setting, were performed dry and indicated a shrinkage. Under moist conditions, these cements probably expand by water absorption. Although useful, physical property tests cannot always identify phenomena that clinical studies can locate.

19. Long-term, large-scale clinical studies were not done at different clinics. Short-term studies with small samples performed at one clinic would not detect this problem, since the problem involves overdrying of the tooth as well.

Chapter 10 Abrasion, Polishing, and Bleaching

1. A material that causes wear of another material through mechanical means.

2. Hardness, particle size and shape, speed and pressure, lubrication.

3. Chalk, rouge, pumice, cuttle, sand, aluminum oxide, silicon carbide, diamond.

4. Little effect; it is too soft to be a good polishing agent for dental porcelain.

5. For esthetic and functional reasons (to retard plaque accumulation).

6. Coarse particles would leave scratches on the polished surface. Avoid contamination of the instruments used and have the patient rinse between the grinding and polishing steps.

7. The tongue can distinguish scratch depths between 20 and 2 µm.

8. (*a*) Pumice, sand, zirconium silicate, and chalk. (*b*) Chalk, dibasic calcium phosphate dihydrate, anhydrous dibasic calcium phosphate, tricalcium phosphate, calcium pyrophosphate, and hydrated alumina. (*c*) Aluminum oxide, silicon carbide, and sand.

9. Degree of staining, toothbrushing habits, soft restorative materials present in the oral cavity, and amount of exposed cementum or dentin.

10. An amalgam restoration should be polished at least 24 hours after placement. Use flour of pumice, extra-fine silex, or tin oxide on a rotating cup, brush, or felt.

11. They are composed of two phases with greatly different hardnesses. A rough surface would be desirable if more composite material or surface glaze had to be added to a previously set composite restorative material.

12. Usually the evidence is based on one observer comparing the affected teeth before and after treatment with an uncalibrated shade guide. Many results are not published.

Chapter 11 Structure and Properties of Metals and Alloys

1. Pure metals have a melting temperature, whereas alloys usually exhibit a melting temperature range. Alloys of eutectic composition are an exception—they melt and solidify at a single temperature.

2. If a casting alloy is incompletely melted or not heated above its melting temperature range, it will not flow into all areas—especially not thin areas—of the investment mold

of a wax pattern. An incomplete casting will result. In the case of soldering, the solder will not flow adequately, and voids may be left in the solder joint.

3. The density of a molten metal is less than that of its crystalline solid, because the atoms pack more closely together in a crystalline solid's crystal lattice than in the disordered liquid state.

4. If more molten liquid cannot flow from the casting button to take up the volume shrinkage in the casting as it solidifies, porosity will result.

5. Each corner atom is shared with eight other unit cells, so one eighth of each corner atom belongs to a unit cell. There are eight corner atoms, so together they contribute one atom to the unit cell. Each face-centered atom is shared between two unit cells, so one half of each face-centered atom belongs to each unit cell. The six face-centered atoms together contribute three atoms to the unit cell. The face-centered cubic unit cell thus contains four atoms.

6. The density is equal to the mass divided by the volume of the unit cell.

$$\text{Density} = \frac{\text{Number of atoms} \times \text{Atomic weight}}{(\text{Lattice parameter})^3}$$

7. Copper, iron, and gold.

8. Work hardening, hardening heat treatment, and a decrease in grain size.

9. Increase the number of grain boundaries (ie, smaller grains); increase the number of dislocations (ie, cold working); or treat with heat to create phase changes to lattices that are more resistant to dislocation motion.

10. Small-grain metals have a higher yield stress and more uniform plastic deformation, which result in a higher ultimate strength.

11. (*a*) The smallest grain visible would equal the resolution of the microscope, ideally 0.5 µm. (*b*) The atoms at the grain boundaries are not as chemically stable because they do not pack together as well as interior atoms of the grain. Different grains etch at different rates because their orientations present planes of atoms of different atomic densities to the polished surface. If the metal is multiphased, the different compositions of the grains will respond differently to the acid etch.

12. The eutectic temperature is 779°C, and the composition is 71.9% Ag and 28.1% Cu.

13. It begins to solidify (liquidus temperature) at 833°C and is completely solidified (solidus temperature) at 779°C.

14. The atomic percentage of silver in Ag_3Sn is 75%: 3 Ag atoms ÷ (3 Ag + 1 Sn) = 0.75. The weight percentage of silver in Ag_3Sn is 73.2%: 3(107.9) ÷ (3[107.9] + 1[118.7]) = 0.732.

15. A crystal lattice indicates the location and periodic spacing of atoms in a crystalline solid. A space lattice indicates the way in which mathematical points can be located in space so that every point has a similar grouping of points surrounding it. This requirement develops a repeat pattern of points that correlates with the periodic table of elements.

16. During the recovery stage, the yield strength decreases only slightly, and the percentage elongation begins to increase. During recrystallization, the yield strength drops rapidly, and the percentage elongation increases rapidly. There is a further small increase in percentage elongation and decrease in yield strength with grain growth.

17. By definition, it takes 1 hour for a metal to recrystallize at its recrystallization temperature; at a higher temperature it would take less time and at a lower temperature it would take more. The melting temperature of iron in degrees Kelvin is 1,535°C + 273°C (1,808 K). The recrystallization temperature in degrees Kelvin is 450°C + 273°C (723 K). The recrystallization temperature divided by the absolute melting temperature is 0.42.

Chapter 12 Dental Amalgams

1. It is best not to alter the trituration conditions because other properties may be degraded. Choose an amalgam that has the working time characteristics desired.

2. Zinc in the presence of moisture decreases the performance of amalgams. Proper moisture control will give a zinc-containing amalgam better performance than a zinc-free system.

3. Yes, fast-setting alloys. Read the instructions for use.

4. The small spherical-shaped particles tend to slip past one another. Less mercury, however, is required for plasticity. These amalgams also require less packing force to condense.

5. Creep is a bad predictor for clinical marginal fracture in high-copper amalgams, but it has some value as a predictor for traditional systems. The best predictor, however, is proof from clinical trials.

6. The primary reason for the sealing/bonding of amalgam restorations is the attempt to reduce postoperative sensitivity seen in teeth restored with some high-copper spherical amalgams.

7. Except for allergic reactions affecting a small segment of the population, there is no credible scientific evidence that dental amalgam restorations cause disease in humans. Environmental concerns regarding mercury in amalgam can be addressed by proper office procedures for handling, dispensing, and waste management.

Chapter 13 Precious Metal Casting Alloys

1. Gold, silver, and the platinum group metals (platinum, palladium, iridium, rhodium, ruthenium, and osmium).

2. Gold, copper, and silver. The platinum metals also contribute some hardening.

3. Type I alloys are used for one-surface restorations that will be subjected to slight stress; type II alloys are for two- and three-surface inlays; type III alloys are for crowns and fixed partial dentures; and type IV alloys are for fixed and removable partial dentures.

4. Iron, tin, and indium.

5. Palladium has a strong whitening effect on the color of gold alloys.

6. Heat for 10 minutes at 700°C followed by water quenching.

7. Heat for 10 minutes at 350°C followed by water quenching or rapid cooling in air. Cooling a casting in a mold to room temperature (bench cooling) will produce hardening, because the alloy remains in the 350°C to 400°C temperature range long enough.

8. Iridium. Smaller grains result in a stronger, more ductile and homogeneous casting.

9. The gold alloys containing iron, indium, and tin are heated from about 700°C to 950°C in air, and then air cooled. The purpose is to burn off organic contamination and produce an adherent oxide for bonding.

10. Palladium, silver, gold, tin, and indium.

11. Ordering is a crystal structure organization in which the atoms of an element (eg, copper) are regularly arranged in a repeating pattern as opposed to a random distribution (ie, disordered).

12. The present theory holds that hardening in gold-copper-silver alloys involves a separation of silver-rich and copper-rich gold phases within the grain structure. Ordering of a gold-copper phase also occurs, but is not as important in these ternary alloys. Silver, therefore, is a hardener when used in proper amounts along with copper.

13. The frequency of tarnish increases as the noble metal content decreases. Laboratory tests indicate that below about 50% palladium or gold, tarnish is very likely.

14. The ductility or percentage elongation measures the degree to which the alloy can be burnished (spread). Other properties involved are hardness and yield strength, which indicate a resistance to burnishing.

15. Silver produces a green discoloration of the porcelain.

Chapter 14 Alloys for Porcelain-Fused-to-Metal Restorations

1. The term *precious* refers to higher-cost alloys. The term *semiprecious* has been applied to alloys that are mixtures of precious and nonprecious ingredients.

2. Nonprecious alloys are composed of nonprecious ingredients, except for small amounts of beryllium. Most are nickel-chromium; some are cobalt-chromium or iron based.

3. Rational selection of a specific alloy should be based on a balanced consideration of cost and intended use. For single crowns, strength and sag resistance are less important than they are for fixed partial dentures. Castability, biocompatibility, tarnish and corrosion resistance, porcelain color, and hardness are usually equally important for both alloy uses. For fixed partial dentures, solder and joining behavior, sag resistance, strength, elastic modulus, and the porcelain's thermal expansion compatibility become increasingly important as the span increases.

4. Excellent clinical working characteristics.

5. Advantages are good clinical working characteristics, excellent strength, and no porcelain color problems. Disadvantages include slightly more difficult melting and casting than with palladium-silver, and some soldering difficulties.

6. Nickel-chromium, cobalt-chromium, and iron-based alloys.
7. Nonprecious alloys offer lower cost, higher hardness (more wear resistance), higher tensile strength, and higher elastic modulus. Elongation is about the same as for precious metals, but is negated by the high yield strength, which makes it difficult or impossible to work the metal. Some nickel-chromium alloys, especially those containing beryllium, have mold-filling abilities that are superior to all other alloy groups, permitting easier casting of thin sections and producing sharp margins on castings.
8. Silver-free alloys containing about 50% gold and 40% palladium. Highly successful commercially, they have favorable yield strength and hardness and higher elastic modulus than high-gold alloys. Cost is comparable to the gold-palladium-silver group. The only disadvantage is thermal expansion incompatibility with some of the higher-expansion porcelains.
9. Strict control of grinding dust (with suction, masks, etc) and screening of patients for possible nickel allergy (eg, pierced ear posts and other jewelry).

Chapter 15 Dental Porcelain

1. Crystalline ceramics have an orderly, repetitive arrangement of atoms. Vitreous ceramics have an amorphous structure without the orderly pattern of a crystal.
2. Alkali ions (ie, Na^+, K^+, Li^+) disrupt the silicate structure to form glasses.
3. Metallic oxides are added for color in dental porcelains.
4. A frit is powdered glass made by fusing the constituents together in a furnace and then quenching and grinding.
5. Sintering involves increasing the density of a powdered mass by bonding at points of contact rather than by melting particles.
6. The driving force for sintering is the reduction of surface area by the force of surface tension. Therefore, a fine particle size and high glass surface tension promote rapid sintering.
7. To reduce porosity created by entrapped air.
8. The porcelain is not heated enough to produce glazing until the final bake in order to limit firing shrinkage. Excessive glazing also produces a rounding of edges.
9. About 30% to 40%.
10. The temperature below which glass becomes very rigid or behaves like a solid.
11. Glasses and other brittle solids fail by crack propagation. Tensile stresses cause cracks to spread, whereas compressive stresses do not.
12. Residual compressive stresses at the surface of a ceramic inhibit surface-crack propagation and increase strength. Tensile stresses at the surface lower strength. Therefore, the location and direction of residual stresses determine their effect on properties.
13. According to the cohesive plateau theory, the maximum measurable bond strength is equal to the cohesive strength of the porcelain (ie, 5,000 psi [35 MPa] in tension).
14. The nature and thickness of the oxide layer formed on alloys are critical to the bond strength. Bonding to pure gold produces only a relatively weak bond. Tin, indium, and iron oxides adhere strongly to a gold-alloy surface, reduce the contact angle, and produce cohesive porcelain fractures.
15. Deduction from scientific theory: Engineering mechanics would predict less failure for stronger materials; however, a full clinical study is still needed. Other factors, including the strength of the outer porcelain layer, will also affect longevity.

Chapter 16 Base Metal Casting Alloys

1. Cobalt-chromium, nickel-chromium, and cobalt-chromium-nickel.
2. Most chromium-type alloys are harder and stronger than conventional gold fixed partial denture alloys. Strength and hardness of some materials are comparable to those of chromium-type removable partial denture alloys.
3. High modulus of elasticity (stiffness) and yield strength (resistance to permanent deformation) suggest the usefulness of chromium-type alloys for the fabrication of long-span fixed appliances.
4. Excessive oxidation of substrate castings inhibits porcelain-to-metal bonding.
5. Proportional limit, offset yield strength, ultimate strength, rupture strength, and elastic modulus of cast titanium alloys are lower than those of chromium-type alloys.

Removable partial denture alloys
1. True: Principal strengthening elements are molybdenum, tungsten, and carbon.
2. False: Nitride inclusions and excessive metallic carbides can cause alloy embrittlement.
3. True: Low density makes chromium-type alloys especially useful for the fabrication of large maxillary appliances. Lighter devices are more resistant to displacement by gravitational forces and are, therefore, less likely to subject abutment teeth to unnecessary stresses.
4. False: Chromium-type removable partial denture alloys are about 30% harder than Type IV golds. Strengths of the chromium-type alloys and Type IV gold alloys, however, are comparable.
5. False: The modulus of elasticity (stiffness) of chromium-type removable partial denture alloys is about twice that of the Type IV golds. Thus, sufficient stiffness can be obtained with the use of relatively thin chromium-type castings.
6. False: Strong oxidizing agents should not be used for cleaning appliances fabricated from chromium-containing alloys.
7. True: Ethyl silicate– or phosphate-bonded investments are required for the casting of alloys with fusion temperatures higher than 1,315°C (2,400°F).
8. True: Casting temperature affects microstructure and mechanical properties.
9. False: The alloys are very hard. Conventional equipment and procedures consume excessive amounts of time and are relatively ineffective.
10. False: Improper design and fit of chromium-type appliances are the major causes of adverse tissue reactions.

Fixed partial denture alloys

1. False: Chromium-type fixed partial denture alloys employ the cobalt-chromium as well as the nickel-chromium system.
2. False: Chromium-type alloys are harder and stronger than conventional gold fixed partial denture alloys. Strength and hardness of some materials are comparable to those of chromium-type removable partial denture alloys.
3. True: High modulus of elasticity and relatively high yield strength (resistance to permanent deformation) suggest the usefulness of chromium-type alloys for the fabrication of long-span fixed appliances.
4. True: The tensile strength and yield strength of some titanium alloys are similar to those of chromium-type fixed partial denture alloys. When compared to chromium-type alloys, modulus of elasticity values for titanium alloys are relatively low.
5. False: Excessive oxidation of a substrate casting can inhibit porcelain-to-metal bonding.
6. False: The biocompatibility of titanium and some titanium alloys is well documented, but the long-term biocompatibility of chromium-type fixed partial denture alloys remains to be determined.

Surgical casting alloys

1. False: The nickel-chromium-cobalt base alloy (Surgical Ticonium) is much softer and much more ductile. The cobalt-chromium–based material (Vitallium) is exceptionally strong and hard.
2. False: Physical and mechanical factors also influence biologic tolerance to alloy implants.
3. True: The lungs, liver, and spleen are principal target organs for metallic ions.
4. True: Large implants are more prone to failure than smaller ones. Large surface areas create spaces between the implant and the tissue that may be transformed into undesirable bursae.
5. True: Complete rejection is characterized by development of fistulae or frank exposure of the implant.

Chapter 17 Casting

1. A wax pattern is used to form a refractory mold for the casting of a molten metal.
2. Wax shrinkage + gold shrinkage = setting expansion + hygroscopic expansion + thermal expansion of the investment + wax expansion.
3. A wax pattern can be made using the direct technique, in which the wax pattern is formed directly on the prepared tooth, or the indirect technique, in which the wax pattern is fabricated on a gypsum replica of the prepared tooth.
4. Geometry of the casting, or more specifically the surface/volume ratio, is the primary factor.
5. A high-expansion form of silica.
6. To increase the setting, hygroscopic, and thermal expansions.
7. High heat, water immersion (low heat–hygroscopic), controlled water added, and phosphate bonded.

8. Phosphate bonded.
9. By varying the amount of the silica sol component of the liquid mixed with the phosphate-bonded investment powder.
10. The sprue is used as a mount for wax pattern, a channel for wax escape during burnout, a channel for filling the mold with molten gold, and a compensation for shrinkage during solidification.
11. To remove oxides, sulfides, and particles of investment that were formed or added during the first melt.
12. Centrifugal, pressure, and pressure/vacuum.
13. These solutions comprise acids or a combination of acid with a HCl base.
14. Cobalt, chromium, nickel, molybdenum, and carbon.
15. Gold alloys possess a relatively low modulus of elasticity and proportional limit. They are relatively soft, and their density is about twice that of the cobalt-chromium alloys.
16. Phosphate-bonded investments and silica-bonded investments.

Chapter 18 Soldering, Welding, and Electroplating

1. Copper will lower the fusion temperature, increase the strength, and make it susceptible to age hardening. Silver is added primarily to improve the free-flowing qualities of the solder.
2. The appliance would probably come apart at the joint during firing of the porcelain because of the high temperatures. In addition, the porcelain near the joint would have a greenish tinge because of the copper in the solder.
3. The fluoride flux is required to remove the chromium oxide coating, which gives the alloy its corrosion resistance. Regular borax flux will not remove chromium oxide.
4. Solder will not wet a surface covered with antiflux. Antiflux can be used to confine the solder to a given region.
5. Graphite from a lead pencil; iron rouge suspended in alcohol.
6. The fineness of the solder should be less than the fineness of the parts.
7. 580-fine.
8. Silver solder has a sufficiently low fusion temperature so that carbide precipitation can be minimized or avoided with proper soldering procedures.
9. Solder will not wet a surface covered with thick casting oxides and organic films. These films must be removed prior to soldering, since the action of the flux is not sufficient to remove them.
10. Investment soldering is used whenever exact positioning of parts is required.
11. Fracture of the sticky wax indicates that the parts have been moved in relationship to each other and that the finished appliance probably will not fit.
12. Preheating eliminates moisture and provides thermal expansion to compensate for the expansion of the metal. Underheating the investment will lead to poor fit of the appliance. Overheating the investment could fracture it,

leading to a poorly fitting appliance, and it could release sulfur, which would contaminate the surface and prevent the flow of solder over the parts.

13. All regions of the appliance adjacent to the joint will be yellowish red.

14. If one part is significantly hotter than the other, the solder will flow to and wet the hot surface and not the other surface.

15. In free-hand soldering, because of the small size of wires, greater care must be exercised to avoid overheating. In addition, wires should be in contact, compared with the 0.1-mm gap distance recommended for investment soldering of larger parts.

16. Diffusion between solder and wire, recrystallization, and grain growth are all possible if a wire is overheated. Overheated stainless steel wires can lead to excessive carbide precipitation.

17. If allowance is not made for the fact that an object at a given temperature will appear much brighter in a dark room than in subdued light, the parts are likely to be too cool for the solder to flow. The lack of flow could mistakenly be attributed to contamination. If the torch is concentrated on the solder, it could become overheated before the parts come to the proper temperature.

18. Surface porosity was probably due to overheating. Excessive use of flux probably resulted in the incorporation of the flux into the solder. The large pore at the center of the joint probably indicates that the parts were in contact in this area.

19. The solder will not wet the oxidized surfaces. If soldering operations are continued, overheating of the work is likely.

20. Oxidation is due to one or more of the following: insufficient flux; improperly adjusted torch; using the oxidizing portion of the flame; and/or removing the flame before soldering operations are completed.

21. A poorly fitting appliance could be caused by one or more of the following: fracturing of the sticky wax, fracture of the investment by improper heating, failure to preheat the investment, and use of a high water/powder ratio for the investment.

22. A flux is required to remove surface oxides and helps to protect the parts and solder from oxidation at soldering temperatures.

23. The large reduction of elongation upon age hardening indicates that the solder has become considerably more brittle. The work is quenched after 5 minutes to prevent it from staying at the age-hardening temperature too long. Waiting 5 minutes allows some hardening, but the increased proportional limit is more important than the slight increase in brittleness.

24. Because the copper parts to be welded and the copper electrodes have similar resistances, the electrodes are likely to be welded to the work.

25. A greater amount of distortion would be required for copper because of its surface oxides. In addition, the stress and energy required for this distortion would be much higher because copper has a higher proportional limit and lower malleability than pure gold.

26. With a laser, the region of heat input can be localized to a very small area, and the time of application can be reduced so the total heat required for melting the metal at the junction is insufficient, when dissipated throughout the parts, to produce a temperature high enough to cause distortion or destruction of the cast.

27. It is, in principle, possible to weld other metals or alloys besides pure gold. In practice, the stresses are considerably higher than those required for pure gold, and in many cases heat is also required to obtain good welds.

28. It would increase the resistance of the contact areas and reduce the current, which varies inversely with the resistance. The heat generated is proportional to the square of the current and only directly proportional to the resistance, so a large reduction in current could make the available heat insufficient to melt the metal.

29. Electroplated dies for fixed partial dentures.

30. Electroplated dies are more abrasion resistant. However, electroplating takes 10 or more hours for completion, requires special equipment and solutions, and may introduce distortions of the impression's surface. Some plating solutions are very toxic and should only be used under a hood.

31. A solution with a high throwing power will produce more uniform plating of an impression and therefore preserve accuracy.

Chapter 19 High-Temperature Investments

1. The reaction time can be altered by changing the temperature of the reacting components (higher temperature results in faster reactions) or by changing the acidic concentration or the amount of water available (lower concentrations of these ingredients result in slower reaction rates).

2. (a) Yes. (b) The temperature may be lowered until the liquid begins to freeze, at which point precipitation of gelled silica hydrate renders the liquid incapable of properly binding investment particles via a gelation process. The temperature of 4.4°C has practical significance, as this is a temperature achieved in the main storage compartment of a refrigerator.

3. To avoid higher costs because of the federal tax on spirits, and to provide an impediment toward consumption by ingestion.

4. Advantages: (1) Rapid setting rate; (2) useful for lower burnout temperatures because much of the expansion is achieved as a result of the setting reaction rather than temperature increase; (3) high green strength; (4) high fired strength, which results in less mold cracking and fewer fins on castings; (5) liquid formed by mixing colloidal silica with water may be used immediately after mixing (which is in contrast to the freshly mixed liquid of ethyl silicate systems that requires an incubation of a few hours to allow the formation of a binding gel when the liquid is mixed with the investment powder).

Disadvantages: (1) The investment powder will react with moisture, imposing limitations on the shelf life of opened containers. (2) High setting expansion is an impediment to using the investment for producing refractory casts that will be used for articulation against "stone" casts (the high expansion results in a cast that will not properly match the opposing cast of stone). (3) High tendency for reaction with nonprecious alloys, which have higher casting temperatures than gold-based alloys, thereby producing oxides that can be difficult to remove from castings. (4) Lower permeability of conventional versions (not the rapid-heat investments) than ethyl silicate bound systems; this results in a higher probability of producing short castings due to entrapment of gasses in the mold. (5) The colloidal silica liquid cannot be shipped under conditions that would result in freezing of the liquid and agglomeration of colloidal silica. (6) Higher-temperature castings (investment temperature higher than 980°C [1,800°F]) have poorer surfaces owing to refractory loss.

5. *Advantages*: (1) High permeability yields sharply defined dental castings. (2) Low setting expansion (contraction) renders refractory partial denture models that may be articulated against stone models. (3) A nearly flat expansion vs temperature curve at high temperature (approx. 1,150°C [2,100°F]) and a low expansion vs time effect at that temperature make possible precise control of total expansion. (4) The investment is more refractory, which results in smoother castings. (5) Lower burnout strength results in easier removal of castings and cleaning of oxides from the casting.
Disadvantages: (1) Limited shelf life of liquid. (2) Substantial waiting period prior to using freshly mixed liquid. (3) Potential of cracking during burnout due to high thermal expansion.

6. The hygroscopic technique to generate the maximum expansion of the investment, thereby helping to compensate for the greater shrinkage of nonprecious alloys as opposed to gold. Rapid-heat investments that expand on mixing and setting might be an alternative.

7. (a) Phosphate-bonded. (b) Ethyl silicate or mixed ethyl silicate, colloidal silica, phosphate-bonded. (c) Phosphate-bonded.

8. (1) Increased colloidal silica for phosphate-bonded systems, increased ethyl silicate or colloidal silica mixed into an ethyl silicate system—these methods increase expansion. (2) Hygroscopic technique (phosphate-bonded). (3) Higher burnout temperatures. (4) Increased soak time. (5) Modification of the grain size of the investment. (6) Alteration of the basic mineral composition of the investment, ie, more cristobalite or increased glass content (ie, glossy quartz).

9. One advantage might be a lower setting shrinkage (possible expansion) than a straight ethyl silicate system. Also, smoother casting surfaces eliminate the need for pattern precoats, because the fine colloidal silica results in sintering of particles on the mold cavity surface and thus smoother finish castings.

10. (a) Use of a properly burned out carbon-filled investment is the best choice for each alloy. Follow the alloy manufacturer's recommendations for burn out of the investment. A carbon mold for the gold alloy reduces oxides on the casting.

(b) For the nonprecious alloy, a noncarbon investment would be advised if control of burnout is difficult, since carbon can interact rapidly with the nonprecious alloys. This may reduce the strength of the PFM bond and could also increase hardness of a nickel-based alloy.

11. The use of rapid-heat phosphate-bonded investments.

Chapter 20 Waxes

1. Paraffin, beeswax, carnauba wax, spermaceti, ceresin.

2. The properties of natural waxes vary with the conditions under which they are produced. For this reason, these waxes are not consistent in their properties. The properties of synthetic waxes are much more uniform, as the manufacturer may impose quality control procedures during their production.

3. Inlay wax: To form inlay, crown, or pontic replicas. Casting wax: Used for thin sections in certain removable and fixed partial denture patterns. Base plate wax: Used in the construction of complete denture patterns.

4. Solidification shrinkage and contraction on cooling to room temperature.

5. Increase temperature and apply force.

6. Heat wax uniformly; invest the pattern without delay; store the uninvested pattern at a low temperature.

7. It must have high flow above oral temperature to reproduce detail of cavity preparation, and it must have low flow at oral temperature to reduce distortion when the pattern is removed.

8. Memory is the return of waxes to their original shapes over time. This produces distortion.

9. Incomplete burnout leaves wax residue, which leads to poor castings from either inclusions or incomplete margins.

Chapter 21 Orthodontic Wires

1. Stainless steel, cobalt-chromium-nickel, β-titanium, and nickel-titanium.

2. Force delivery characteristics, elastic working range, ease of manipulation by permanent deformation to desired shapes, capability of joining individual segments to fabricate more complex appliances, corrosion resistance and biocompatibility in the oral environment, and cost. The beta-titanium and nickel-titanium archwires are much more expensive than the traditional stainless steel alloys, but they offer unique properties that should be carefully considered when selecting wires.

3. The composition and structure of the wire alloy, which determine the elastic modulus, and the wire segment geometry—cross-section shape and size (moment of inertia) and the length.

4. Excellent clinical corrosion resistance in the oral environment, excellent formability, and low cost.

5. A cobalt-chromium-nickel alloy very similar in appearance, physical properties, and joining characteristics to stainless steel wires, but with a much different composition and considerably greater heat treatment response. Available in four tempers: soft, ductile, semiresilient, and resilient.

6. The two commercially available products have very similar compositions: titanium, 78% to 79%; molybdenum, 11%; zirconium, 6% to 7%; and tin, 4%. The addition of alloying elements to pure titanium causes the body-centered cubic β polymorphic phase to be retained at room temperature, rather than the hexagonal close-packed α phase, which results in excellent formability or the capability for permanent deformation.

7. An intermediate force delivery between stainless steel or cobalt-chromium-nickel and nickel-titanium wires, excellent formability, and true weldability. Because of their lower elastic modulus, β-titanium archwires more nearly fill the bracket slots, as compared to stainless steel or cobalt-chromium-nickel archwires. The ductility allows arches or segments with complicated loop configurations, which are not possible with nickel-titanium wires.

8. Special techniques are required for permanent bending, and the wires cannot be bent over a sharp edge or into a complete loop. The wires cannot be soldered or welded but must be joined by a mechanical crimping procedure.

9. The complex proprietary strategies involve the amount of cold work and the heat-treatment temperatures used during wire processing, along with varying the alloy composition. The latter may involve slight variations in the relative atomic percentages of nickel and titanium, in addition to the incorporation of slight amounts of other alloying elements such as copper and chromium. For the shape-memory orthodontic wires, the austenite-finish temperature, where the transformation from martensitic NiTi to austenitic NiTi is completed, must be at the temperature of the oral environment.

Chapter 22 Endodontic Materials

1. (c) K-file.
2. (a) Access, biomechanical instrumentation, and obturation.
3. (a) They work best by rotation.
4. (d) EDTA.
5. (b) Spreader.

Chapter 23 Implant and Bone Augmentation Materials

1. A working definition of osseointegration is a direct structural and functional connection between ordered, living bone and the surface of a load-carrying implant.
2. Commercially pure titanium, titanium alloy (Ti-6Al-4V), bioactive glasses and glass ceramics, and calcium phosphate ceramics.
3. Surgical technique, bone quality, minimization of interfacial motion, and surface chemistry, among other factors.
4. Materials and material processing; mechanisms of implant-tissue attachment; mechanical properties; implant design; loading type; tissue properties; stress analysis; initial stability and mechanisms of enhancing osseointegration; biocompatibility of the implant materials; surface chemistry, mechanics, and bone-bonding ability of the implant.

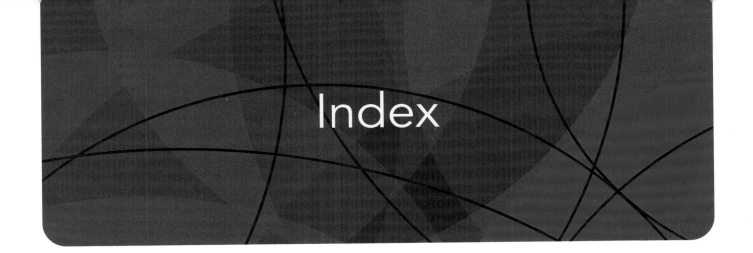

Index